T0195406

The Unofficial Guide to Radiology

SECOND EDITION

EDITION
2

The Unofficial Guide to Radiology

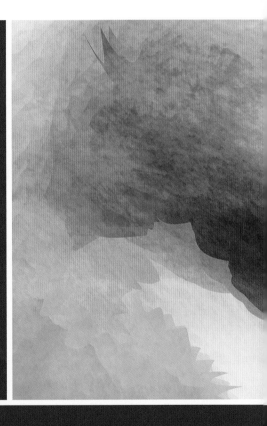

Volume and Series Editor
Zeshan Qureshi BM, BSc (Hons), MSc, MRCPCH,
FAcadMEd, MRCPS (Glasg)
Paediatric Registrar
London Deanery
United Kingdom

ELSEVIER

© 2024, Elsevier, Ltd. All rights reserved.

First edition 2014

No part of this publication may be reproduced or transmitted in any form or by any means, electronic or mechanical, including photocopying, recording, or any information storage and retrieval system, without permission in writing from the publisher. Details on how to seek permission, further information about the Publisher's permissions policies and our arrangements with organizations such as the Copyright Clearance Center and the Copyright Licensing Agency, can be found at our website: www.elsevier.com/permissions

This book and the individual contributions contained in it are protected under copyright by the Publisher (other than as may be noted herein).

Notices

Practitioners and researchers must always rely on their own experience and knowledge in evaluating and using any information, methods, compounds or experiments described herein. Because of rapid advances in the medical sciences, in particular, independent verification of diagnoses and drug dosages should be made. To the fullest extent of the law, no responsibility is assumed by Elsevier, authors, editors or contributors for any injury and/or damage to persons or property as a matter of products liability, negligence or otherwise, or from any use or operation of any methods, products, instructions, or ideas contained in the material herein.

ISBN: 978-0-443-10914-0

Content Strategist: Trinity Hutton
Content Project Manager: Tapajyoti Chaudhuri
Design: Hitchen Miles
Marketing Manager: Deborah J. Watkins

Printed in Poland.

Last digit is the print number: 9 8 7 6 5 4 3 2 1

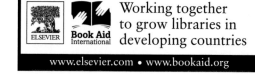

Contents

For reference, the X-rays are also all listed by diagnosis and clinical signs in 'Case Index'.

Series Editor Foreword

The Unofficial Guide to Medicine is not just about helping students study, it is also about allowing those that learn to take back control of their own education. Since its inception, it has been driven by the voices of students, and through this, democratised the process of medical education, blurring the line between learners and teachers.

Medical education is an evolving process, and the latest iteration of our titles has been rewritten to bring them up to date with modern curriculums, after extensive deliberation and consultation. We have kept the series up to date, incorporating new guidelines and perspectives from a wide range of students, junior doctors and senior clinicians. There is greater consistency across the titles, more illustrations, and through these and other changes, I hope the books will now be even better study aids.

These books though are a process of continual improvement. By reading this book, I hope that you not only get through your exams but also consider contributing to a future edition. You may be a student now, but you are also the future of medical education.

I wish you all the best with your future career and any upcoming exams.

Zeshan Qureshi
November 2022

Preface

Almost every patient has some form of medical imaging performed during their investigations and management. The commonest form of imaging, and the modality which all doctors should be able to interpret, remains the X-ray. This important aspect of radiology is therefore the main focus of the book. Other imaging modalities are specialised investigations interpreted by radiologists. However, medical students, doctors, nurses, physician's associates and surgeons need to understand what these tests involve, when they are indicated and contraindicated, and how to best request them. Therefore, these aspects are also covered in the book.

Despite its universal importance, X-ray interpretation is often an overlooked subject in the medical school curriculum, which many medical students and junior doctors find difficult and daunting.

The keys to interpreting X-rays are having a systematic method for assessing the X-ray and getting lots of practice at looking at and presenting X-rays. Occasionally, there may be a complex X-ray you find difficult, or a subtle finding you overlook, but that's what keeps radiologists in a job, so do not worry about it.

The '4 Ds' are a useful framework for X-ray interpretation which underpins the approach used in this book. First, you need to **Detect** and **Describe** the abnormalities on the X-ray. You then need to form a **Differential diagnosis** based on clinical and X-ray findings before **Deciding** what further imaging and management is required.

There are lots of radiology textbooks available, but I do not think there is one which is ideally suited for teaching medical students and junior doctors. Many have small, often poor-quality images. Radiology is a visual subject and therefore such images are difficult to use to demonstrate key clinical findings. This is confounded by the fact that the findings are usually only described in a figure below the image, and it is often difficult to know exactly what part of the image corresponds to which finding! Another fundamental problem with many radiology textbooks is that they deal with X-rays in isolation. In reality, X-rays are part of the clinical assessment and management of patients, and thus, they should be taught in a clinical context.

The content, layout and approach used in this book are designed to make it as useful and clinically relevant as possible:

- Over 200 large, high-quality radiological images are used throughout the book and important findings are annotated on the images to highlight the key points and findings to the reader.
- The chest, abdominal and orthopaedic X-ray chapters contain step-by-step approaches to interpreting and presenting X-rays.
- Each of these chapters also covers 20 common and important X-ray cases/diagnoses. They are labelled as 'Case X' to not give away the diagnosis, but at the end of the book there is a list of all the diagnoses.
- The X-rays are presented in the context of a clinical scenario. The reader is asked to 'present their findings' before turning over the page to reveal a model X-ray report accompanied by a fully annotated version of the X-ray. This encourages the reader to look at the X-ray thoroughly, as if working on a ward, and come to their own conclusions about the X-ray findings and any further management required before seeing the answers.
- To further enhance the clinical relevance, each case has five clinical and radiology-related multiple-choice questions with detailed answers. These are aimed to test core knowledge needed for exams and working life, and illustrate how the X-ray findings will influence patient management.
- The bonus X-ray chapter provides over 50 further X-ray cases to help consolidate the reader's knowledge and provide an opportunity to practise the skills they have learnt.
- Five chapters are devoted to other important imaging investigations: CT, MRI, USS, nuclear medicine and fluoroscopy. These cover the details of what the examinations entail, their common indications, contraindications and key imaging findings. There is also a dedicated chapter on interventional radiology.
- The content is in line with the Royal College of Radiologists' Undergraduate Radiology Curriculum, making it up to date and relevant to today's students and junior doctors.

With this textbook, we hope you will become more confident and competent in these radiology competencies, both in exams and in clinical practice, and we also hope that this is just the beginning. We want you to get involved, this textbook has been a collaboration with junior doctors and students just like you. You have the power to contribute something valuable to medicine; we welcome your suggestions and would love for you to get in touch.

Acknowledgements

Thank you to the following contributors for their contribution to the first edition:
Mark Rodrigues
Jonathan Rodrigues

Bijan Hedayati
Amanda Cheng
Kabir Varghese

Abbreviations

A&E	accident and emergency
AAA	abdominal aortic aneurysm
ABCDE	Airway, Breathing, Circulation, Disability, and Exposure
ACE	angiotensin converting enzyme
ACJ	acromioclavicular joint
ADEM	acute disseminated encephalomyelitis
ADH	antidiuretic hormone
AIN	anterior interosseous nerve
AMPLE	Allergies, Medications, Past illness/Pregnancy history, Last meal
AMT	abbreviated mental test
ANCA	antineutrophil cytoplasmic antibodies
AO	Arbeitsgemeinschaft für Osteosynthesefragen
AP	anterior to posterior
ATLS	Advanced Trauma Life Support
AV	arteriovenous
AVN	avascular necrosis
AVPU	Alert, responds to Voice, responds to Pain, Unresponsive scale
AXR	abdominal X-ray
BTS	British Thoracic Society
CABG	coronary artery bypass graft
CBD	common bile duct
CCAM	congenital cystic adenoid malformation
CHRIST	Crystals, Rheumatoid arthritis and other inflammatory arthropathies, Infection, Synovial pathology and Trauma
cm	centimetre
COPD	chronic obstructive pulmonary disease
CRITOE	Capitellum, Radial head, Medial/Internal epicondyle, Trochlear, Olecranon, External/Lateral epicondyle
CPAP	continuous positive airway pressure ventilation
CPPD	calcium pyrophosphate dehydrate disease
CRP	C-reactive protein
CSF	cerebrospinal fluid
CT	computed tomography
CTPA	computed tomography pulmonary angiogram
DDH	developmental dysplasia of the hip
DEXA	dual energy X-ray absorptiometry
DHS	dynamic hip screw
DIPJ	distal interphalangeal joint
DMSA	dimercaptosuccinic acid
DRUJ	distal radioulnar joint
DTPA	diethylenetriaminepentaacetic acid
DVT	deep venous thrombosis
DWI	diffusion-weighted image
ECG	electrocardiogram
ED	emergency department
ENT	ear, nose and throat
ERCP	endoscopic retrograde cholangiopancreatography
ESR	erythrocyte sedimentation rate

ESWL	extracorporeal shock wave lithotripsy
ET	endotracheal
EVAR	endovascular aneurysm repair
FAST	focused assessment with sonography in trauma
FBC	full blood count
FDL	flexor pollicis longus
FDP	flexor digitorum profundus
FDS	flexor digitorum superficialis
FLAIR	fluid attenuation inversion recovery
FOOSH	falls onto an outstretched hand
FPS	flexor pollicis longus
G	gauge
g/L	grams per litre
G&S	group and save
GCS	Glasgow coma scale
GI	gastrointestinal
GTN	glyceryl trinitrate
HAS	human serum albumin
HIDA	hepatobiliary iminodiacetic acid
HIP	heparin-induced thrombocytopaenia
HLA	human leukocyte antigen
HPOA	hypertrophic pulmonary osteoarthropathy
HRCT	high-resolution CT
HRT	hormone replacement therapy
HU	Hounsfield unit
IP	interphalangeal
IRMER	Ionising Radiation [Medical Exposure] Regulations
ITP	idiopathic thrombocytopenic purpura
ITU	intensive treatment unit
IU	international unit
IUCD	intrauterine contraceptive device
IV	intravenous
IVC	inferior vena cava
IVU	intravenous urogram
JVP	jugular venous pressure
kg	kilogram
KUB	kidneys, urethra, bladder
LDH	lactate dehydrogenase
LFT	liver function test
LIF	left iliac fossa
LLL	left lower lobe
LUL	left upper lobe
m	metre
MAG3	mercaptoacetyltriglycine
MCPJ	metacarpophalangeal joint
MDP	methylene disphosphonate
MDT	multidisciplinary team
MIRP	minimally invasive retroperitoneal pancreatic necrosectomy
mm	millimetre
mmHg	millimetres of mercury
mmol/L	millimoles per litre
MRA	magnetic resonance angiography

MRCP	magnetic resonance cholangiopancreatography	**RML**	right middle lobe
MRI	magnetic resonance imaging	**RUL**	right upper lobe
MRSA	methicillin-resistant *Staphylococcus aureus*	**RUQ**	right upper quadrant
mSv	millisieverts	**SCIWORA**	spinal cord injury without radiological abnormality
MTPJ	metatarsophalangeal joint	**SHO**	senior house officer
NAI	nonaccidental injury	**SI**	sacroiliac
NG	nasogastric	**SiADH**	syndrome of inappropriate antidiuretic hormone
NICE	National Institute of Health and Care Excellence	**SLE**	systemic lupus erythematosus
NSAID	nonsteroidal antiinflammatory drug	**SMA**	superior mesenteric artery
OA	osteoarthritis	**SMV**	superior mesenteric vein
PA	posterior to anterior	**SP**	spinous process
PaCO$_2$	partial pressure of carbon dioxide	**STIR**	short tau inversion recovery
PaO$_2$	partial pressure of oxygen	**SUFE**	slipped upper femoral epiphysis
PE	pulmonary embolus	**TB**	tuberculosis
PEA	pulseless electrical activity	**THR**	total hip replacement
PEG	percutaneous endoscopic gastrostomy	**TNF**	tumour necrosis factor
PET	positron emission tomography	**TNM**	tumour, nodes, metastases
PFO	patent foramen ovale	**U&Es**	urea and electrolytes
PICC	peripherally inserted central catheter	**USS**	ultrasound scan
PIN	posterior interosseous nerve	**VACTERL**	Vertebral, Anorectal, Cardiac, Tracheal, Oesophageal, Renal, Limb anomalies
PIPJ	proximal interphalangeal joint		
PR	per rectum	**VQ**	ventilation/perfusion
RICE	rest, ice, compression, elevation	**VTE**	venous thromboembolism
RLL	right lower lobe	**β-hCG**	beta human chorionic gonadotropin

Contributors

EDITOR

Zeshan Qureshi, BM, BSc (Hons), MSc, MRCPCH, FAcadMEd, MRCPS (Glasg)
Paediatric Registrar, London Deanery, United Kingdom

AUTHORS

Cindy Chew, MBChB, MRCS, MSc (Research), FRCR, FEGAR, PhD
Honorary Clinical Professor, Director of Imaging & Anatomy, University of Glasgow, Scotland

Consultant Radiologist, University Hospital Hairmyres, NHS Lanarkshire, Scotland

Nishaanth Dalavaye, BSc (Hons)
Medical student, Faculty of Medicine, Imperial College London, United Kingdom

Medical student, Cardiff University School of Medicine, Cardiff University, United Kingdom

Bryan Dalton, MRCPI, MD, BE (Hons)
Radiology Specialist Registrar, St James's Hospital, Dublin, Ireland

Christopher Gee, MBChB, MSc, FRCSEd (Tr&Orth), MFSTEd
Interim Clinical Director and Consultant Orthopaedic Surgeon, NHS Golden Jubilee Glasgow, Scotland

Honorary Senior Clinical Lecturer, University of Glasgow, Scotland

Education Lead for the West of Scotland Orthopaedics Rotation

Anita Saigal, BM (Medicine), BSc (Biomedical Sciences), MRCP
Respiratory Registrar and Clinical Research Fellow, Thoracic Department, Royal Free Hospital, London, United Kingdom

Erin Visser, MB BCh BAO, BSc HKIN (Hons)
School of Medicine, Trinity College Dublin, Ireland

Intern doctor, University Hospital Waterford, Waterford, Ireland

Introduction

Zeshan Qureshi

WHAT ARE X-RAYS?

X-rays, like light, radio waves and microwaves, are a type of electromagnetic radiation. They are the most energetic type of electromagnetic radiation and whilst they have particle-like properties, they are composed of packets of energy called photons. Together, these features mean X-rays can pass through the body.

X-rays are produced when electrons, released from a heated metal filament, are suddenly stopped by a metal 'target' (Fig. 1.1). The filament and 'target' are contained within a vacuum inside glass housing. There is a difference in electrical potential energy between the filament (negatively charged) and 'target' (positively charged), which accelerates the electrons towards the 'target'. The vacuum ensures these

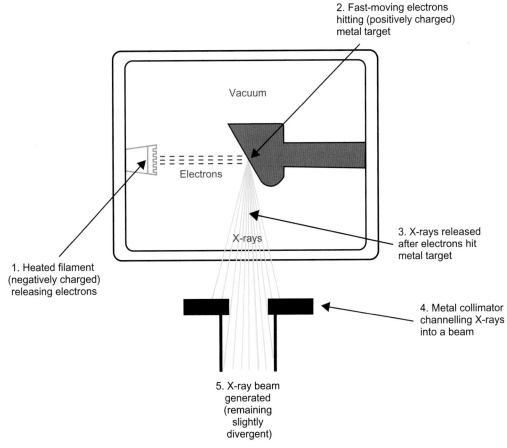

2. Fast-moving electrons hitting (positively charged) metal target

Vacuum

Electrons

1. Heated filament (negatively charged) releasing electrons

X-rays

3. X-rays released after electrons hit metal target

4. Metal collimator channelling X-rays into a beam

5. X-ray beam generated (remaining slightly divergent)

Fig. 1.1 Diagram showing X-ray production.

fast-moving electrons are not slowed by air molecules, and they hit the 'target' at approximately half the speed of light. This high energy interaction results in the production of X-rays. Metal sheets, known as collimators, are used to channel the resultant X-rays into a beam. This can be directed towards the body part being imaged.

IMAGE PRODUCTION

In simple terms, X-rays can either pass straight through the body or get absorbed by the tissues. The proportion of X-rays absorbed is roughly proportional to the density of the material they are passing through. For example, bone will absorb a higher proportion of X-rays than fat, and metal more than bone. The X-rays which pass through the body are detected by a detector plate. The more X-rays detected in a particle spot on the plate, the more intense the signal produced. Thus, the proportions of X-rays transmitted through different parts of the body being imaged are detected by the detector plate and result in an X-ray image.

Another way to think of it is to image a torch shining on an object and producing a shadow on a wall. The light from the torch is analogous to the X-ray beam. The object represents the body part being imaged and the shadow cast on the wall represents the image (this is an over simplification as the hand will block all of the light but not all of the X-rays would be absorbed).

> **❶ KEY POINT**
>
> A higher dose of X-rays is needed to go through parts of the body composed of thicker or denser tissues, resulting in a higher radiation dose to the patient. For example, an abdominal X-ray, which has to travel through multiple layers of soft tissue within the abdominal cavity, requires a higher dose of radiation than a chest X-ray (the chest is largely composed of gas within the lungs which absorbs relatively few X-rays).

DENSITIES

The denser a tissue, the more X-rays it will absorb. There will be fewer corresponding X-rays hitting the detector plate, leading to a radiopaque (whiter) area in the resultant X-ray image. The body has four main tissue densities discernible on X-ray (Fig. 1.2). Bone is the densest tissue and is represented by white on the image, whilst gas is the least dense and appears black (also known as radiolucent). Soft tissues, such as muscle, are light grey, and fat is dark grey. Metal and contrast material absorb even more X-rays than bone and appear as bright white. The level of greyness not only relates to the type of tissue, but also its thickness (thicker tissues absorb more X-rays and are thus

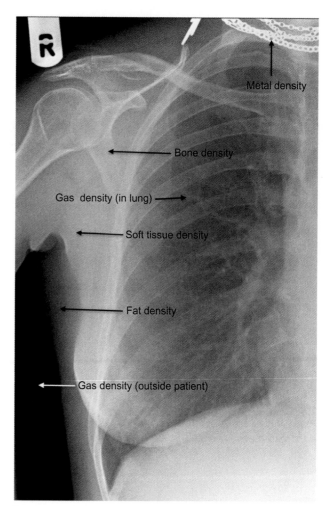

Fig. 1.2 The main densities on X-ray.

whiter) and any other structures/tissues which are in front or behind (the mediastinum is very white on X-ray as there are multiple layers of soft tissue as well as the sternum anteriorly and vertebrae posteriorly).

MAGNIFICATION

As mentioned earlier, collimation is used to produce a narrow beam of X-rays; however, even with this, the X-ray beam is still divergent. The divergent nature of the beam means there is some magnification of structures on an X-ray image and this magnification increases as the distance from the structure to the detector plate increases. Therefore, as illustrated in Fig. 1.3, an anteroposterior (AP) chest X-ray will result in significantly more magnification of the heart compared with a posteroanterior (PA) X-ray. This makes accurate assessment of the heart size more difficult on an AP chest X-ray.

The edges of structures which are further from the detector plate are also less well defined.

The torch example mentioned earlier helps to highlight these two points. As with an X-ray beam, the beam of light from a torch is divergent. If you shine the torch at your hand, with your hand held close to a wall,

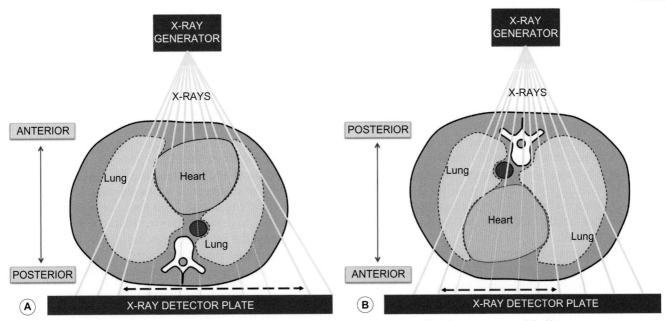

Fig. 1.3 The effect of projection on magnification of the heart on chest X-rays. The divergent nature of the X-ray beam has been exaggerated to highlight this point. **(A)** With an anteroposterior (AP) chest X-ray, the heart is further from the X-ray detector plate. Therefore, there is a significant amount of magnification *(dashed arrow)* due to the divergent nature of the X-ray beam. **(B)** In contrast, a posteroanterior (PA) chest X-ray results in very little magnification of the heart as the heart is located closer to the X-ray detector plate.

you will see the shadow produced is roughly the same size of your hand (i.e. there is little magnification) and the edges are crisp. Now if you do the same thing with your hand held further from the wall you will notice that the shadow of your hand increases in size (magnification) and the edges are less well defined.

HAZARDS

Due to their high energy, X-rays can have detrimental effects on tissues. X-rays have sufficient energy to expel an electron from an atom, resulting in the formation of an ion (X-rays are therefore a type of ionising radiation). This ionisation process can result in the formation of free radicals and cause changes in molecular structures such as DNA, RNA and enzymes. These changes can result in two types of effect.

Deterministic effects are the result of cell death and do not occur unless a threshold level of radiation exposure has been exceeded (the rate of radiation exposure (amount of radiation in a given time period) is also important). Skin erythema, hair loss and cataract formation are all examples of deterministic effects.

Stochastic effects are due to cell transformation/mutation and can lead to cancer induction or genetic abnormalities. Such effects occur by chance and whilst their risk rises with radiation dose, they can occur at any radiation level (i.e. unlike deterministic effects, there is no threshold level of exposure that needs to be achieved). There is a lag period of many years between radiation exposure and the occurrence of stochastic effects. Children's organs are the most radiosensitive because they are growing. Additionally, children have a long period to live (they are likely to live long enough for a stochastic effect to occur – this is not true for elderly patients). These facts make children the patient group most at risk from stochastic effects.

LEGISLATION

Due to the potential hazards of radiation exposure, there is legislation in the UK (Ionising Radiation (Medical Exposure) Regulations 2022 (IRMER)) which governs the use of X-rays. This legislation applies to anybody who can request imaging which involves ionising radiation.

The person who requests the X-ray needs to supply sufficient clinical information to justify the radiation exposure to the patient. The justification is usually made by a radiologist or radiographer depending on the examination requested (radiographers can usually justify limb, chest and abdominal X-rays, whereas a radiologist usually justifies CT scans and other advanced radiology techniques). The higher the dose of an investigation, the harder it is to justify. Therefore, a finger X-ray requires less justification than an abdominal X-ray, which is turn needs less than a CT scan.

The referrer should have access to recommended referral criteria. The hospital in which you work should provide these criteria. In the UK, these usually take the form of the Royal College of Radiologists 'Making the Best Use of Clinical Radiology' guidelines (https://www.rcr.ac.uk/guidelines), which are available on paper or as a smartphone app (iRefer).

PREGNANCY

Additional measures are required for women of child-bearing age undergoing X-rays of the abdomen/pelvis, due to the risks to any potential foetus (imaging of other body parts will have a very low radiation dose to the foetus). An alternative imaging technique which does not use ionising radiation, such as ultrasound or magnetic resonance imaging (MRI), should be considered if such patients are or could be pregnant or their period is late (negative pregnancy tests can be inaccurate, especially if performed very early). This information will be ascertained by the radiographers but it is good practice for the doctor or person requesting the test to ask as well.

There may not be an appropriate alternative imaging option, in which case the risks of radiation to the foetus must be weighed against the potential benefits to the mother. Senior clinicians and radiologists should make such decisions.

REQUESTING IMAGING

The following are parts of the radiology request form which will need to be completed:
- Patient name.
- Date of birth.
- Sex.
- Hospital number.
- Ward/location.
- Type of scan being requested.
- Clinical details.
- Pregnancy status.
- Referrer details (name and contact number).
- For more advanced scanning, additional details may be required, e.g. renal function (important if intravenous (IV) contrast is to be given). MRI scans usually also necessitate a safety checklist to ensure that no contraindications (e.g. the presence of certain pacemakers) are missed.

> ❶ KEY POINT
>
> Radiology requests are often now electronic with many of the basic details (such as demographics and ward location) entered automatically. It is imperative you select the correct patient on the computer when requesting a radiological investigation. This sounds obvious but on a busy ward it is easy to accidentally fill out a radiology request for the wrong patient, resulting in the wrong patient being scanned and (potentially) exposed to radiation.

The clinical details on a request for an imaging test fulfil several roles:
- It is important to ensure the correct patient is scanned. Therefore, the patient details (name, age, date of birth, hospital number, ward location, etc.) are important.
- Under the IRMER legislation discussed earlier, the clinical details must be sufficient to justify an examination if it involves ionising radiation. Think about using scoring systems such as the STONE score for ureteric stones to help you with this.
- The most appropriate test will depend on the clinical findings and likely differential diagnosis. Therefore, to ensure that the correct imaging is performed, it is important that the clinical details on the request are completed as accurately as possible with the pertinent clinical findings, relevant past medical history, the likely differential diagnosis and any specific questions which you want the imaging to answer.
- The clinical details provided help the radiologist to interpret the imaging. It is helpful to mention any relevant past medical or surgical history and any previous imaging the patient may have had.

> ❶ KEY POINT
>
> Providing good clinical details when requesting imaging will help ensure the right patient gets the right test and aid interpretation of the images by the reporting radiologist.

Take the example of a patient with acute abdominal pain. There is a wide differential diagnosis for this and the appropriate imaging investigations depend on the likely diagnoses.
- If the patient has right upper quadrant pain and with localised peritonism, they will require an abdominal ultrasound to assess for gallstones and cholecystitis.
- If they have flank pain, no peritonism but microscopic haematuria, they may have renal colic and a noncontrast CT would be appropriate.
- If the patient has left iliac fossa pain and peritonism with elevated inflammatory markers, they may have diverticulitis and a contrast-enhanced CT (portal venous phase) would be helpful.
- If they have a significant cardiovascular past medical history and present very unwell with severe abdominal pain and a raised lactate, then ischaemic bowel may be high on the list of differentials and a contrast-enhanced CT (arterial and portal venous phases) may be appropriate.
- If the patient has recently had a colectomy and primary anastomosis, then rectal contrast may be useful to identify an anastomotic leak.
- A female patient with suprapubic pain and normal inflammatory markers may have a gynaecological cause for their pain, such as an ovarian cyst, and therefore a pelvic ultrasound would be the best initial investigation.

These are just a few examples of possible scenarios and we hope they highlight how accurate clinical information will help the radiology department determine what imaging test(s) is/are most appropriate, which will ultimately help in the diagnosis and management of the patient.

WHEN AND HOW TO DISCUSS A PATIENT WITH RADIOLOGY

A lot of doctors will be able to tell you about the difficult, and sometimes frightful, experiences they have had when trying to discuss a potential scan, so the following are a few tips to help you.

Some radiology departments require the clinical team to discuss most advanced imaging requests, whereas in others, this is not necessarily the case, as the clinical request form may be deemed sufficient. In either case, it is important to discuss:

- Patients who require urgent scans (to make the radiology team aware, allowing them to prioritise their workload appropriately).
- Patients requiring scans out of hours (as there may not be anybody in the radiology department to pick up the paper/electronic request).
- Complicated patients (as it may not be possible to convey the complexity and clinical questions clearly on the written request form).
- Patients in whom you are not sure what test is the most appropriate.
- Scan reports which are unclear or do not answer the clinical question which was asked.

Discussions can be held over the phone or in person. Radiologists generally appreciate face-to-face discussions about patients or scans; however, this may not be possible (e.g. if the radiologist is not on site) or practical (e.g. you are managing an acutely unwell patient).

It is important to have sufficient information about a patient before making a referral. What clinical question needs answering? Remember: the duty radiologist is often a consultant radiologist, who will have a wealth of experience and knowledge, but even with their knowledge, they cannot help you if cannot give them the relevant patient information.

The age and sex are important to give an idea about which differential diagnoses are most likely, whilst the other details are required to ensure the correct patient is scanned, and to allow any previous imaging to be accessed.

- **The reason for the scan** – unfortunately 'because my consultant wants it' is not a good enough reason for scanning a patient! You need to know the patient's current clinical presentation, relevant past medical history, the working differential diagnosis and clinical question to be answered. It is important to know about any relevant blood test results, including the renal function (renal failure may preclude use of IV contrast) and previous imaging.
- **The reason why a scan is required urgently or out of hours** (if appropriate). It is important to understand how the results of the scan will alter the management of the patient, particularly if the scan is to be performed out of hours. Patients may require a scan, but if the results are not going to influence the immediate management out of hours, then the scan can usually be postponed until the next day. For example, a CT head may be appropriate to look for cerebral metastases in a patient with metastatic cancer who has developed increasing confusion over the last 2 weeks; however, this does not need to be performed out of hours as the results are unlikely to change the immediate management. In contrast, if a patient has acute onset confusion after a fall and reduced consciousness, they could have an intracranial bleed. In this case, the scan may influence the immediate management (the patient may need urgent surgical intervention) and therefore should be performed out of hours.
- **The most senior clinician who has assessed the patient**. Patients should usually be discussed with and reviewed by senior clinicians prior to requesting scans, particularly CT and MRI scans.

❗ KEY POINTS

1. Discussing potential scans should not be like ordering a drink at a coffee shop! Say you want to 'request' a scan rather than 'order' a scan. It's even better to say you 'would like to ask the radiologist's opinion about what imaging would be most appropriate'.
2. Treat discussions with radiology like a referral to another clinical speciality; know the patient in question (their presentation, relevant past medical history, previous imaging, etc.) and understand what clinical question needs answering.

Key points to know before discussing a potential scan with radiology are:
- **Basic patient details** – name, date of birth, age, sex, hospital number, which ward the patient is on, etc.

❗ KEY POINT

Often the decision to request a scan is made during a busy ward round and the exact reason is not necessarily clear. It is important to clarify with the registrar or consultant on the ward round exactly what clinical question they want answered by the scan. If you don't know, you won't be able to justify it to the radiology department, and will end up asking your seniors later in the day, therefore delaying the scan.

❗ KEY POINT

Try and request scans at the start of the day. This gives the radiology department time to triage their workload for the day and increases the likelihood that your scan will be done on the day it is requested.

Chest X-rays

Nishaanth Dalavaye and Anita Saigal

Chapter Outline

This introduction to the chapter is aimed at providing a systematic framework for approaching chest X-rays. Further details and examples of the specific X-ray findings discussed next are covered more extensively in the example cases later in the chapter and in the bonus X-ray chapter.

In this book we look only at frontal chest X-rays (PA and AP X-rays), as these account for almost all chest X-rays performed. The lateral chest X-ray is not commonly performed and has been largely replaced by CT.

> **❶ KEY POINT**
>
> Systematic approach to chest X-rays
> 1. Projection
> 2. Patient details
> 3. Technical adequacy
> 4. Obvious abnormalities
> 5. Systematic review of the X-ray
> 6. Review areas
> 7. Summary

PROJECTION (AP/PA)

The projection of a chest X-ray can affect its appearance and interpretation. The two possible projections for a frontal chest X-ray are the anteroposterior (AP) and the posteroanterior (PA) and should be marked as such on the chest X-ray.

The PA X-ray requires the patient to be able to stand (or sit on a stool). This is the standard projection, so if there is no annotation stating otherwise, you can assume the X-ray is PA.

- AP X-rays provide a less comprehensive assessment than PA X-rays due to the effects of magnification and scapulae position (Fig. 2.1). They are usually only performed in patients that are difficult to mobilise.

- If you are asked to justify why an X-ray is PA, remember that in PA X-rays, the patient's arms are positioned in such a way that the scapulae are pulled almost fully out of the lung fields. In AP X-rays, this positioning is not possible, and the scapulae are projected further over the lungs.

PATIENT DETAILS

- It is important to ensure you are looking at the correct X-ray from the correct patient.
- The patient's details will be on the X-ray (unless anonymised for an exam).
- State the name, age/date of birth, gender and the date on which the X-ray was taken.
- The age and gender of the patient are useful for formulating your differential diagnosis.

> **❶ KEY POINT**
>
> It is imperitive to compare the current X-ray with previous X-rays and imaging to see if there is any new acute pathology or deterioration in chronic pathology.

TECHNICAL QUALITY

- Check that the X-ray includes the thorax (both lung apices, the lateral sides of the ribcage and both costophrenic angles). Important pathology can be missed if the entire thorax is not imaged.
- It is important to assess RIP – Rotation, Inspiration, Penetration.

ROTATION

- The heads of the clavicles (medial ends) should be equidistant from the spinous processes of the vertebral bodies. If they are not, the X-ray film is classed as rotated.

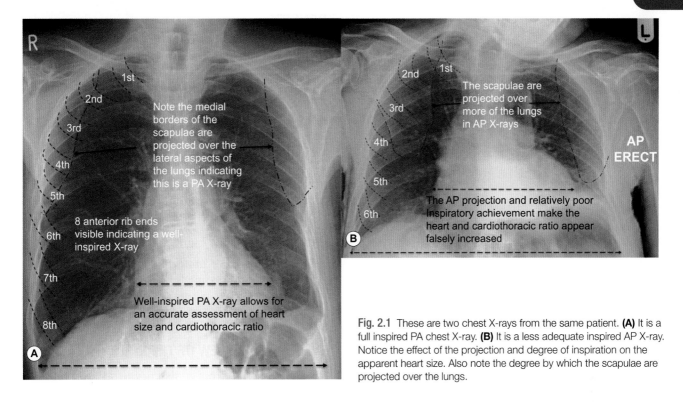

Fig. 2.1 These are two chest X-rays from the same patient. **(A)** It is a full inspired PA chest X-ray. **(B)** It is a less adequate inspired AP X-ray. Notice the effect of the projection and degree of inspiration on the apparent heart size. Also note the degree by which the scapulae are projected over the lungs.

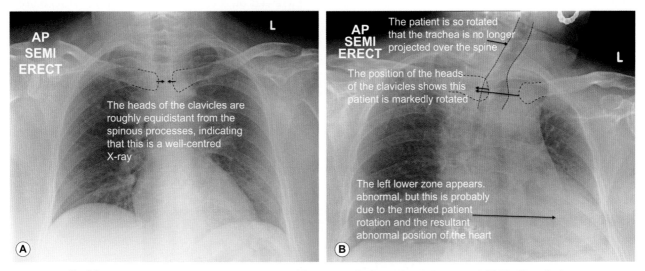

Fig. 2.2 These are two X-rays from the same patient. **(A)** The X-ray film is not classified as rotated. **(B)** The X-ray film is markedly rotated, which has resulted in an apparent left lower zone consolidation. This appearance is likely caused by the abnormally positioned cardiac shadow, and a repeat X-ray, with the patient well centred, should be obtained.

- Rotation can erroneously give the impression of mediastinal shift or lung pathology (Fig. 2.2).

INSPIRATION

- PA and AP X-rays are taken in held deep inspiration. Count the ribs to assess for inspiratory effort.
- You should count down to the lowest rib crossing through the diaphragm. Six anterior ribs or ten posterior ribs indicate adequate inspiratory effort.
- Fewer ribs indicate a poorly inspired X-ray. This may be due to the timing of the X-ray, or because the patient is unable to take and hold a deep breath (due to pain, abnormal breathing pattern or confusion). Poorly inspired X-rays can cause crowding of the lung markings at the bases and create an impression of consolidation or other pathology. Additionally, the heart may appear falsely enlarged (see Fig. 2.1).
- A greater number of ribs together with flattened diaphragms, indicate hyperinflation due to airway obstruction, such as COPD.

PENETRATION

- The X-ray is adequately penetrated if you can just see the vertebral bodies behind the heart.

- 'Underpenetrated' means that you cannot see behind the heart and 'overpenetrated' means that you will be able to see the vertebral bodies very clearly.
- Over- and underpenetration can obscure or obliterate significant findings, particularly in the lungs.
- This is less of a problem with the advent of digital viewers which allow the X-ray 'windows' to be manipulated.

> **! KEY POINT**
>
> Rotated, poorly inspired or under/overpenetrated X-rays can hinder accurate assessment. These technical factors must be taken into consideration when assessing the X-ray.

OBVIOUS ABNORMALITIES

If you can see obvious abnormalities, say so and describe them.

LUNG INVOLVEMENT

- Determine which lung is involved (right or left) and specify the location (upper, middle, or lower zone). If possible, identify the lobe(s) affected. CT can locate abnormalities more accurately.

SIZE AND SHAPE

- Is it focal or diffuse, rounded or spiculated, well or poorly demarcated?

DENSITY

Describe the density of an abnormality in relation to the normal surrounding tissue, e.g. if the abnormality is in the lung, compare it to the normal lung; if in the bone, compare it with other bony structures.

If the abnormality is denser (i.e. whiter) than the normal tissue, you can say that there is increased opacification or density; if less dense (i.e. blacker), say there is increased lucency or reduced density.

TEXTURE

You should assess whether the abnormality has a uniform or heterogeneous appearance.

OTHER FEATURES

- If there are other abnormalitiess such as air bronchograms or fluid levels, then mention these as well.
- Are there other abnormalities, such as volume change, bony abnormalities or surgical clips?

SYSTEMATIC REVIEW OF THE X-RAY (FIG. 2.3)

- Initially assess from a distance to see differences in lung shadowing/obvious masses. Most X-rays are viewed on a computer so zoom out maximally for your initial inspection.
- After that, reassess from close-up to look for subtle abnormalities.
- A useful system to ensure you do NOT miss areas is ABCDD (Airway, Breathing, Circulation, Diaphragm/Delicates).
- Lastly, comment on man-made abnormalities, e.g. externally placed lines, pacemakers, a nasogastric (NG) tube.

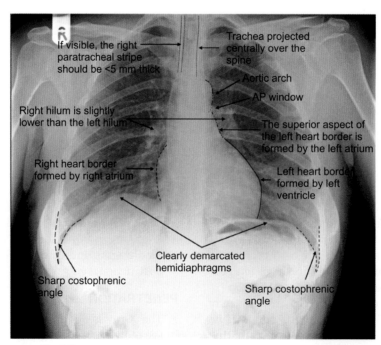

Fig. 2.3 A normal PA chest X-ray demonstrating the normal anatomy.

A – AIRWAY

- Is the trachea central or deviated due to rotation or other pathology?
- Is the trachea pulled to one side (from volume loss, such as lobar or lung collapse) or pushed away (from increased volume such as a large pleural effusion, tension pneumothorax or mediastinal mass)?

B – BREATHING

- Start in the apices and work down to the costophrenic angles, comparing both lungs for differences.
- Ensure that you inspect the entire lung, including the apices, hila and costophrenic angles.
- The left hilum should never be lower than the right. If this is the case, you must look for volume loss either pulling the right hilum up or pulling the left hilum down.
- Both hila should be the same density and have no lumps or convex margins.
- Look around the edge of the lungs, assessing for pneumothoraces which can be subtle at the lung apices.

C – CARDIAC AND MEDIASTINUM

- Assess the heart size. Cardiomegaly is defined by the maximal transverse cardiac diameter being greater than 50% of the maximal transverse internal thoracic diameter (cardiothoracic ratio). This is accurately assessed on a well-inspired PA X-ray due to the effects of magnification on AP (see Fig. 2.1). However, it is still important to assess cardiac size on an AP X-ray – if it is normal on the AP, then it will be normal on the PA; conversely, if it is grossly enlarged on the AP, it is likely to be enlarged on the PA X-ray.
- The cardiac and mediastinal borders should be clearly visible. If this is not the case, you must consider pathology in the adjacent lung.
- The mediastinum and heart should be positioned over the thoracic vertebra. If this is not the case, you must first check that the patient is not rotated. Then you must assess for volume change in the lungs (volume loss pulling structures towards the abnormal side or increased volume pushing them away). Marginal mediastinal shift can be observed if the margins of the thoracic vertebral bodies can be clearly seen beyond the cardiac and mediastinal contours on a well-centred X-ray.
- Mediastinum widening may be due to technical factors (e.g. AP projection), vascular structures (e.g. unfolding of the thoracic aorta or aortic dissection), masses (mediastinal tumours or lymph node enlargement) or haemorrhage (e.g. ruptured aorta). The clinical findings in such cases are important, as the causes are difficult to determine on X-ray. CT can be used for further assessment.
- The right paratracheal stripe is useful to assess, if visible. It is composed of the soft tissue between the right lung medial wall and the right wall of the trachea. It is visible in 50% to 60% of X-rays and should measure <5mm in diameter. If it is thickened, it is commonly due to lymph node enlargement.
- The aortopulmonary window is another area to assess for lymph node enlargement. This is located between the aortic arch and the left pulmonary artery. If this is not the case, you must consider lymph node enlargement.
- You should assess the mediastinum for presence of gas within it (pneumomediastinum). This appears as linear lucencies projected over the mediastinum. These often extend into the neck and may be associated with surgical emphysema (Fig. 2.4).
- It is important to remember that a large portion of the left lower lobe is behind the heart. The cardiac shadow should be of uniform density. If this is not the case, you must consider retrocardiac pathology (consolidation, lobar collapse or a mass). This can be difficult to assess due to the overlying cardiac shadow. Inverting the image often makes any abnormalities more visible (Fig. 2.5).

D – DIAPHRAGM

- Both hemidiaphragms should be visible and upwardly convex. Flattening of a hemidiaphragm suggests lung hyperexpansion, as seen in air trapping with COPD, or tension pneumothoraces.
- The right hemidiaphragm is normally slightly higher than the left due to the mass effect of the adjacent liver. If this is not the case, you must consider whether one of the hemidiaphragms is being abnormally pulled up or pushed down.

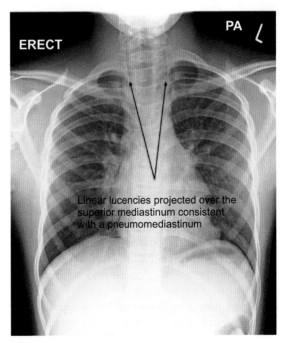

Fig. 2.4 PA chest X-ray showing linear lucencies projected over the upper mediastinum. Their location and appearances are consistent with a pneumomediastinum. There may also be evidence of gas within the soft tissues (surgical emphysema) or pericardium (pneumopericardium).

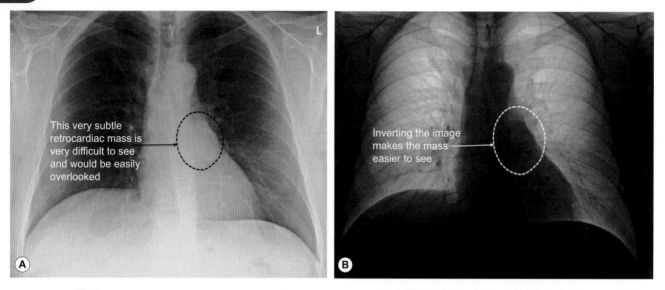

Fig. 2.5 (A) This X-ray looks normal on initial viewing; however, closer inspection of the review areas reveals a very subtle retrocardiac mass, which will be located in the medial aspect of the lower lobe. **(B)** This abnormality is much easier to see if the X-ray is inverted.

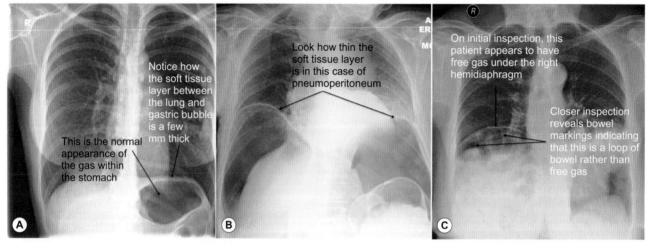

Fig. 2.6 These three X-rays show how difficult it can be to diagnose free subdiaphragmatic gas. **(A)** It is a normal chest X-ray with gas in the stomach. We know the gas is within the stomach, as it is under the left hemidiaphragm, and the soft tissue rim overlying the gas is a few millimetres thick, as it consists of the stomach wall and adjacent diaphragm. **(B)** Contrast that appearance to the centre X-ray, which shows a large pneumoperitoneum. In this case, the soft tissue rim between the lung and abdomen is very thin, as it solely represents the diaphragm. **(C)** Is a mimic of free subdiaphragmatic gas. In this case, inspection of the area below the right hemidiaphragm reveals bowel markings. These appearances are due to interposition of a loop of bowel between the liver and right hemidiaphragm and is known as Chilaiditi's sign.

- Remember that the lungs extend behind the diaphragms, so you need to look for lung pathology through the hemidiaphragms. Again, inverting the image can make such pathology more obvious.
- Look for free air under the diaphragm. This can be difficult, as the gastric bubble and bowel loops can have a similar appearance (Fig. 2.6).
- The costophrenic angles should be sharp. If not, there may be pleural fluid or other pathology present.

D – DELICATES

- Assess the bones. Look at the ribs for fractures or bone destruction. Assess the rib spaces, which should be roughly equal. Narrowing can be seen with volume loss in the underlying lung. Review the rest of the imaged skeleton for fractures or destructive bone lesions.
- Look at the soft tissues for evidence of surgical emphysema (gas (black areas) in the soft tissues) and previous surgery (surgical clips, mastectomy).

LINES (FIG. 2.7)

- An ET tube should have its tip proximal to the carina. Problems can arise if it is inserted too far and the tip enters a bronchus. This will result in collapse of the non-ventilated lung.

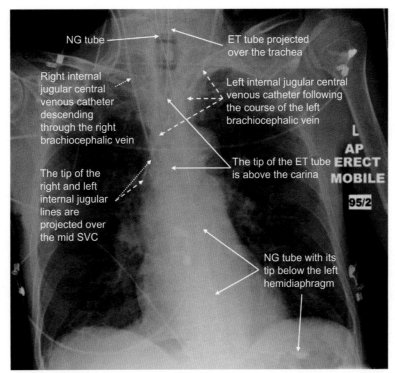

Fig. 2.7 An AP chest X-ray demonstrating satisfactorily positioned endotracheal tube, right and left internal jugular central lines and NG tube. Note that the right internal jugular line descends straight down the right side of the mediastinum (as it travels through the right brachiocephalic vein), whereas the left-sided central line passes diagonally across the mediastinum (as it travels through the left brachiocephalic vein). The tips of both of the lines should be projected over the mid or lower superior vena cava.

- NG tubes should lie below the left hemidiaphragm in the stomach. Problems include misplacement into the lungs, or the tip lying within the distal oesophagus.
- Central lines tips should be seen in the mid to lower superior vena cava. Complications include misplacement and a pneumothorax.

REVIEW AREAS

Double-check the following areas, since pathology is easily overlooked at these sites on initial viewing (Fig. 2.8):
- Apices
- Hila
- Behind the heart
- Costophrenic angles
- Below the diaphragm

SUMMARY

- Summarise your findings and give a differential list. Think about the history and clinical examination as well as the X-ray findings when making your differential diagnosis.
- Say whether you would like to review previous imaging if you think this would help.
- Suggest further investigations, including imaging, which may be useful.
- Suggest a management plan for the patient.

> **❶ KEY POINT**
>
> Remember you are looking at a chest X-ray, not a lung X-ray. Ensure you assess all of the X-ray, including the soft tissues, bones such as the clavicles, scapulae and visible humeri, and the upper abdomen.

SPECIFIC FINDINGS ON CHEST X-RAY

PNEUMONIA

- Dense or patchy consolidation, usually unilateral.
- May contain air bronchograms (air-containing bronchioles running through consolidated lung).
- In the lower zones, pneumonia may be difficult to distinguish from pleural effusions, so both should be on your differential list (remember there can be an associated parapneumonic effusion).
- The silhouette sign is useful for locating which lobe of the lung the pathology is located (Fig. 2.9). Normally, there is a sharp border between the aerated lung and the soft tissues of the heart and diaphragm. This is due to the large differences in the number of X-rays attenuated by the soft tissues (a relatively high proportion of X-rays) and the lung (relatively few X-rays).
- If there is consolidation, the normally aerated lung is replaced by fluid or pus. This attenuates X-rays to a similar extent to the heart and diaphragms. The sharp border between the lung and these structures

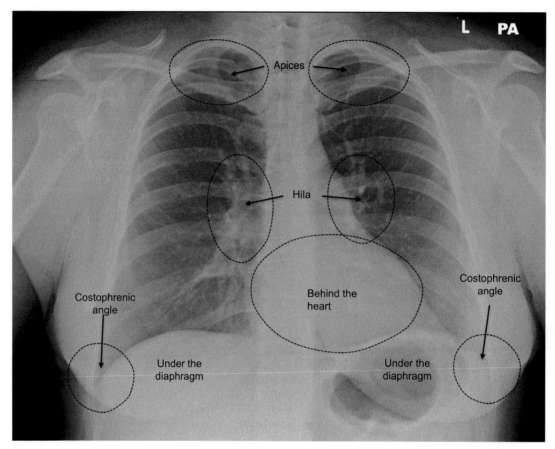

Fig. 2.8 The common chest X-ray review areas. Remember to add to this list any sites where you commonly overlook pathology.

is thus lost if lobar consolidation abuts these soft tissues.

- It is necessary to know which lobes contact the heart and diaphragmatic borders in order to be able to use the silhouette sign:
  - Diaphragms: left and right lower lobes
  - Right heart border: right middle lobe
  - Left heart border: lingula (part of the left upper lobe)
- Remember that pathology can affect more than one lobe.
- It is not always possible to identify in which lobe pathology is located. In these cases, describe it as affecting the 'upper, middle or lower zone'.

PLEURAL EFFUSIONS

- Look for blunting of the costophrenic angles, a homogeneous opacification and a fluid level manifesting as a meniscus (Fig. 2.10).

PULMONARY OEDEMA

ABCDEF can be used as an aide-mémoire for the features of pulmonary oedema (Fig. 2.11). Usually only some of these X-ray signs are present, and the diagnosis is made in conjunction with the clinical picture:

- A: Alveolar and interstitial shadowing
- B: Kerley B lines (little white horizontal lines usually in the lateral lower edges)

- C: Cardiomegaly (Cardiothoracic ratio of greater than 50% on a PA X-ray)
- D: Upper lobe venous blood Diversion (prominent upper lobe vasculature relative to the lower zones)
- E: Effusions
- F: Fluid in the horizontal fissure

PNEUMOTHORAX

- Air within the pleural space (Fig. 2.12).
- Loss of lung markings in the peripheral lung field. You may also identify a discrete lung edge.
- With a simple pneumothorax, there is no mediastinal shift. In contrast, a tension pneumothorax results in tracheal/mediastinal deviation away from the pneumothorax, and flattening of the ipsilateral dome of the diaphragm. A tension pneumothorax should never be diagnosed by a chest X-ray! It is a medical emergency and should be diagnosed clinically and treated immediately with needle thoracocentesis.

❶ KEY POINT

Inverting the imaging can make pneumothoraces more obvious.

LOBAR COLLAPSE (FIG. 2.13)

- Look for loss of volume

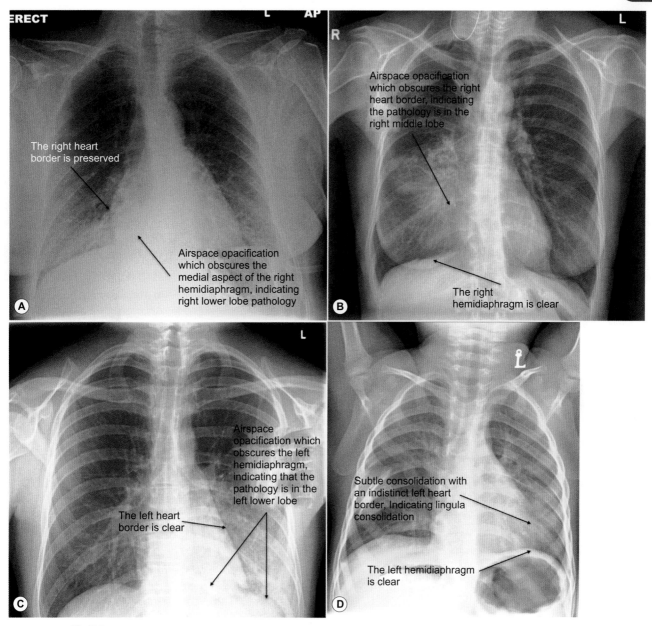

Fig. 2.9 X-rays demonstrating consolidation and the silhouette sign. **(A)** Shows loss of the medial aspect of the right hemidiaphragm but a clear right heart border, indicating right lower lobe consolidation. **(B)** Shows an indistinct right heart border with preservation of the right hemidiaphragm, in keeping with right middle lobe consolidation. **(C)** Shows a clear left heart border but loss of the left hemidiaphragm, consistent with left lower lobe consolidation. **(D)** The bottom right X-ray shows loss of the left heart border but a clear left hemidiaphragm, indicating consolidation within the lingula.

- A raised hemidiaphragm ipsilaterally
- Tracheal and mediastinal shift towards the collapsed side
- Displacement of the hila
- Narrowing of the space between the ribs compared to the opposite side

Left Upper Lobe (LUL) Collapse
Veil sign – the whole lung field looks like it is covered by a veil. This can be difficult to appreciate. Luftsichel sign is sometimes seen – radiolucency in the left upper zone, around the aortic arch, due to compensatory hyperinflation of the left lower lobe.

Left Lower Lobe (LLL) Collapse
Sail sign – sharp line like the edge of a sail at the same angle as the left heart border – giving the impression of a double left heart border. The medial left hemidiaphragm will be indistinct and the left heart border clear.

Right Upper Lobe (RUL) Collapse
Increased opacification in the right upper zone with a raised horizontal fissure (usually has a concave border). The abnormality is well demarcated by the horizontal fissure. Golden's S sign is present if there is an associated right hilar mass.

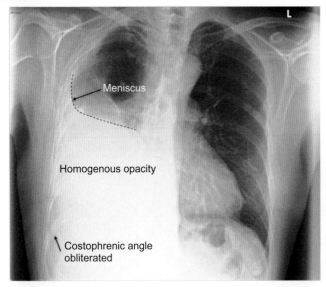

Fig. 2.10 A large right homogeneous opacity which fills most of the right hemithorax. The right costophrenic angle has been obliterated, and a meniscus is present. These findings are consistent with a large right-sided pleural effusion.

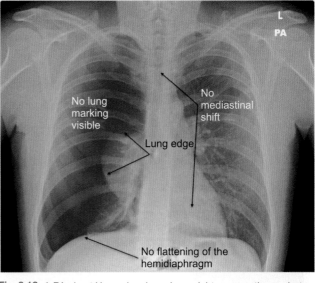

Fig. 2.12 A PA chest X-ray showing a large right pneumothorax, but no evidence of tension.

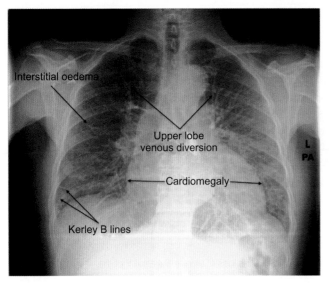

Fig. 2.11 This PA chest X-ray shows interstitial oedema and Kerley B lines, cardiomegaly and upper lobe venous diversion. No pleural effusions are evident, but the findings are in keeping with pulmonary oedema.

Right Middle Lobe (RML) Collapse

This is the most difficult lobar collapse to detect on chest X-ray. Look for horizontal fissure depression and an indistinct right heart border. CT is much better for detecting middle lobe collapses.

Right Lower Lobe (RLL) Collapse

Sail sign – similar to the appearance of a left lower lobe collapse. The medial part of the right hemidiaphragm will be indistinct, while the right heart border is clear.

> ❗ KEY POINT
>
> A right middle lobe collapse can be very subtle on a frontal chest X-ray. A lateral chest X-ray will help confirm the diagnosis; however, nowadays a CT is often performed for confirmation and to identify the cause.

You can use the checklist in Table 2.1 to assess the chest X-rays shown in this chapter. You should practise using this checklist in the various chest X-ray cases (Cases 2.1–2.20).

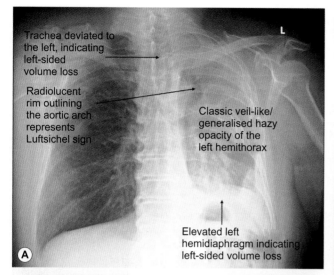

Trachea deviated to the left, indicating left-sided volume loss

Radiolucent rim outlining the aortic arch represents Luftsichel sign

Classic veil-like/ generalised hazy opacity of the left hemithorax

Elevated left hemidiaphragm indicating left-sided volume loss

(A)

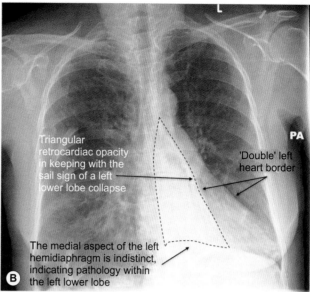

Triangular retrocardiac opacity in keeping with the sail sign of a left lower lobe collapse

'Double' left heart border

The medial aspect of the left hemidiaphragm is indistinct, indicating pathology within the left lower lobe

(B)

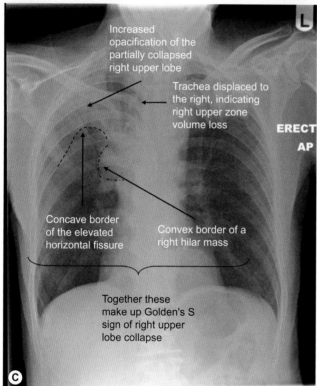

Increased opacification of the partially collapsed right upper lobe

Trachea displaced to the right, indicating right upper zone volume loss

ERECT AP

Concave border of the elevated horizontal fissure

Convex border of a right hilar mass

Together these make up Golden's S sign of right upper lobe collapse

(C)

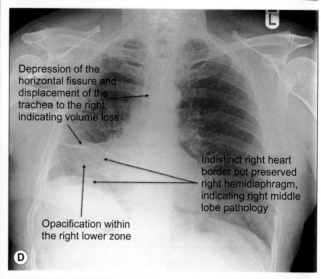

Depression of the horizontal fissure and displacement of the trachea to the right, indicating volume loss

Indistinct right heart border but preserved right hemidiaphragm, indicating right middle lobe pathology

Opacification within the right lower zone

(D)

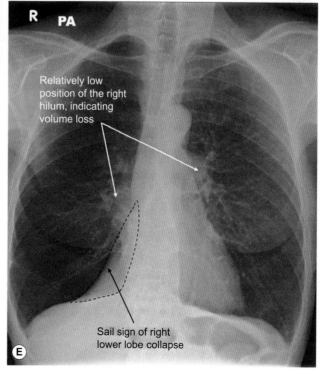

R PA

Relatively low position of the right hilum, indicating volume loss

Sail sign of right lower lobe collapse

(E)

Fig. 2.13 **(A)** Left upper lobe collapse with the veil and Luftsichel signs. **(B)** A left lower lobe collapse with a sail sign and apparent double left heart border. **(C)** A right upper lobe collapse and Golden's S sign. **(D)** Right middle lobe collapse. **(E)** Right lower lobe collapse with a sail sign.

TABLE 2.1	Checklist for Systematic Interpretation of a Chest X-ray	
Technical Aspects		
Check patient details (name, date of birth, hospital number)		✓
Check the date of the X-ray		✓
Identify the projection of the X-ray		✓
Assess technical quality of X-ray (rotation, inspiration, penetration)		✓
Obvious Abnormalities		
Describe any obvious abnormality		✓
Site (lung and zone/lobe)		✓
Size (if relevant)		✓
Shape (if relevant)		✓
Density		✓
Systematic Review of the X-ray		
Position of trachea		✓
Assessment of lungs		✓
Size and appearance of hila		✓
Assess for cardiomegaly		✓
Assess cardiac and mediastinal borders and cardiophrenic angles		✓
Position and appearance of hemidiaphragms		✓
Evidence of pneumoperitoneum (free air under the diaphragm)		✓
Assess the imaged skeleton		✓
Assess the imaged soft tissues (e.g. surgical emphysema, mastectomy)		✓
Comment on iatrogenic abnormalities		✓
Look at review areas (apices, hila, behind the heart, costophrenic angles, under the diaphragm)		✓
Summary		
Present findings		✓
Review relevant previous imaging if appropriate		✓
Provide a differential diagnosis where appropriate		✓
Suggest appropriate further imaging/investigations if relevant		✓

CASE EXAMPLES

CASE **2.1**

An 18-year-old presents with sudden-onset right-sided chest pain and shortness of breath. As part of his workup he undergoes a chest X-ray.

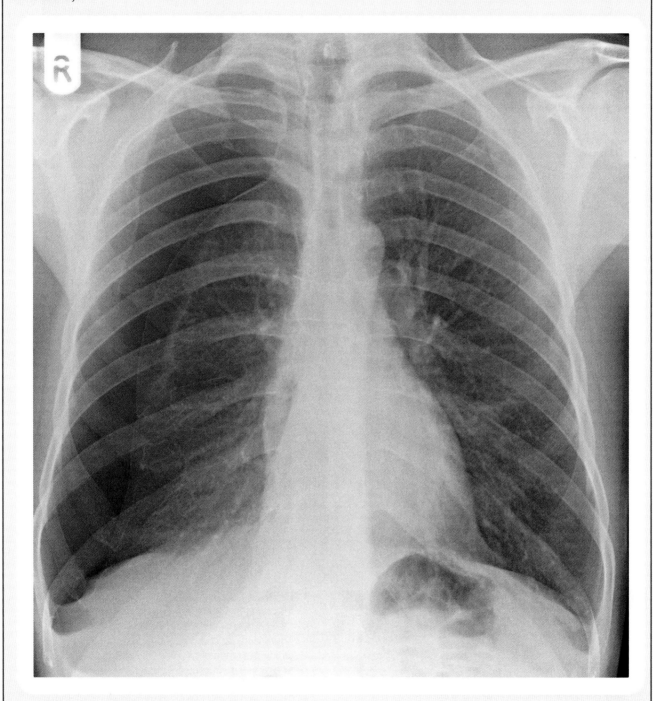

Continue

CASE **2.1**   *Contd.*

ANNOTATED X-RAY

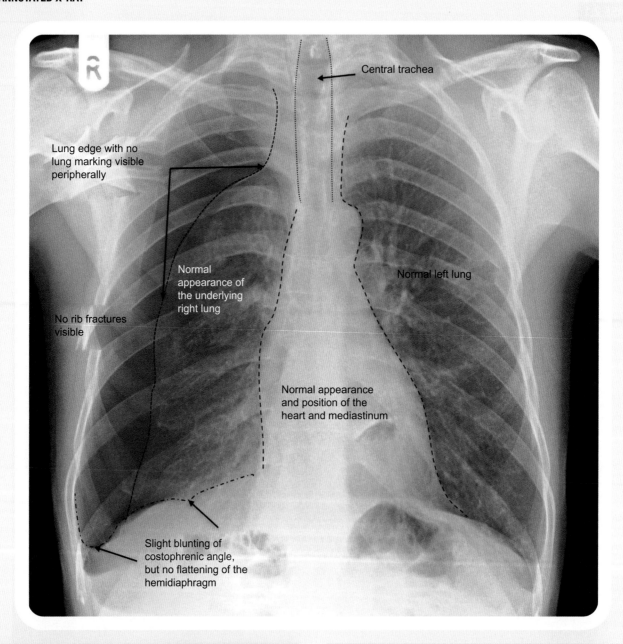

Central trachea

Lung edge with no
lung marking visible
peripherally

Normal
appearance of
the underlying
right lung

Normal left lung

No rib fractures
visible

Normal appearance
and position of the
heart and mediastinum

Slight blunting of
costophrenic angle,
but no flattening of the
hemidiaphragm

PRESENT YOUR FINDINGS

- This is a PA chest X-ray of an adult.
- There are no identifying markings – I would like to ensure that this is the correct patient, and to check when the X-ray was taken.
- The patient is slightly rotated; this is otherwise a technically adequate X-ray with adequate penetration and good inspiratory effort. No important areas are cut off at the edges of the film.
- There is an obvious abnormality in the right hemithorax: a line can clearly be seen with absence of lung markings beyond it, in keeping with a lung edge.
- The aerated right lung is otherwise normal in appearance.
- The trachea and mediastinum are not deviated, and the right hemidiaphragm is not flattened.

- Reviewing the rest of the film, the left lung is normal.
- The heart is not enlarged, heart borders are clear and there is no abnormality visible behind the heart.
- There is minor blunting of the costophrenic angles which may represent small volumes of pleural effusion.
- The hemidiaphragms are clear.
- There is no free air under the diaphragm.
- There are no soft tissue abnormalities or fractures; in particular, no rib fractures are visible.

IN SUMMARY – This chest X-ray shows a large right pneumothorax. There is no evidence of associated tension. There is no underlying cause discernible on this X-ray, suggesting that this is a primary spontaneous pneumothorax.

QUESTIONS

1. Which of the following are risk factors for a primary spontaneous pneumothorax?
   A) Male sex
   B) Smoking
   C) COPD
   D) Trauma
   E) Marfan syndrome

2. Which of the following clinical findings would be supportive of a large simple right-sided pneumothorax?
   A) Central trachea. Dull percussion and reduced air entry on the right side of the chest
   B) Central trachea. Dull percussion with bronchial breathing and crackles on the right side of the chest
   C) Central trachea. Hyperresonant percussion and reduced air entry on the right side of the chest
   D) Central trachea. Hyperresonant percussion and reduced air entry on the left side of the chest
   E) Trachea deviated to the left. Hyperresonant percussion and reduced air entry on the right side of the chest. Hypotensive, tachycardic

3. Which of the following are appropriate differential diagnoses for a patient who presents with sudden breathlessness?
   A) Pulmonary embolism
   B) Pneumothorax
   C) Pneumonia
   D) Heart failure
   E) Anaphylaxis

4. Which of the following is the most appropriate initial imaging investigation in a patient suspected of having a simple pneumothorax?
   A) Erect PA chest X-ray
   B) PA and lateral chest X-rays
   C) Expiratory chest X-ray
   D) Supine chest X-ray
   E) CT

5. Which of the following is the most appropriate management option for a previously healthy patient with a small, asymptomatic primary pneumothorax?
   A) Conservative management and discharge the patient
   B) Conservative management with outpatient follow-up
   C) Admit for conservative management, high-flow oxygen and monitoring
   D) Aspirate as much of the pneumothorax as possible
   E) Chest drain insertion

Continue

CASE 2.1 *Contd.*

ANSWERS TO QUESTIONS

1. Which of the following are risk factors for a primary spontaneous pneumothorax?

The correct answers are **A) Male sex and B) Smoking**. A pneumothorax is the presence of air or gas within the pleural space. The gas separates the visceral and parietal pleura and can lead to the compression of the adjacent lung. Pneumothoraces can be considered as:

- Primary spontaneous (no cause is identified)
- Secondary spontaneous (occur in the setting of lung disease)
- Traumatic (either blunt or penetrating)
- Iatrogenic (such as after lung biopsy or central line or pacemaker insertion)

  A) Male sex – Correct. As mentioned earlier, primary spontaneous pneumothoraces occur in patients without underlying lung disease or trauma. The precise cause of these pneumothoraces is uncertain. There is some evidence that they are due to the rupture of small subpleural blebs (small, air-filled cysts just under the visceral pleura). Patients are typically tall, slim young men. Other risk factors for primary spontaneous pneumothoraces include smoking and family history.

  B) Smoking – Correct. Smoking is a recognised risk factor for primary spontaneous pneumothoraces.

  C) COPD – Incorrect. COPD is a risk factor for pneumothoraces. However, it is classified as a secondary cause. Patients who have extensive emphysema and large bullae are most at risk, as these are thin-walled, air-containing structures which are prone to rupture. Most pneumothoraces (>70%) are secondary. In addition to COPD, there are many other lung pathologies which can increase the risk of a secondary pneumothorax, including airway disorders (such as asthma/interstitial lung disease), infections (such as TB/necrotising pneumonia/*Pneumocystis jirovecii*), systemic connective tissue disorders (such as Marfan syndrome/Ehlers–Danlos syndrome/rheumatoid arthritis) and lung cancer.

  D) Trauma – Incorrect. Trauma is a well-established cause of a pneumothorax. However, it does not cause a spontaneous pneumothorax. Blunt trauma can result in rib fractures which tear the lung surface, whereas penetrating trauma can injure the lung surface directly. In addition to air, there may be blood in the pleural space, resulting in a haemopneumothorax. A horizontal air-fluid level is a useful clue to the presence of both air and fluid in the pleural space (remember that a pleural effusion will usually have a curving meniscus rather than a completely horizontal upper margin).

  E) Marfan syndrome – Incorrect. Marfan syndrome is a systemic connective tissue disorder which is known to increase the risk of secondary pneumothoraces. It is considered a risk factor for secondary, not primary spontaneous pneumothoraces.

KEY POINT

Most pneumothoraces are secondary, and a variety of lung and systemic disorders can be implicated. Spontaneous primary pneumothoraces typically occur in young, slim, tall male smokers.

2. Which of the following clinical findings would be supportive of a large simple right-sided pneumothorax?

The correct answer is **C) Central trachea. Hyperresonant percussion and reduced air entry on the right side of the chest**.

Accurate clinical assessment is a key part of clinical practice and is commonly assessed in examinations. It is important to know the different combinations of clinical findings associated with a pneumothorax, a pleural effusion, lobar collapse and pneumonia. Briefly, the chest examination should follow the pattern of inspection, palpation, percussion and auscultation. Look for symmetrical shape and chest expansion. Assess the position of the mediastinum (trachea and apex beat) and assess for chest expansion. Percuss and auscultate both lungs. Assessing routine observations, such as oxygen saturations and blood pressure, is also important.

A) Central trachea. Dull percussion and reduced air entry on the right side of the chest – Incorrect. This combination of findings is suggestive of a right-sided pleural effusion. With a pleural effusion you would expect to find reduced chest expansion, a very dull/stony dull percussion note, absent or reduced breath sounds, reduced vocal resonance and no added sounds on the side of the effusion. With large effusions there may be a shift of the mediastinum to the contralateral side.

B) Central trachea. Dull percussion and bronchial breathing and crackles on the right side of the chest – Incorrect. This combination of clinical findings is in keeping with a right-sided pneumonia. Typically, there is reduced chest expansion, dull percussion, bronchial breathing with added crackles and increased vocal resonance in pneumonia.

C) Central trachea. Hyperresonant percussion and reduced air entry on the right side of the chest – Correct. These findings are consistent with a simple right pneumothorax. You would expect to find reduced chest expansion, hyperresonant percussion and absent breath sounds, with no added sounds on the side of the pneumothorax. There should be no mediastinal shift.

D) Central trachea. Hyperresonant percussion and reduced air entry on the left side of the chest – Incorrect. These findings would be in keeping with a simple left-sided pneumothorax.

E) Trachea deviated to the left. Hyperresonant percussion and reduced air entry on the right side of the chest. Hypotensive, tachycardic – Incorrect. This combination of clinical findings is worrying and should raise your suspicions of a tension pneumothorax. In addition to the usual findings associated with a simple pneumothorax, there is mediastinal shift to the contralateral side and evidence of significantly impaired ventilation and circulation (hypoxia, cyanosis, hypotension, tachycardia, reduced consciousness level). Tension pneumothoraces are a medical emergency and need urgent treatment (there is a case covering tension pneumothorax in more detail later in the chapter).

❗ KEY POINTS

1. Patients with a small pneumothorax may have few if any findings on clinical examination. Chest X-ray is a more sensitive test for identifying a pneumothorax, particularly a small pneumothorax.
2. Not all patients have classic findings on history and examination. It is important to use your clinical findings to request appropriate investigations, such as blood tests and a chest X-ray, to help narrow your differential diagnosis.

3. Which of the following are appropriate differential diagnoses for a patient who presents with sudden breathlessness?
   The correct answers are **A) Pulmonary embolism, B) Pneumothorax and E) Anaphylaxis**.
   There is a wide range of pathologies which can cause breathlessness. These include respiratory conditions, cardiac diseases and systemic problems. It is important to be able to formulate an appropriate differential diagnosis from the history and examination to guide suitable investigations and initial management. Establishing the time frame of the onset of breathlessness is very helpful in formulating your differential diagnosis. Sudden onset refers to breathlessness that develops over seconds and can result from PE, pneumothorax, anaphylaxis and inhaled foreign bodies. Dyspnoea associated with pneumonia, heart failure, metabolic acidosis and exacerbations of asthma or COPD tends to develop more slowly. Other conditions, such as interstitial lung disease and anaemia, have a much more chronic onset.
   A) Pulmonary embolism – Correct. PE can cause very sudden breathlessness. Other symptoms include pleuritic chest pain and dizziness. Clinical examination of the chest often reveals no abnormal signs. There may be a swollen limb, suggesting an underlying deep venous thrombosis. The patient may have had recent surgery or have other risk factors present, such as being on the oral contraceptive pill, a recent flight, being at risk of an underlying malignancy or a genetic prothrombotic tendency.
   B) Pneumothorax – Correct. A pneumothorax often results in a sudden onset of breathlessness and pleuritic chest pain. There may be a history of an underlying lung condition (see question 1 for examples of conditions which predispose to secondary pneumothoraces) or trauma. The constellation of clinical findings associated with a pneumothorax is discussed in question 2.

C) Pneumonia – Incorrect. Pneumonia and other infections are common causes of breathlessness; however, the onset of breathlessness is usually more subacute, occurring over hours rather than seconds. Other symptoms include a productive cough with sputum production and fever.
D) Heart failure – Incorrect. The onset of heart failure is more insidious. Patients may also complain of orthopnoea and paroxysmal nocturnal dyspnoea. There may be a previous history of cardiac disease. Clinical examination may demonstrate an elevated jugular venous pulse and pleural effusions.
E) Anaphylaxis – Correct. Anaphylaxis is a systemic and life-threatening allergic reaction. It usually occurs shortly after contact with the allergen (previous sensitisation to the allergen is required). Symptoms develop rapidly over minutes and include facial swelling, wheezing, breathlessness, urticaria and, potentially, shock. Urgent management using the ABCDE approach and administration of intramuscular adrenaline is required.

❗ KEY POINT

Use the history and examination findings to help formulate a differential diagnosis to guide appropriate investigations and management. But remember that some patients, such as those presenting with anaphylaxis, may need urgent treatment before you will be able to complete a full history and examination. In these patients, use the ABCDE approach to assessment and management.

4. Which of the following is the most appropriate initial imaging investigation in a patient suspected of having a simple pneumothorax?
   The correct answer is **A) Erect PA chest X-ray**.
   The chest X-ray is the first-line imaging modality for suspected simple pneumothoraces. Imaging has a key role in confirming the diagnosis of a pneumothorax, assessing its size and excluding other differential diagnoses. There are various different types of chest X-ray, which are discussed next.
   A) Erect PA chest X-ray – Correct. The standard method for imaging pneumothoraces is an erect PA chest X-ray performed during inspiration. This provides an accurate and reliable assessment for a pneumothorax. A well-inspired PA X-ray allows a better assessment of the lungs and cardiac contours compared to an AP or expiratory X-ray. The key finding on a chest X-ray is displacement of the lung edge (visceral pleura) away from the chest wall, with no lung markings visible peripheral to this.
   B) PA and lateral chest X-rays – Incorrect. The lateral chest X-ray can provide helpful information if a pneumothorax is not visible on the PA X-ray. However, it is not part of routine practice.
   C) Expiratory chest X-ray – Incorrect. Expiratory X-rays may make a subtle pneumothorax

Continue

more readily visible. However, they are not performed in the first instance.

D) Supine chest X-ray – Incorrect. Pneumothoraces can be very subtle and difficult to identify on supine chest X-rays, as the air collects anteriorly, and there may not be a clearly discernible lung edge as seen in an erect X-ray. Supine chest X-rays are thus not performed routinely. Instead they are reserved for trauma patients who cannot be safely moved. Features suggestive of a pneumothorax on a supine chest X-ray include a sharply outlined dome of the hemidiaphragm, a deep lateral costophrenic sulcus and a hyperlucent upper quadrant of the abdomen (due to the lucent gas within the pleural space overlying the upper abdomen).

E) CT – Incorrect. Whilst CT is the most sensitive and specific test for a pneumothorax, its high-radiation dose (approximately equivalent to 400 chest X-rays!) and the satisfactory accuracy of standard PA chest X-rays mean CT is not the first-line imaging modality for suspected pneumothoraces. It is reserved for patients in whom there is continued suspicion of a pneumothorax but no evidence on a chest X-ray, or for assessing trauma patients. CT also provides the most reliable assessment of pneumothorax size.

❗ KEY POINTS

1. Remember that your environment can affect how easy or difficult it is to interpret X-rays. For example, a brightly lit room, with glare and a low-resolution ward monitor, may make it difficult or impossible to identify a small pneumothorax. Optimise your chance of picking up pathology by using diagnostic quality workstations in a dark room.
2. Pneumothoraces can be difficult to see on chest X-rays. Inverting the image can make the lung edge more obvious.
3. Always check the apices on an erect chest X-ray and around the lung bases on a supine chest X-ray for evidence of a pneumothorax.

5. Which of the following is the most appropriate management option for a previously healthy patient with a small, asymptomatic primary pneumothorax?
   The correct answer is **B) Conservative management with outpatient follow-up**.
   A) Conservative management and discharge the patient – Incorrect. Whilst asymptomatic (not

breathless) patients with a small (<2 cm) spontaneous primary pneumothorax can be safely managed conservatively with analgesia. It is important to arrange for the patient to be reviewed in the outpatient clinic in 2 to 4 weeks. This is to ensure that the patient has not deteriorated and the pneumothorax has not increased in size. Patients should be followed up with the respiratory team until complete resolution of their pneumothorax has occurred. Patients should also be instructed to return to hospital if they develop symptoms.

B) Conservative management with outpatient follow-up – Correct. See earlier. The patient should be instructed to return immediately if they experience symptoms to identify those patients with enlarging pneumothoraces. All patients with a pneumothorax should avoid air travel until a week following complete resolution on a chest X-ray. Smoking cessation should be advised in all patients as it increases risk of further pneumothoraces. Diving should be permanently avoided in most patients who have had a pneumothorax unless preventative surgery has been performed.

C) Admit for conservative management, high-flow oxygen and monitoring – Incorrect. If the patient is not breathless and has a small primary spontaneous pneumothorax, they can usually be managed safely as an outpatient; admission to hospital and high-flow oxygen is not required. In contrast, symptomatic patients with a small (<2 cm) secondary pneumothorax should be admitted, treated with high-flow oxygen (if necessary) and monitored for 24 hours. Supplementary oxygen not only improves hypoxaemia, but also increases the speed at which a pneumothorax resolves.

D) Aspirate as much of the pneumothorax as possible – Incorrect. Patients with a large and/or symptomatic primary or secondary pneumothorax need active management. Needle aspiration, using a 14- to 16-G needle, is as effective as chest drain insertion but reduces length of hospital stay and morbidity. These procedures should be performed in the safe triangle in the mid-axillary region. If, following needle aspiration, the patient's symptoms have improved and the pneumothorax is <2 cm in size, then no further intervention is required at that stage. If, however, this is not the case, the patient may require a chest drain (repeat needle aspiration should not be performed).

E) Chest drain insertion – Incorrect. Small bore (<14 F) chest drains are indicated in patients who do not improve following needle aspiration and those with bilateral or tension pneumothoraces.

❗ KEY POINTS

1. The size of the pneumothorax is one of the parameters used in deciding appropriate treatment. A large pneumothorax is defined by a rim of >2 cm between the lung margin and chest wall, measured at the level of the hilum. If this rim is <2 cm the patient has a small pneumothorax.
2. Patients admitted with a pneumothorax should be reviewed by a respiratory physician within 24 hours.
3. Pleurodesis is a procedure in which the pleural space is obliterated (either chemically or surgically) and can be used in patients who suffer with recurrent pneumothoraces.

 IMPORTANT LEARNING POINTS

- A pneumothorax is a collection of air in the pleural space.
- It can be primary, secondary to underlying lung disease, related to trauma, or related to medical procedures.
- Typical clinical features of a simple pneumothorax include reduced chest expansion, hyperresonant percussion and reduced air entry ipsilaterally, without evidence of mediastinal shift or cardiovascular compromise.
- The erect PA chest X-ray is the first-line investigation for suspected pneumothorax; however, CT is the gold standard.
- Treatment depends on whether the patient is symptomatic, the size of the pneumothorax and the presence of underlying lung disease.

CASE 2.2

A 48-year-old man is brought to A&E hypotensive and tachycardic. There is a preceding history of sudden-onset left-sided pleuritic chest pain following blunt trauma to the chest.

The patient is rushed through to X-ray for an urgent chest X-ray as part of his assessment.

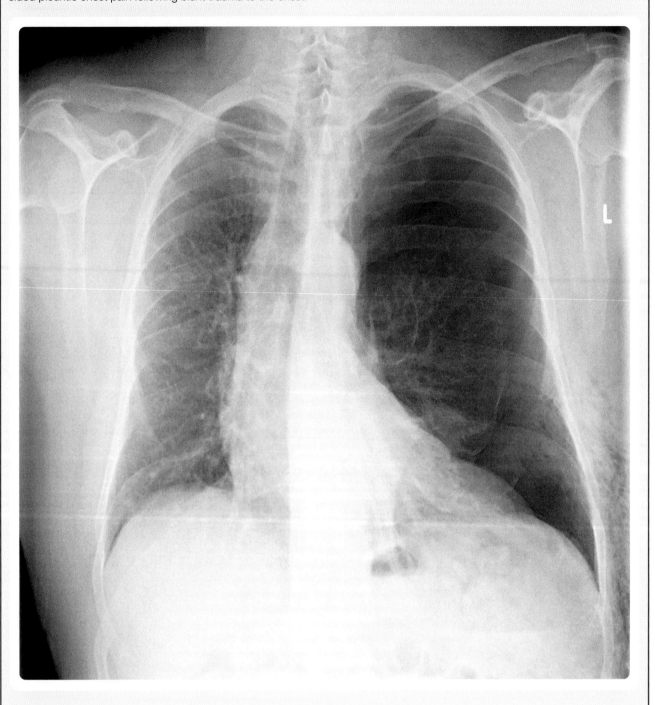

ANNOTATED X-RAY

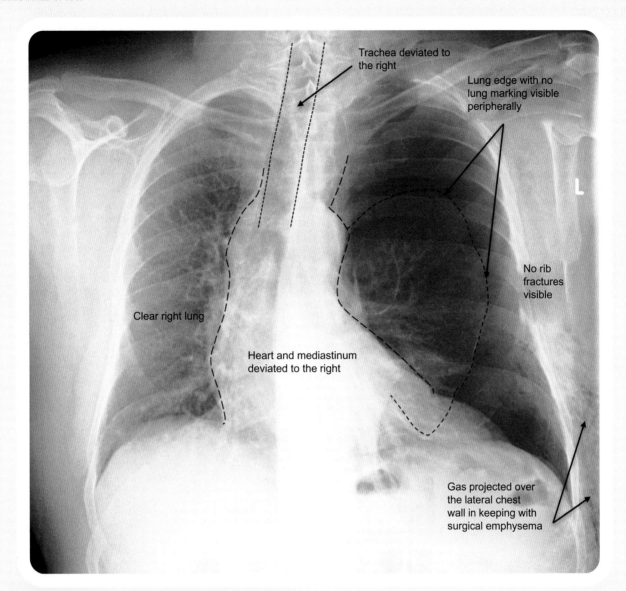

Trachea deviated to the right

Lung edge with no lung marking visible peripherally

L

No rib fractures visible

Clear right lung

Heart and mediastinum deviated to the right

Gas projected over the lateral chest wall in keeping with surgical emphysema

🔍 PRESENT YOUR FINDINGS

- This is a PA chest X-ray of an adult.
- There are no identifiers on the X-ray. I would like to ensure that it is the correct patient and to check the date and time when it was taken.
- It is a technically adequate X-ray: the patient is not rotated, there is good inspiratory achievement and adequate penetration. There are no important areas cut off at the edges of the X-ray.
- The important radiological signs demonstrated include a lung edge in the left hemithorax beyond which no lung markings are visible. Additionally, there is marked trachea and mediastinal shift to the contralateral (right) side. These features are consistent with a left-sided tension pneumothorax.
- Gas can be seen projected over the soft tissues of the lower left lateral chest wall, in keeping with surgical emphysema.

- The right lung is clear.
- The costophrenic angles and hemidiaphragms are sharply demarcated.
- There is no free subdiaphragmatic gas.
- There is no evidence of rib fractures or bony abnormality.
- Apart from the surgical emphysema, the soft tissues are normal.

IN SUMMARY – This chest X-ray shows a left tension pneumothorax. I would urgently review the patient, commence high-flow oxygen and perform needle decompression of the pneumothorax in the left 2nd intercostal space in the mid-clavicular line. Technically, this chest X-ray should never have been performed and the patient should have been treated on clinical grounds initially.

Continue

CASE **2.2**   *Contd.*

QUESTIONS

1. Which of the following is/are correct regarding a tension pneumothorax?
   A) It occurs when air is trapped in the pleural space under negative pressure
   B) It occurs because the damaged lung acts as a ball valve mechanism, letting air into the pleural cavity but not back in to the lung
   C) This is the most common type of pneumothorax
   D) A simple pneumothorax can become a tension pneumothorax
   E) Mechanical ventilation is a useful treatment option in tension pneumothoraces to expand the lung

2. Which of these clinical features is/are associated with a tension pneumothorax?
   A) Hypoxia
   B) Tachycardia and hypotension
   C) Reduced jugular venous pulse
   D) Reduced consciousness
   E) Deviation of the trachea and apex beat towards the side of the pneumothorax

3. What is the most appropriate immediate management option in a patient suspected to have a tension pneumothorax?

A) Urgent departmental PA chest X-ray to confirm the diagnosis followed by needle decompression
B) Urgent portable AP chest X-ray to confirm the diagnosis followed by needle decompression
C) Urgent needle decompression
D) Urgent respiratory review and chest drain insertion
E) Urgent intubation and ventilation

4. Which X-ray features indicate a tension rather than simple pneumothorax?
   A) A large pneumothorax
   B) The presence of rib fractures
   C) Mediastinal deviation away from the side of the pneumothorax
   D) Elevation of the ipsilateral hemidiaphragm
   E) Flattening of the ipsilateral hemidiaphragm

5. What is the definitive management of a tension pneumothorax following needle decompression?
   A) No further management needed
   B) Admit for high-flow oxygen and close monitoring
   C) Admit for supplementary oxygen and chest drain insertion
   D) Aspiration of the pneumothorax
   E) Urgent surgical pleurodesis

ANSWERS TO QUESTIONS

1. Which of the following is/are correct regarding a tension pneumothorax?

The correct answers are **B) It occurs because the damaged lung acts as a ball valve mechanism, letting air into the pleural cavity but not back in to the lung and D) A simple pneumothorax can become a tension pneumothorax**.

A tension pneumothorax can be defined as a pneumothorax that results in significant compromise to the respiratory and/or cardiovascular system. It is a medical emergency that should be diagnosed clinically – waiting for a chest X-ray to make the diagnosis can be fatal.

A) It occurs when air is trapped in the pleural space under negative pressure – Incorrect. The air trapped within the pleural space is under positive pressure in a tension pneumothorax, whereas in a simple pneumothorax this is not the case. With inspiration, the thorax expands, reducing the thoracic pressure in relation to atmospheric pressure. This normally results in air being drawn into the airways and alveoli. The opposite occurs in expiration. With a tension pneumothorax, the damaged lung acts as a one-way valve mechanism. During inspiration, air is drawn into the lungs, and into the pleural space through the damaged part of the lung. However, on expiration this air within the pleural space cannot escape back into the lung. With every breath, more air is drawn into the pleural space, resulting in positive pressure within the pleural space. As the pressure increases, the mediastinal structures, including the great vessels and heart, are displaced to the opposite side, resulting in respiratory and/or cardiovascular compromise.

B) It occurs because the damaged lung acts as a ball valve mechanism, letting air into the pleural cavity but not back into the lung – Correct. See answer A for more details.

C) They are the most common type of pneumothorax – Incorrect. Simple pneumothoraces are much more common than tension pneumothoraces. However, patients with a tension pneumothorax can become very unstable and may potentially die if not managed appropriately in a timely manner. Therefore, although tension pneumothoraces are rare, it is important to consider and recognise a tension pneumothorax clinically in collapsed/unwell patients.

D) A simple pneumothorax can become a tension pneumothorax – Correct. A simple pneumothorax can be converted into a tension pneumothorax if the patient undergoes positive pressure ventilation. Air is forced through the damaged lung into the pleural space, causing it to collect under pressure. Mechanical ventilation can also cause a tension pneumothorax without the presence of a preexisting simple pneumothorax. Recognising a tension pneumothorax in a patient being ventilated can be difficult because the effects of sedation may mask the symptoms and signs. However, it should be considered if there is sudden deterioration in a ventilated patient.

E) Mechanical ventilation is a useful treatment option in tension pneumothoraces to expand the lung – Incorrect. See answer D for more details.

❗ KEY POINTS

1. Tension pneumothoraces should be recognised clinically and treated. You should never see a chest X-ray with a tension pneumothorax in clinical practice.
2. Consider a tension pneumothorax in any ventilated patient who suddenly deteriorates.

2. Which of these clinical features is/are associated with a tension pneumothorax?

The correct answers are **A) Hypoxia, B) Tachycardia and hypotension and D) Reduced consciousness**.

The clinical findings associated with a tension pneumothorax are caused by the raised intrapleural pressure. As the pressure increases due to the one-way valve mechanism, there is compression of the ipsilateral lung and deviation of the mediastinum to the contralateral side. This can compress the opposite lung and the great vessels (superior and inferior vena cava, pulmonary vessels and (to a lesser extent) the aorta), compromising respiratory function and cardiac output.

A) Hypoxia – Correct. As the pneumothorax enlarges, alveoli collapse, and the gas exchange surface area reduces. In addition, cardiac output is compromised by pressure on the great vessels from the displaced mediastinum.

B) Tachycardia and hypotension – Correct. Displacement of the mediastinum causes kinking of the inferior and superior vena cava. This impairs blood flow to the right atrium, compromising cardiac output. The persistently high intrathoracic pressure from air trapped in the pleural space under positive pressure contributes to reduced venous return and reduction in cardiac output, causing hypotension and resultant tachycardia.

C) Reduced jugular venous pulse – Incorrect. Raised intrathoracic pressure and kinking of the superior vena cava result in and increased jugular venous pulse. Elevated jugular venous pressure, hypotension and tachycardia can also present in cardiac tamponade. Remember that in hypovolaemia there will be tachycardia, hypotension and a reduced jugular venous pulse.

D) Reduced consciousness – Correct. The reduced cardiac output can cause decreased consciousness from the resultant reduction in blood flow to the brain (and brainstem in particular), and chest pain secondary to reduced perfusion of the coronary arteries. It can lead to cardiac arrest. Tension pneumothorax is one of the reversible causes of PEA cardiac arrest, which should be excluded (four 'T's of reversible causes of PEA: toxins, tamponade, thrombosis and tension pneumothorax. Four 'H's of reversible causes of PEA:

Continue

hypovolaemia, hypoxia, hyper/hypokalaemia and hypothermia).

E) Deviation of the trachea and apex beat towards the side of the pneumothorax – Incorrect. Due to the positive pressure within the ipsilateral pleural space and hemithorax, the mediastinum will be displaced to the opposite side (assessed by the position of the trachea and apex beat).

❗ KEY POINT

The clinical features of a tension pneumothorax are a result of increased pressure within the pleural cavity. If left untreated, the respiratory and cardiovascular compromise can result in a loss of consciousness and cardiac arrest (tension pneumothorax is one of the four 'T's of reversible causes of a cardiac arrest).

3. What is the most appropriate immediate management option in a patient suspected to have a tension pneumothorax?
   The correct answer is **C) Urgent needle decompression**.
   A tension pneumothorax can be rapidly fatal. It is a medical emergency which should be clinically diagnosed, with urgent appropriate management instigated.
   A) Urgent departmental PA chest X-ray to confirm the diagnosis followed by needle decompression – Incorrect. A tension pneumothorax is a clinical diagnosis. The patient needs to be stabilised with urgent needle decompression in the 2nd intercostal space in the midclavicular line. Waiting for a chest X-ray (even a portable AP X-ray) can have catastrophic consequences for the patient.
   B) Urgent portable AP chest X-ray to confirm the diagnosis followed by needle decompression – Incorrect. See answer A for more details.
   C) Urgent needle decompression – Correct. The approach to any unwell patient should be the same – assessing and correcting life-threatening abnormalities using the ABCDE approach in the first instance. If a tension pneumothorax is clinically suspected, then the patient should have urgent needle decompression. This involves inserting a cannula (14 G) into the pleural space on the affected side to allow the trapped air to escape. The common site for needle decompression is the 2nd intercostal space in the midclavicular line. Needle decompression is used to convert a tension pneumothorax into a simple pneumothorax. The patient will still require treatment of the underlying pneumothorax.
   D) Urgent respiratory review and chest drain insertion – Incorrect. A tension pneumothorax is initially managed with emergency needle decompression, not chest drain insertion. A chest drain will, however, be required as part of the definitive management of the pneumothorax.
   E) Urgent intubation and ventilation – Incorrect. Positive pressure ventilation will make the tension pneumothorax worse by increasing the pressure within the

pleural space. It can also convert a simple pneumothorax into a tension pneumothorax. It is therefore not part of the initial management. If a patient with a tension pneumothorax requires ventilation, they must have a chest drain inserted first.

❗ KEY POINT

Urgent needle decompression is used to convert a tension pneumothorax into a simple pneumothorax. Remember that the patient will still require treatment of the underlying pneumothorax.

4. Which X-ray features indicate a tension rather than simple pneumothorax?
   The correct answers are **C) Mediastinal deviation away from the side of the pneumothorax and E) Flattening of the ipsilateral hemidiaphragm**.
   Although in theory you should never see a tension pneumothorax on a chest X-ray, it is useful to know what findings are in keeping with a tension rather than simple pneumothorax. These findings relate to the effects of raised intrapleural pressure.
   A) A large pneumothorax – Incorrect. Tension pneumothoraces tend to be large due to the one-way valve effect. However, simple pneumothoraces can also be large. Size alone is not a reliable distinguisher between a tension and simple pneumothorax.
   B) The presence of rib fractures – Incorrect. Rib fractures can result in both simple and tension pneumothoraces and therefore cannot be used to differentiate between the two.
   C) Mediastinal deviation away from the side of the pneumothorax – Correct. Raised intrapleural pressure in tension pneumothoraces will result in deviation of the mediastinum away from the side of the pneumothorax. In a well-centred X-ray, the trachea should lie over the spinous processes of the vertebral bodies, most of the cardiac shadow should be projected to the left of the spine, and the thoracic vertebral bodies should not be visible beyond the cardiac silhouette.
   D) Elevation of the ipsilateral hemidiaphragm – Incorrect. The raised intrapleural pressure will cause flattening of the ipsilateral hemidiaphragm.
   E) Flattening of the ipsilateral hemidiaphragm – Correct. See answer D.

❗ KEY POINTS

1. Chest X-ray signs of tension include mediastinal displacement away from the pneumothorax and flattening of the hemidiaphragm on the side of the pneumothorax.
2. Remember that patient rotation can make the normal mediastinum appear displaced on a chest X-ray.

5. What is the definitive management of a tension pneumothorax following needle decompression?
   The correct answer is **C) Admit for supplementary oxygen and chest drain insertion**.

As previously discussed, the initial management of a tension pneumothorax is needle decompression. Once this has been performed, the remaining pneumothorax (which is no longer under tension) will need definitive treatment.

A) No further management needed – Incorrect. Needle decompression relieves the tension but does not definitively treat the underlying pneumothorax. Further management is therefore required.

B) Admit for high-flow oxygen and close monitoring – Incorrect. Both supplementary oxygen and close monitoring are required; however, patients with a tension pneumothorax will require definitive treatment of the pneumothorax. The British Thoracic Society recommends chest drain insertion in these patients.

C) Admit for supplementary oxygen and chest drain insertion – Correct. Supplementary oxygen i) treats hypoxia and ii) has a therapeutic effect in reducing the size of the pneumothorax. The chest drain definitively treats the pneumothorax. It is connected to an underwater seal to prevent backflow of air or fluid into the pleural space. It should be monitored for swinging of the underwater seal during inspiration to ensure the drain is patent. Chest drains are usually inserted in the 'safe triangle'. The anatomic borders of the 'safe triangle' are formed anteriorly by the lateral border of the pectoralis major, laterally by the lateral border of the latissimus dorsi, and inferiorly by the line of the 5th intercostal space. Follow-up X-ray will determine when the pneumothorax has resolved, and guide drain removal.

D) Aspiration of the pneumothorax – Incorrect. Aspiration is not recommended as a definitive treatment for large pneumothoraces or tension pneumothoraces.

E) Urgent surgical pleurodesis – Incorrect. Pleurodesis means sticking the visceral and parietal pleura together and obliterating the pleural space, preventing further pneumothoraces. Pneumothoraces can usually be treated without surgery; however, indications for surgical intervention include unexpanded lung despite treatment with a chest drain, bilateral pneumothoraces, recurrent episodes of pneumothorax and a pneumothorax in a high-risk patient (diver or pilot).

IMPORTANT LEARNING POINTS

- A tension pneumothorax causes significant respiratory and/or cardiovascular compromise due to increased intrapleural pressure.
- It is a medical emergency which should be diagnosed clinically and managed initially with urgent needle decompression.
- Definitive treatment of the pneumothorax involves chest drain insertion.
- You should never see a chest X-ray showing a tension pneumothorax (as it should have been treated with needle decompression prior to imaging). However, its features include contralateral displacement of the mediastinum, and flattening of the ipsilateral hemidiaphragm.

CASE **2.3**

An asymptomatic 25-year-old male has a chest X-ray for an overseas work visa.

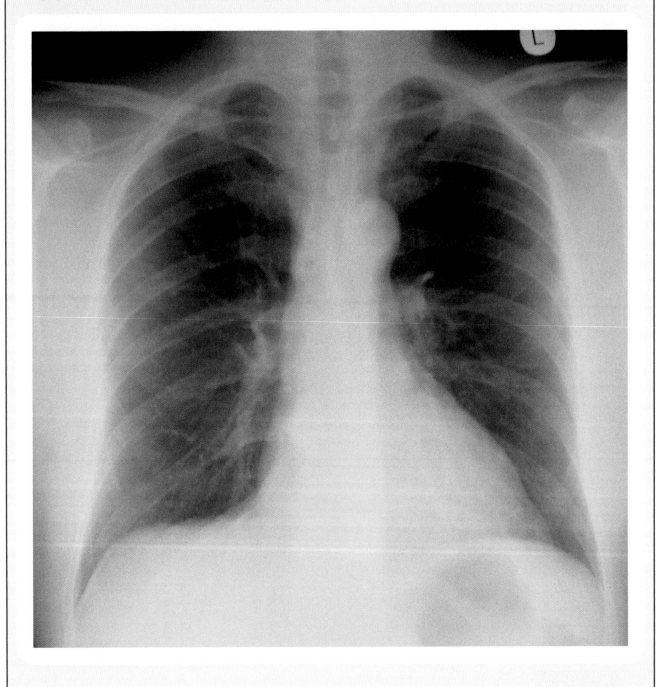

ANNOTATED X-RAY

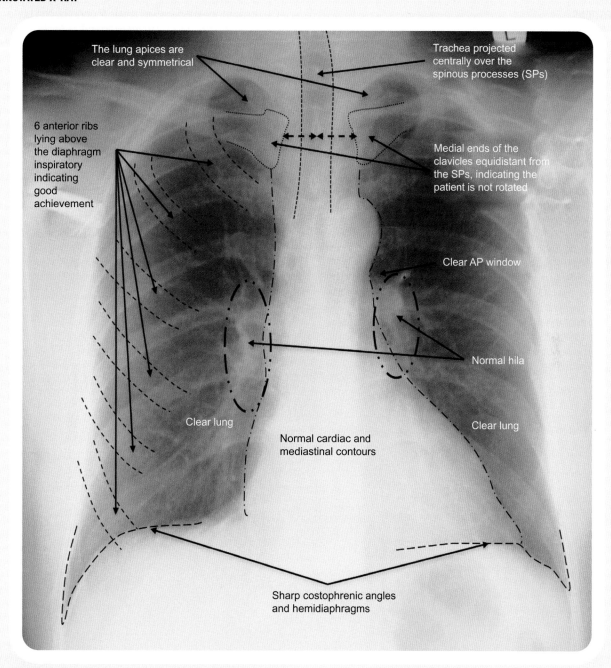

The lung apices are clear and symmetrical

Trachea projected centrally over the spinous processes (SPs)

6 anterior ribs lying above the diaphragm inspiratory indicating good achievement

Medial ends of the clavicles equidistant from the SPs, indicating the patient is not rotated

Clear AP window

Normal hila

Clear lung

Clear lung

Normal cardiac and mediastinal contours

Sharp costophrenic angles and hemidiaphragms

🔍 PRESENT YOUR FINDINGS

- This is a PA chest X-ray of an adult.
- There are no identifying markings. I would like to ensure that this is the correct patient and to check the date and time when the X-ray was taken.
- Apart from being slightly underpenetrated, this is a technically adequate X-ray – the patient is not rotated and has made a good inspiratory effort. There are no important areas cut off at the edges of the film.
- There are no obvious abnormalities on the X-ray.
- The trachea is central.

- The lungs are clear, with no masses, nodules, consolidation or collapse visible.
- The heart is not enlarged, and the cardiac and mediastinal contours are normal.
- Both hemidiaphragms and the costophrenic angles are clearly demarcated.
- No free subdiaphragmatic gas is seen.
- There is no abnormality of the imaged soft tissues or skeleton.

IN SUMMARY – This is a normal chest X-ray.

Continue

CASE 2.3   *Contd.*

QUESTIONS

1. Which of the following are appropriate indications for a chest X-ray?
   A) Upper respiratory tract infection
   B) Preoperative chest X-ray in a healthy 35-year-old undergoing an elective hernia repair
   C) Suspected PE
   D) Acute chest pain
   E) Acute abdominal pain

2. Which of the following statements regarding chest X-ray radiation dose is/are correct?
   A) Chest X-rays do not involve the use of ionising radiation
   B) Chest X-rays use ionising radiation, but the dose is negligible
   C) Chest X-rays use ionising radiation, and the dose is similar to 3 days of background radiation
   D) Chest X-rays use ionising radiation, and the dose is similar to an abdominal X-ray
   E) Frontal (AP or PA) and lateral chest X-rays expose the patient to the same dose of radiation

3. Which of the following is/are correct regarding a normal chest X-ray?
   A) The right ventricle forms the right heart border
   B) The left ventricle forms the left heart border
   C) The aortopulmonary window is formed by the aorta and the right main pulmonary artery
   D) The left hemidiaphragm should not be higher than the right
   E) The left hilum may be higher than the right

4. Which of the following statements is/are correct regarding the normal cardiothoracic ratio?
   A) The width of the heart and the width of the chest should be measured at the same level
   B) The cardiothoracic ratio is best measured on the PA chest X-ray
   C) No comment regarding the heart size can be made on AP chest X-ray
   D) The normal cardiothoracic ratio is less than 50% in the paediatric population
   E) An enlarged cardiothoracic ratio is pathognomonic of cardiomegaly

5. Subtle pathology may be commonly missed in which of the following locations on a chest X-ray?
   A) Apices
   B) Hila
   C) Retrocardiac position
   D) Middle zones of the lungs
   E) Below the domes of the diaphragm

ANSWERS TO QUESTIONS

1. Which of the following are appropriate indications for a chest X-ray?

   The correct answers are **C) Suspected PE, D) Acute chest pain and E) Acute abdominal pain**.

   The chest X-ray is a simple, straightforward examination with a wide range of indications. However, there are certain situations in which it is not required. 'Making the best use of clinical radiology services' is within the Royal College of Radiologists' guidelines for requesting imaging investigations. These guidelines describe the appropriate imaging for various pathologies. They are now available as a Smartphone/Tablet app (iRefer).

   A) Upper respiratory tract infection – Incorrect. This is not an indication for a chest X-ray. Such infections are usually viral, and chest signs are often absent. In contrast, a chest X-ray may be useful in patients with signs of a lower respiratory tract infection to confirm the diagnosis and identify any complications, such as abscess formation or lobar collapse. Follow-up chest X-ray 4 to 6 weeks after treatment of the pneumonia can be used to ensure resolution.

   B) Preoperative chest X-ray in a healthy 35-year-old undergoing an elective hernia repair – Incorrect. Routine preoperative chest X-rays in patients <60 years old undergoing non-cardiothoracic surgery are not usually required. Indeed, the value of routine preoperative chest X-rays in those >60 years old is limited, as there is a low yield for detecting pathology. Preoperative chest X-rays are indicated in those undergoing cardiothoracic surgery, or if there are symptoms or signs of cardiorespiratory disease.

   C) Suspected PE – Correct. In patients with a suspected PE, a chest X-ray should be the initial imaging modality. Its role is primarily to exclude other differential diagnoses, such as pneumonia, lobar collapse or pneumothorax. A chest X-ray is also helpful in enabling interpretation if the patient goes on to have ventilation/perfusion or CTPA imaging to confirm or refute the presence of a PE. Remember, a normal chest X-ray does not exclude a PE.

   D) Acute chest pain – Correct. Acute chest pain can have a wide differential diagnosis. A chest X-ray is helpful for excluding pathologies, such as pneumothorax or pneumonia. There may be evidence of other differential diagnoses or complications related to ischaemic heart disease, such as cardiomegaly or pulmonary oedema.

   E) Acute abdominal pain – Correct. An erect chest X-ray is useful for identifying free subdiaphragmatic gas (pneumoperitoneum), which in the context of acute abdominal pain is indicative of a perforated viscus.

> ❗ KEY POINT
>
> There is a wide range of indications for chest X-rays. Other indications which have not been mentioned include congenital heart disease, suspected heart failure, pleural effusion, haemoptysis and after insertion of certain lines/devices (endotracheal tube, central line, pacemaker, NG tubes, chest drain) to check that they are in the correct position.

2. Which of the following statements regarding chest X-ray radiation dose is/are correct?

   The correct answer is **C) Chest X-rays use ionising radiation, and the dose is similar to 3 days of background radiation**.

   X-rays are a form of ionising radiation and have the potential to damage tissues. It is therefore necessary for medical staff requesting X-rays to have an understanding of the dose involved and the potential hazards to the patient.

   A) Chest X-rays do not involve the use of ionising radiation – Incorrect. X-rays are a form of ionising radiation. Ultrasound and MRI do not use ionising radiation.

   B) Chest X-rays use ionising radiation, but the dose is negligible – Incorrect. Chest X-rays are low-dose investigations, but no exposure to ionising radiation can be described as negligible. This is because ionising radiation can cause stochastic effects, such as cancer induction, which are related to chance rather than cumulative radiation dose. Although these effects are more likely at higher doses, there is no lower dose cut-off below which cancer cannot be induced by radiation.

   C) Chest X-rays use ionising radiation and the dose is similar to 3 days of background radiation – Correct. Relative to other X-ray examinations, such as abdominal, spine or pelvic X-rays, the chest X-ray uses a relatively low dose of radiation. The typical dose of a frontal chest X-ray is 0.02 mSv (millisieverts). To put this into context, this is approximately equivalent to 3 days of natural background radiation or a 6-hour flight.

   D) Chest X-rays use ionising radiation, and the dose is similar to an abdominal X-ray – Incorrect. Abdominal X-rays use 30 to 50 times the dose that a chest X-ray does. This is because the chest is largely composed of gas-filled alveoli, which absorb relatively few X-rays, whereas a higher dose is needed to penetrate the many layers of soft tissues in the abdominal cavity.

   E) Frontal (AP or PA) and lateral chest X-rays expose the patient to the same dose of radiation – Incorrect. The lateral chest X-ray uses approximately twice the dose of a frontal chest X-ray. This is due to the increased amount of soft tissues and the lung X-ray beams have to travel through before reaching the X-ray plate (X-rays have to travel through the chest wall muscles of the axilla, both lungs and the mediastinum on the lateral view, whereas on the frontal view the X-rays pass through the anterior and posterior chest walls, which are thinner, and travel through one lung or the mediastinum, rather than lateral X-rays which have to travel through both lungs and the mediastinum).

Continue

CASE 2.3 *Contd.*

❶ KEY POINTS

1. It is useful to have an idea of the amount of radiation associated with X-ray examinations, and be able to put them into a context a patient is likely to understand (Table C2.3.1).

Table C2.3.1   Ionising Radiation Doses of Different X-rays

EXAMINATION	DOSE (mSv)	APPROXIMATE EQUIVALENT DOSE AS BACKGROUND RADIATION
Frontal chest X-ray	0.02 (3 days background)	3 days radiation
Abdominal X-ray	0.7	100 days
Pelvis X-ray	0.7	100 days
Lumbar spine	1.0	150 days (AP and lateral)

2. Under UK IR(ME)R 2000 legislation (Ionising radiation (Medical Exposure) Regulations 2000), each investigation that exposes a patient to ionising radiation must be justified. When making a request for an X-ray, CT, nuclear medicine examination or fluoroscopy study, the referrer must provide enough clinical information to justify the examination. Examinations involving a low dose, such as limb X-rays, are easier to justify than high-dose examinations, such as CT.

3. X-rays and other forms of ionising radiation can result in two types of damage. One form of harm is due to cumulative damage to cells within tissues. These are known as DETERMINISTIC EFFECTS and include skin erythema, hair loss and cataracts. There are cellular repair mechanisms which can repair such damage, and these deterministic effects therefore do not occur below a threshold dose (the threshold dose varies between different tissues and organs). If the tissues are exposed to radiation dose(s) above the threshold, these repair mechanisms can be overwhelmed, resulting in cell death and the deterministic effects. Whilst the threshold dose is never reached with most diagnostic investigations, there are cases of these effects occurring after very long interventional cardiology or neuroradiology cases with prolonged fluoroscopic exposure.
The other type of damage caused by ionising radiation is due to the random chance of radiation resulting in a genetic mutation. These are known as STOCHASTIC effects. Carcinogenesis is the most important stochastic effect and occurs through mutations in tumour suppressor genes and oncogenes. There is no threshold dose for stochastic effects to occur (they can occur after one exposure), but they are more likely with increasing doses of radiation (you can win the lottery with just one ticket, but you are much more likely to do so if you buy more tickets).

3. Which of the following is/are correct regarding a normal chest X-ray?
The correct answers are **B) The left ventricle forms the left heart border, D) The left hemidiaphragm should not be higher than the right and E) The left hilum may be higher than the right**.
It is important to understand the normal anatomy and relationships on a chest X-ray to allow you to interpret abnormalities correctly.

A) The right ventricle forms the right heart border – Incorrect. Knowledge of the structures constituting the cardiac and mediastinal contours is important for both examinations and clinical work. The upper right side of the mediastinum is formed initially by the right brachiocephalic vein, which then forms the superior vena cava. The right heart border is composed of the right atrium. The inferior IVC can often be seen inferiorly merging with the right atrium. The left side of the mediastinum (from superior to inferior) is formed by mediastinal fat, the arch of the aorta, the aortopulmonary window, the left atrium and left ventricle. Remember that the right ventricle lies anteriorly and therefore does not form one of the heart borders on the frontal chest X-ray.

B) The left ventricle forms the left heart border – Correct. See answer A for more details.

C) The aortopulmonary window is formed by the aorta and the right main pulmonary artery – Incorrect. The aortopulmonary window is a gap between the aorta and the left main pulmonary artery which is visible on the frontal chest X-ray as well as on CT. It predominantly contains fat, but also lymph nodes, the left recurrent laryngeal nerve and the remnants of the ligamentum arteriosum. It is of importance because it is a commonly overlooked site of lymph node enlargement. On the frontal chest X-ray, the aortopulmonary window should be empty; if it is not, then one should suspect enlarged lymph nodes filling in the aortopulmonary window. This is an important finding on the chest X-ray, but the X-ray is often nonspecific. CT provides more detailed assessment of the aortopulmonary window, as well as of the rest of the mediastinum and lungs.

D) The left hemidiaphragm should not be higher than the right – Correct. The right hemidiaphragm should be at the same level as or slightly higher than the left, due to slight elevation caused by the adjacent liver. It is abnormal if the left is higher than the right or the right significantly higher than the left. Causes of a raised hemidiaphragm include phrenic nerve injury (surgery or tumour), pain-related causes (rib fractures, pneumonia, PE), abdominal masses, subphrenic collections or effusions and pleural tumours. Both hemidiaphragms should be curved and clearly demarcated. The costophrenic angles should be sharply demarcated – pleural effusions or pleural thickening can cause blunting of these angles.

E) The left hilum may be higher than the right – Correct. The left hilum should be as high as or higher than the right. If this is not the case, then one must suspect that there has been volume loss somewhere in the lung. For example, a right upper lobe collapse would elevate the right hilum, or a left lower lobe collapse would lower the left hilum. Both hila should be of equal density. Increased size and density of a hilum raises the suspicion of a hilar mass or hilar lymphadenopathy.

❗ KEY POINTS

1. Knowing what a normal chest X-ray looks like is a key part of learning radiology. Without knowing what is normal, one cannot recognise what is abnormal.
2. Not all normal chest X-rays look the same. Try to look at as many X-rays as possible so you get a feel for the range of normality.

4. Which of the following statements is/are correct regarding the normal cardiothoracic ratio?
The correct answer is **B) The cardiothoracic ratio is best measured on the PA chest X-ray**.
The cardiothoracic ratio is used to assess whether there is cardiomegaly. It is the maximum transverse diameter of the heart divided by the maximum internal thoracic diameter. Its measurement can be affected by the projection of the X-ray, degree of inspiration and patient rotation.
A) The width of the heart and the width of the chest should be measured at the same level – Incorrect. The definition of the cardiothoracic ratio is the maximal transverse diameter of the heart divided by the maximal transverse diameter of the thorax. The chest is often widest at its inferior aspect, and this is where the measurement for thoracic diameter should be made. The heart should be measured transversely, not obliquely.
B) The cardiothoracic ratio is best measured on the PA chest X-ray – Correct. In an AP X-ray, the X-ray detector plate is farther from the heart than in a PA X-ray. As there is some divergence of the X-ray beams, this difference means the cardiac shadow is magnified somewhat in the AP projection.
C) No comment regarding the heart size can be made on an AP chest X-ray – Incorrect. Although the cardiothoracic ratio can only be reliably calculated on a PA chest X-ray, the heart size should be assessed on every chest X-ray, even AP X-rays – if the cardiothoracic ratio is normal on an AP projection, then it will be normal on a PA projection!
D) The normal cardiothoracic ratio is less than 50% in the paediatric population – Incorrect. A cardiothoracic ratio of less than 50% on a well-inspired, nonrotated PA chest X-ray is considered normal in adults. In children, the heart is normally slightly larger relative to the chest, and a ratio of 55% to 60% is often used as the cut-off for normality.

E) An enlarged cardiothoracic ratio is pathognomonic of cardiomegaly – Incorrect. Limited inspiratory achievement by the patient will cause a spuriously increased cardiothoracic ratio – the anterior aspect of at least six ribs should lie above the hemidiaphragm in a well-inspired X-ray. Patient rotation can alter the cardiothoracic ratio – look at the medial ends of the clavicles and their relative positions to the spinous processes of the vertebral bodies to assess whether the patient is rotated. Even when an increased cardiothoracic ratio is confirmed on a technically adequate X-ray, there are a variety of causes of it other than cardiomegaly, such as pericardial effusions and cardiac masses.

❗ KEY POINTS

1. It is very important to recognise the projection of the chest X-ray when assessing the heart size. AP X-rays lead to magnification of the cardiac silhouette and therefore cannot be used to assess the cardiothoracic ratio accurately. A rough assessment of the cardiac size can still be made, however.
2. The degree of inspiration and patient rotation must also be taken into account when assessing the cardiothoracic ratio.
3. Assessment of serial examinations is more useful than a one-off measurement, as an increase in the cardiac diameter of greater than 2 cm on serial PA chest X-rays suggests cardiac enlargement (even if the cardiothoracic ratio is less than 50%).

5. Subtle pathology may be commonly missed in which of the following locations on a chest X-ray?
The correct answers are **A) Apices, B) Hila, C) Retrocardiac position and E) Below the domes of the diaphragm**.
Review areas are parts of an X-ray in which pathology is commonly overlooked. Once you have finished looking at an X-ray, go back and look specifically at the review areas to make sure you have not overlooked anything. For chest X-rays, there are five review areas (the costophrenic angles in addition to those listed earlier); however, everyone is different – do not be afraid to add your own review areas if there are specific parts of the X-ray in which you tend to overlook pathology.
A) Apices – Correct. The apices are one of the five main review areas on the chest X-ray. Pathology is commonly missed here because of their location at the upper edge of the X-ray and the fact that there are usually multiple overlying shadows from the clavicles and 1st ribs. A useful tip is to compare one side to the other – they should both appear similar, with a similar density. Abnormalities that can occur include tumours, such as a Pancoast tumour, and small apical pneumothoraces.
B) Hila – Correct. The hila are complex structures made of pulmonary arteries, pulmonary veins, bronchi and lymph nodes, making them difficult to assess.

Continue

CASE 2.3   *Contd.*

Remember that both hila should have the same density and be similar in size. If one is denser than the other, then consider whether there is a hilar mass or lymph node enlargement. The left hilum should not be lower than the right – if this is not the case, then look at the rest of the X-ray for evidence of volume loss. Abnormalities which occur at the hila include tumours, enlarged lymph nodes and enlarged vessels.

C) Retrocardiac position – Correct. Remember that there is lung behind the cardiac shadow on a chest X-ray. This is difficult to assess due to the overlying cardiac silhouette, and pathology is often overlooked. The cardiac shadow should be the same density throughout. If there are parts that are more dense, then consider whether there is pathology lurking behind the heart. Also, the hemidiaphragms should be clearly visible all the way to the middle of the X-ray. If this is not the case, then there may be pathology, such as consolidation or collapse, in the lower lobes. Invert the X-ray to allow subtle differences in density to become more obvious.

D) Middle zones of the lungs – Incorrect. The middle zones of the lung are usually well assessed due to their central location and few overlying structures. They are not, therefore, one of the common review areas.

E) Below the domes of the diaphragm – Correct. The lung continues behind the hemidiaphragms. Pathology in this part is often overlooked, as it is at the lower edge of the X-ray and partly obscured by the diaphragms. Try inverting the X-ray to clarify any abnormalities in these areas. Masses, consolidation or effusions may be seen in this review area.

❶ KEY POINTS

1. Personalise the review areas to suit your assessment style. If there are particular parts of the chest X-ray you often overlook, then make a conscious effort to review them again at the end of your assessment.
2. Sometimes inverting the X-ray clarifies pathology that was not initially obvious.
3. Remember to look at the bones, soft tissues and upper abdomen. Pathology on the peripheries of the X-ray film, such as shoulder dislocations or surgical emphysema, is easily overlooked if not consciously searched for.

IMPORTANT LEARNING POINTS

- Chest X-rays use a relatively small dose of radiation and have a wide range of indications.
- Knowledge of the normal appearance and anatomy of the chest X-ray is important for appreciating and interpreting pathology.
- The projection of the X-ray, inspiratory effort and rotation of the patient can affect what the X-ray looks like and may mimic pathology. Take these into account when assessing any chest X-ray.
- Remember to look at your review areas and the edge of the X-ray carefully during your assessment.

CASE **2.4**

An 83-year-old non-binary person presents with shortness of breath and weight loss. Clinical examination reveals reduced air entry in the right upper zone. As part of their assessment, he has a chest X-ray performed.

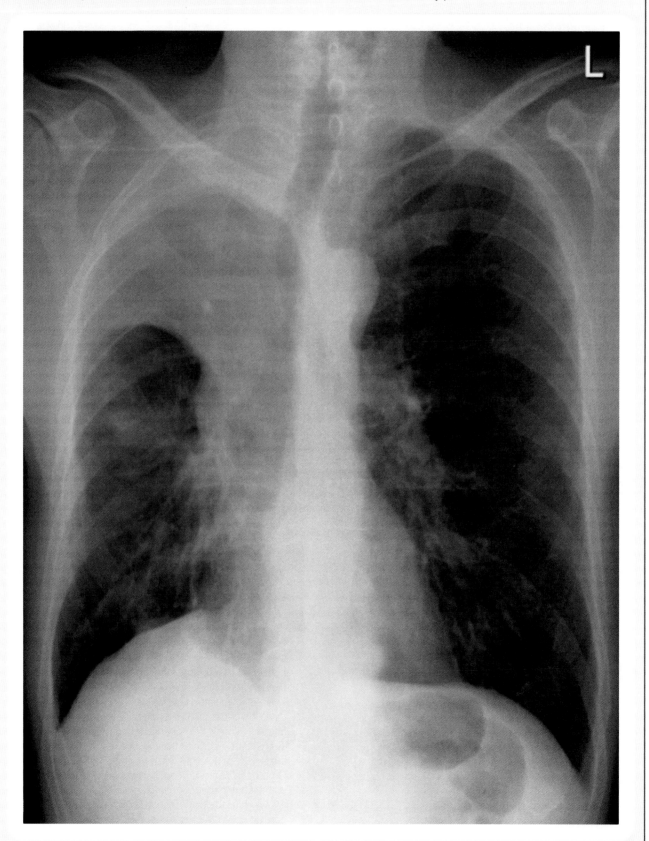

Continue

CASE **2.4** *Contd.*

ANNOTATED X-RAY

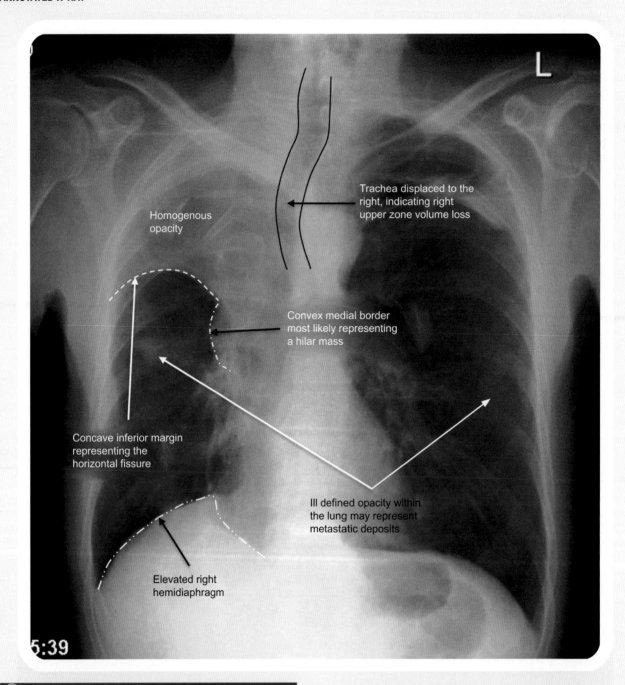

Trachea displaced to the right, indicating right upper zone volume loss

Homogenous opacity

Convex medial border most likely representing a hilar mass

Concave inferior margin representing the horizontal fissure

Ill defined opacity within the lung may represent metastatic deposits

Elevated right hemidiaphragm

L

5:39

🔍 **PRESENT YOUR FINDINGS**

- This is a PA chest X-ray of an adult.
- There are no patient identifier markings. I would like to ensure that this is the correct patient and to check the time and date when the X-ray was taken.
- It is a technically adequate film: it has adequate penetration and there are no important areas cut off at the edges of the film. The patient is not rotated, and there is good inspiratory achievement.
- The most striking abnormality is in the right upper zone, in which there is homogenous increased density and the lower border is a sharply defined curvilinear line formed by the horizontal fissure. There is a prominent soft tissue density at the medial aspect of the

horizontal fissure at the right hilum, representing the Golden S sign.
- There is associated volume loss in the right lung, with deviation of the trachea and cardiac contour to the right and elevation of the right hilum and hemidiaphragm.
- There is an ill-defined opacity in the right midzone. The remainder of the right lung is clear.
- On the left, there is possibly a subtle ill-defined opacity in the left midzone. The left lung is otherwise clear.
- Allowing for the position of the mediastinum, the cardiac contour is unremarkable.
- There is no free subdiaphragmatic gas.
- No obvious abnormality in the imaged soft tissues or bones.

IN SUMMARY – This chest X-ray shows a classic partially collapsed right upper lobe with the Golden S sign, highly suggestive of a central tumour causing the obstruction. There are also a couple of ill-defined opacities in the right and left midzones. These, in combination with the clinical information, make an underlying malignancy high on the list of differential diagnoses. Further investigation with CT is warranted.

QUESTIONS

1. Which of the following is/are correct regarding the clinical presentation of a lobar collapse?
   A) It may be associated with weight loss
   B) It may result in dyspnoea
   C) It can be asymptomatic
   D) Clinical examination will reveal a dull percussion note over the collapsed lobe
   E) A central trachea and nondisplaced apex beat on clinical examination reliably exclude the diagnosis

2. Which of the following is/are causes of lobar collapse?
   A) Bronchiectasis
   B) Bronchogenic tumour
   C) Hilar lymph node enlargement
   D) Inhaled foreign body
   E) Mucous plug

3. Which of the following chest X-ray features is/are in keeping with volume loss in the upper lobe of the left lung?
   A) Right hilum higher than the left hilum
   B) Deviation of the trachea to the left
   C) Elevated left hemidiaphragm
   D) Crowding of the left-sided ribs
   E) Elevated horizontal fissure

4. Which chest X-ray sign may be found in a right upper lobe collapse?
   A) Fleischner's sign
   B) Golden's S sign
   C) Sail sign
   D) Luftsichel sign
   E) Veil-like opacity

5. Which of the following regarding the further investigation and management of a lobar collapse is/are correct?
   A) A lateral chest X-ray is mandatory to confirm the diagnosis
   B) All patients need a CT to confirm the diagnosis and exclude malignancy
   C) All patients require bronchoscopy
   D) Chest physiotherapy may be helpful
   E) Antibiotics and a repeat chest X-ray are indicated for all patients

Continue

CASE 2.4 *Contd.*

ANSWERS TO QUESTIONS

1. Which of the following is/are correct regarding the clinical presentation of a lobar collapse?

   The correct answers are **A) It may be associated with weight loss, B) It may result in dyspnoea, C) It can be asymptomatic and D) Clinical examination will reveal a dull percussion over the collapsed lobe**.

   Lobar collapse can present with clinical features relating directly to the collapse or to the underlying pathology. History and clinical examination are very useful for diagnosing lobar collapse, although imaging will confirm or refute the diagnosis.

   A) It may be associated with weight loss – Correct. There are a variety of causes of lobar collapse (see question 2), and the patient may present with signs and symptoms of the cause rather than the collapse itself. The most worrisome aetiology is an underlying bronchogenic tumour which may have caused unintentional weight loss, a chronic cough or haemoptysis in the preceding weeks/months.

   B) It may result in dyspnoea – Correct. The partial or complete collapse of a lobe has a detrimental effect on the respiratory function. The presence and severity of dyspnoea depends on the degree of collapse and the patient's underlying lung function.

   C) It can be asymptomatic – Correct. Lobar collapse can occur acutely and present with a relatively sudden onset of symptoms. Conversely, the collapse may develop over weeks or months, for example due to a slow growing tumour compressing or obstructing the bronchus. The patient may even be asymptomatic, with the collapse diagnosed incidentally on a chest X-ray.

   D) Clinical examination will reveal a dull percussion note over the collapsed lobe – Correct. Lobar collapses will classically cause reduced chest expansion, dull percussion, reduced or absent breath sounds and increased vocal resonance over the collapsed lobe. The increased vocal resonance is caused by the fact that solid structures (i.e. the airless lung) are better conductors of sound than gases. However, remember that patients very rarely present in the classic way!

   E) A central trachea and nondisplaced apex beat on clinical examination reliably exclude the diagnosis – Incorrect. The position of the upper mediastinum is assessed clinically by examining the position of the trachea relative to the clavicular heads. The lower mediastinum is assessed by feeling for the position of the apex beat. Whilst the volume loss associated with a lobar collapse should deviate the mediastinum towards the collapse, it is not always easy to identify this clinically. In addition, lower lobe collapse may not necessarily cause superior mediastinal shift and vice versa. Finally, if the collapse is associated with a pleural effusion, volume can appear maintained.

❗ KEY POINTS

1. Lobar collapses may by asymptomatic or present with clinical features due to the collapse itself or the underlying aetiology.
2. Clinical assessment is helpful but imaging will confirm or refute the diagnosis.

2. Which of the following is/are causes of lobar collapse?

   The correct answers are **B) Bronchogenic tumour, C) Hilar lymph node enlargement, D) Inhaled foreign body and E) Mucous plug**.

   Lobar collapse develops due to partial or complete obstruction of the supplying bronchus. This can be due to intraluminal, luminal or extraluminal causes. Obstruction of the bronchus prevents ventilation of the distal lung. The air which is already in that part of the lung is gradually reabsorbed into the blood stream or diffuses to other lung segments in cases of subsegmental collapse via the pores of Kohn (interalveolar connections). Collapse can occur at any level of the bronchial tree (main, lobar or segmental bronchus).

   A) Bronchiectasis – Incorrect. Bronchiectasis is permanent dilatation of the bronchi and bronchioles, relative to their accompanying pulmonary artery. There are many causes of bronchiectasis but focal bronchiectasis can result from recurrent infection. Bronchiectasis itself does not cause lobar collapses; however, some pathologies, such as inhaled foreign body that initially result in lobar collapse can eventually result in bronchiectasis following the initial insult. Bronchiectatic lung is prone to mucous plugging and secondary subsegmental collapse.

   B) Bronchogenic tumour – Correct. Bronchogenic tumours can cause extrinsic compression of a bronchus or may originate in an endobronchial position, leading to intrinsic obstruction. Such patients are likely to have risk factors for lung cancer, as well as having a more insidious presentation. Treatment of the underlying tumour may help resolve the collapse.

   C) Hilar lymph node enlargement – Correct. Pathological hilar lymph node enlargement, e.g. from malignant infiltration, may result in extrinsic compression of a bronchus and subsequent lobar collapse. Reactive lymphadenopathy in the context of pulmonary infections does not usually result in lobar collapse.

   D) Inhaled foreign body – Correct. An inhaled foreign body can become lodged in a bronchus, leading to distal collapse. The right lower lobe is most commonly affected by inhaled foreign bodies, due to the relatively wide, vertical and straight course of the right main bronchus compared to the left. Such patients may need the foreign body removed under bronchoscopy.

   E) Mucous plug – Correct. A mucous plug can cause luminal obstruction of a single bronchus or multiple bronchi. Mucous plugging can be seen in asthmatics and postoperative patients. Treatment with chest physiotherapy to dislodge the plug may be helpful. A good way to see examples of lobar collapse is to review the chest X-rays of intubated patients on the intensive treatment unit (ITU). It is important to review the positioning of the endotracheal tube in any intubated patient – it should lie approximately 4 cm above the carina. If the tube is misplaced, it may result in iatrogenic lobar collapse of the nonventilated lung/lobes.

❶ KEY POINT

The clinical presentation gives a clue to the likely underlying cause of a lobar collapse. In middle-aged to elderly smokers, bronchial carcinoma must be high on the list of differentials. In asthmatics, think of mucous plugging, and in children consider an inhaled foreign body. Postoperative patients may develop collapse due to mucous plugging or a misplaced endotracheal tube.

3. Which of the following chest X-ray features is/are in keeping with volume loss in the upper lobe of the left lung?
   The correct answers are **B) Deviation of the trachea to the left, C) Elevated left hemidiaphragm and D) Crowding of the left-sided ribs**.
   Volume loss, in addition to increased opacification, is an important feature of a lobar collapse. It is important to be able to assess for volume loss on a chest X-ray to help differentiate collapse from other pathologies such as consolidation and pleural effusions, all of which cause increased opacification. As you might expect, loss of volume in the chest distorts the normal anatomy, and it is this distortion of normal for which we must look.
   A) Right hilum higher than the left hilum – Incorrect. The left hilum should normally be at the same level as or higher than the right hilum. Volume loss in the left upper lobe should cause the left hilum to be even higher than the right. Causes of the right hilum being higher than the left include volume loss in the right upper lobe (pulling the right hilum up relative to the normally positioned left hilum) or left lower lobe (pulling the left hilum down relative to the normally positioned right hilum).
   B) Deviation of the trachea to the left – Correct. Assessing the position of the mediastinum is a useful way to determine volume loss. The trachea represents the upper mediastinum and should be central over the spinous processes of the thoracic vertebral bodies in a well-centred X-ray. Deviation of the trachea to the left can be caused by loss of volume on the left (e.g. collapse of part or all of the left lung) or increased volume on the right, pushing it over (e.g. due to a pleural effusion or tension pneumothorax).
   C) Elevated left hemidiaphragm – Correct. Normally, the left hemidiaphragm is lower than or at the same level as the right. If it is higher than the right hemidiaphragm, this implies volume loss in the left hemithorax or increased volume in the right, leading to depression of the right hemidiaphragm (e.g. right-sided tension pneumothorax).
   D) Crowding of the left-sided ribs – Correct. The spacing between the posterior aspects of the ribs should be equal and symmetrical. Loss of volume in the left upper lobe may cause crowding of the left-sided ribs.
   E) Elevated horizontal fissure – Incorrect. Volume loss in the right upper lobe will cause elevation of the horizontal fissure. However, this question related to volume loss in the left upper lobe, and there is no horizontal fissure in the left lung!

❶ KEY POINT

It is important to assess whether the patient is rotated before commenting on the relative position of the trachea, heart and the rest of the mediastinum. Patient rotation can result in apparent mediastinal deviation – do not get caught out!

4. Which chest X-ray sign may be found in a right upper lobe collapse?
   The correct answer is **B) Golden S sign**.
   In addition to volume loss, there are a few classic chest X-ray appearances and signs which are useful for diagnosing lobar collapses. The appearances of the lobar collapses differ due to the manner in which each lobe collapses.
   A) Fleischner's sign – Incorrect. Fleischner's sign is a chest X-ray finding associated with pulmonary emboli. It represents visible dilatation of a pulmonary artery proximal to an obstructing PE. Westermark's sign is another chest X-ray sign in pulmonary emboli and represents focal oligaemia (reduced blood flow) distal to the PE. Both these signs are rare; remember that most patients with a PE have a normal chest X-ray.
   B) Golden S sign – Correct. As the right upper lobe collapses, the horizontal fissure moves superomedially. If the right upper lobe collapse is caused by a central mass, it usually has a typical X-ray appearance. The lateral portion of the horizontal fissure is concaved inferiorly, while the medial aspect, due to the central mass, is convexed inferiorly. This gives the horizontal fissure an S-shape. It is known as the Golden S sign.
   C) Sail sign – Incorrect. The sail sign on a chest X-ray is found in lower lobe collapses (right- and left-sided collapses). It is formed by the oblique fissure, which moves posteromedially as the lower lobe collapses. As it rotates, the oblique fissure is seen in profile and forms the well-defined lateral margin of the sail. On the left, the sail sign gives the impression of a double left heart border. Other findings in lower lobe collapses include depression of the ipsilateral hilum, indistinct medial aspect of the ipsilateral hemidiaphragm and the obscuring of the lateral margin of the adjacent vertebrae.
   D) Luftsichel sign – Incorrect. Luftsichel is German for 'air crescent'. In some cases of left upper lobe collapse, the hyperinflated apical segment of the left lower lobe comes to lie between the collapsed lung and the aortic knuckle. This crescent-shaped air lucency around the aortic knuckle is known as the Luftsichel sign.
   E) Veil-like opacity – Incorrect. Left upper lobe collapse is one of the more difficult diagnoses to make on a chest X-ray. The Luftsichel sign is not frequently seen; instead, there may be only a slight increase in opacification of the left hemithorax compared with the right. This is often described as a veil-like opacification, and occurs because the left upper lobe collapses anteriorly, so there is diffuse increase in opacity throughout most of the left hemithorax. In addition, the left heart border may be obscured, and the left hilum elevated.

Continue

CASE **2.4**   *Contd.*

❶ KEY POINT

In addition to volume loss, the different lobar collapses have characteristic appearances: Golden's S sign in right upper lobe collapse, veil-like opacification and the Luftsichel sign in the left upper lobe, and the sail sign in lower lobe collapses. A middle lobe collapse can be very difficult to detect on chest X-ray – the right heart border will be indistinct, and you may be able to see a depressed horizontal fissure. The right hilum and hemidiaphragm should appear normal.

5. Which of the following regarding the further investigation and management of a lobar collapse is/are correct?
   The correct answer is **D) Chest physiotherapy may be helpful**.
   The further investigation and management of a lobar collapse is determined by the likely underlying aetiology.

   A) A lateral chest X-ray is mandatory to confirm the diagnosis – Incorrect. Whilst a lateral chest X-ray may be useful for confirming the diagnosis, it is not routinely required. If there is persisting doubt over the diagnosis, a CT may be a more useful imaging option.

   B) All patients need a CT to confirm the diagnosis and exclude malignancy – Incorrect. CT with multiplanar reformatting (looking at the images in axial, sagittal and coronal planes) can clearly show lobar collapses. It also provides an assessment of the underlying cause. In a cohort of patients in whom cancer is the suspected aetiology, a CT is an appropriate investigation; however, CT is not routinely required in patients who are likely to have a collapse secondary to mucous plugging or a foreign body. Instead, a follow-up chest X-ray to ensure resolution of the collapse is appropriate.

   C) All patients require bronchoscopy – Incorrect. Bronchoscopy is a therapeutic option in patients with an inhaled foreign body. It may also be used diagnostically in patients with a malignant aetiology to obtain a tissue diagnosis via biopsy, brushings and washing. It is not, however, required for all patients with a lobar collapse.

   D) Chest physiotherapy may be helpful – Correct. Chest physiotherapy may be useful to expel a mucous plug which has caused a lobar collapse. It is particularly useful in postoperative patients who may not be able to inspire fully due to pain and are therefore at risk of developing atelectasis and collapse.

   E) Antibiotics and a repeat chest X-ray are indicated for all patients – Incorrect. If there is no evidence of associated infection, patients with a lobar collapse do not routinely require antibiotics. A follow-up chest X-ray to ensure resolution of collapse is usually helpful.

❶ KEY POINT

The investigation and management of lobar collapses is directed by the underlying aetiology.

👥 IMPORTANT LEARNING POINTS

- Lobar collapse has a variety of causes.
- The patient may present with features related to the collapse itself or to the underlying aetiology.
- Clinical assessment helps to identify the most likely underlying cause of the collapse and guides further investigations.
- There are general (e.g. volume loss) and specific (e.g. sail or Golden S sign) chest X-ray findings in lobar collapse.
- CT provides a more accurate assessment of the collapse and its cause than does chest X-ray, but is not required in all cases of collapse.
- Management is determined by the underlying cause.

CASE 2.5

A 45-year-old woman presents with right-sided pleuritic chest pain and shortness of breath to the medical assessment unit. As part of her assessment, you request a chest X-ray.

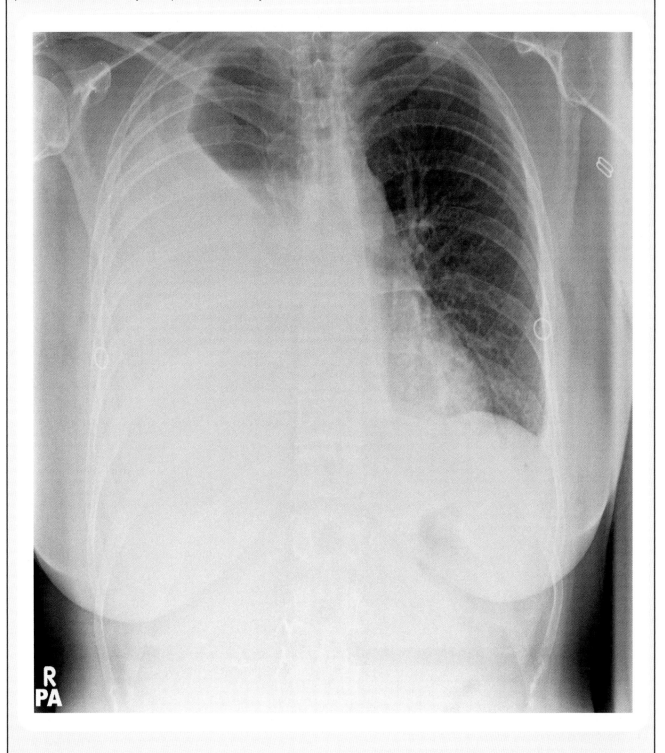

Continue

CASE 2.5   *Contd.*

ANNOTATED X-RAY

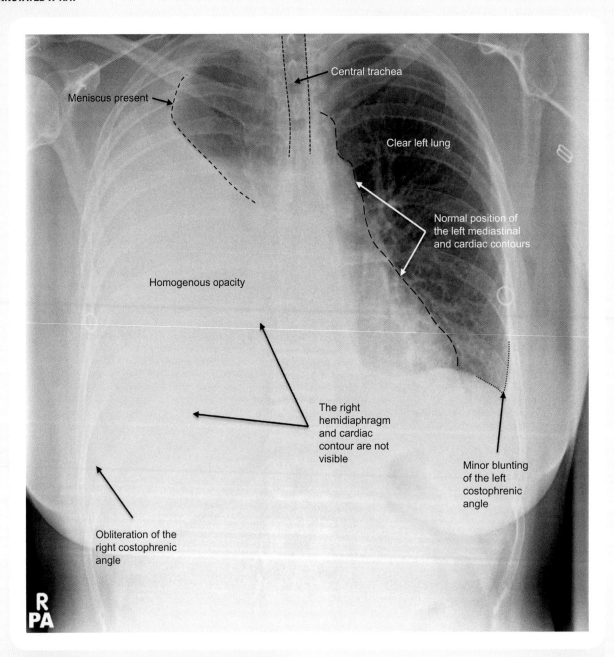

Central trachea

Meniscus present

Clear left lung

Normal position of the left mediastinal and cardiac contours

Homogenous opacity

The right hemidiaphragm and cardiac contour are not visible

Minor blunting of the left costophrenic angle

Obliteration of the right costophrenic angle

R
PA

🔍 PRESENT YOUR FINDINGS

- This is a PA chest X-ray of an adult woman.
- It has been anonymised, and the date and time of the examination have been removed. I would like to confirm these details before proceeding.
- The X-ray is technically adequate. The patient is not rotated, and the X-ray is well inspired and penetrated. No important areas have been cut off at the edges.
- The most striking abnormality is homogeneous opacification of most of the right hemithorax. It obliterates the right costophrenic angle, and both the right hemidiaphragm and the right-sided cardiac contour are

indistinct from this density. There is evidence of a meniscus laterally. There are no discernible air bronchograms in this area.
- The aerated right lung is clear. No pneumothorax is present.
- The trachea and heart are central.
- The left lung field is normal. There is minor blunting of the left costophrenic angle, which may represent a small left-sided pleural effusion.
- There is no free subdiaphragmatic gas.
- No skeletal abnormality, and in particular no rib fracture, has been identified.
- The visible soft tissues are unremarkable.

IN SUMMARY – The chest X-ray demonstrates a large right-sided pleural effusion, and a small left-sided effusion. I would like to review any previous X-rays to determine whether this is a new finding. The differential diagnosis of bilateral pleural effusions is wide and needs to be considered in the clinical context. Further imaging with ultrasound would be warranted if diagnostic or therapeutic thoracocentesis is being considered.

QUESTIONS

1. Which of the following is/are recognised clinical signs or symptoms of a pleural effusion?
   A) Pleuritic chest pain
   B) Stony dull percussion note
   C) Bronchial breathing
   D) Decreased breath sounds
   E) Displacement of the trachea to the ipsilateral side
2. Which of the following is/are features of an exudate in pleural fluid analysis?
   A) pH <7.2
   B) Protein >35 g/L
   C) Glucose <3.3 mmol/L
   D) Pleural fluid lactate dehydrogenase (LDH): serum LDH ratio >0.6
   E) Pleural fluid protein: serum protein ratio <0.5
3. Which of the following is/are causes of an exudative pleural effusion?
   A) Pneumonia
   B) Meigs syndrome
   C) Acute pancreatitis
   D) Pulmonary infarction
   E) TB
4. Which of the following investigations is/are often performed in the assessment of a pleural effusion?
   A) Chest X-ray
   B) Chest ultrasound
   C) Echocardiogram
   D) CTPA
   E) MRI (thorax)
5. Regarding pleural fluid aspiration/intercostal drain insertion for pleural effusions, which of the following is/are correct?
   A) These procedures should be guided by ultrasound
   B) The Seldinger technique is commonly performed to place chest drains
   C) When draining an effusion, the drain tip is often placed in a basal position
   D) Large effusions can be drained quickly without any adverse effect relating to rapid drainage
   E) A postprocedure chest X-ray is required after intercostal drain insertion

Continue

CASE **2.5** *Contd.*

ANSWERS TO QUESTIONS

1. Which of the following is/are recognised clinical signs or symptoms of a pleural effusion?

The correct answers are **A) Pleuritic chest pain, B) Stony dull percussion note and D) Decreased breath sounds**.

The classic clinical signs of a patient with a large pleural effusion include tachypnoea and decreased chest expansion on the affected side. If large enough, the effusion can exert a mass effect and cause a degree of tracheal deviation away from the effusion. The percussion note is stony dull. Upon auscultation, there is an absence of breath sounds. Occasionally, crepitations may be heard just above the effusion where there is some adjacent atelectatic lung.

A) Pleuritic chest pain – Correct. Pleural effusions may simply present with shortness of breath. However, depending on the aetiology, there may be associated pleuritic chest pain.

B) Stony dull percussion note – Correct. The classic percussion note in a patient with a pleural effusion is said to be stony dull.

C) Bronchial breathing – Incorrect. Bronchial breathing and increased vocal resonance are associated with lung parenchymal consolidation and not pleural effusion.

D) Decreased breath sounds – Correct. Fluid in the pleural space displaces the aerated lung. Consequently, there is an absence of breath sounds overlying the area of the effusion.

E) Displacement of the trachea to the ipsilateral side – Incorrect. If large enough, there may be displacement of the trachea to the contralateral side (away from the effusion).

❗ KEY POINT

There are specific clinical signs associated with a pleural effusion. Lower lobe collapse can present with similar clinical findings to an effusion, with reduced chest expansion, dull percussion note and decreased air entry. Look for evidence of volume loss to help identify collapse and distinguish between the two pathologies. Characterising the percussion note as stony dull (in effusion), rather than just dull (in collapse), can be very difficult. You should interpret the clinical findings in conjunction with the history and relevant investigation findings.

2. Which of the following is/are features of an exudate in pleural fluid analysis?

The correct answer is **A) pH <7.2, B) Protein >35 g/L, C) Glucose <3.3 mmol/L and D) Pleural fluid lactate dehydrogenase: serum LDH ratio >0.6**.

Analysis of a sample of pleural fluid is important to help determine the aetiology of a unilateral pleural effusion. The fluid should be assessed in terms of macroscopic appearances, cytology, clinical chemistry and, occasionally, immunology and microbiology culture and sensitivity. Distinguishing an exudate from a transudate helps to limit the differential diagnosis.

A) pH <7.2 – Correct. A pH <7.2 is specific for an exudate but not sensitive, i.e. a pH >7.2 does not exclude an exudate as a cause of the effusion, but if the pH is <7.2 it invariably confirms an exudate. Certain exudative effusions can give low pH values, such as empyema, malignancy, TB, rheumatoid arthritis and systemic lupus erythematosus.

B) Protein >35 g/L – Correct. Protein concentration <25 g/L is consistent with a transudate and >35 g/L is consistent with an exudate. Light's criteria must be applied in these situations to determine if the fluid is truly a transudate or exudate.

C) Glucose <3.3 mmol/L – Correct. Like a low pH, pleural fluid glucose <3.3 mmol/L is seen in certain exudates such as empyema, malignancy, TB, rheumatoid arthritis and systemic lupus erythematosus. However, it is not a sensitive finding.

D) Pleural fluid LDH: serum LDH ratio >0.6 – Correct. Exudates often have elevated LDH. Comparing the pleural fluid LDH level with the serum LDH level enables an LDH ratio to be calculated, which is more accurate than looking at absolute LDH levels in the pleural fluid.

E) Pleural fluid protein: serum protein ratio <0.5 – Incorrect. It is important to take a contemporaneous plasma sample at the time of pleural tap to help classify pleural fluid samples with protein concentrations between 25 and 35 g/L. The amount of protein in the pleural fluid relative to the plasma is important because the patient might be in a catabolic state, with low levels of protein synthesis. However, if the pleural fluid: serum protein ratio is >0.5 (not <0.5), then this implies leakage of protein into the pleural fluid and is suggestive of an exudate.

❗ KEY POINTS

1. Always send a contemporaneous sample of blood to be analysed for glucose, protein and LDH in conjunction with the pleural aspirate to enable interpretation of potentially ambiguous biochemical results from the pleural sample alone.

2. The fluid is an exudate if it meets one or more of Light's criteria, which include:
   - Pleural fluid protein: serum ratio >0.5
   - Pleural fluid: serum LDH ratio >0.6
   - Pleural fluid LDH more than 2/3 the upper limit of serum LDH

3. Which of the following is/are causes of an exudative pleural effusion?

The correct answers are **A) Pneumonia, C) Acute pancreatitis, D) Pulmonary infarction and E) TB**.

There are multiple causes of pleural effusions. It is important to know common causes of transudates and exudates. Although the macroscopic appearance of the pleural fluid can sometimes imply the presence of an exudate (blood-stained, turbid, etc.), the protein content of the sample is the key value in distinguishing an exudate from a transudate.

A) Pneumonia – Correct. A pleural effusion can result from a pneumonic process in the adjacent lung. This is termed a parapneumonic effusion. If the effusion does not resolve or there is persistent pyrexia, the possibility of super-added infection of the effusion needs to be considered – i.e. an empyema.

B) Meigs syndrome – Incorrect. Meigs syndrome is the association of a transudative pleural effusion (usually right sided) with benign ovarian fibroma and ascites. It is a rare cause of a pleural effusion in routine clinical practice, but an exam favourite!

C) Acute pancreatitis – Correct. Pleural effusions are not uncommon in cases of acute pancreatitis, especially if the episode is severe. The fluid is an exudate, and the aetiology can be confirmed by measuring the concentration of amylase in the pleural sample, which will usually be elevated.

D) Pulmonary infarction – Correct. Pulmonary infarction classically results in a blood-stained pleural effusion, which is an exudate.

E) TB – Correct. TB causes an exudate pleural effusion, most commonly seen in cases of primary TB infection. Other indicators of this aetiology are very low pleural glucose concentrations and a predominance of lymphocytes in the sample. Culturing of TB from pleural fluid is only successful in approximately 20% of cases.

❶ KEY POINT

In general, transudates are due to increased venous pressure or hypoproteinaemia. Exudates are the result of increased leakiness of pleural capillaries due to infection, inflammatory processes or neoplasia (Table C2.5.1).

Table C2.5.1   The Major Differences Between Transudate And Exudate Pleural Effusions

FEATURES	TRANSUDATE	EXUDATE
pH	>7.2 (NB exudates can also be >7.2)	Can vary, but <7.2 is specific for exudate
Protein (Pleural fluid: serum protein)	<25 g/L (<0.5)	>35 g/L (>0.5)
Glucose	[a]Not discriminatory	[a]<3.3 mmol/L
Pleural fluid LDH	Less than 2/3 the upper limit of normal serum LDH	Greater than 2/3 the upper limit of normal serum LDH

Table C2.5.1   The Major Differences Between Transudate And Exudate Pleural Effusions

FEATURES	TRANSUDATE	EXUDATE
Causes	**Raised venous pressure** (cardiac failure, constrictive pericarditis) **Hypoproteinaemia** (cirrhosis, nephrotic syndrome, malabsorption, protein losing enteropathy) **Hypothyroidism**	**Infection** (pneumonia, TB) **Inflammation** (pulmonary infarction, rheumatoid arthritis, systemic lupus erythematosus (SLE)) **Malignancy** (primary or secondary lung tumours, lymphoma, mesothelioma)

[a]Some types of exudative effusions, such as empyema, TB and malignancy, can cause a low glucose level, but this is not a sensitive method for distinguishing transudates from exudates.
NB Cytology and culture and sensitivity are also commonly performed on samples of pleural fluid to aid diagnosis.

4. Which of the following investigations is/are often performed in the assessment of a pleural effusion? The correct answers are **A) Chest X-ray, B) Chest ultrasound, C) Echocardiogram and D) CTPA**.
A variety of imaging modalities can detect fluid in the pleural cavity. However, deciding on an appropriate investigation depends on your index of suspicion of the underlying aetiology.

A) Chest X-ray – Correct. A chest X-ray is routinely performed in patients with suspected pleural effusion. Approximately 200 mL of pleural fluid is required to produce an abnormal PA chest X-ray. However, only approximately 50 mL of pleural fluid is necessary to blunt the posterior costophrenic angle on a lateral chest X-ray.

B) Chest ultrasound – Correct. Ultrasound is a common and useful investigation of a pleural effusion. It is more accurate than chest X-ray at estimating the volume of fluid. Ultrasound-guided aspiration is recommended as a safe and accurate method of obtaining pleural fluid. Furthermore, ultrasound is better than CT at demonstrating fibrous septations within the effusion, which is important because, if fibrous septations are present, the effusion may not resolve without specific treatment to break down the loculations, e.g. intrapleural streptokinase or surgical decortication.

C) Echocardiogram – Correct. In the appropriate clinical setting, performing an echocardiogram to assess left ventricular function would be an important investigation to perform. Although pleural effusions in the

Continue

CASE **2.5**   *Contd.*

context of heart failure are often bilateral, unilateral effusions can also occur.

D) CTPA – Correct. CT pulmonary angiography may be performed in the investigation of a suspected PE and pulmonary infarction as a cause of an effusion. A CT scan can help determine the presence of lung malignancy and distinguish between benign and malignant pleural thickening.

E) MRI (thorax) – Incorrect. Although pleural fluid can be readily demonstrated on MRI and certain centres may perform MRI (thorax) in patients with suspected mesothelioma, its role in the routine clinical assessment of pleural effusions has not been established at present.

5. Regarding pleural fluid aspiration/intercostal drain insertion for pleural effusions, which of the following is/are correct?

The correct answers are **A) These procedures should be guided by ultrasound, B) The Seldinger technique is commonly performed to place chest drains, C) When draining an effusion, the drain tip is often placed in a basal position and E) A postprocedure chest X-ray is required**.

A) These procedures should be guided by ultrasound – Correct. The British Thoracic Society advises that pleural aspiration and pleural drain insertion should be guided by ultrasound. This permits accurate assessment of the pleural effusion and can help to minimise complications, such as injury to adjacent abdominal organs (liver or spleen).

B) The Seldinger technique is commonly performed to place chest drains – Correct. The Seldinger technique is a common method for insertion of a small bore chest drain. This involves placement of a guide wire into the pleural cavity, dilatation of the tract (made by the guide wire) using a dilator along the wire and, finally, placing the drain over the wire before removing the guide wire. Large bore chest drains in surgical emergencies (e.g. severe chest trauma or ruptured oesophagus) are often placed with a surgical cut-down technique.

C) When draining an effusion, the drain tip is often placed in a basal position – Correct. It is desirable to position the drain tip inferiorly to drain a pleural effusion, as the fluid collects in the direction of gravity, and superiorly to drain a pneumothorax, as the air within the pleural space tends to rise superiorly within the thorax.

D) Large effusions can be drained quickly without any adverse effect relating to rapid drainage – Incorrect. Care should be taken when draining a large pleural effusion. Rapid drainage of large collections can result in reexpansion pulmonary oedema in the previously collapsed adjacent lung.

E) A postprocedure chest X-ray is required after intercostal drain insertion – Correct. A chest X-ray following intercostal drain insertion is mandatory to exclude the introduction of a pneumothorax and to check the position of the drain.

> ❗ KEY POINT
>
> Previously, pleural intervention was performed blindly, with only clinical examination as a guide. With the widespread availability, chest ultrasound is required prior to performing any pleural procedure.

IMPORTANT LEARNING POINTS

- A pleural effusion simply indicates fluid in the pleural cavity. It does not distinguish among the types of fluid (e.g. blood = haemothorax, pus = empyema/pyothorax, chyle = chylothorax), or the aetiology.
- The chest X-ray is often the first procedure performed in the investigation of a pleural effusion. Look for any potential clues to help determine the aetiology (e.g. displaced rib fractures raise the possibility of a haemothorax; a lung mass suggests a malignant cause).
- Determining the pleural fluid's protein content is the key parameter in distinguishing a transudate from an exudate and helps to narrow the differential diagnosis.
- Pleural procedures should always be ultrasound-guided, by an appropriately trained practitioner, to reduce the risk of complications.

CASE 2.6

A 54-year-old man, who is a lifelong smoker, attends with unintentional weight loss, a persistent cough and haemoptysis. A chest X-ray is performed.

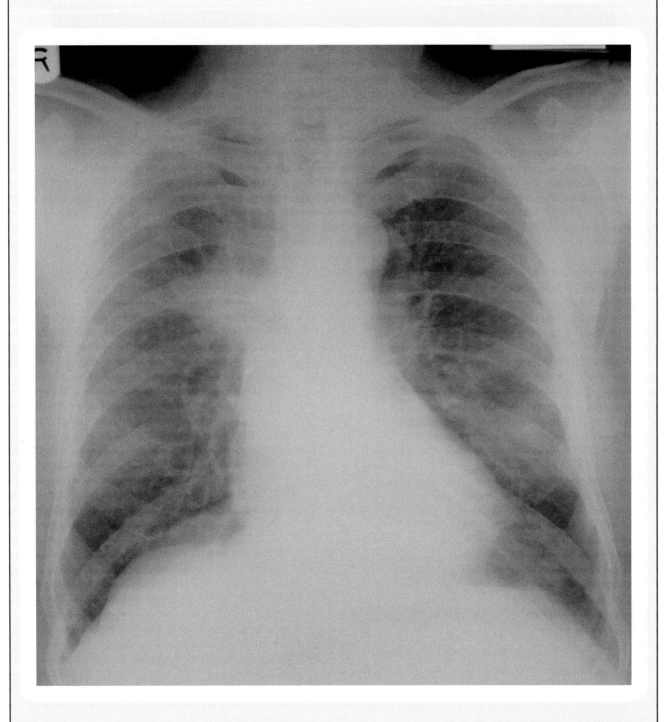

Continue

CASE **2.6**   *Contd.*

ANNOTATED X-RAY

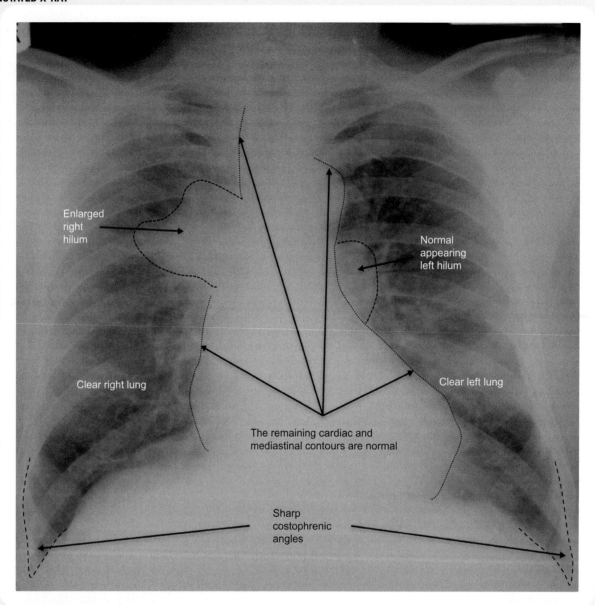

Enlarged right hilum

Normal appearing left hilum

Clear right lung

Clear left lung

The remaining cardiac and mediastinal contours are normal

Sharp costophrenic angles

🔍 PRESENT YOUR FINDINGS

- This is a PA chest X-ray of an adult.
- There are no patient identifiers on the X-ray. I would like to ensure that this is the correct patient and to check the time and date when the X-ray was taken.
- The patient is not rotated and the X-ray is well inspired. The X-ray is slightly underpenetrated, but still diagnostic. There are no important areas cut off at the edges of the X-ray.
- The most striking abnormality is a circular opacity projected over the right hilar region. It is ill-defined, homogenously dense and measures approximately 4 cm in diameter.
- The rest of the lungs appear clear; in particular, there is no associated lobar collapse or consolidation.
- There is no evidence of pleural effusions.

- The trachea is central.
- The remaining mediastinal contours, including the left hilum, are unremarkable.
- The heart is not enlarged, and the cardiac contours are well defined.
- There is no free subdiaphragmatic gas.
- There is no obvious abnormality of the imaged bones and soft tissues.

IN SUMMARY – This chest X-ray shows a right hilar mass and, given the clinical history, bronchial carcinoma should be considered. The rest of the X-ray is unremarkable, with no associated distal collapse or consolidation or other masses visible. Urgent further imaging and referral to the lung cancer multidisciplinary meeting are advised.

QUESTIONS

1. Which of the following is/are causes of haemoptysis?
   A) Lung cancer
   B) Pulmonary infections
   C) Haemopneumothorax
   D) Mallory–Weiss tear
   E) Pulmonary infarction
2. Which of the following is/are causes of a hilar mass?
   A) Bronchogenic carcinoma
   B) TB
   C) Sarcoidosis
   D) Pulmonary artery enlargement
   E) Lymphoma
3. Which of the following is/are recognised paraneoplastic manifestations of lung cancer?
   A) SIADH
   B) Guillain–Barré syndrome
   C) ADEM
   D) HPOA
   E) Myasthenia (Lambert–Eaton syndrome)

4. In addition to bone, primary bronchogenic lung carcinoma commonly metastasises to which of the following organs?
   A) Brain
   B) Liver
   C) Stomach
   D) Ovary
   E) Adrenals
5. What would be the next radiological investigation in a patient with the above chest X-ray?
   A) Lateral chest X-ray to localise the abnormality
   B) CT of the chest and abdomen
   C) MRI of the thorax
   D) PET scan
   E) Radiolabelled white cell scan to confirm or refute infection as a cause

Continue

ANSWERS TO QUESTIONS

1. Which of the following is/are causes of haemoptysis?
The correct answers are **A) Lung cancer, B) Pulmonary infections and E) Pulmonary infarction**.
Haemoptysis is the coughing up of blood or blood-stained sputum. It should be distinguished from haematemesis, which is vomiting up blood from the gastrointestinal tract. There are many different causes of haemoptysis, some of which can be sinister in nature, requiring urgent investigation and treatment. Clinical assessment, in combination with blood tests and imaging findings, helps differentiate the various causes. Other relatively rare causes of haemoptysis not mentioned in the questions include bronchiectasis, Granulomatosis with polyangiitis, Goodpasture syndrome and arteriovenous malformations.

A) Lung cancer – Correct. Bronchial malignancy must be considered when a patient presents with haemoptysis. The history should enquire about smoking history, associated weight loss and a persistent cough. The chest X-ray is often the initial investigation and may reveal a mass. However, a normal chest X-ray does not exclude malignancy, and CT should be performed if there is significant clinical concern.

B) Pulmonary infections – Correct. Infections are a frequent cause of haemoptysis. Clinically, the patient usually presents with fever, purulent sputum and breathlessness. Blood tests will usually show elevated inflammatory markers. Chest X-ray findings and sputum cultures help confirm the aetiology. Certain pathogens are more likely to result in haemoptysis – for example, rusty-coloured, blood-stained sputum is classically seen in pneumococcal infections.

C) Haemopneumothorax – Incorrect. A pneumothorax usually presents with pain and breathlessness, but does not cause haemoptysis. A haemopneumothorax results if there is associated bleeding, but as the bleeding is into the pleural space and not the bronchial tree, haemoptysis will not result.

D) Mallory–Weiss tear – Incorrect. A Mallory–Weiss tear is a mucosal tear in the distal oesophagus that characteristically results from repeated forceful vomiting. It can result in haematemesis, rather than haemoptysis. Large upper gastrointestinal tract haemorrhage can result in apparent haemoptysis if the patient aspirates vomited blood and then subsequently coughs up the blood products, but haematemesis is the overwhelming clinical presentation in these scenarios.

E) Pulmonary infarction – Correct. Pulmonary embolic disease can result in ischaemia and subsequent pulmonary infarction. Although the lung receives most of its blood supply from the pulmonary arteries, there are also bronchial arteries that contribute, so pulmonary infarction does not occur in all cases of PE. The clinical features include dyspnoea, pleuritic chest pain and risk factors for venous thromboembolism. There may be clinical or ultrasound evidence of a deep vein thrombosis. The chest X-ray features are often non-specific, although a peripheral wedge of consolidation reflecting infarcted lung may be present. This is known as a Hampton hump. The diagnosis is confirmed with either CT pulmonary angiography or a ventilation/perfusion scan.

❗ KEY POINT

The first step in assessing a patient with suspected haemoptysis is to clarify from the patient whether they are experiencing haemoptysis or haematemesis, as the differential diagnoses, subsequent investigations and treatments are different.

2. Which of the following is/are causes of a hilar mass?
The correct answers are **A) Bronchogenic carcinoma, B) TB, C) Sarcoidosis, D) Pulmonary artery enlargement and E) Lymphoma**.
The hila consist of the bronchi, pulmonary vessels (arteries and veins) and lymph nodes. The hilar point is defined as the angle between the upper lobe pulmonary vein and the lower lobe pulmonary artery. Pathology arising from any of these structures can result in an apparent hilar mass. The clinical assessment, results of blood tests and X-ray findings may help identify the underlying cause. CT is very helpful for assessing the hila and can distinguish between masses/lymph nodes and vascular enlargement.

A) Bronchogenic carcinoma – Correct. A central bronchogenic carcinoma can present as a hilar mass. CT is helpful for further investigation; however, it may be difficult to differentiate a central tumour from an enlarged lymph node (s) even on CT.

B) TB – Correct. TB is becoming increasingly common in the developed world. It is most frequently seen in immigrants from high-risk areas, patients of low socioeconomic status and the immunocompromised. Enlarged lymph nodes are most commonly seen in the primary infection. Other features at this stage include consolidation and effusions. With secondary infection (reactivation) there is consolidation, scarring and/or cavitation, with upper zone predilection. Lymphadenopathy is uncommon at this stage.

C) Sarcoidosis – Correct. Sarcoidosis is a systemic granulomatous disease that most frequently affects the lungs. It frequently causes hilar (and right paratracheal) lymph node enlargement. There may rarely be eggshell calcification of the lymph nodes (peripheral calcification which is best appreciated on CT). Other findings on the chest X-ray can include lung nodules, reticulonodular opacification and pulmonary fibrosis.

D) Pulmonary artery enlargement – Correct. One of the hallmarks of pulmonary artery hypertension is enlargement of the main pulmonary arteries with rapid tapering of the peripheral vessels. Calcification of the pulmonary arteries is a late but pathognomonic feature.

Causes of pulmonary artery hypertension can be precapillary, such as left-to-right shunts, chronic pulmonary emboli and interstitial fibrosis, or postcapillary, including left ventricular failure and mitral stenosis which result in pulmonary venous hypertension with secondary pulmonary artery hypertension. CTPA is often performed in cases of suspected pulmonary artery hypertension to confirm the pulmonary artery enlargement and identify a possible cause.

E) Lymphoma – Correct. Lymphoma is a haematological malignancy that usually results in solid tumour deposits within lymphoid tissue (lymph nodes and spleen). It should be considered in the differential diagnosis of a patient with a hilar mass/masses.

KEY POINTS

1. Secondary effects from a central tumour or enlarged lymph nodes include obstruction of the bronchi leading to distal consolidation and/or collapse.
2. The differential diagnosis for bilateral hilar lymph node enlargement includes sarcoidosis, infection such as TB, malignancy including lymphoma and metastases and inorganic dust disease, such as silicosis.

3. Which of the following is/are recognised paraneoplastic manifestations of lung cancer?
The correct answers are **A) SIADH, D) HPOA and E) Myasthenia (Lambert–Eaton syndrome)**.
Paraneoplastic syndromes are non-metastatic distant effects of a cancer. They are caused by the hormones and cytokines excreted by the tumour, as well as the body's immune response against the cancer. Of the lung cancers, paraneoplastic features are most commonly seen with small cell lung cancer, especially the inappropriate secretion of antidiuretic and adrenocorticotrophic hormones. Squamous cell cancer can cause hypercalcaemia via parathyroid-related peptide production. Any lung cancer can produce the neurological syndromes. Other paraneoplastic syndromes not mentioned in the questions include carcinoid syndrome, gynaecomastia, polyneuropathy, cerebellar degeneration, polymyositis and dermatomyositis.

A) SIADH – Correct. The syndrome of inappropriate antidiuretic hormone causes excess antidiuretic hormone secretion from the posterior pituitary gland, resulting in hyponatraemia and fluid overload. It can be caused by a variety of conditions including small cell lung cancer, subarachnoid haemorrhage, pneumonia and lung abscesses. Any patient with unexplained hyponatraemia should be considered for a chest X-ray in the first instance to look for pulmonary causes of SIADH. Treatment includes management of the underlying causes and fluid restriction.

B) Guillain–Barré syndrome – Incorrect. This is an acute peripheral polyneuropathy which results in an ascending paralysis. It is caused by an autoimmune response to foreign antigens, such as campylobacter or cytomegalovirus infection. It is not a paraneoplastic condition.

C) ADEM – Incorrect. This is a postinfective autoimmune-mediated demyelinating process which affects the central nervous system. It is similar to multiple sclerosis, but, unlike multiple sclerosis, the patient usually recovers. It is not a paraneoplastic syndrome.

D) HPOA – Correct. This consists of finger clubbing and inflammation of the periosteum of the long bones, with expansion of the bone at the wrists and ankles. The patients may complain of wrist and ankle joint pain. It can be primary or secondary to lung cancer, lung abscesses and bronchiectasis. X-rays will show long, smooth periosteal reaction at the metaphyses and diaphyses of the long bones. Classically, there is sparing of the epiphyses.

E) Myasthenia (Lambert–Eaton syndrome) – Correct. This is a rare autoimmune disorder in which antibodies affect the neuromuscular junction, leading to peripheral weakness. Small cell lung cancer is the most common cause.

4. In addition to bone, primary bronchogenic lung carcinoma commonly metastasises to which of the following organs?
The correct answers are **A) Brain, B) Liver and E) Adrenals**.
Patients with lung cancers often have metastatic disease at the time of presentation, especially those with small cell lung cancer.

A) Brain – Correct. The brain is a common site to which lung cancer may metastasise. Brain metastases may be asymptomatic or can cause various different signs and symptoms. These may be related directly to the metastasis or result from secondary effects such as associated cerebral oedema and hydrocephalus, and include headache, nausea and vomiting, focal neurological deficits, papilloedema and seizures. CT (ideally contrast enhanced) is commonly used to identify brain metastases. MRI can also be used and has a higher sensitivity.

B) Liver – Correct. The liver is another common site for metastatic disease from lung cancer. Again, the patient may be asymptomatic. Alternatively, there may be pain, jaundice, ascites or abnormal liver function tests. Ultrasound and CT are commonly used to assess the liver, with CT being more accurate.

C) Stomach – Incorrect. Although there have been cases of lung cancers spreading to the stomach, it is a very rare site for metastatic disease.

D) Ovaries – Incorrect. Lung cancer does not usually metastasise to the ovaries. A common examination topic is the Krukenberg tumour which is the name given to metastases within the ovary/ovaries. The primary cancers responsible are most commonly located in the gastrointestinal tract, such as the stomach, and also the breast.

E) Adrenals – Correct. Lung cancer is one of the most common cancers to metastasise to the adrenal glands.

KEY POINT

A useful memory aid to remember the common sites of metastasis from lung cancer is 'Lung cancer loves to BLAB'. BLAB stands for brain, liver, adrenals and bones.

Continue

5. What would be the next radiological investigation in a patient with the earlier mentioned chest X-ray?
The correct answer is **B) CT of the chest and abdomen**.

Staging of a cancer is an important part of the assessment. It helps determine which treatment is most appropriate and gives an indication of prognosis. Most tumours are staged using the TNM (Tumour, Node and Metastasis) system. Imaging must therefore assess all three of these parameters.

A) Lateral chest X-ray to localise the abnormality – Incorrect. A lateral chest X-ray can be performed to help clarify the findings of a frontal chest X-ray; however, they are not routinely performed in the UK these days, as CT provides a better assessment and is readily available.

B) CT of the chest and abdomen – Correct. CT is the mainstay of noninvasive staging. It allows an accurate assessment of the chest. The primary tumour can be assessed (location, size and relation to other structures, such as the mediastinum or chest wall). Lymph node enlargement (hilar, mediastinal, supraclavicular, axillary, abdominal) can be identified. The abdomen is also routinely imaged to look for the presence of metastatic deposits, especially in the liver, adrenal glands and bones. Patients with lung cancer and clinical features of brain metastases should also have a CT of the head.

C) MRI of the thorax – Incorrect. MRI is used to assess chest wall invasion in superior sulcus (Pancoast) tumours. It provides a better assessment of the soft tissues and bones than CT. It also has a role in the assessment of suspected malignant cord or cauda equina compression; however, in this patient with a hilar mass, there is no current established role for MRI in the staging process.

D) PET scan – Incorrect. PET is a nuclear medicine imaging technique (further details about PET scanning can be found in Chapter 9). It is most commonly performed with a glucose analogue and therefore identifies cells, such as tumours, that have increased metabolism. In contrast to CT, which provides anatomical information, PET provides a metabolic assessment. When combined with CT, it can be useful to detect metastases and lymph node involvement.

PET is not a routine part of staging of every patient with lung cancer; it is currently used for further assessment in patients being considered for radical surgery or radical radiotherapy. Causes of false positives include infection and inflammation, such as sarcoidosis, whereas false negatives include small tumour deposits and certain tumour types, e.g. carcinoid.

E) Radiolabelled white cell scan to confirm or refute infection as a cause – Incorrect. A white cell scan is another nuclear medicine scan in which white blood cells are labelled with a radioactive tracer and reinjected into the patient. It is used to identify occult infections. It is not part of the staging of lung cancer. Infection as a cause of the anomalies appearing on this chest X-ray would be excluded by correlating with the patient's history, inflammatory markers and response to antibiotics.

KEY POINTS

1. The staging and management of cancers is complex, and patients and the results of their investigations are often discussed at a multidisciplinary team meeting.
2. The mainstay for most tumour staging is CT. However, other modalities are also used, as described earlier.

IMPORTANT LEARNING POINTS

- Haemoptysis has a range of causes, some of which, such as lung cancer, are sinister and require urgent investigation and treatment.
- A hilar mass may be due to enlargement of any of the structures which constitute the hilum, e.g. a central bronchogenic carcinoma, lymphadenopathy or pulmonary arterial enlargement.
- Lung cancer can present with features directly related to metastases, or to paraneoplastic syndromes.
- The liver, adrenals, brain and bone are the most common sites for lung cancer metastases.
- Staging of lung cancer is important in helping to select the most appropriate treatment and in estimating prognosis. CT is the main imaging modality for staging; however, PET and MRI play roles in staging for specific patients.

CASE **2.7**

An 81-year-old male smoker presents with a chronic cough, weight loss, left arm pain and a left Horner syndrome. A chest X-ray is performed as part of his assessment.

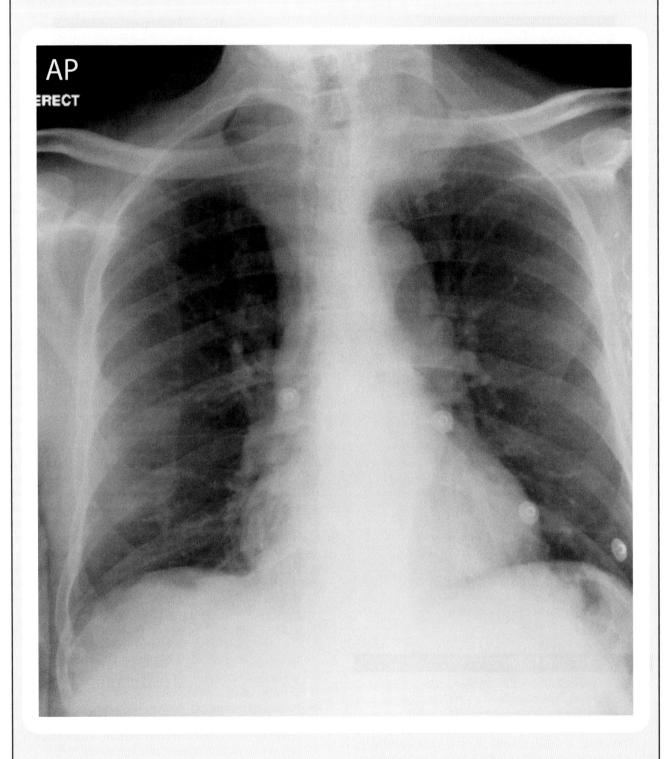

Continue

CASE **2.7** *Contd.*

ANNOTATED X-RAY

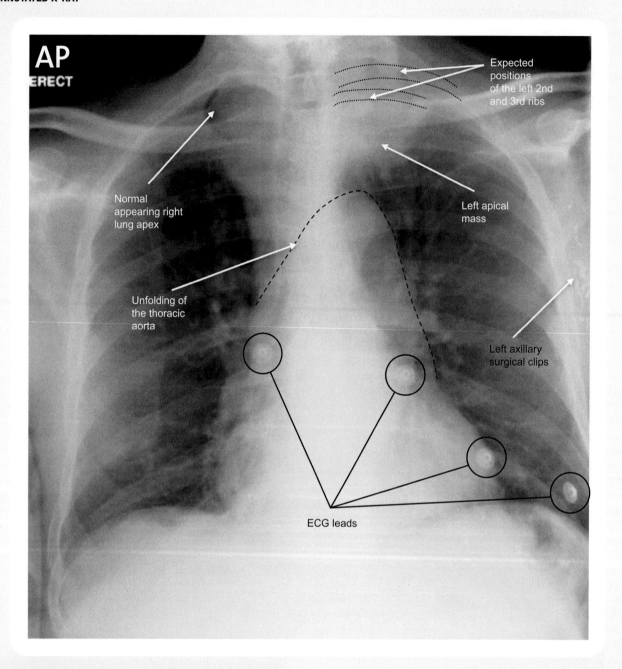

AP
ERECT

Expected
positions
of the left 2nd
and 3rd ribs

Normal
appearing right
lung apex

Left apical
mass

Unfolding of
the thoracic
aorta

Left axillary
surgical clips

ECG leads

🔍 **PRESENT YOUR FINDINGS**

- This is an erect AP chest X-ray of an adult.
- There are no patient identifiers on the X-ray. I would like to ensure that this is the correct patient and to check the time and date when the X-ray was taken.
- The patient is slightly rotated. There is good inspiratory achievement, and although the X-ray is slightly under-penetrated, it is still diagnostic. However, the left costo-phrenic angle has not been included. It is thus technically inadequate, but sufficient to show the pertinent diagnosis.
- The most obvious abnormality is the asymmetry of the apices. There is a homogenous mass at the left apex which obscures the left side of the superior

mediastinum. The posterior aspects of the 2nd and 3rd left ribs are not visible, suggesting bone destruction.
- The right apex appears normal.
- Reviewing the rest of the X-ray, one sees that the tra-chea is central. The rest of the lungs are clear, with no collapse, consolidation or other masses visible. There is no obvious pleural effusion, although the left costo-phrenic angle has not been included. There is unfolding of the thoracic aorta. The cardiac contours are clear.
- There is no free subdiaphragmatic gas.
- The rest of the imaged skeleton appears unremarkable.
- There are surgical clips projected over the left axilla, in keeping with previous axillary lymph node clearance.

IN SUMMARY – This chest X-ray shows a left apical mass with associated rib destruction. Appearances are highly suggestive of malignancy, that of either a primary lung tumour (Pancoast or superior sulcus tumour), or of metastatic disease, given the evidence of previous surgery to the left axilla. Further imaging with CT is warranted.

QUESTIONS

1. Which of the following is/are features of Horner syndrome?
   A) Exophthalmos
   B) Miosis
   C) Partial ptosis
   D) Hyperhidrosis
   E) Down and out eye
2. Which of the following is/are recognised causes of Horner syndrome?
   A) Multiple sclerosis
   B) Carotid artery dissection
   C) Cervical rib
   D) Pancoast tumour
   E) Cavernous sinus thrombosis
3. A Pancoast tumour can cause which of the following clinical signs/symptoms?
   A) Arm pain
   B) Wasting of the small muscles of the hand
   C) Lower lobe collapse
   D) Facial swelling
   E) Hoarseness
4. Which imaging modality provides the most accurate assessment of the local involvement of a Pancoast tumour?
   A) PA and lateral chest X-rays
   B) Ultrasound
   C) CT
   D) PET scan
   E) MRI
5. Regarding the treatment of Pancoast tumours, which of the following is/are correct?
   A) Surgery is never curative
   B) Radiotherapy is an option
   C) Chemotherapy is an option
   D) Brachytherapy is an option
   E) Stenting of the superior vena cava is sometimes necessary

Continue

CASE **2.7**   *Contd.*

ANSWERS TO QUESTIONS

1. Which of the following is/are features of Horner syndrome?
The correct answers are **B) Miosis and C) Partial ptosis**.
Horner syndrome is due to disruption of the cervical or thoracic sympathetic chain of the autonomic nervous system. The clinical signs associated with Horner syndrome are found on the same side as the pathological lesion.

A) Exophthalmos – Incorrect. Exophthalmos refers to anterior bulging of the eye out of the orbit and indicates that there is a retro-orbital mass effect. There are a variety of causes, including inflammation (Grave disease, orbital cellulitis, orbital pseudotumour), malignancy (lymphoma, meningioma), carotid-cavernous fistula and trauma. Horner syndrome is not a cause. In Horner syndrome, patients may have apparent enophthalmos (the impression that the eye is sunk into the orbit) due to the partial ptosis which can also occur.

B) Miosis – Correct. Miosis refers to constriction of the pupil. The autonomic nervous system is involved in the photomotor reflex (the response of the iris to light). Sympathetic fibres lead to dilatation of the pupil, whereas the parasympathetic system causes constriction (miosis). Therefore disruption to the sympathetic system (in this case by thoracic tumour invasion) leads to unopposed parasympathetic stimulation and resultant miosis.

C) Partial ptosis – Correct. Ptosis refers to drooping of the eyelid. Ptosis has a variety of causes, including trauma, inflammation and neurological abnormalities. The superior tarsal muscle (supplied by sympathetic fibres) works with the levator palpebrae superioris muscle (supplied by cranial nerve III) to retract the upper eye lid. Disruption to the sympathetic supply in Horner syndrome leads to loss of function of the superior tarsal muscle, but not levator palpebrae superioris, resulting in a partial (rather than total) ptosis.

D) Hyperhidrosis – Incorrect. Horner syndrome causes hypohidrosis (reduced sweating, due to damage to the sympathetic nerve fibres), affecting the ipsilateral side of the face; it does not cause hyperhidrosis.

E) Down and out eye – Incorrect. The autonomic nervous system is not involved in the innervation of the extraocular muscles. The oculomotor nerve (cranial nerve III) supplies all of the extraocular muscles except for superior oblique (cranial nerve IV) and lateral rectus (cranial nerve VI). A lesion affecting cranial nerve III results in the classic down and out eye due to the unopposed action of the superior oblique and lateral rectus muscles.

❗ KEY POINT

Classically, Horner syndrome results in miosis, partial ptosis and anhidrosis. In children with Horner syndrome, there may also be a difference in the colour of the eyes (heterochromia) due to altered pigmentation of the iris which occurs with loss of the sympathetic supply.

2. Which of the following is/are recognised causes of Horner syndrome?
The correct answers are **A) Multiple sclerosis, B) Carotid artery dissection, C) Cervical rib, D) Pancoast tumour and E) Cavernous sinus thrombosis**.
The sympathetic chain starts in the hypothalamus and travels down through the brainstem and cervical cord to the T1 level before exiting the central nervous system and travelling back up towards the head and face, alongside the carotid artery and through the cavernous sinus. Horner syndrome can occur from disruption at any point in the cervical or thoracic sympathetic chain. Lesions can be classed as central (involving the hypothalamic tract in the brainstem and cervical cord), preganglionic or postganglionic. Therefore the initial differential diagnosis of Horner syndrome can be wide.

A) Multiple sclerosis – Correct. Multiple sclerosis is a relapsing and remitting demyelinating disorder that affects the central nervous system. If it affects the central part of the sympathetic chain, it can result in Horner syndrome.

B) Carotid artery dissection – Correct. The sympathetic chain travels back up to the head alongside the carotid artery. Dissection of the carotid artery can disrupt these sympathetic fibres.

C) Cervical rib – Correct. A cervical rib may impinge on the preganglionic segment of the sympathetic chain.

D) Pancoast tumour – Correct. A Pancoast tumour could invade through the apex of the lung into the surrounding soft tissues and affect the sympathetic chain.

E) Cavernous sinus thrombosis – Correct. The postganglionic segment of the sympathetic chain travels through the cavernous sinus with the carotid artery. Pathology at this site, such as a cavernous sinus thrombosis, can cause a partial Horner syndrome.

❗ KEY POINTS

Horner syndrome can be caused by a variety of different pathologies. Clinical assessment is essential to narrow this differential diagnosis and guide appropriate imaging. Imaging options include a chest X-ray +/– CT chest (to look for a Pancoast tumour or cervical rib), CT or MRI of the head (to look for central causes such as infarcts, tumours or demyelination in the brainstem or cervical cord) and CT or MRI angiography of the carotid arteries if a carotid artery dissection is considered.

3. A Pancoast tumour can cause which of the following clinical signs/symptoms?
The correct answers are **A) Arm pain, B) Wasting of the small muscles of the hand, D) Facial swelling and E) Hoarseness**.
A Pancoast tumour is a tumour at the apex of the lung. It is defined by its location rather than pathology, although it is most commonly a squamous cell carcinoma. It is also known as a superior sulcus tumour.

Pancoast tumours often result in destruction of the overlying ribs and invade the adjacent soft tissues. They can lead to a variety of symptoms, depending on which structures are affected. Structures at risk include the brachial plexus, subclavian vessels, brachiocephalic vein, and superior vena cava, recurrent laryngeal nerve, vagus nerve, phrenic nerve and the sympathetic ganglion.

A) Arm pain – Correct. Invasion into the chest wall and brachial plexus can result in chest wall pain and pain radiating into the arm and hand.

B) Wasting of the small muscles of the hand – Correct. The lower nerve roots and fibres of the brachial plexus are most at risk, due to their proximity to the lung apex. Damage to these fibres by a Pancoast tumour typically results in weakness and loss of function in the small muscles of the hand (which are predominately supplied by C8 and T1 nerve roots).

C) Lower lobe collapse – Incorrect. A Pancoast tumour is a tumour located at the apex of the lung, in the upper lobe. It is therefore unlikely to cause collapse of a lower lobe. Related enlarged hilar lymph nodes could, however, lead to extrinsic compression of the lower lobe bronchus, with resultant collapse.

D) Facial swelling – Correct. Compression or infiltration of the superior vena cava by a tumour can result in facial swelling, cyanosis and dilatation of the superficial veins of the head and neck.

E) Hoarseness – Correct. The recurrent laryngeal nerve, a branch of the vagus nerve, supplies the vocal cords and may be damaged by a lung tumour, particularly a Pancoast tumour. It enters the thorax, looping around the aortic arch on the left and the subclavian artery on the right before travelling cranially along the trachea and oesophagus to the larynx. The left recurrent laryngeal nerve is more prone to injury, due to its longer route around the aortic arch.

❗ KEY POINTS

1. A Pancoast tumour can cause a variety of symptoms and signs, some of which, such as wasting of the hand muscles and arm pain, are distant from the site of pathology.
2. Pancoast tumours are difficult to identify at an early stage, as they can often initially be asymptomatic. By the time a patient has developed any of the earlier mentioned clinical features, the tumour will have invaded locally into the surrounding blood vessels and nerves and will usually be inoperable.

4. Which imaging modality provides the most accurate assessment of the local involvement of a Pancoast tumour?
The correct answer is **E) MRI**.
A Pancoast tumour is staged like any other lung cancer. However, the degree of soft tissue invasion and local involvement needs to be carefully assessed to help determine appropriate management.

A) PA and lateral chest X-rays – Incorrect. The chest X-ray is often the first modality which identifies the Pancoast tumour. There may be evidence of overlying rib destruction, but the chest X-ray does not provide enough information to assess local involvement accurately. Also, remember that the apex of the lung is a notoriously difficult area to assess on chest X-rays due to its position near the edge of the film and the overlying clavicle and ribs. It is easy to overlook pathology at this site; therefore the apices of the lung should be one of your review areas for a chest X-ray.

B) Ultrasound – Incorrect. Ultrasound does not have a role in staging lung cancer. The soft tissue component of the tumour may be visible on ultrasound, but it is not usually possible to visualise the tumour completely and assess its effects on the surrounding structures. Ultrasound is, however, very useful for assessing the patency of blood vessels, such as the superior vena cava or subclavian vessels, which may be compressed by the tumour. Ultrasound may identify pathological supraclavicular lymph nodes, which, if histologically confirmed, up-stage the disease to N3 disease, which is inoperable.

C) CT – Incorrect. Contrast-enhanced CT is the main imaging modality for staging lung cancer. It can show whether there are other suspicious nodules within the lungs, and whether there are enlarged lymph nodes or distant metastatic deposits. It can also assess bony and soft tissue involvement; however, MRI is superior for these, and better in the case of Pancoast tumour.

D) PET scan – Incorrect. PET is reserved for lung cancer patients who are considered for surgical resection or radical radiotherapy. Its role is mainly to identify occult sites of distant disease. It does not have the spatial resolution required to assess the local involvement of a Pancoast tumour accurately. Combining PET with CT (PET/CT) leads to greater spatial resolution.

E) MRI – Correct. MRI provides the best assessment of the soft tissues, including chest wall invasion and vascular or brachial plexus involvement. Tumour infiltration into bone can also be identified. It takes longer to acquire than a CT and is therefore much more prone to movement and respiratory artefact; however, it provides superior visualisation of the soft tissues.

❗ KEY POINT

Pancoast tumours are staged like any other lung cancer, using the TNM system (primarily with CT). Local involvement into the chest wall and surrounding structures is best assessed with MRI.

5. Regarding the treatment of Pancoast tumours, which of the following is/are correct?
The correct answers are **B) Radiotherapy is an option, C) Chemotherapy is an option and E) Stenting of the superior vena cava is sometimes necessary**.
The management of a Pancoast tumour is often difficult due to its proximity to/involvement with adjacent blood vessels and nerves. Despite these challenges, treatment can be curative in some patients; however, many patients present once the disease has spread to an

Continue

CASE **2.7** *Contd.*

extent for which there is no curative option. In such patients, there may be palliative procedures which can be helpful.

A) Surgery is never curative – Incorrect. Surgical resection with curative intent is possible in patients with early localised disease. However, many patients have locally advanced or nodal or distant metastatic disease at presentation. Surgery is not usually considered in such patients.

B) Radiotherapy is an option – Correct. Patients undergoing surgical resection may undergo preoperative, neoadjuvant chemoradiotherapy to shrink the tumour. Chemotherapy or radiotherapy can also be used palliatively to shrink the tumour and provide pain relief.

C) Chemotherapy is an option – Correct. See answer B for further details.

D) Brachytherapy is an option – Incorrect. Brachytherapy is a form of internal radiotherapy in which the radiation source is placed within the tumour itself. It is most commonly used in prostate, cervical and some skin cancers. It is not used for lung cancer or Pancoast tumours.

E) Stenting of the superior vena cava is sometimes necessary – Correct. Endovascular stenting of the superior vena cava may be required in patients who have developed superior vena cava obstruction due to tumour compression. In such patients, a metallic stent is usually left inside the superior vena cava to help maintain its patency and restore venous return.

Steroids and radiotherapy can also help with superior vena cava obstruction.

❶ KEY POINT

The treatment of Pancoast tumours is often difficult due to the proximity of blood vessels and nerves, as well as the stage of disease at presentation. Preoperative chemoradiotherapy followed by surgery can be curative in certain patients, although for many palliative treatment is more appropriate.

IMPORTANT LEARNING POINTS

- Pancoast tumours are a rare type of lung cancer which arise in the lung apex.
- Clinical features often relate to the tumour's involvement in surrounding nerves and blood vessels.
- The brachial plexus, sympathetic chain, recurrent laryngeal, phrenic and vagus nerves are all at risk.
- Horner syndrome may occur with a Pancoast tumour, but there are a variety of other possible causes – the imaging required is guided by the clinical assessment.
- The lung apex is a difficult area to assess on the chest X-ray – it should be one of your review areas.
- Staging is primarily with CT, although MRI provides a better assessment of local involvement.
- Treatment can be pursued with curative intent but is often palliative.

CASE 2.8

A 60-year-old male patient presents with cough, weight loss and haematuria. As part of his investigation, a chest X-ray is performed.

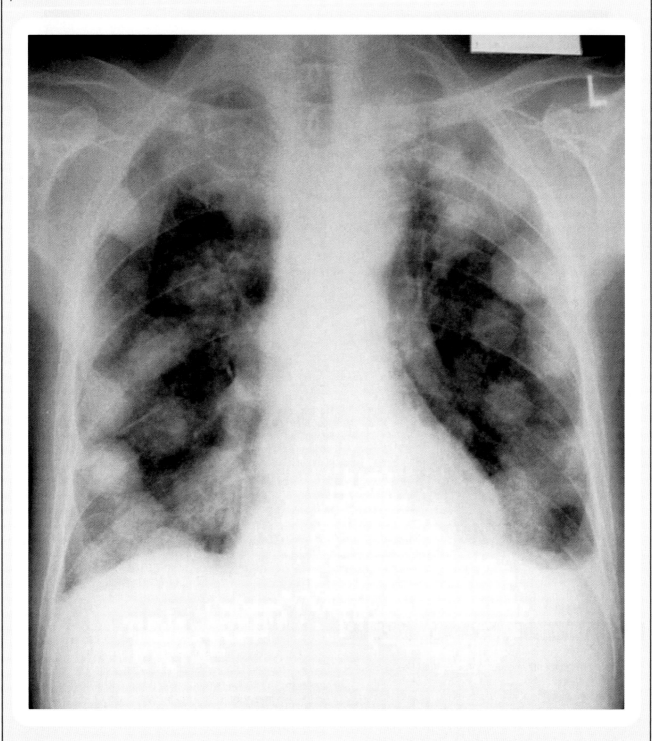

Continue

CASE 2.8 *Contd.*

ANNOTATED X-RAY

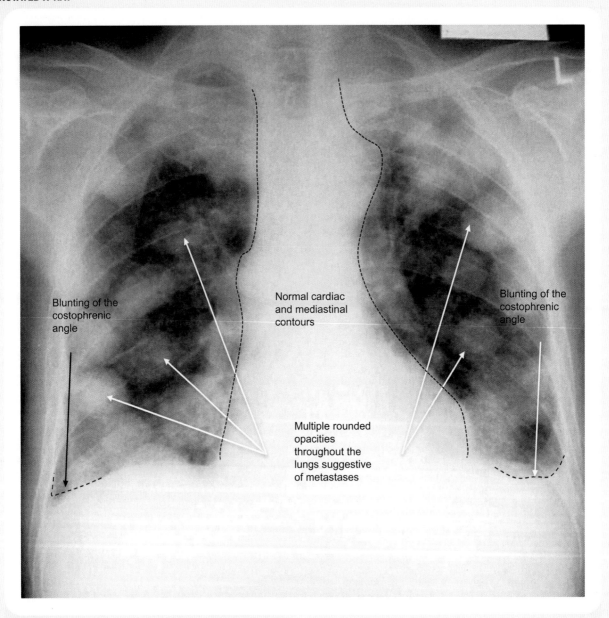

Blunting of the costophrenic angle

Normal cardiac and mediastinal contours

Blunting of the costophrenic angle

Multiple rounded opacities throughout the lungs suggestive of metastases

🔍 PRESENT YOUR FINDINGS

- This is a PA chest X-ray of an adult.
- There are no identifying markings. I would like to ensure that this is the correct patient and to check the date and time when the X-ray was taken.
- The patient is not rotated and has made a good inspiratory effort. The X-ray is slightly underpenetrated, but otherwise technically adequate. No important areas have been cut off.
- The most striking abnormality is the multiple round opacities throughout the lungs that are suggestive of 'cannonball' metastases.
- There is blunting of the costophrenic angles, more marked on the left, which may represent small pleural effusions.

- The trachea is central.
- The heart is not enlarged, and the cardiac and mediastinal contours are normal.
- There is no collapse or consolidation.
- Both hemidiaphragms are clearly demarcated.
- No free subdiaphragmatic gas is seen.
- There is no abnormality of the imaged soft tissues or skeleton.

IN SUMMARY – This chest X-ray shows multiple round opacities throughout both lungs. The radiological findings, combined with clinical history, are most in keeping with multiple pulmonary metastases.

QUESTIONS

1. Pulmonary metastases may present with which of the following signs/symptoms?
   A) Asymptomatic
   B) Dysphagia
   C) Haemoptysis
   D) Pneumothorax
   E) Lobar collapse

2. Which of the following is/are pathways of metastatic spread of tumour to the lungs?
   A) Haematogenous
   B) Lymphatic
   C) Direct extension
   D) Transcoelomic
   E) Pleural

3. Which of the following is/are differential(s) for multiple pulmonary nodules/masses?
   A) Abscesses
   B) TB

C) Sarcoidosis
D) Pulmonary metastases
E) Emphysema

4. Which of the following cancers is least likely to be the primary tumour in a 70-year-old woman with pulmonary metastases?
   A) Wilm tumour
   B) Melanoma
   C) Breast cancer
   D) Renal cell carcinoma
   E) Colorectal cancer

5. Which of the following imaging modalities is/are commonly used to assess for pulmonary metastases?
   A) Ultrasound
   B) PET-CT
   C) Chest X-ray
   D) CT
   E) MRI thorax

Continue

CASE **2.8** *Contd.*

ANSWERS TO QUESTIONS

1. Pulmonary metastases may present with which of the following signs/symptoms?

   The correct answers are **A) Asymptomatic, C) Haemoptysis, D) Pneumothorax and E) Lobar collapse**.

   Pulmonary metastases can be asymptomatic or present with a variety of symptoms and clinical signs.

   A) Asymptomatic – Correct. In patients with metastatic cancer, the predominant symptoms are usually related to the primary tumour or constitutional symptoms due to the disseminated disease. Pulmonary metastases are most commonly asymptomatic and are only identified when imaging of the chest (either as part of staging or for another reason) is performed.

   B) Dysphagia – Incorrect. Dysphagia is usually caused by endoluminal obstruction (foreign body), oesophageal mucosal pathology (tumours, strictures, webs) or extraluminal compression (retrosternal goitre, mediastinal malignancy and lymphadenopathy, aortic aneurysm, hiatus hernia). Pulmonary metastases are usually confined to the lung and therefore unlikely to cause dysphagia.

   C) Haemoptysis – Correct. Haemorrhage into the alveolar system from pulmonary metastases can result in haemoptysis.

   D) Pneumothorax – Correct. Pneumothorax is a rare but recognised complication of pulmonary metastases, which most commonly occurs with sarcomatous metastases.

   E) Lobar collapse – Correct. Compression of a bronchus or bronchiole by pulmonary metastases can result in distal collapse and/or consolidation.

❶ KEY POINT

Pulmonary metastases can result in a variety of clinical findings; however, most commonly they are asymptomatic and only identified on imaging of the chest, e.g. for staging.

2. Which of the following is/are pathways of metastatic spread of tumour to the lungs?

   The correct answers are **A) Haematogenous, B) Lymphatic and E) Pleural**.

   As with metastases to any organ, there are a variety of routes through which tumour cells can spread into the lung. The route of spread is determined by the location and pathological characteristics of the primary tumour.

   A) Haematogenous – Correct. Haematogenous spread is the most common route, usually via the pulmonary arteries. Tumours with a rich vascular supply, such as renal cell carcinoma, sarcomas and testicular cancers, are most likely to spread this way.

   B) Lymphatic – Correct. The lymphatic system is the most common route for spread of adenocarcinoma, such as breast, lung, colon and gastric cancer. It can result in the typical appearance of lymphangitis

carcinomatosis. On X-ray, this appears as interlobular septal thickening with a reticulonodular pattern. CT is much more sensitive at identifying interlobular septal thickening.

   C) Direct extension – Incorrect. Although direct invasion can result in tumour spreading into the lung, it is not strictly speaking a form of metastatic spread, but local extension. Tumours which arise in organs adjacent to the lungs, such as oesophageal or thyroid cancer, or intrathoracic metastases, such as mediastinal lymph nodes or rib deposits, can extend directly into the lungs.

   D) Transcoelomic – Incorrect. Transcoelomic spread refers to the spread of tumour cells throughout the peritoneal surfaces of the abdominal and pelvic cavities. A Krukenberg tumour (metastatic malignancy in the ovary, usually from a gastric primary) is an example of transcoelomic spread.

   E) Pleural – Correct. Spread within the pleural cavity usually results in deposits located in its most dependent part (the posterior and basal aspects).

❶ KEY POINT

The haematogenous route is the most common mechanism for pulmonary metastases, followed by lymphatic spread.

3. Which of the following is/are differential(s) for multiple pulmonary nodules/masses?

   The correct answers are **A) Abscesses, B) TB, C) Sarcoidosis and D) Pulmonary metastases**.

   Multiple pulmonary nodules are usually the result of haematogenous spread and can be caused by a variety of conditions. The clinical findings and results of other investigations (blood tests, microbiology, further imaging) will usually allow the diagnosis to be made. Other causes of multiple pulmonary nodules, in addition to the answers mentioned earlier, include rheumatoid nodules, silicosis and Granulomatosis with polyangiitis.

   A) Abscesses – Correct. Infection by a number of different pathogens can result in the development of multiple nodules and abscesses. Commonly implicated pathogens include Staphylococcus, Klebsiella and Legionella. Abscesses may appear solid (fluid filled) or can contain an air-fluid level. Infective symptoms and supporting blood and microbiology results can help identify infection as the underlying cause.

   B) TB – Correct. Haematogenous spread of TB can result in miliary TB, with numerous small nodules throughout the lungs.

   C) Sarcoidosis – Correct. Sarcoidosis is a systemic granulomatous disease that most commonly affects the lungs. A variety of possible conditions may be reflected on chest X-ray, including a normal state, bilateral hilar lymphadenopathy, pulmonary opacities (reticulonodules or large nodules) and pulmonary fibrosis. Serum ACE levels may be elevated. Biopsy is the gold standard for diagnosis.

D) Pulmonary metastases – Correct. As already discussed, pulmonary metastases can spread via a number of different routes and can result in multiple pulmonary nodules or masses. CT may be indicated to identify a primary tumour.

E) Emphysema – Incorrect. Emphysema results in destruction of the lung parenchyma, with enlargement of the airspaces distal to the terminal bronchiole. X-ray findings include hyperinflated lungs (flattened hemidiaphragms and more than seven anterior ribs) and reduced attenuation of the lung parenchyma. Large cystic areas (bullae) may form, but multiple nodules/masses would suggest an alternative or additional diagnosis.

❗ KEY POINT

There are various causes of multiple pulmonary nodules/masses. The history, clinical examination and results of blood tests and other radiology examinations usually point to the underlying causes. Occasionally, a biopsy of one of the nodules may be required.

4. Which of the following cancers is least likely to be the primary tumour in a 70-year-old woman with pulmonary metastases?

The correct answer is **A) Wilm tumour**.

Any cancer can metastasise to the lungs (all of the options in this question commonly cause pulmonary metastases); however, the likely primary tumour is determined largely by the age and sex of the patient.

A) Wilm tumour – Correct. Wilm tumour is a malignancy of the kidneys. Whilst it has a strong propensity to spread to the lungs, it occurs predominantly in children and very rarely affects adults. Therefore it would be a very uncommon cause of pulmonary metastases in an elderly woman.

B) Melanoma – Incorrect. The lung is a common site for malignant melanoma metastases. Other frequent sites include the brain, bone and liver.

C) Breast cancer – Incorrect. Breast cancer often spreads to the lungs. It can spread via the lymphatic route, leading to lymphangitis carcinomatosis, which is often unilateral (ipsilateral to the breast cancer).

D) Renal cell carcinoma – Incorrect. Renal cell carcinomas are highly vascular tumours which spread via the haematogenous route. They are increasingly common with advancing age and can result in multiple large pulmonary ('cannon ball') metastases – as seen in this case.

E) Colorectal cancer – Incorrect. The incidence of colorectal cancer increases with age. This tumour commonly spreads to the liver and lung.

❗ KEY POINT

Pulmonary metastases are common, and the primary tumour is often known. If, however, the site of the primary tumour is unknown, the patient's age and sex will help point to likely sites. In an elderly woman, examination of the breasts and CT of the abdomen and pelvis will often reveal the underlying cancer.

5. Which of the following imaging modalities is/are commonly used to assess for pulmonary metastases?

The correct answers are **C) Chest X-ray and D) CT**.

The imaging used to stage metastatic disease in different cancers is determined by the likelihood of metastases and their common locations. Assessment for lung metastases can be performed by chest X-ray, CT, PET-CT or no imaging at all, depending on the underlying cancer and the clinical scenario. Lung metastases are often multiple and usually peripheral. In addition, metastases are often at the bases of the lung, reflecting the blood flow through the lungs.

A) Ultrasound – Incorrect. Ultrasound waves do not travel well through gas-filled structures. Therefore ultrasound is not a useful modality for imaging the lung parenchyma. It is, however, commonly used for assessing the size, location and character of pleural effusions, which may have a malignant aetiology.

B) PET-CT – Incorrect. PET-CT is a radionuclide imaging technique which most commonly assesses glucose uptake in the body. It can therefore assess the metabolic activity of lesions, helping to differentiate malignant lesions (increased metabolism) from benign. However, there can be false-negative results (small nodule or diabetic patient) and false-positive results (inflammatory nodules). It is also associated with a relatively high-radiation dose. It is therefore not used as the first-line staging modality for assessing the lung; instead, it is used more as a problem-solving tool for assessing indeterminate nodules, masses and lymph nodes.

C) Chest X-ray – Correct. The chest X-ray is a cheap and fast investigation with a very low radiation dose. It can often show large pulmonary metastases; however, it has a relatively low sensitivity for small metastases. A normal chest X-ray thus does not exclude lung metastases, and if there is ongoing clinical suspicion, a CT should be considered.

D) CT – Correct. CT has much higher spatial resolution compared with the other imaging modalities. It can assess size, location, number and position of pulmonary nodules/masses. CT is therefore very sensitive in detecting pulmonary metastases. The size of the nodule, its appearance (calcification, cavitation) and its rate of growth, along with the presence of enlarged lymph nodes, can all help determine whether a nodule is likely to be malignant. However, some nodules will remain indeterminate on CT, and further assessment with PET-CT or biopsy may be needed.

E) MRI thorax – Incorrect. MRI has a lower spatial resolution than CT, takes longer to perform, is more prone to respiratory and movement artefact and is less-readily available. It is therefore not commonly used for staging the lungs. Even in children, who are more sensitive to the detrimental effects of ionising radiation, chest X-ray and CT are more frequently used than MRI for staging the lungs. MRI is better than CT for assessing chest wall invasion from a lung tumour, such as a Pancoast tumour.

Continue

CASE **2.8**   *Contd.*

❗ KEY POINT

CT of the chest is the most commonly used investigation for staging the lungs. Although CT has a very high sensitivity for pulmonary metastases, it does have limited specificity, and other imaging, such as PET-CT, may be helpful in certain circumstances. Some patients may need to have a biopsy (either percutaneous, endobronchial or open) to confirm the nature of an indeterminate pulmonary nodule.

IMPORTANT LEARNING POINTS

- Lung metastases can result in a variety of different signs and symptoms; however, they are often asymptomatic.
- The differential diagnosis of multiple pulmonary nodules on chest X-ray is wide. Clinical assessment and the results of blood tests can help identify the underlying cause.
- Most tumours can metastasise to the lungs, but in adults, breast, colorectal and renal cancers are common primaries.
- CT is often the imaging modality of choice for assessing pulmonary metastases.

CASE 2.9

A 30-year-old Afro-Caribbean man presents with a dry cough. He also complains of a purple rash on his legs. A chest X-ray is performed as part of his assessment.

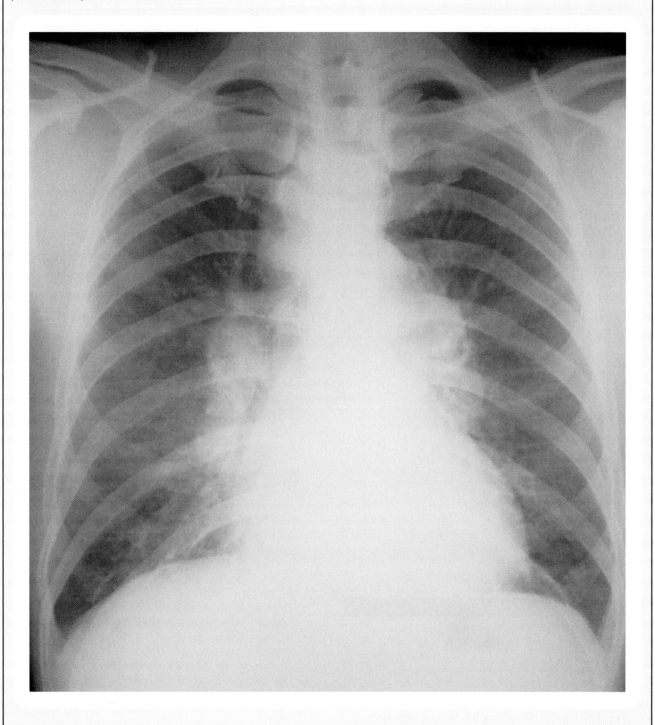

Continue

CASE **2.9** *Contd.*

ANNOTATED X-RAY

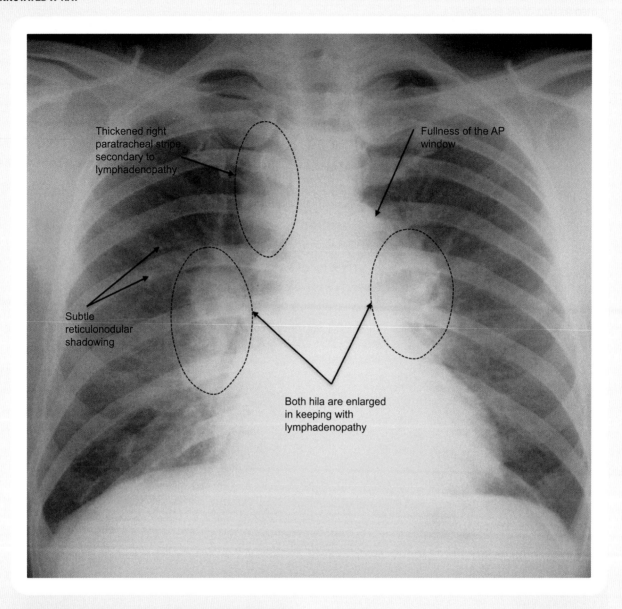

Thickened right paratracheal stripe secondary to lymphadenopathy

Fullness of the AP window

Subtle reticulonodular shadowing

Both hila are enlarged in keeping with lymphadenopathy

🔍 PRESENT YOUR FINDINGS

- This is a PA chest X-ray of an adult.
- The film has been anonymised, but I would like to confirm the patient's name and date of birth and the date and time when the study was performed before proceeding.
- There is minor patient rotation, and the X-ray is slightly underpenetrated. Otherwise, the study is technically adequate, with a good inspiratory achievement and no important areas cut off.
- The most striking abnormality is increased soft tissue density at both hila and in the right paratracheal region, with widening of the right paratracheal stripe. There is also soft tissue fullness within the aortopulmonary window.
- There is some subtle reticulonodular shadowing in the lung parenchyma in the perihilar regions.
- No other abnormality within the lungs is visible.
- The cardiac contours are clear.
- There is no free subdiaphragmatic gas.
- The visualised skeleton and soft tissues are normal.

IN SUMMARY – This chest X-ray demonstrates bilateral hilar and right paratracheal lymphadenopathy, with evidence of an interstitial lung process. Given the history, sarcoidosis is the most likely diagnosis. I would like to review any previous X-rays to assess for disease progression.

QUESTIONS

1. Regarding lymphadenopathy on chest X-ray, which of the following statements is/are correct?
   A) Lymphadenopathy should be considered if the right paratracheal stripe is thicker than 5 mm
   B) The hilar point consists of the region in which the upper lobe pulmonary veins and lower lobe pulmonary arteries cross
   C) Lymphoma should be considered in the differential diagnosis of bilateral hilar lymphadenopathy
   D) Splaying of the carina raises the possibility of subcarinal lymphadenopathy
   E) A normal chest X-ray excludes clinically relevant lymphadenopathy

2. Regarding sarcoidosis, which of the following statements is/are correct?
   A) The peak incidence occurs in the 20- to 40-year-old age group
   B) There is a female preponderance
   C) It more commonly affects individuals of Afro-Caribbean descent
   D) The presence of caseating granulomas on histology is characteristic
   E) It is a multisystem disease

3. Which of the clinical findings is/are compatible with a diagnosis of sarcoidosis?
   A) Hypercalcaemia
   B) Hypercalciuria
   C) Raised serum ACE
   D) Positive Heaf test
   E) Restrictive lung disease

4. Which of the following is/are recognised clinical presentations of sarcoidosis?
   A) Asymptomatic, incidental finding on chest X-ray
   B) Dry cough
   C) Erythema multiforme
   D) Lupus pernio
   E) Uveitis

5. Regarding the radiological features of sarcoidosis, which of the following statements is/are correct?
   A) The 1, 2, 3 sign may be present on chest X-ray
   B) Reticulonodular shadowing alone is less advanced disease than reticulonodular shadowing and bilateral hilar lymphadenopathy
   C) There may be evidence of lymph node calcification
   D) Fissural nodularity may be seen on CT
   E) Lung fibrosis can result

Continue

CASE **2.9** *Contd.*

ANSWERS TO QUESTIONS

1. Regarding lymphadenopathy on chest X-ray, which of the following statements is/are correct?

   The correct answers are **A) Lymphadenopathy should be considered if the right paratracheal stripe is thicker than 5 mm, B) The hilar point consists of the region in which the upper lobe pulmonary veins and lower lobe pulmonary arteries cross, C) Lymphoma should be considered in the differential diagnosis of bilateral hilar lymphadenopathy and D) Splaying of the carina raises the possibility of sub-carinal lymphadenopathy**.

   The differential diagnosis for bilateral hilar lymphadenopathy includes lymphoma, TB and sarcoidosis. However, remember that hilar enlargement can arise from any structure within the hilum, such as lymph nodes, pulmonary vessels or a proximal bronchial tumour.

   A) Lymphadenopathy should be considered if the right paratracheal stripe is thicker than 5 mm – Correct. A thin stripe of soft tissue is normally seen alongside the right side of the trachea. However, anything >5 mm in thickness should be viewed suspiciously for lymphadenopathy.

   B) The hilar point consists of the region in which the upper lobe pulmonary veins and lower lobe pulmonary arteries cross – Correct. There should be a sharp angle between these structures. Any lumps or convexity to the hilum should raise suspicion of pathology. The positions of the hila are also important, as they provide an indication of volume loss. The left hilum should never be lower than the right. If the left hilum is lower, you must consider whether there is volume loss in the left lower lobe (pulling the left hilum down) or right upper lobe (pulling the right hilum up). Understanding the anatomical basis for the chest X-ray appearance can help identify subtle abnormalities.

   C) Lymphoma should be considered in the differential diagnosis of bilateral hilar lymphadenopathy – Correct. Lymphoma is in the differential diagnosis for widespread mediastinal lymphadenopathy.

   D) Splaying of the carina raises the possibility of subcarinal lymphadenopathy – Correct. Mass effect from an enlarged subcarinal lymph node can cause splaying of the carina on a chest X-ray. Left atrial enlargement is another cause of splaying of the carina, in which case there is often an accompanying double right heart shadow.

   E) A normal chest X-ray excludes clinically relevant lymphadenopathy – Incorrect. The limitations of the chest X-ray need to be understood. A normal chest X-ray does not necessarily exclude clinically relevant lymphadenopathy, and if there are convincing clinical symptoms (e.g. weight loss and night sweats – ?lymphoma), the patient should proceed to CT. Lymphadenopathy relates to the appearance of the nodes, as well as to their size. Nodes within normal size limits can still have abnormal appearances consistent with lymphadenopathy – this is frequently demonstrated when functional imaging (e.g. PET scans) is combined with anatomical imaging (e.g. CT) for staging certain malignancies.

❗ KEY POINTS

1. Assessing for mediastinal lymphadenopathy on a chest X-ray can be difficult, not least because there is a wide spectrum of normal hilar appearances due to composite and vascular shadows. Knowing where the normal hilar points should be found and what they should look like will help you spot any abnormality. Review of previous X-rays is useful to assess for subtle changes. Fortunately, there is always the contralateral side to assess for comparison (but this may not be helpful in the case of bilateral hilar lymphadenopathy!).

2. Beware of differential densities between the hila – the dense hilum (where one hila is denser than the other) is a sign which warrants further investigation to exclude lymphadenopathy, even if there is no definite abnormal mass discernible.

2. Regarding sarcoidosis, which of the following statements is/are correct?

   The correct answers are **A) The peak incidence occurs in the 20- to 40-year-old age group, B) There is a female preponderance, C) It more commonly affects individuals of Afro-Caribbean descent and E) It is a multisystem disease**.

   Sarcoidosis is a multisystem granulomatous disorder of unknown aetiology. Initially, the disease tends to affect the lungs, skin or lymph nodes; however, it can affect multiple other organs. It generally affects adults between the ages of 20 and 40. Afro-Caribbeans are more frequently and more severely affected than the White population, particular with extrathoracic manifestations of the disease (see question 4 for more details).

   A) The peak incidence occurs in the 20- to 40-year-old age group – Correct.

   B) There is a female preponderance – Correct.

   C) It more commonly affects individuals of Afro-Caribbean descent – Correct.

   D) The presence of caseating granulomas on histology is characteristic – Incorrect. The presence of caseating granulomas on histology is characteristic of TB. Sarcoidosis is a granulomatous disease, but the granulomas are noncaseating.

   E) It is a multisystem disease – Correct. In addition to the lung, sarcoidosis can affect the eye, skin, heart and central nervous system.

❗ KEY POINT

Being familiar with the demographic of patients more prone to developing sarcoidosis will help you remember it in your differential diagnosis. This is especially important during medical examinations!

3. Which of the clinical findings is/are compatible with a diagnosis of sarcoidosis?

The correct answers are **A) Hypercalcaemia, B) Hypercalciuria, C) Raised serum ACE and E) Restrictive lung disease**.

No individual finding is pathognomonic for sarcoidosis. The diagnosis is often made by consensus of clinical history, radiographic findings and biochemical results.

A) Hypercalcaemia – Correct. The inflammatory cells within granulomas can activate vitamin D. This in turn can result in hypercalcaemia and hypercalciuria; however, the body's compensatory mechanisms mean these biochemical abnormalities occur in <10% of patients with sarcoidosis.

B) Hypercalciuria – Correct. In conjunction with hypercalcaemia, patients may also have increased urinary excretion of calcium in a 24-hour urine assessment.

C) Raised serum ACE – Correct. Some patients with sarcoidosis may have elevated levels of serum ACE.

D) Positive Heaf test – Incorrect. A positive Heaf test is suggestive of TB, not sarcoidosis.

E) Restrictive lung disease – Correct. Advanced pulmonary sarcoidosis involves the development of pulmonary infiltrates and fibrosis causing thickening of the pulmonary interstitium. This can lead to restrictive lung disease that can be confirmed on spirometry.

❗ KEY POINT

There are a variety of biochemical findings which support the diagnosis of sarcoidosis, but none of them is highly sensitive and specific.

4. Which of the following is/are recognised clinical presentations of sarcoidosis?

The correct answers are **A) Asymptomatic, incidental finding on chest X-ray, B) Dry cough, D) Lupus pernio and E) Uveitis**.

There are multiple nonpulmonary manifestations of sarcoidosis, involving the eyes, lacrimal and salivary glands, central nervous system, skin and heart.

A) Asymptomatic, incidental finding on chest X-ray – Correct. Up to 20% to 40% of cases of sarcoidosis may be diagnosed incidentally after a routine chest X-ray in patients without any symptoms.

B) Dry cough – Correct. History of a dry cough is typical of sarcoidosis. Other pulmonary symptoms include dyspnoea, reduced exercise tolerance and sometimes even chest pain.

C) Erythema multiforme – Incorrect. Erythema nodosum is associated with sarcoidosis. Painful, purple raised lesions are found typically on the shins. It may be part of Lofgren syndrome, which is an acute form of sarcoidosis consisting of bilateral hilar lymphadenopathy, fever polyarthritis and erythema nodosum. It has a good prognosis, often resolving spontaneously.

Erythema multiforme consists of target lesions and is often seen in drug reactions or with mycoplasma infection, but not with sarcoidosis.

D) Lupus pernio – Correct. Lupus pernio is an indurate violaceous rash affecting the nose and cheeks and is associated with sarcoidosis. Patients with sarcoidosis and lupus pernio often have a worse prognosis, and the disease is less likely to resolve completely.

E) Uveitis – Correct. Uveitis has a recognised association with sarcoidosis. In fact, some patients may present to an ophthalmologist initially, who should request a chest X-ray. Symptoms of uveitis include blurred vision, photophobia, redness, floaters and pain.

❗ KEY POINT

Sarcoidosis is a multisystem disorder. Some patients are asymptomatic, some develop acute symptoms but recover fully and some develop chronic disease.

5. Regarding the radiological features of sarcoidosis, which of the following statements is/are correct?

The correct answers are **A) The 1, 2, 3 sign may be present on chest X-ray, C) There may be evidence of lymph node calcification, D) Nodularity affecting the fissures on CT may be seen and E) Lung fibrosis can result**.

Radiology is useful in the diagnosis and monitoring of patients with sarcoidosis. You should familiarise yourself with the sarcoidosis staging on radiological imaging, as it has prognostic indications and is an easy examination question.

A) The 1, 2, 3 sign may be present on chest X-ray – Correct. This sign is also known as Garland's triad and consists of right paratracheal, right hilar and left hilar lymph node enlargement.

B) Reticulonodular shadowing alone is less advanced disease than reticulonodular shadowing and bilateral hilar lymphadenopathy – Incorrect. Reticulonodular shadowing alone is consistent with stage III disease, whereas reticulonodular shadowing and bilateral hilar lymphadenopathy represent stage II disease.

C) There may be evidence of lymph node calcification – Correct. Lymph node calcification is usually a feature in longstanding disease. The pattern of calcification can vary from punctate (tiny dots), through amorphous (lumps with no specific shape), to eggshell-like (thin peripheral rim of calcification).

D) Fissural nodularity may be seen on CT – Correct. This is a classic CT appearance of sarcoidosis.

E) Lung fibrosis can result – Correct. Linear bands of fibrosis typically radiate laterally and superiorly from the hila.

Continue

CASE 2.9   *Contd.*

KEY POINTS

- Stage 0 – Normal chest X-ray
  - 5% to 10% of patients at presentation
- Stage I – Hilar or mediastinal lymphadenopathy only
  - 45% to 65% of patients at presentation
  - 60% have complete resolution
- Stage II – Lymphadenopathy and parenchymal disease
  - 25% to 30% of patients at presentation
- Stage III – parenchymal disease only
  - 15% of patients at presentation
- Stage IV – pulmonary fibrosis
  - End-stage

IMPORTANT LEARNING POINTS

- Identifying lymphadenopathy on a chest X-ray can be difficult. A good understanding of the normal anatomical structures at the hilar points and an appreciation of the wide range of normality will help.
- Beware of the unilateral dense hilum – aim to exclude lymphadenopathy or a proximal bronchial tumour.
- Sarcoidosis is a multisystem disease in which clinical history and signs, radiological and biochemical findings are important in confirming the diagnosis.
- Remember the chest X-ray staging of sarcoidosis – it has prognostic implications.

CASE **2.10**

The parents of a 2-year-old child are concerned that their daughter has swallowed an object and present to the Emergency Department. A chest X-ray is performed.

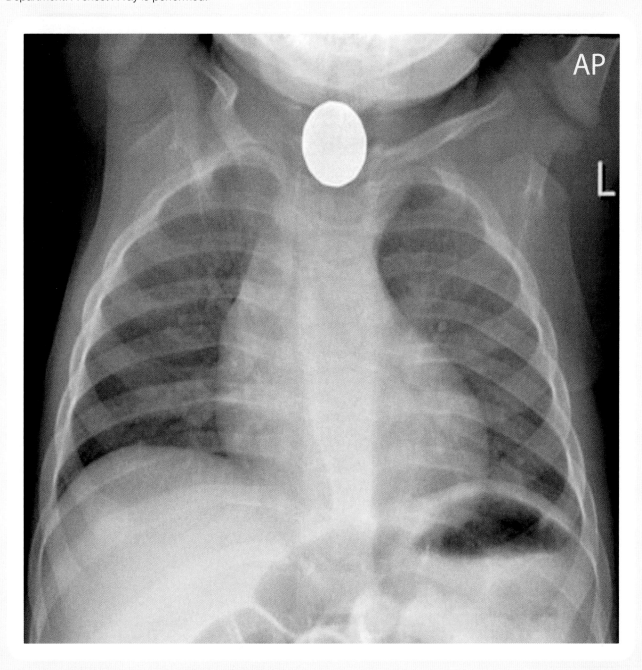

Continue

CASE **2.10** *Contd.*

ANNOTATED X-RAY

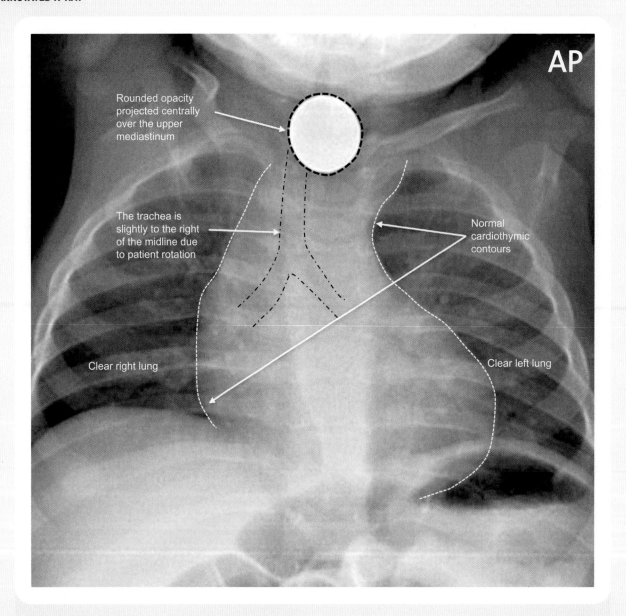

Rounded opacity projected centrally over the upper mediastinum

The trachea is slightly to the right of the midline due to patient rotation

Normal cardiothymic contours

Clear right lung

Clear left lung

AP

PRESENT YOUR FINDINGS

- This is an AP chest X-ray of a child.
- The film has been anonymised, but I would like to check the name and date of birth of the subject and confirm the time and date when the X-ray was taken before proceeding.
- The patient is slightly rotated, but the X-ray is adequately inspired and penetrated, displaying the abnormality.
- The most striking abnormality is a well-defined circular radio-opaque entity projected over the superior aspect of the mediastinum.
- The trachea is projected slightly to the right of the midline due to patient rotation. The cardiomediastinal contours are unremarkable. Normal thymic shadow.

- There is no evidence of lobar/lung hyperexpansion or collapse. No pneumothorax or pleural effusion.
- There is no free subdiaphragmatic gas.
- The visualised skeleton and soft tissues are unremarkable.

IN SUMMARY – This chest X-ray demonstrates a circular radio-opaque foreign body, consistent with a metallic coin, projected over the superior mediastinum. Its position is consistent with impaction of the ingested coin within the oesophagus at the level of the aortic arch. I would discuss the case with a gastroenterologist for endoscopic removal.

QUESTIONS

1. Regarding suspected ingestion of a coin by a child, which of the following is/are correct?
   A) The chest X-ray should include the neck
   B) An abdominal X-ray should be performed if the object cannot be visualised on the chest X-ray
   C) Hand-held metal detectors may be an alternative to performing X-rays
   D) Serial abdominal X-rays to monitor the transition of the object are required
   E) An object lodged within the oesophagus can potentially lead to mediastinitis

2. Regarding suspected ingestion of sharp or potentially poisonous foreign bodies, which of the following is/are correct?
   A) A frontal chest X-ray should be the first radiographic imaging performed
   B) A circular radio-opaque foreign body with lucent rim is suggestive of a button/disc battery
   C) If a button battery is demonstrated on abdominal X-ray, the X-ray should be repeated every 24 hours
   D) If there is suspicion of ingestion of a sharp object, the role of the abdominal X-ray is to confirm or exclude the presence of the object
   E) CT may be required

3. Which of the following is/are a recognised appearance of an inhaled foreign body on chest X-ray in an otherwise healthy child?
   A) Normal appearances
   B) Right lower lobe collapse
   C) Hyperexpansion
   D) Rib fracture from coughing
   E) Complete whiteout of one hemithorax

4. Regarding immediate management of a choking 2 year old child who is conscious and not able to cough, which of the following statements is/are correct?
   A) Five rescue breaths should be performed
   B) Five back blows should be performed
   C) Five chest thrusts should be performed
   D) Cardiopulmonary resuscitation should be performed
   E) High flow oxygen via a non-rebreather should be given

5. Regarding retrieval of inhaled foreign bodies identified on chest X-rays, which of the following is true?
   A) All foreign bodies are eventually coughed out
   B) Nasendoscopy and bronchoscopy are usually successful in retrieving the foreign body
   C) A foreign body never gets trapped long enough to need removal
   D) Thoracoscopy is often used
   E) Mediastinoscopy is an alternative to bronchoscopy

Continue

CASE **2.10**   *Contd.*

ANSWERS TO QUESTIONS

1. Regarding suspected ingestion of a coin by a child, which of the following is/are correct?

    The correct answers are **A) The chest X-ray should include the neck, C) Hand-held metal detectors may be an alternative to performing X-rays and E) An object lodged within the oesophagus can potentially lead to mediastinitis**.

    British coins are inert, and there is no danger to a child if an ingested coin lies within the stomach or intestine. In cases of suspected coin ingestion, a chest X-ray should be performed first. In countries in which coins are potentially poisonous, a chest X-ray, followed by an abdominal X-ray if the chest X-ray is negative, would be appropriate.

    A) The chest X-ray should include the neck – Correct. The chest X-ray should be extended to include the neck, as foreign bodies can be lodged in the cervical portion of the oesophagus. If the ingested foreign body is small and inert/blunt, like a British coin, then no further imaging is required (see B for further details).

    B) An abdominal X-ray should be performed if the object cannot be visualised on the chest X-ray – Incorrect. If the coin is not demonstrated on the chest X-ray, it is assumed to be either below the diaphragm in the gastrointestinal tract, or that the patient never ingested the object in the first place. If the coin is below the diaphragm (and it is inert, like UK coins), it is harmless and should pass spontaneously.

    C) Hand-held metal detectors may be an alternative to performing X-rays – Correct. Some advocate the use of hand-held metal detectors in the investigation of ingested metallic coins. If the coin can be demonstrated to be below the level of the diaphragm with a metal detector, then there is an argument for not proceeding to perform any form of X-ray, as the coin must be within the gastrointestinal tract.

    D) Serial abdominal X-rays to monitor the transition of the object are required – Incorrect. It is not necessary to track the transit of a coin through the gastrointestinal tract with serial abdominal X-rays. This would expose the child to a significant radiation dose in the pursuit of no relevant clinical information.

    E) An object lodged within the oesophagus can potentially lead to mediastinitis – Correct. The narrowest parts of the gastrointestinal tract are within the oesophagus, and so this is the site at which foreign bodies are most likely to become lodged. Objects stuck within the oesophagus can lead to erosion of the mucosa, which can cause abscess formation or even mediastinitis. If a foreign body reaches the stomach, it is unlikely to get stuck, and as long as it is small and inert/blunt, it will not cause the patient any harm.

❶ KEY POINT

In cases of ingested small inert/blunt objects, such as coins, it is appropriate to perform a single frontal chest X-ray, including the neck, in children. No further radiographic imaging is usually justified, as once the foreign body is distal to the stomach it is unlikely to become stuck.

2. Regarding suspected ingestion of sharp or potentially poisonous foreign bodies, which of the following is/are correct?

    The correct answer is **A) A frontal chest X-ray should be the first radiographic imaging performed, B) A circular radio-opaque foreign body with lucent rim is suggestive of a button/disc battery, C) If a button battery is demonstrated on abdominal X-ray, the X-ray should be repeated every 24 hours, D) If there is suspicion of ingestion of a sharp object, the role of the abdominal X-ray is to confirm or exclude the presence of the object and E) CT may be required**.

    Unlike inert, blunt objects, sharp or potentially poisonous foreign bodies still pose a risk to the patient if they are in the gastrointestinal tract below the diaphragm. Consequently, if the chest X-ray is negative in such cases, then an abdominal X-ray is indicated. The role of imaging in these cases is to confirm or exclude the presence of such entities.

    A) A frontal chest X-ray should be the first radiographic imaging performed – Correct. If the chest X-ray is clear, then an abdominal X-ray should be performed.

    B) A circular radio-opaque foreign body with lucent rim is suggestive of a button/disc battery – Correct. This is the classic appearance of a button/disc battery. It is important to recognise this foreign body because most modern batteries contain sodium or potassium hydroxide, which is corrosive. The contents of the batteries may leak out in the gastrointestinal tract, with the potential to cause serious harm.

    C) If a button battery is demonstrated on abdominal X-ray, the X-ray should be repeated every 24 hours – Correct. It is important to track an ingested button battery with serial abdominal X-rays. If there is the suggestion of delayed transition/hold up or disintegration, then endoscopic or surgical removal needs to be considered.

    D) If there is suspicion of ingestion of a sharp object, the role of the abdominal X-ray is to confirm or exclude the presence of the object – Correct. This is the role of imaging in the case of suspected ingestion of sharp objects.

    E) CT may be required – Correct. Occasionally, both the abdominal X-ray and chest X-ray will be normal in the case of an ingested sharp foreign body. If there is clinical concern, CT may be indicated. Remember that certain sharp foreign bodies, such as toothpicks, are not radio-opaque on X-ray.

❶ KEY POINT

The investigation pathway depends on whether the ingested foreign body is sharp/poisonous or inert and blunt. In cases of the former, an abdominal X-ray is indicated if the chest X-ray is normal. In the latter case, if the chest X-ray (including the neck) is normal, you can be reassured.

3. Which of the following is/are a recognised appearance of an inhaled foreign body on chest X-ray in an otherwise healthy child?
The correct answers are **A) Normal appearances, B) Right lower lobe collapse, C) Hyperexpansion and E) Complete whiteout of one hemithorax**.
It is important to realise that there are a variety of different chest X-ray appearances compatible with an inhaled foreign body in an otherwise healthy child.
A) Normal appearances – Correct. An inhaled foreign body may result in normal radiographic appearances, particularly if the foreign body is not radio-opaque. If there is ongoing clinical concern, direct visualisation with nasendoscopy/bronchoscopy is required.
B) Right lower lobe collapse – Correct. The right main bronchus runs a more inferior course than the left main bronchus, which runs more laterally. As a result, foreign bodies are more likely to become impacted in the right main bronchus, resulting in right middle or lower lobe collapse. However, any form of collapse may potentially occur.
C) Hyperexpansion – Correct. An inhaled foreign body can act as a ball valve in a bronchus, causing hyperexpansion (air can enter into the lobe/lung during inspiration, but the foreign body prevents it from leaving during expiration). Occasionally, an expiratory phase chest X-ray is performed to exploit this phenomenon. The hyperexpanded area implies the site of the underlying obstruction.
D) Rib fracture from coughing – Incorrect. In an otherwise healthy child, vigorous coughing should not result in rib fractures. All chest X-rays in children should be scrutinised for the presence of acute, healing or previous rib fractures, which may be an indicator of nonaccidental injury.
E) Complete whiteout of one hemithorax – Correct. Proximal obstruction of one of the main bronchi by an inhaled foreign body can result in whiteout of a hemithorax.

! KEY POINT

A normal chest X-ray is not necessarily reassuring in cases of suspected inhaled foreign body. If there is ongoing clinical concern, direct visualisation with bronchoscopy may be required.

4. Regarding immediate management of a choking 2 year old child who is conscious and not able to cough, which of the following statements is/are correct?
The correct answer is **B) 5 back blows should be performed.**
As part of the paediatric basic life support algorithm according to Resuscitation Council (UK), management of choking in children depends on whether the child is conscious and whether they can cough.
A) Five rescue breaths should be performed – Incorrect. In children who have choked on an object and are unconscious, the most important management step is to give five breaths via mouth-to-mouth. CPR should also be commenced if there are no signs of life. In this question, the patient was conscious so rescue breaths are not indicated.
B) Five back blows should be performed – Correct. The first step in the management of choking in children is to encourage the patient to cough. If the patient had an effective cough, then they hopefully can dislodge the obstruction. Patients should be observed to see if their cough becomes ineffective. This patient's cough is not effective so five back blows should be performed instead. If the back blows fail, then abdominal thrusts can be performed. Abdominal thrusts are also known as the Heimlich manoeuvre. If the obstruction has not cleared, then emergency help must be called. The five back blows and abdominal thrusts should be repeated to clear the obstruction until help arrives. If the object causing the obstruction is visible, then McGill forceps may also be used to remove the object.
C) Five chest thrusts should be performed – Incorrect. If back blows fail initially, then abdominal thrusts should be performed in patients older than 1 year old. In small infants that are aged less than 1 years old, chest thrusts should be performed instead of abdominal thrusts.
D) Cardiopulmonary resuscitation should be performed – Incorrect. Cardiopulmonary resuscitation (CPR) is performed if a patient has no pulse and has insufficient or no respiratory effort. This patient is still conscious, so CPR is not indicated and the choking algorithm should instead be followed.
E) High flow oxygen via a non-rebreather should be given – Incorrect. This patient is suffering airway compromise due to choking, therefore the airway problem should be addressed as per the ABCDE assessment. Oxygen therapy, instead, forms part of the management of breathing and so is not yet appropriate.

! KEY POINT

Choking is very common in young children who frequently put things in their mouths. Their small airway diameter means it is more readily occluded compared to adolescents and adults. The level of airway obstruction in a choking child is indicated by how effective their cough is and whether they are conscious.

5. Regarding retrieval of inhaled foreign bodies identified on chest X-rays, which of the following is true?
The correct answer is **B) Nasendoscopy and bronchoscopy are usually successful in retrieving the foreign body**.
Once a foreign body is identified, it is important to understand the next step in management in order to remove the foreign body safely.
A) All foreign bodies are eventually coughed out – Incorrect. Occasionally, a foreign body will be coughed out, but this is not always the case.

Continue

CASE 2.10   *Contd.*

B) Nasendoscopy and bronchoscopy are usually successful in retrieving the foreign body – Correct. Nasendoscopy and bronchoscopy can provide direct visualisation of the foreign body and are usually successful in retrieving it.

C) A foreign body never gets trapped long enough to need removal – Incorrect. Foreign bodies can occasionally get trapped for long periods of time and therefore need removal. Focal downstream bronchiectasis is a recognised complication of longstanding obstruction and recurrent infection from an impacted foreign body.

D) Thoracoscopy is often used – Incorrect. Thoracoscopy involves inserting a camera into the pleural space. It is therefore unlikely to be of benefit in removing an object stuck within the lumen of the bronchial tree.

E) Mediastinoscopy is an alternative to bronchoscopy – Incorrect. Mediastinoscopy involves making an incision in the suprasternal notch region and examining the mediastinum with a video camera from within the chest. It is not an alternative to bronchoscopy, as it does not permit access to the bronchial tree.

❶ KEY POINT

In the emergency setting, management of a choking child should proceed along the paediatric basic life support algorithm. Otherwise, nasendoscopy and/or bronchoscopy are employed.

IMPORTANT LEARNING POINTS

- Foreign bodies can become stuck within the respiratory or gastrointestinal tracts.
- Inhaled foreign bodies often need to be removed, as do ingested sharp/poisonous ones. In contrast, a small, inert/blunt foreign body which has been swallowed will usually transit through the patient without causing any problems as long as it has cleared the oesophagus. An ingested inert/blunt foreign body will need to be removed if it becomes stuck within the oesophagus.
- Regarding investigation of ingested foreign bodies in children, the type of foreign body guides the initial investigation; chest X-ray in the case of small, blunt objects (including coins), and chest X-ray +/− abdominal X-ray in the case of sharp or potentially poisonous objects.
- A normal chest X-ray does not exclude an inhaled foreign body.
- In cases of suspected impacted fish or chicken bones, look for direct and indirect prevertebral soft tissue swelling and retropharyngeal gas) evidence of a foreign body.

CASE **2.11**

A 77-year-old presents with purulent cough, fever and shortness of breath. A chest X-ray is performed.

Continue

CASE **2.11** *Contd.*

ANNOTATED X-RAY

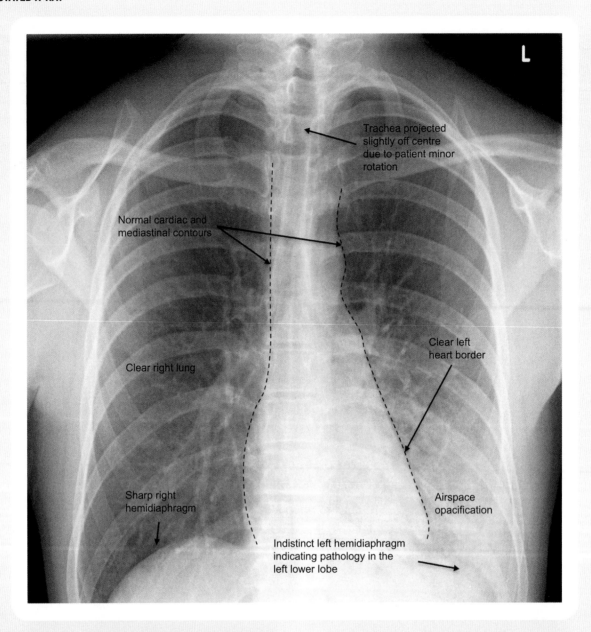

Trachea projected slightly off centre due to patient minor rotation

Normal cardiac and mediastinal contours

Clear left heart border

Clear right lung

Airspace opacification

Sharp right hemidiaphragm

Indistinct left hemidiaphragm indicating pathology in the left lower lobe

🔍 **PRESENT YOUR FINDINGS**

- This is a PA chest X-ray of an adult.
- It has been anonymised. I would like to ensure that this is the correct patient, and to check the date and time when the X-ray was taken.
- The patient is slightly rotated, there is good inspiratory achievement and the X-ray is adequately penetrated. However, the costophrenic angles have not been included, and therefore it is a technically inadequate X-ray.
- The most striking abnormality is the airspace opacification in the left lower zone, in keeping with consolidation. The left heart border is clearly defined; however, the left hemidiaphragm is not visible, indicating that the pathology is in the left lower lobe.

- It is not possible to exclude a small effusion, as the costophrenic angle has not been included on the X-ray; however, there is no large effusion.
- The trachea is central (allowing for the patient rotation).
- The cardiac and mediastinal contours are normal.
- The right lung is clear.
- The imaged thoracic skeleton and soft tissues are normal.

IN SUMMARY – This chest X-ray demonstrates left lower lobe consolidation. Given the clinical details, it is likely infective in aetiology and represents lobar pneumonia. I would advise a follow-up chest X-ray in 4 to 6 weeks, following appropriate antibiotic therapy, to ensure resolution.

QUESTIONS

1. Which of the following is/are causes of consolidation on a chest X-ray?
   A) Pulmonary oedema
   B) Pulmonary haemorrhage
   C) Proteinaceous fluid
   D) Infection
   E) Tumour

2. A patient presents with a clinical diagnosis of pneumonia and their chest X-ray shows consolidation obscuring the right heart border and medial part of the right hemidiaphragm. Which lobe or lobes are affected?
   A) Right upper lobe
   B) Right middle lobe
   C) Right lower lobe
   D) Right middle and lower lobes
   E) Not able to say with certainty

3. What is the commonest pathogen responsible for community-acquired pneumonia?
   A) *Staphylococcus aureus*
   B) *Streptococcus pneumoniae*
   C) *Haemophilus influenza*
   D) *Legionella pneumophila*
   E) *Mycoplasma pneumoniae*

4. Which of the following is a scoring system for community-acquired pneumonia?
   A) Gleason score
   B) Rockall score
   C) Nottingham prognostic index
   D) Modified Glasgow prognostic criteria
   E) CURB-65 score

5. Which of the following is/are complications of pneumonia?
   A) Pleural effusion
   B) Empyema
   C) Bronchiectasis
   D) Pneumothorax
   E) Deep vein thrombosis

Continue

CASE **2.11**   *Contd.*

ANSWERS TO QUESTIONS

1. Which of the following is/are causes of consolidation on a chest X-ray?

   The correct answers are **A) Pulmonary oedema, B) Pulmonary haemorrhage, C) Proteinaceous fluid, D) Infection and E) Tumour**.

   Consolidation refers to any pathological process that fills the alveoli. Consolidation is often thought to be synonymous with infection. However, there are a variety of other causes of consolidation. Therefore the terms *pneumonia* and *consolidation* should not be used interchangeably. The clinical scenario and X-ray features may help to differentiate the cause of the consolidation. Other causes of consolidation not listed in this question include aspiration (food, water). In addition to infective pneumonia, there are a variety of less common noninfective pneumonias, which include cryptogenic organising pneumonia and chronic eosinophilic pneumonia.

   A) Pulmonary oedema – Correct. Alveoli filled with water (oedema) can cause consolidation. Pulmonary oedema is associated with cardiomegaly, upper lobe venous diversion, pleural effusions and Kerley B lines. Most often, pulmonary oedema is cardiogenic in aetiology. However, there are noncardiogenic causes of pulmonary oedema, such as fluid overload, renal impairment and neurogenic. Remember that cardiogenic oedema can occur with a normal-sized heart in very acute conditions such as acute myocardial infarction or acute mitral valve regurgitation.

   B) Pulmonary haemorrhage – Correct. Alveoli filled with blood can cause consolidation. Trauma is the most common cause. Other causes include bleeding disorders, Goodpasture syndrome, Henoch–Schönlein purpura, vasculitis and pulmonary infarction.

   C) Proteinaceous fluid – Correct. Proteinaceous fluid within the alveoli is another cause of consolidation. Alveolar proteinosis is a rare disorder in which excessive protein and lipid-rich surfactant is produced, resulting in litres of sputum being produced daily.

   D) Infection – Correct. Infective pneumonia is the most common cause of consolidation. An air bronchogram can be present and is formed when the air-containing bronchiole is surrounded by consolidated lung. Remember that early pneumonia affecting the bronchi and bronchioles (bronchopneumonia) can be difficult to identify on a chest X-ray.

   E) Tumour – Correct. Tumour cells may fill the alveoli, resulting in consolidation on the chest X-ray. Bronchoalveolar carcinoma and lymphoma are the commonest cancers to give this appearance. Consolidation that does not improve following appropriate treatment (usually antibiotics for suspected infection) should thus raise the possibility of a neoplastic cause, due either to malignancy consolidation or an obstructive proximal bronchogenic carcinoma.

❗ KEY POINT

Consolidation refers to filling of alveoli with products of pathology, typically pus (infection), blood (pulmonary haemorrhage), cells (tumour), water (pulmonary oedema) or protein (alveolar proteinosis). Whilst infection is by far the commonest cause of consolidation, the two terms are not synonymous.

2. A patient presents with a clinical diagnosis of pneumonia and their chest X-ray shows consolidation obscuring the right heart border and medial part of the right hemidiaphragm. Which lobe or lobes are affected?

   The correct answer is **D) Right middle and lower lobes**.

   The silhouette sign is useful for locating in which lobe of the lung pathology is located. In normal cases, there is a sharp border between aerated lung and the soft tissues of the heart and diaphragm. This is due to the large differences in the amount of X-ray attenuated by the soft tissues (relatively high proportion of X-rays) and the lung (relatively few X-rays).

   If there is consolidation, the normally aerated lung is replaced by fluid or pus. This attenuates X-rays to an extent similar to that of the heart and diaphragms. The usually sharp border between the lung and these structures is thus lost if there is consolidation in the lobe abutting these soft tissues. Loss of this sharp border is referred to as loss of the silhouette sign.

   A) Right upper lobe – Incorrect. Right upper lobe pathology does not result in a silhouette sign. There may be an abrupt inferior border in right upper lobe consolidation due to the confines of the horizontal fissure.

   B) Right middle lobe – Incorrect. Pathology in the right middle lobe alone would obscure the heart border, but not the hemidiaphragm.

   C) Right lower lobe – Incorrect. Pathology in the right lower lobe alone would obscure the right hemidiaphragm, but not the right heart border.

   D) Right middle and lower lobes – Correct. Since both the right heart border and part of the hemidiaphragm are obscured, the consolidation must be in both the right middle (heart border) and lower (hemidiaphragm) lobes.

   E) Not able to say with certainty – Incorrect. The silhouette sign allows us to identify within which lobe the consolidation is located. Remember that there may still be pathology within a lobe without evidence of a silhouette sign if the pathology is not in contact with a border. In such cases, it is not possible to assess reliably where the pathology is, and it is useful to describe it as upper, middle or lower zone (rather than lobe). An example of this would be a lesion in the left midzone but not in contact with the left heart border. It may be in the upper lobe, lingula or the apical segment of the left lower lobe.

❶ KEY POINTS

1. The right middle lobe lies against the right heart border; the right lower lobe against the right hemidiaphragm; the lingula (part of the left upper lobe) abuts the left heart border; and the left lower lobe is in contact with the left hemidiaphragm.
2. If the silhouette sign is not present, then describe the pathology as affecting the upper, middle or lower zone/s of the lung.
3. The silhouette sign is not specific to consolidation – other intrathoracic pathology such as masses can also result in loss of a silhouette.

3. What is the commonest pathogen responsible for community-acquired pneumonia?
   The correct answer is **B) *Streptococcus pneumoniae***.
   Knowledge of the most likely pathogen causing pneumonia is useful to help guide empirical antibiotic treatment. Other factors, such as patient demographics, severity and local antibiotic resistance patterns, should also be taken into account.
   A) *S. aureus* – Incorrect. *S. aureus* is an uncommon cause of community-acquired pneumonia, accounting for less than 5% of cases. It often occurs in patients with other debilitating illness, is often preceded by an influenza infection and has a high mortality. It (including MRSA) is more commonly a cause of hospital-acquired pneumonia. Radiologically, it can cause multilobar bronchopneumonia, cavitation, abscesses and effusions/empyemas.
   B) *S. pneumoniae* – Correct. *S. pneumoniae* is the commonest cause of community-acquired pneumonia, accounting for 30% to 50% of cases. It is particularly common in middle-aged patients. It can cause lobar or bronchopneumonia on a chest X-ray. In children it can result in round pneumonia, which, as the name suggests, is mass-like consolidation.
   C) *H. influenzae* – Incorrect. *H. influenzae* occurs most commonly in children, patients with COPD and immunocompromised adults. It usually leads to a bronchopneumonia, particularly in the lower lobes.
   D) *L. pneumophila* – Incorrect. Legionella usually occurs in middle-aged and older patients. It is frequently spread from infected water sources (e.g. air conditioning units). Patients may be hyponatraemic and hypoalbuminaemic and have deranged liver function tests. Chest X-ray classically shows initial peripheral consolidation, which becomes dense lobar consolidation with bulging pleural fissures. It is associated with a 20% mortality rate.
   E) *M. pneumonia* – Incorrect. *M. pneumoniae* tends to affect children and young adults, accounting for about 10% of community-acquired pneumonia. It occurs in epidemics. Most are mild, but it can occasionally result in haemolytic anaemia, Guillain–Barré syndrome and Stevens–Johnson syndrome. It causes diffuse lower lobe reticular opacification or consolidation.

❶ KEY POINTS

1. The X-ray features of pneumonia often do not reliably distinguish among the different pathogens. Blood and sputum cultures are the best way to do this, supplemented with screening urine for legionella and pneumococcal antigen, but even then a pathogen is not always isolated.
2. Ideally, cultures (blood and sputum) should be taken prior to starting antibiotics. However, antibiotics should not be delayed to allow this. Even if cultures are taken, the initial antibiotic choice will have to be empirical and made without knowing the culture results, because these may take days. Knowledge of the most likely organism is thus important. Hospitals often produce guidelines for the most appropriate antibiotic for certain patient groups.
3. The causes, and therefore treatments, of community- and hospital-acquired pneumonia vary. This question relates to community-acquired pneumonia. Hospital-acquired pneumonia refers to pneumonia occurring at least 48 hours after admission to hospital. These patients are more likely to be infected with Gram-negative bacteria or *S. aureus*.

4. Which of the following is a scoring system for community-acquired pneumonia?
   The correct answer is **E) CURB-65 score**.
   Scoring systems can be useful to stratify patients based on clinical findings and results of investigations into groups with varying prognoses.
   A) Gleason score – Incorrect. The Gleason score is a pathology-based scoring system used for prostate cancer.
   B) Rockall score – Incorrect. The Rockall score is used to identify patients at risk of adverse outcome following acute nonvariceal upper gastrointestinal haemorrhage.
   C) Nottingham prognostic index – Incorrect. The Nottingham prognostic index helps determine prognosis following surgery for breast cancer.
   D) Modified Glasgow prognostic criteria – Incorrect. Glasgow prognostic criteria are used to help stratify patients with acute pancreatitis.
   E) CURB-65 score – Correct. CURB-65 is a validated prognostic scoring system which is used to assess severity and predict mortality in patients with community-acquired pneumonia. It comprises five different parameters:
   C = new-onset confusion (abbreviated mental test <8 or drop by 2 or more from baseline)
   U = urea >7 mmol/L
   R = respiratory rate ≥30 breaths per minute
   B = blood pressure (<90 mmHg systolic or <60 mmHg diastolic)
   65 = ≥65 years of age
   Each parameter is worth 1 point. The higher the score the more severe the community-acquired pneumonia and the higher the predicted 30-day mortality (a score of 0 = <1% risk of death, 5 = >55% risk of death). It can be used to identify those with severe community-acquired pneumonia who will need admission, closer monitoring and possibly critical care input.

Continue

CASE 2.11   *Contd.*

❗ KEY POINT

CURB-65 relates to community-acquired (not hospital-acquired) pneumonia. It is a simple scoring system which can predict prognosis. All patients with community-acquired pneumonia should have a CURB-65 score calculated. The score will guide antibiotic therapy, and whether high dependency care should be considered.

5. Which of the following is/are complications of pneumonia?
   The correct answers are **A) Pleural effusion, B) Empyema, C) Bronchiectasis, D) Pneumothorax and E) Deep vein thrombosis**.
   In 90% of patients, pneumonia resolves within 4 weeks. However, you should be aware that a variety of complications can occur. Other complications not listed in the question earlier include lung abscess, bronchopleural fistula, acute respiratory distress syndrome and ectopic abscess formation. Nonclearance of pneumonia may be due to antibiotic resistance, the wrong choice of antibiotics, an obstructing tumour causing postobstructive pneumonitis or recurrent infection.
   A) Pleural effusion – Correct. Parapneumonic effusions are relatively common. They are initially exudative and free flowing but can become fibropurulent with loculations. They usually resolve with treatment of the underlying pneumonia.
   B) Empyema – Correct. Empyema refers to pus in the pleural space, or a pleural effusion in which an organism can be identified. They are usually postinfective, but can be secondary to trauma or surgery. Their development progresses from an exudative collection (treated with antibiotics) to a fibropurulent phase (treated with percutaneous drainage) to become fibrinous (treated with surgery) finally. Contrast-enhanced CT helps diagnosis (pleural fluid collection with thickened, enhancing pleura which can contain gas). Ultrasound may show a complex pleural fluid collection with echogenic debris, gas and loculations.
   C) Bronchiectasis – Correct. Bronchiectasis is permanent dilatation of the bronchi. It can be caused by a variety of factors, best split into congenital (rare),

obstructive and postinfective (common). Recurrent infections are one of the commonest causes. Remember that bronchiectasis can also result in recurrent pneumonias. Also remember that bacterial and viral infections can cause reversible (rather than permanent) bronchial dilatation.
   D) Pneumothorax – Correct. Infections are a relatively rare cause of pneumothorax. Lung abscesses, necrotic pneumonias and lung infarcts due to septic emboli may cause a pneumothorax.
   E) Deep vein thrombosis – Correct. Pneumonias and other infections can increase the risk of venous thromboembolism. Therefore it is important to consider venous thromboembolism prophylaxis is these patients.

❗ KEY POINT

Most pneumonias respond to treatment; however, there is a range of complications which can occur. It is important to be familiar with the potential complications so that they can be recognised promptly and treated accordingly.

👥 IMPORTANT LEARNING POINTS

- The term 'consolidation' refers to any pathological process that fills the alveoli; it is not specific to infection (although this is the commonest cause).
- The silhouette sign can be useful for identifying the location of intrathoracic pathology.
- *S. pneumoniae* is the commonest cause of community-acquired pneumonia, whereas hospital-acquired pneumonias tend to be caused by Gram-negative bacilli or *S. aureus*. However, the chest X-ray findings are not a reliable way of identifying the underlying organism.
- CURB-65 is a clinical scoring system for assessing severity and predicting mortality in community-acquired pneumonia.
- Most patients respond well to treatment; however, there are a variety of complications associated with pneumonia, such as empyema, bronchiectasis, pneumothorax, deep vein thrombosis, lung collapse, atrial fibrillation and respiratory failure.

CASE 2.12

A 30-year-old woman, who is 1 week post caesarean section, presents with right-sided pleuritic chest pain and shortness of breath. She has a preceding history of right calf swelling and discomfort. As part of her investigation, you request a chest X-ray.

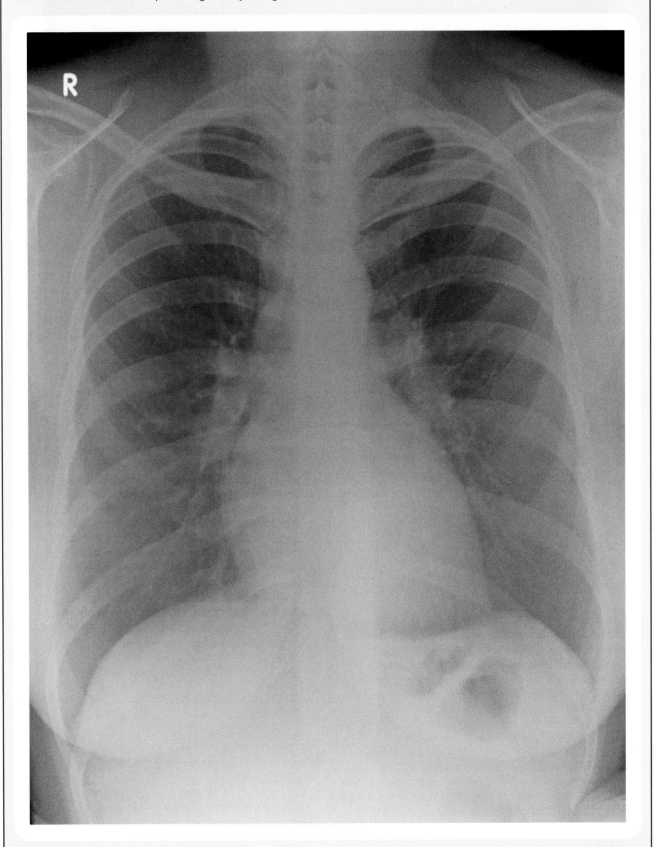

Continue

CASE 2.12   *Contd.*

ANNOTATED X-RAY

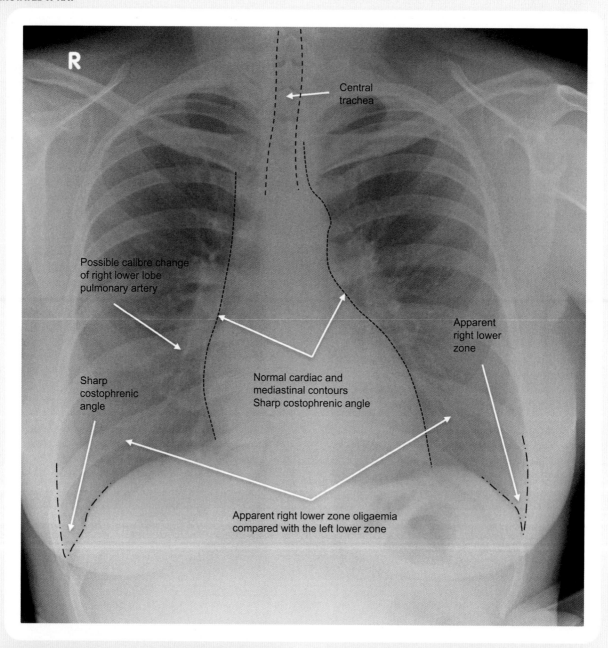

Central trachea

Possible calibre change of right lower lobe pulmonary artery

Apparent right lower zone

Sharp costophrenic angle

Normal cardiac and mediastinal contours
Sharp costophrenic angle

Apparent right lower zone oligaemia compared with the left lower zone

🔍 **PRESENT YOUR FINDINGS**

- This is a PA chest X-ray of an adult woman.
- It has been anonymised, and the date and time of the examination have been removed. I would like to confirm the patient's identify and examination details before proceeding.
- The patient is slightly rotated. Otherwise, the X-ray is technically adequate, with satisfactory inspiration and penetration.
- There is no striking abnormality on the X-ray.
- The trachea is central, the lungs and pleural spaces are clear and the hilar points are preserved. The heart is not enlarged, and the cardiac and mediastinal contours are clear.
- There is a possible subtle finding of an abrupt change in calibre of the right lower lobe pulmonary artery with

reduced perfusion peripherally (darkened lung fields representing reduced blood flow).
- There is no free subdiaphragmatic gas.
- No abnormality within the imaged soft tissues or bone is demonstrated.

IN SUMMARY – There is no striking abnormality on this chest X-ray. The subtle finding of change in calibre of the right lower lobe pulmonary artery may represent Westermark's sign, which can be seen in pulmonary embolic disease. Regardless, given the history, I am concerned that this patient has had a veno-thromboembolism and requires urgent investigation to confirm or refute this. There is no radiographic evidence of pulmonary infarction at present.

QUESTIONS

1. Which of the following is/are recognised risk factors for pulmonary embolism (PE)?
   A) Malignancy
   B) Major abdominal surgery
   C) Lower limb fracture
   D) Factor VIII deficiency
   E) HRT

2. Which of the following statements is/are correct regarding the initial investigation of a patient with a suspected PE?
   A) A negative D-Dimer excludes a PE
   B) CRP confirms infection, rather than PE, as the cause of the symptoms
   C) If a chest X-ray demonstrates a pleural effusion, then no further investigations are required, as a cause for the patient's symptoms has been demonstrated
   D) S1 Q3 T3 is the most common ECG finding in patients with PE
   E) The chest X-ray may demonstrate consolidation

3. Which of the following statements is/are correct regarding the radiological investigation of pregnant patients with suspected PE?
   A) If a lower limb Doppler ultrasound confirms the presence of a DVT, then no further investigation is required
   B) A CTPA exposes the foetus to the highest radiation dose

   C) A V/Q scan (ventilation/perfusion nuclear scan) is contraindicated because the nuclear medicine pharmaceuticals are potentially teratogenic
   D) A chest X-ray should not be performed because it cannot diagnose a PE and simply represents additional exposure to radiation
   E) Performing an echocardiogram has no role in the investigation of suspected PE

4. Which of the following statements is/are correct regarding the potential treatment of patients with confirmed PE?
   A) Thrombolysis may be required
   B) Patients on low-molecular-weight heparin should have a regular full blood count
   C) Direct-acting oral anticoagulants are routinely used for long-term anticoagulation
   D) All patients with a proximal DVT of the lower limb should have an IVC filter
   E) Warfarin is initially prothrombotic

5. Which of the following is/are recognised potential complications of DVT or PE?
   A) Pulmonary artery hypertension
   B) Right ventricular dysfunction
   C) Ischaemic stroke
   D) Pulmonary AV fistula formation
   E) Chronic calf pain and swelling

Continue

CASE **2.12**   *Contd.*

ANSWERS TO QUESTIONS

1. Which of the following is/are recognised risk factors for PE? The correct answers are **A) Malignancy, B) Major abdominal surgery, C) Lower limb fracture and E) HRT**.

There are multiple risk factors for veno-thromboembolic disease. The majority of risk factors are acquired. However, there are some genetic conditions which confer a procoagulant state; these include Factor V Leiden deficiency, Protein C deficiency and Protein S deficiency. Factor VIII deficiency is otherwise known as haemophilia A and is a bleeding diathesis.

A) Malignancy – Correct. Malignancy is a risk factor. If a patient does not have a known malignancy and develops an unprovoked pulmonary embolism, further assessment should be considered. This may include physical examination, chest X-ray, blood tests, urinalysis, CT and, in women, mammography.

B) Major abdominal surgery – Correct. Major abdominal surgery is a risk factor. Prophylactic anticoagulants are often given to such patients, especially if there has been prolonged abdominopelvic surgery for malignancy. The benefits of potentially preventing a life-threatening PE usually outweigh the risks of increased bleeding risk in the postoperative period, but this should be an individual judgement.

C) Lower limb fracture – Correct. Lower limb fracture is a risk factor, as such patients are particularly prone to developing DVT. They may require surgical fixation or a period of immobility in a cast. Remember that patients who fracture long bones such as their femur are also at risk of fat embolism from bone marrow.

D) Factor VIII deficiency – Incorrect. Factor VIII deficiency is haemophilia A and confers an increased bleeding risk to the patient.

E) HRT – Correct. The oestrogenic effects of hormone replacement therapy for treatment of perimenopausal symptoms increase the risk of veno-thromboembolism.

❶ KEY POINT

All patients admitted to hospital should be assessed for their individual risk of developing a DVT or PE, and appropriate prophylactic measures should be taken accordingly. Prophylactic measures can range from encouraging activity to compression stocking through to prophylactic low-molecular-weight heparin administration. Each hospital will have its own guidelines. Familiarise yourself with your institution's protocols.

2. Which of the following statements is correct regarding the initial investigation of a patient with a suspected PE? The correct answer is **E) The chest X-ray may demonstrate consolidation**.

The exclusion of a PE is a common clinical question faced by medical and surgical teams, and a clear understanding of the pathophysiology behind the condition helps clarify the investigative rationale. The Wells score is a widely used tool to assess the likelihood of a patient having a PE. The parameters of the Well's score are based on risk factors for PE. If the Wells score is more than 4, this indicates a PE is likely and a CTPA should be arranged immediately. If the Wells score is 4 or less, then a PE may be less likely and a D-Dimer test may aid decision making.

A) A negative D-Dimer excludes a PE – Incorrect. D-Dimer levels are often requested in patients with suspected PE. It is a measure of thrombus breakdown products and is a useful test, but only in particular circumstances. D-Dimer levels are raised in a variety of conditions and are not specific to PE. A negative D-Dimer only implies that a PE is unlikely in patients with low pretest probability, i.e. they have an unremarkable history and physical examination. In these patients, an alternative diagnosis should be considered. However, in all other patients, further investigations are still warranted, depending on the clinical level of suspicion. Consequently, a D-Dimer should only be requested in patients in whom PE is low on the differential diagnosis list which can be indicated by a low Wells score. Blindly performing D-Dimer levels on all patients with chest pain is not useful and a waste of resources.

B) A raised CRP confirms infection, rather than PE, as the cause of the symptoms – Incorrect. CRP is a sensitive marker of inflammation. It is often incorrectly thought to be synonymous with infection, but noninfectious inflammatory conditions can cause CRP levels to rise. A PE with resultant pulmonary infarction will result in an elevated CRP.

C) If a chest X-ray demonstrates a pleural effusion, then no further investigations are required as a cause for the patient's symptoms has been demonstrated – Incorrect. Although a pleural effusion can be the cause of pleuritic chest pain, only rarely can the underlying cause of the effusion be confirmed on chest X-ray. Pleural effusions can complicate PEs, especially if there is associated pulmonary infarction. Consequently, if the chest X-ray demonstrates a pleural effusion in a patient with a convincing clinical presentation for a PE, further investigations are warranted to exclude an underlying PE.

D) S1 Q3 T3 is the most common ECG finding in patients with PE – Incorrect. S1 Q3 T3 is commonly described in medical textbooks as the characteristic ECG finding in PE. However, it is not very common in clinical practice. ECG evidence of right heart strain (e.g. right axis deviation +/– T wave inversion in the anterior leads) is also recognised. The most common ECG finding in patients with PE, however, is a sinus tachycardia.

E) The chest X-ray may demonstrate consolidation – Correct. Consolidation may represent an area of pulmonary infarction, in the correct clinical context. The characteristic appearance of infarct is a wedge-shaped opacity in the periphery of the lung abutting the pleural surface. This is referred to as Hampton hump.

KEY POINT

You should be familiar with the common findings of routinely requested investigations in patients with suspected PE. The chest X-ray is primarily used to exclude other causes of breathlessness and chest pain, such as a pneumothorax. The chest X-ray is typically normal in patients with a PE. However, a unilateral pleural effusion may be present. Hampton hump (peripheral consolidation) and Westermark's sign (change in calibre of a pulmonary artery with peripheral hypovolaemia are rarely seen. D-Dimers only have a role in the low pretest probability subgroup of patients with suspected PE.

3. Which of the following statements is/are correct regarding the radiological investigation of pregnant patients with suspected PE?
   The correct answer is **A) If a lower limb Doppler ultrasound confirms the presence of a DVT, then no further investigation is required**.
   The most commonly performed investigation nowadays in patients with suspected pulmonary embolism is the CTPA. This is not without risks, as it exposes the patient to ionising radiation and intravenous (IV) contrast medium, which can cause contrast-induced nephropathy in patients with renal impairment. Pregnancy is a procoagulant state. Clinicians are not infrequently presented with a pregnant patient with a suspected PE. A clear imaging rationale is required in such cases.
   A) If a lower limb Doppler ultrasound confirms the presence of a DVT then no further investigation is required – Correct. In pregnancy, avoiding ionising radiation is the desired end point. Consequently, if Doppler ultrasound demonstrates an above knee DVT then there is no clear benefit in performing any further investigation, provided the patient is stable, because the treatment for a DVT is the same as for a PE.
   B) A CTPA exposes the foetus to the highest radiation dose – Incorrect. A CTPA does involve ionising radiation. However, the scan field can be limited to the proximal pulmonary arteries and CT scanner settings can be adjusted to minimise the dose. The foetus within the pelvis actually receives relatively little radiation from a CTPA. The main concern is exposure of the patient's mammary tissue, which is exquisitely radiosensitive in pregnancy and postpartum to radiation, leading to an increased risk of subsequent breast cancer. A V/Q scan is thus preferred. A V/Q scan, however, actually exposures the foetus to a greater dose of radiation than CTPA, because the radioactive tracer is excreted via the renal tract and the foetus is thus at risk as the trace accumulates in the bladder.
   C) A V/Q scan (ventilation/perfusion nuclear scan) is contraindicated because the nuclear medicine pharmaceuticals are potentially teratogenic – Incorrect. A V/Q scan involves injecting a radionuclide and inhaling a different radionuclide. The lung should be both ventilated and perfused. If there is an area of the lung with lack of perfusion but maintained ventilation, then PE should be suspected. The nuclear medicine pharmaceuticals used in V/Q scans are not known to be teratogenic. The dose from this investigation can

be minimised in pregnancy by using half the normal dose of the perfusion radiopharmaceutical. In addition to pregnancy, V/Q scans may be a preferred modality to CTPA for diagnosing PE in patients with renal insufficiency or contrast allergy.
   D) A chest X-ray should not be performed because it cannot diagnose a PE and simply represents additional exposure to radiation – Incorrect. A chest X-ray is important to perform, even though it cannot diagnose PE. Firstly, it may demonstrate a completely different cause for the suspected symptoms, e.g. pneumothorax. Secondly, if the chest X-ray is normal, then a V/Q scan can be performed. If the chest X-ray is abnormal, a V/Q will be difficult to interpret, and a low-dose CTPA may be advised instead.
   E) Performing an echocardiogram has no role in the investigation of suspected PE – Incorrect. An echocardiogram can be performed at the bedside and can confirm or refute the presence of acute right heart strain, which may be present in patients with massive PE and haemodynamic compromise.

KEY POINTS

1. When investigating pregnant patients with suspected pulmonary embolism, a potential protocol would involve bilateral lower limb Doppler. If the Doppler shows a DVT, treat the DVT (which will also treat any potential PE).
2. If the Doppler is normal, perform a chest X-ray.
3. If the chest X-ray is normal, consider a low-dose V/Q study. If the chest X-ray is abnormal, and a PE is still suspected, consider a low-dose CTPA.

4. Which of the following statements is/are correct regarding the potential treatment of patients with confirmed PE?
   The correct answers are **A) Thrombolysis may be required, B) Patients on low-molecular-weight heparin should have a regular full blood count, C) Direct-acting oral anticoagulants are routinely used for long-term anticoagulation and E) Warfarin is initially prothrombotic**.
   The mainstay of treatment for patients with confirmed PE is anticoagulation. Treatment should be tailored to the individual, depending on the aetiology of the PE and potential contraindications.
   A) Thrombolysis may be required – Correct. Massive PE can result in haemodynamic instability, and is a recognised cause of a PEA cardiac arrest. In these circumstances, thrombolysis should be considered. There is a significant bleeding risk with thrombolysis hence it should only be used when the benefits outweigh the risks. An embolectomy to mechanically retrieve the embolus may also be considered in patients with a massive PE and where interventional radiology facilities are available.
   B) Patients on low-molecular-weight heparin should have a regular full blood count – Correct. Low molecular-weight heparin (LMWH) is commonly used as PE prophylaxis and whilst patients are being established on warfarin. A rare but important complication of heparin is the development of

Continue

CASE **2.12** *Contd.*

heparin-induced thrombocytopaenia (HIP), which should be monitored with regular full blood counts. Other heparin-based anticoagulation options such as unfractionated heparin may also be used depending on local hospital guidelines.

C) Direct-acting oral anticoagulants are routinely used for long-term anticoagulation – Correct. Direct-acting oral anticoagulants (DOACs) have become the preferred long-term anticoagulation option for patients presenting with PE. Commonly used DOACs include apixaban and rivaroxaban. Unlike warfarin, these drugs do not require regular monitoring of coagulation parameters or require initial treatment with LMWH. Other advantages of these drugs over warfarin include fixed dosing, fewer drug-drug interactions and a lower risk of intracranial bleeding. The duration of anticoagulation for PE varies depending on whether the PE was provoked or unprovoked, the location of the PE, bleeding risk and whether the underlying risk factor has been removed. Patients who have had a provoked PE and have only transient risk factors (e.g. recent surgery) only need three months of anticoagulation usually. Patients with an unprovoked PE, those with more durable risk factors for PE (e.g. active cancer, thrombophilia), and those with recurrent PE should be considered for anticoagulation beyond 3 months. For this reason, and because Warfarin takes a few days to reach stable therapeutic levels, patients should be covered with heparin whilst commencing warfarin.

D) All patients with a proximal DVT of the lower limb should have an IVC filter – Incorrect. Patients with proximal DVT of the lower limb are at risk of PE, but should simply receive anticoagulation. IVC filter placement is largely reserved for patients who cannot be safely anticoagulated – a common scenario for indication of an IVC filter is a patient with proximal DVT awaiting pelvic surgery for gynaecological malignancy, or patients who have had recurrent PEs despite therapeutic anticoagulation.

E) Warfarin is initially prothrombotic – Correct. Warfarin is prothrombotic in the first few days of treatment. For this reason, and because Warfarin takes a few days to reach stable therapeutic levels, patients should be covered with heparin whilst commencing warfarin.

❶ KEY POINT

The mainstay of treatment of PE is subcutaneous anticoagulation. The choice of anticoagulation includes low-molecular weight heparin whilst the patient is established on (LMWH), direct oral-acting anticoagulants (DOAC), unfractionated heparin (UFH) and warfarin. If there is clinical suspicion of PE, and there are no contraindications, empirically commencing therapeutic dose low-molecular weight heparin is often performed whilst definitive diagnosis with CTPA is awaited. DOACs have become the mainstay choice for long-term anticoagulation.

5. Which of the following is/are recognised potential complications of DVT or PE?

The correct answers are **A) Pulmonary artery hypertension, B) Right ventricular dysfunction, C) Ischaemic stroke and E) Chronic calf pain and swelling**.

The most serious acute complication of a PE is death. If patients survive the acute episode, there are potential chronic complications that need to be considered.

A) Pulmonary artery hypertension – Correct. PEs may fail to lyse, and may instead organise within the pulmonary arteries as pulmonary webs and chronic thrombi. This can lead to pulmonary artery hypertension.

B) Right ventricular dysfunction – Correct. Right ventricular dysfunction can occur acutely in massive pulmonary emboli, but also in cases of recurrent or chronic PEs.

C) Ischaemic stroke – Correct. This is a difficult question. Patients with a patent foramen ovale (PFO) between the atria are at risk of right to left shunting of venous thrombi. These can then enter the arterial circulation and result in an ischaemic stroke (the so-called paradoxical embolus). A bubble echocardiogram is the investigation of choice to exclude a PFO.

D) Pulmonary arteriovenous (AV) fistula formation – Incorrect. Pulmonary AV fistula formation is not a recognised complication of acute or chronic PEs.

E) Chronic calf pain and swelling – Correct. Patients with DVTs can develop a postthrombotic syndrome consisting of chronic calf pain, swelling, rash and sometimes ulceration.

❶ KEY POINT

The mainstay of treatment of PE is subcutaneous low-molecular-weight heparin whilst the patient is established on warfarin. If there is clinical suspicion of PE, and there are no contraindications, commencing therapeutic dose low-molecular-weight heparin is often performed whilst definitive diagnosis with CTPA is awaited.

IMPORTANT LEARNING POINTS

- In suspected PE, the chest X-ray is mainly used to exclude other differential diagnoses and is most commonly normal in patients with PE.
- The most common ECG finding is a sinus tachycardia.
- D-Dimer levels are only useful in patients with low pre-test probability of PE.
- CTPA is the mainstay of investigation for patients with suspected PE nowadays.
- Pregnant women are at risk of PE and require extra consideration in their diagnostic pathways.
- Treat patients with suspected PE promptly to reduce mortality and be mindful of the potential complications during follow-up.

CASE 2.13

A 70-year-old man presents with chest pain, shortness of breath and cough productive of pink, frothy sputum. He has a past medical history significant for hypertension and diabetes, and he is a lifelong smoker. You request a chest X-ray as part of his assessment.

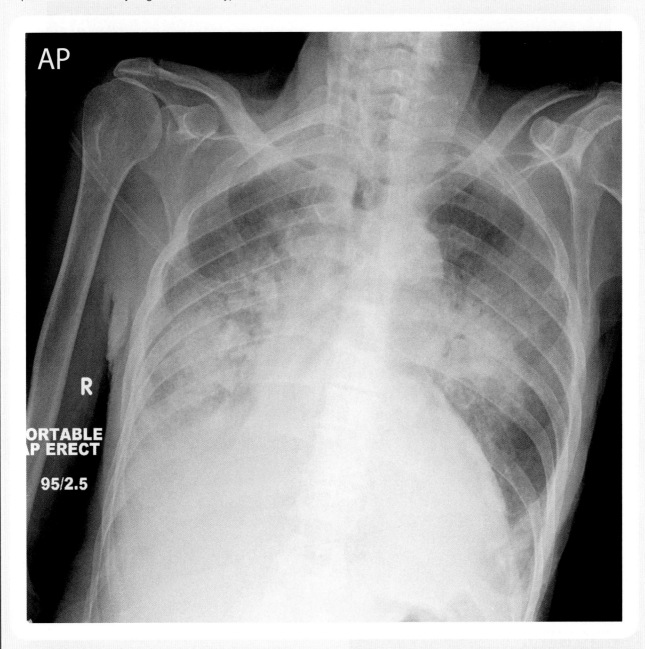

Continue

CASE **2.13**   *Contd.*

ANNOTATED X-RAY

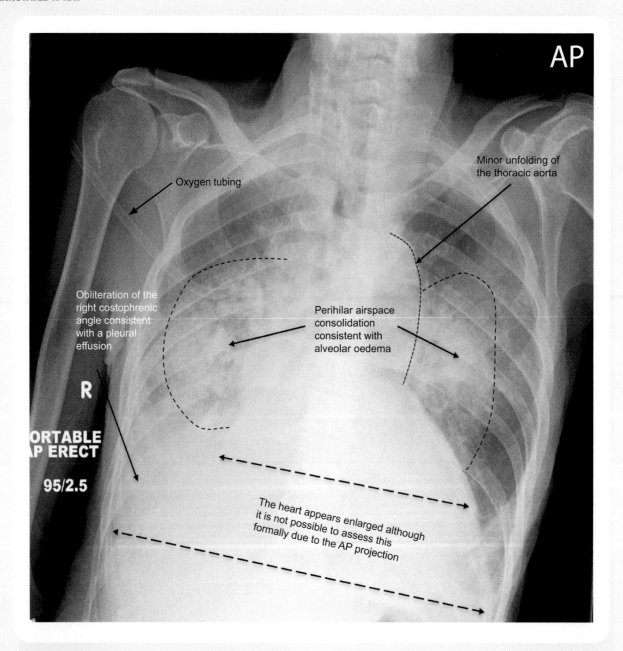

AP

Minor unfolding of
the thoracic aorta

Oxygen tubing

Obliteration of the
right costophrenic
angle consistent
with a pleural
effusion

Perihilar airspace
consolidation
consistent with
alveolar oedema

R

ORTABLE
P ERECT

95/2.5

The heart appears enlarged although
it is not possible to assess this
formally due to the AP projection

🔍 **PRESENT YOUR FINDINGS**

- This is an AP chest X-ray of an adult.
- It has been anonymised, and the date and time of the examination have been removed. I would like to confirm these details before proceeding.
- Penetration is adequate. The patient is rotated, and there is a suboptimal inspiratory achievement. The left costophrenic angle has not been fully imaged. Therefore this is a technically inadequate chest X-ray.
- The most striking abnormality is the bilateral, patchy, perihilar airspace opacification.
- Even allowing for the AP projection and associated magnification, the heart appears enlarged; however, I would like to confirm this on a PA X-ray.

- There is a moderate size right pleural effusion. The left costophrenic angle has not been imaged so a left-sided effusion cannot be excluded.
- There is unfolding of the thoracic aorta.
- No other significant abnormality is demonstrated.
- Review of the imaged skeleton and soft tissues is unremarkable.

IN SUMMARY – This chest X-ray demonstrates perihilar 'bat's wing' consolidation in keeping with alveolar oedema. This, in combination with the cardiomegaly and pleural effusions, suggests that congestive cardiac failure is the likely aetiology. Given the patient's chest pain, I would arrange an urgent ECG and cardiac markers to exclude an acute coronary syndrome.

QUESTIONS

1. Which of the following is/are clinical features of congestive cardiac failure?
   A) Elevated jugular venous pressure
   B) Bibasal crepitations on auscultation of the chest
   C) Orthopnoea
   D) Pulsatile hepatomegaly
   E) Pulsus paradoxus

2. Regarding the features of congestive cardiac failure on a chest X-ray, which of the following statements is/are correct?
   A) Thin horizontal lines in the periphery of the lungs, particularly in the lung bases, which extend to the pleural surface are suggestive of Kerley A lines
   B) Cardiothoracic ratio >50% on PA chest X-ray is consistent with cardiomegaly
   C) Cardiomegaly cannot be diagnosed on an AP chest X-ray
   D) Bilateral pleural effusions may be seen
   E) Prominence of the upper lobe pulmonary veins is a feature of elevated venous pressure

3. Which of the following is/are recognised causes of pulmonary oedema?
   A) Pulmonary artery hypertension secondary to pulmonary embolism
   B) Bilateral renal artery stenosis
   C) Significant central nervous system insult
   D) Anuric renal failure
   E) Acute mitral regurgitation

4. Which of the following is/are routinely performed in the assessment of congestive cardiac failure?
   A) ECG
   B) Chest X-ray
   C) Troponin
   D) Echocardiogram
   E) Brain natriuretic peptide

5. Which of the following is/are a potential symptomatic treatment in a patient with severe cardiogenic pulmonary oedema?
   A) Beta-blocker
   B) Diuretics
   C) CPAP
   D) GTN infusion
   E) Intraaortic balloon pump

Continue

CASE 2.13 *Contd.*

ANSWERS TO QUESTIONS

1. Which of the following is/are clinical feature of congestive cardiac failure?

The correct answers are **A) Elevated jugular venous pressure, B) Bibasal crepitations on auscultation of the chest, C) Orthopnoea and D) Pulsatile hepatomegaly**.

A) Elevated jugular venous pressure – Correct. Since the internal jugular vein drains directly into the right atrium and contains no valves, it can be used to gauge right atrial pressure. The jugular venous pressure is elevated in congestive cardiac failure.

B) Bibasal crepitations on auscultation of the chest – Correct. Bibasal crepitations that do not clear upon coughing may represent pulmonary oedema. There may also be clinical evidence of pleural effusions (stony dull percussion note and absent breath sounds).

C) Orthopnoea – Correct. Patients with congestive cardiac failure often develop marked shortness of breath when lying flat. In chronic cases of heart failure, patients may admit to requiring multiple pillows to sleep at night, or even to resorting to sleeping upright in a chair. Paroxysmal nocturnal dyspnoea occurs when a patient is awoken from sleep with shortness of breath and can occur in heart failure.

D) Pulsatile hepatomegaly – Correct. In patients with severe congestive cardiac failure, tricuspid valve incompetence can occur. This can be manifest as pulsatile hepatomegaly. There may be associated ascites and peripheral oedema.

E) Pulsus paradoxus – Incorrect. Pulsus paradoxus refers to a fall in systolic blood pressure >10 mmHg on inspiration. It is a sign of pericardial disease, such as pericardial tamponade and constrictive pericarditis. It is not a feature of congestive cardiac failure.

❗ KEY POINT

Heart failure is a common condition which should be recognised early so that prompt symptomatic and prognostic treatment can be instigated. The New York Health Association classifies the severity of heart failure based on patient symptoms:

I   Cardiac disease but no symptoms or limitation in normal physical activity

II   Mild symptoms and slight limitation during normal activity

III Marked limitation in activity due to symptoms, even during less-than-normal activity and comfortable only at rest

IV Severe limitations with symptoms at rest

2. Regarding the features of congestive cardiac failure on a chest X-ray, which of the following statements is/are correct?

The correct answers are **B) Cardiothoracic ratio >50% on PA chest X-ray is consistent with cardiomegaly, D) Bilateral pleural effusions may be seen and E) Prominence of the upper lobe pulmonary veins is a feature of elevated venous pressure**.

There are a variety of clues on the chest X-ray that can help with diagnosis. Look for evidence of midline sternotomy wires, coronary artery by-pass graft clips, metallic cardiac valve prostheses and pacemakers. All of these suggest significant cardiac past medical history which, in turn, impacts on how you interpret the current X-ray.

A) Thin horizontal lines in the periphery of the lungs, particularly in the lung bases, which extend to the pleural surface are suggestive of Kerley A lines – Incorrect. This description refers to Kerley B lines, which represent interlobular septal thickening due to interstitial oedema, and are seen in congestive cardiac failure. They are typically <1 cm long. Beware of mentioning the eponymous name in an examination scenario, as some examiners may ask you to tell them about Kerley A lines (longer lines coursing from the hila out to the lung periphery) and Kerley C lines (short, fine lines throughout the lungs with a reticular appearance) too! It is often safer simply to state that there is evidence of interstitial or interlobular septal thickening.

B) Cardiothoracic ratio >50% on PA chest X-ray is consistent with cardiomegaly – Correct. This is the definition of cardiomegaly in an adult on PA chest X-ray.

C) Cardiomegaly cannot be diagnosed on an AP chest X-ray – Incorrect. AP projected chest X-rays are subject to magnification of the mediastinum. However, this does not mean that no assessment of the cardiac silhouette can be made at all. For example, if the cardiothoracic ratio is normal on a magnified AP X-ray, it will also definitely be normal on a PA X-ray. In this scenario, cardiomegaly is excluded. Likewise, if the cardiac silhouette is grossly enlarged, with the left heart border approximating the left lateral chest wall, that the heart is likely to be enlarged (even on an AP chest X-ray).

D) Bilateral pleural effusions may be seen – Correct. Bilateral pleural effusions are a feature of congestive cardiac failure which is often discernible on chest X-ray.

E) Prominence of the upper lobe pulmonary veins is a feature of elevated venous pressure – Correct. Prominence of the upper lobe pulmonary veins is a feature of elevated pulmonary venous and left atrial pressure. This is most commonly seen with left-sided heart failure and mitral valve disease.

❗ KEY POINTS

1. There are different grades of cardiogenic pulmonary oedema which increase in severity:
   - Grade 1 = Vascular redistribution (upper lobe venous diversion, i.e. increased size of the upper lobe pulmonary blood vessels relative to the lower lobes)
   - Grade 2 = Interstitial oedema (Kerley lines, perivascular oedema and pleural effusions)
   - Grade 3 = Alveolar oedema (airspace opacification)

2. When pulmonary oedema is present, look for evidence of previous cardiac intervention, cardiomegaly, pleural effusions and upper lobe pulmonary diversion to support the notion that the aetiology is cardiac. Some, albeit limited, assessment of the cardiac silhouette is possible on the AP projected chest X-ray.

3. Which of the following is/are recognised causes of pulmonary oedema?

The correct answers are **B) Bilateral renal artery stenosis, C) Significant central nervous system insult, D) Anuric renal failure and E) Acute mitral regurgitation**.

It is important to realise that there are several other causes of pulmonary oedema in addition to congestive cardiac failure.

A) Pulmonary artery hypertension secondary to pulmonary embolism – Incorrect. Acute right heart strain can result from acute pulmonary embolism. Chronic pulmonary emboli can result in pulmonary artery hypertension. Neither of these conditions, however, will result in pulmonary oedema.

B) Bilateral renal artery stenosis – Correct. Pulmonary oedema is a recognised complication of bilateral renal artery stenosis.

C) Significant central nervous system insult – Correct. A significant central nervous system insult can result in neurogenic pulmonary oedema.

D) Anuric renal failure – Correct. The inability to excrete urine in anuric renal failure puts the patient at increased risk of developing pulmonary oedema, which will not respond to conventional pulmonary oedema treatment and often requires haemofiltration or haemodialysis.

E) Acute mitral regurgitation – Correct. Whilst left ventricular dysfunction is the most common cause of cardiogenic pulmonary oedema, acute mitral regurgitation can result from infarction of the site of papillary muscle insertion, and this is a recognised cause of pulmonary oedema.

❗ KEY POINTS

1. Pulmonary oedema can be caused by a variety of different conditions.
   - Cardiogenic – Left ventricular failure and mitral regurgitation. There are various congenital heart conditions, such as hypoplastic left heart syndrome, that can cause cardiogenic pulmonary oedema in neonates.
   - Renal – Renal failure or volume overload.
   - Lung injury – Neurogenic shock, septic shock, fat embolism, aspiration, drowning, inhalation of noxious gases.
2. Often the clinical situation will point to the underlying aetiology. It is important to make this distinction, as conventional heart failure treatment may not be appropriate or successful in these patients. As a guide, remember that in noncardiac cases of pulmonary oedema, cardiomegaly is not usually present; however, this is not an absolute distinction between cardiac and noncardiac causes, as pulmonary oedema from acute cardiac failure may also involve a normal-sized heart.

4. Which of the following is/are routinely performed in the assessment of congestive cardiac failure?

The correct answers are **A) ECG, B) Chest X-ray and D) Echocardiogram**.

The investigation of congestive cardiac failure revolves around confirming the diagnosis and then determining whether there is a treatable underlying aetiology, such as coronary artery disease.

A) ECG – Correct. An ECG should be performed in all patients who present with suspected congestive cardiac failure. This may demonstrate evidence of ischaemia (ST changes) or previous infarction (Q waves). A potentially important cardiac arrhythmia may be demonstrated. Consider the use of continuous ECG monitoring.

B) Chest X-ray – Correct. A chest X-ray is a readily available investigation and can help confirm the diagnosis and assess for the degree of pulmonary oedema. Although the best diagnostic quality X-rays result from radiology departmental PA X-rays, patients in cardiac failure can be very unwell and potentially unstable; in these cases, a portable chest X-ray can often answer the pertinent clinical questions.

C) Troponin – Incorrect. Heart failure itself is a recognised cause of a troponin rise. In this scenario (with chest pain) a baseline admission troponin can be useful to help interpret the delayed level. Significant elevation in the later sample supports the diagnosis of acute coronary syndrome. In general, however, heart failure in and of itself is not an indication for performing a troponin. Take the example of a young patient with known aortic stenosis who has no cardiac risk factors and develops pulmonary oedema with no chest pain. This is unlikely to be an acute coronary syndrome, and therefore doing a troponin (which might be mildly elevated due to heart failure) can be misleading.

D) Echocardiogram – Correct. An echocardiogram is a useful investigation which can be performed at the bedside. Impaired left ventricular function and evidence of regional wall motion abnormalities are important pieces of clinical information. This will diagnose left ventricular failure and give an assessment of the severity.

E) Brain natriuretic peptide – Correct. Brain natriuretic peptide (BNP) is a protein released by cardiac myocytes in response to excessive stretching or being overworked. A raised BNP is used to establish the diagnosis of heart failure. Conditions other than heart failure which may raise BNP levels include diabetes, sepsis, hypoxaemia, kidney disease and liver cirrhosis. It has a high negative predictive value hence a negative test should warrant investigation into others causes of a patient's symptoms.

Continue

CASE **2.13**   *Contd.*

❗ KEY POINT

Patients in severe congestive cardiac failure are very unwell. Appropriate treatment should be instigated whilst investigations are being arranged. Early senior review should occur. Consider transferring the patient to the coronary care unit for monitoring and treatment. A portable (rather than departmental) chest X-ray may be required.

5. Which of the following is/are a potential symptomatic treatment in a patient with severe cardiogenic pulmonary oedema?

There is extensive evidence behind the treatment of heart failure. Several of the treatments have prognostic benefit, but not necessarily symptomatic benefit.

The correct answer is **B) Diuretics, C) Continuous positive airways pressure ventilation, D) Glyceryl trinitrate infusion and E) Intraaortic balloon pump**.

A) Beta-blocker – Incorrect. Beta-blockers are contraindicated in patients with unstable cardiac failure. However, there is a role for beta-blockers in cardiac failure patients as it has been shown to improve prognosis. Small doses of cardioselective beta-blockers may be introduced once the patient is stable and the medication carefully titrated to optimal dose.

B) Diuretics – Correct. Diuretics promote negative fluid balance and reduce cardiac preload. The intravenous route is preferred in the acute situation to facilitate the effect. Continuous diuretic infusions can be beneficial.

C) Continuous positive airways pressure ventilation – Correct. CPAP is a proven treatment in cases of acute pulmonary oedema that fail to respond to conventional pharmacological therapies.

D) Glyceryl trinitrate infusion – Correct. GTN can be administered sublingually in the first instance before a GTN infusion is set up. It helps reduce cardiac afterload. GTN is contraindicated in patients with fixed cardiac output, e.g. severe aortic stenosis. The patient's blood pressure should be carefully monitored in case hypotension develops.

E) Intraaortic balloon pump – Correct. An intraaortic balloon pump is an invasive treatment of cardiogenic shock. The balloon is placed in the descending thoracic aorta, usually via access through the femoral artery at the groin. It inflates during diastole to maximise coronary artery perfusion pressure, and deflates in systole, so that the distal arterial blood supply is not compromised. Deflating the balloon also creates a vacuum effect due to the empty space created. This reduces the afterload and increases cardiac output.

❗ KEY POINT

In addition to the pharmacological management of congestive cardiac failure, there are several key nursing interventions, such as ensuring that the patient sticks to an appropriate fluid restriction, that fluid balance and patient weight are accurately documented to determine the efficacy of the treatment, and implementing salt restriction. In addition, regular monitoring of the patient's renal profile and electrolytes is important, as the diuretic treatment can have deleterious effects, such as hypokalaemia, which can cause arrhythmias.

👥 IMPORTANT LEARNING POINTS

- A useful mnemonic for the chest X-ray features of congestive cardiac failure is ABCDEF. A: Alveolar and interstitial shadowing; B: Kerley B lines (little white horizontal lines usually in the lateral lower edges of the lung); C: Cardiomegaly; D: Upper lobe venous blood Diversion; E: Effusions; and F: Fluid in the horizontal fissure.
- Look for evidence to support a cardiac cause, e.g. midline sternotomy wires, CABG clips, pacemaker, etc.
- Symptomatic treatment should be instigated promptly in patients with severe congestive cardiac failure and should continue alongside subsequent investigations.

CASE 2.14

A 40-year-old female presents with severe, acute abdominal pain. On examination, she is pyrexial, tachycardic and peritonitic. An erect chest X-ray is performed as part of her assessment.

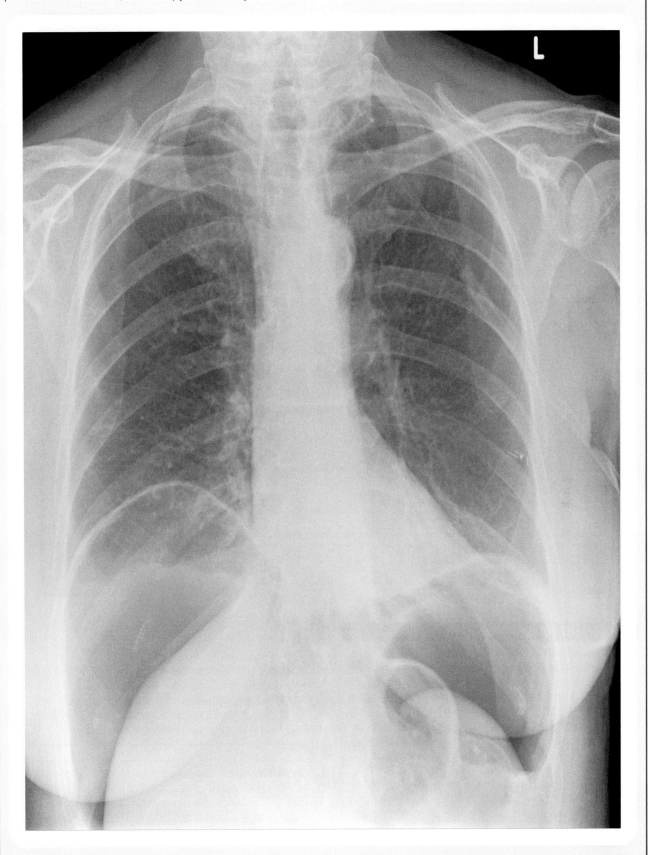

Continue

CASE **2.14**   *Contd.*

ANNOTATED X-RAY

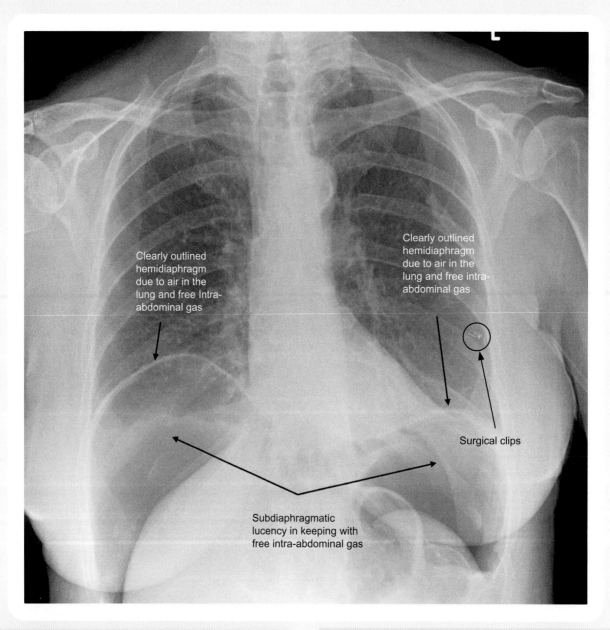

Clearly outlined hemidiaphragm due to air in the lung and free Intra-abdominal gas

Clearly outlined hemidiaphragm due to air in the lung and free intra-abdominal gas

Surgical clips

Subdiaphragmatic lucency in keeping with free intra-abdominal gas

🔍 PRESENT YOUR FINDINGS

- This is a PA chest X-ray of an adult.
- There are no identifiable patient data on the X-ray. I would like to confirm the patient's name and date of birth, and the date and time when the X-ray was taken, before making any further assessment.
- The patient is slightly rotated, and the right costo-phrenic angle has not been fully included. Otherwise, it is a technically adequate X-ray (there is adequate penetration and inspiration).
- The most striking abnormality is the marked radiolu-cency below the diaphragm. Both hemidiaphragms are clearly demarcated. These findings are consistent with a large pneumoperitoneum.
- The trachea is central.

- The heart size and the cardiac and mediastinal contours are normal.
- The lungs are clear.
- No pleural effusions are visible, although none of the right costophrenic angle has been imaged.
- Bones and visualised soft tissues are normal.
- There are surgical clips projected over the left lower zone, in keeping with previous breast surgery.

IN SUMMARY – The appearance of this erect chest X-ray is consistent with a large volume of free subdiaphragmatic gas. Given the clinical presentation, I suspect the underlying cause is a perforated viscus, and an urgent surgical review is required.

QUESTIONS

1. Regarding pneumoperitoneum, which of the following statements is/are true?
   A) Free air will not be identifiable in up to 20% to 30% of cases on erect chest X-ray
   B) This can represent a surgical emergency, and the general surgeons must be contacted immediately because there may be a perforated viscus
   C) As little as 1 mL of free intraperitoneal gas can be identified on a left lateral decubitus abdominal X-ray
   D) The pneumoperitoneum should be aspirated, and then a follow-up erect chest X-ray performed to see if it has resolved
   E) CT scan is better than plain X-rays at identifying free intraperitoneal gas

2. Which of following imaging modalities can detect free intraperitoneal gas?
   A) Erect chest X-ray
   B) Supine abdominal X-ray
   C) CT scan
   D) Radionuclide HIDA scan
   E) PET scan

3. Which of the following is/are causes of pneumoperitoneum on erect chest X-ray?
   A) Perforated colonic diverticulum
   B) Perforated peptic ulcer
   C) Appendicitis
   D) Recent laparotomy
   E) Cholecystitis

4. Which of the following statements regarding pneumoperitoneum is/are correct?
   A) Rigler's sign is the visualisation of bowel loops due to intraluminal gas
   B) Chilaiditi syndrome is a cause of pseudopneumoperitoneum and can simulate free intraperitoneal gas
   C) Pneumoperitoneum can be secondary to water skiing
   D) Inflammatory bowel disease can lead to pneumoperitoneum
   E) Some ingested foreign bodies such as batteries can cause bowel perforation

5. Which of the follow is/are correct regarding postoperative pneumoperitoneum?
   A) Post-laparoscopy pneumoperitoneum usually resolves within 24 to 48 hours in children, and 7 days in adults
   B) It can be due to a leaking surgical anastomosis
   C) Antibiotics are always necessary
   D) It may occur with gas-forming peritonitis
   E) It can be due to air from a healthy colostomy

Continue

CASE 2.14 *Contd.*

ANSWERS TO QUESTIONS

1. Regarding pneumoperitoneum, which of the following statements is/are true?

The correct answers are **A) Free air will not be identifiable in up to 20% to 30% of cases on erect chest X-ray, B) This can represent a surgical emergency, and the general surgeons must be contacted immediately because there may be a perforated viscus, C) As little as 1 mL of free intraperitoneal gas can be identified on a left lateral decubitus abdominal X-ray and E) CT scan is better than plain X-rays at identifying free intraperitoneal gas**.

The erect chest X-ray is often the first-line investigation performed in patients with suspected perforation to look for the presence of free intraperitoneal gas. However, it is important to realise that this investigation is not 100% sensitive, and a normal erect chest X-ray does not exclude a pneumoperitoneum. If clinical concern persists, a CT is commonly performed.

A) Free air will not be identifiable in up to 20% to 30% of cases on erect chest X-ray – Correct. Usually if a chest X-ray is requested for possible perforation, then the radiographer will try to ensure that the patient has been sitting upright for about 10 minutes prior to the X-ray, so that any free intraperitoneal gas will rise up and collect beneath the hemidiaphragms, most often the right hemidiaphragm. There are situations in which the chest X-ray will not be able to detect free intraperitoneal gas. Firstly, the patient's condition may prevent him or her from sitting upright for the required length of time, if, for example, they are in severe pain or in hypotensive shock. Also, in some cases, the free intraperitoneal gas may be localised around the perforated viscus, due to a reactive inflammatory response causing a 'contained perforation'; it will therefore not be able to disseminate throughout the abdomen. In these cases, the clinical signs of perforated intraabdominal viscus are an important guide to prompting further investigation with CT.

B) This can represent a surgical emergency, and the general surgeons must be contacted immediately because there may be a perforated viscus – Correct. The presence of subdiaphragmatic gas is not synonymous with a perforated viscus, as there are a variety of causes. However, with a clinical history of abdominal pain and examination findings of peritonism, free subdiaphragmatic gas on erect chest X-ray is highly likely to represent a perforated viscus. In this case, urgent referral to the general surgeons is required.

C) As little as 1 mL of free intraperitoneal gas can be identified on a left lateral decubitus abdominal X-ray – Correct. If a pneumoperitoneum cannot be demonstrated on an erect chest X-ray, then, if the patient can tolerate it, they can be asked to lie down on their left side for 10 minutes, and a lateral decubitus abdominal X-ray can be performed. This will allow enough time for the free gas to rise up to the right side of the peritoneal cavity and thus be seen on the abdominal X-ray. As little as 1 mL of free intraperitoneal gas has been identified as a small radiolucency adjacent to the liver on the X-ray using this technique. However, with the advent of CT scanning, this practice is used less frequently, although it may still be of use in the paediatric population.

D) The pneumoperitoneum should be aspirated and then a follow-up erect chest X-ray performed to see if it has resolved – Incorrect. This is not done – do not confuse pneumoperitoneum with pneumothorax! If there is free intraperitoneal gas, then the cause of this should be sought and treated. Even if there is pneumoperitoneum secondary to laparoscopic CO_2 insufflation or laparotomy, the gas is usually absorbed within 7 days by adults and 24 hours in children. The free gas is not aspirated unless it is part of an abscess cavity that is being treated by percutaneous drainage.

E) CT scan is better than plain X-rays at identifying free intraperitoneal gas – Correct. CT scans will detect tiny locules of free intraperitoneal gas not visible on other imaging modalities. Sometimes radiologists review the CT scan of the abdomen on settings aimed to maximise the contrast between air and soft tissues to help spot tiny locules of free gas (lung windows).

❗ KEY POINT

Although most radiographers should identify that a chest X-ray request for possible perforation will require the patient to be sitting up, as a referrer, you should always specify that you would like an erect chest X-ray. You will have assessed the patient – are they able to sit upright for at least 10 minutes? If not, they are likely to be very unwell, and you should seek urgent senior review and consider moving straight to CT as your investigation of choice.

2. Which of the following imaging modalities can detect free intraperitoneal gas?

The correct answers are **A) Erect chest X-ray, B) Supine abdominal X-ray and C) CT scan**.

X-rays and CT scans are the mainstay investigations for detecting free intraperitoneal gas.

A) Erect chest X-ray – Correct. The free intraperitoneal gas usually collects beneath the diaphragm, most commonly the right hemidiaphragm.

B) Supine abdominal X-ray – Correct. The free intraperitoneal gas can be seen as Rigler's sign or the Football sign (children). Other features of intraperitoneal gas include outlining the falciform ligament and small radiolucent triangles of gas outside the bowel (see the abdominal X-ray chapter for further details).

C) CT scan – Correct. CT scan has a high sensitivity for detecting free intraperitoneal gas and is often requested by surgeons to confirm their clinical diagnosis and determine the site of perforation prior to operating.

D) Radionuclide HIDA scan – Incorrect. This is used to look for biliary atresia in neonates with conjugated hyperbilirubinaemia who do not have an identifiable gallbladder on ultrasound scan. It can also be used in the investigation of acute cholecystitis, although this is not routine.

E) PET scan – Incorrect. PET uses 18-Fluorodeoxyglucose, a glucose analogue taken up by cancer cells, to detect malignancy; it is not a useful test to identify free intraperitoneal gas.

> **❗ KEY POINT**
>
> Investigations which are readily available and quick to perform are important in cases of suspected perforation, because, often, definitive treatment needs to be undertaken urgently.

3. Which of the following is/are causes of pneumoperitoneum on erect chest X-ray?

The correct answers are **A) Perforated colonic diverticulum, B) Perforated peptic ulcer, C) Appendicitis and D) Recent laparotomy**.

You should remember that the presence of free subdiaphragmatic gas is not synonymous with a perforated viscus. However, this is often the most serious cause and should always be considered.

A) Perforated colonic diverticulum – Correct. Colonic diverticula are acquired herniations of the bowel mucosa and submucosa through the muscle layers of the bowel wall and are more prevalent in developed countries in which the aetiology is linked to a low-fibre diet. Diverticulitis results from inflamed diverticula, which are prone to perforation. Additionally, the presence of diverticula increases the risk of iatrogenic perforation if the patient undergoes a colonoscopy, because the scope can inadvertently enter one of the blind-ending thin-walled diverticula.

B) Perforated peptic ulcer – Correct. A perforated peptic ulcer is a serious condition in which an ulcer (a breech in a mucosal surface of the gastrointestinal tract) erodes so deeply that a hole forms in the wall. This is a surgical emergency. Remember that the majority of the duodenum, except the proximal aspect of the first part, is retroperitoneal. Consequently, the free gas from a perforated duodenal ulcer will often be contained within the retroperitoneum rather than spreading throughout the peritoneal cavity, and may not be readily discernible on erect chest X-ray.

C) Appendicitis – Correct. An inflamed appendix is prone to rupture, which essentially represents another example of a 'hole in the bowel'.

D) Recent laparotomy – Correct. Postlaparotomy or laparoscopic surgery, there is often some free gas remaining within the peritoneal cavity, and this is gradually absorbed – usually more quickly in children than adults.

E) Cholecystitis – Incorrect. Simple cholecystitis is not a cause of pneumoperitoneum. Even in complex cases of gallbladder empyema when the gallbladder can perforate, the result is usually biliary peritonitis. No pneumoperitoneum will occur, as the gallbladder and biliary tree contains bile, not gas.

> **❗ KEY POINT**
>
> Free subdiaphragmatic gas on erect chest X-ray is not always due to a perforated hollow viscus. Even when it is due to perforation, it is not possible to determine whether there has been an upper gastrointestinal (GI) or lower GI perforation. Most patients will have a CT prior to surgery to help determine the aetiology and plan the surgical approach.

4. Which of the following statements regarding pneumoperitoneum is/are correct?

The correct answers are **B) Chilaiditi syndrome is a cause of pseudopneumoperitoneum and can simulate free intraperitoneal gas, C) Pneumoperitoneum can be secondary to water skiing, D) Inflammatory bowel disease can lead to pneumoperitoneum and E) Some ingested foreign bodies such as batteries can cause bowel perforation**.

This question highlights some of the more obscure causes of pneumoperitoneum. Although they are less common in clinical practice, they are favourite topics for examiners.

A) Rigler's sign is the visualisation of bowel loops due to intraluminal gas – Incorrect. Rigler's sign refers to the clear definition of the bowel wall on an X-ray and is due to the presence of both intra- and extraluminal air. The contrast in densities among intraluminal gas, soft tissue of the bowel wall and extraluminal gas can make both sides of the bowel wall clearly visible. In normal patients, only the internal bowel wall is usually visible.

B) Chilaiditi syndrome is a cause of pseudopneumoperitoneum and can simulate free intraperitoneal gas – Correct. Chilaiditi syndrome is due to the large bowel having a long and mobile mesentery, allowing the bowel to move and interpose itself between the right hemidiaphragm and the right lobe of the liver. This presence of bowel beneath the right hemidiaphragm can simulate free intraperitoneal gas because of the radiolucency of its intraluminal gas. The presence of haustral bowel markings confirms this diagnosis. It is often an incidental finding in normal individuals. The clinical scenario also helps differentiate this appearance from a pneumoperitoneum. If there is ongoing concern, a CT will provide a definite answer.

C) Pneumoperitoneum can be secondary to water skiing – Correct. During water skiing, air can enter the peritoneal cavity transvaginally in females. It then passes into the uterus and fallopian tubes when water is forced at high pressure into the perineal region during this activity. Pneumoperitoneum can subsequently result. It is a very rare cause of pneumoperitoneum and should be near the bottom of your differential list.

D) Inflammatory bowel disease can lead to pneumoperitoneum – Correct. Inflamed bowel is oedematous and more friable than normal bowel, making it more easily prone to perforation.

Continue

E) Some ingested foreign bodies such as batteries can cause bowel perforation – Correct. Ingested batteries should ideally be removed as soon as possible, as they contain corrosive material that can leak into the bowel and cause irritation of the bowel wall with perforation. Sometimes ingested batteries also set up a current across the bowel wall, leading to damage and perforation.

❶ KEY POINTS

1. Rigler's sign consists of well-defined bowel loops due to intra- and extraluminal gas. Its presence on an abdominal X-ray can help confirm the diagnosis of pneumoperitoneum.
2. Chilaiditi syndrome is a pneumoperitoneum mimic. It occurs when large bowel is interposed between the right hemidiaphragm and the right lobe of the liver. The clinical condition of the patient and the presence of bowel markings usually help to differentiate this from a pneumoperitoneum.

5. Which of the follow is/are correct regarding postoperative pneumoperitoneum?

The correct answers are **A) Post-laparoscopy pneumoperitoneum usually resolves within 24 to 48 hours in children and 7 days in adults, B) It can be due to a leaking surgical anastomosis and D) It may occur with gas-forming peritonitis**.

The presence of free subdiaphragmatic gas is common on postoperative X-rays. It is important to recognise when this becomes abnormal in order to help identify a complication.

A) Post-laparoscopy pneumoperitoneum usually resolves within 24 to 48 hours in children and 7 days in adults – Correct. The gas used in laparoscopy is usually CO_2, and this is rapidly absorbed from the peritoneal cavity. This occurs more quickly in children than in adults.

B) It can be due to a leaking surgical anastomosis – Correct. There is usually some air that remains in the peritoneal cavity following abdominal surgery.

However, if there is a leaking surgical anastomosis, then larger quantities of gas can escape from the bowel into the peritoneal cavity; this can occur outside of the time frame for the normal postoperative pneumoperitoneum.

C) Antibiotics are always necessary – Incorrect. If there is bacterial contamination of the peritoneal cavity with sepsis, then antibiotics will be necessary. In other causes of a postoperative pneumoperitoneum, antibiotics are not required. Incorrect use of antibiotics contributes to unnecessary antibiotic resistance and can lead to complications such as pseudomembranous colitis from *Clostridium difficile*. Each clinical case should be judged individually and should take into account benefits/risks.

D) It may occur with gas-forming peritonitis – Correct. Some gas-forming organisms (e.g. Clostridium perfringens) may lead to gas production and accumulation in the peritoneal cavity.

E) It can be due to air from a healthy colostomy – Incorrect. A healthy colostomy should not allow air to leak into the peritoneal cavity.

❶ KEY POINT

It is very useful to include the information that the patient has had a recent operation on the clinical request to highlight this to the reporting radiologist.

👥 IMPORTANT LEARNING POINTS

- There are various causes of free intraperitoneal gas, but a perforated viscus is the commonest and most significant cause.
- An erect chest X-ray is often the first investigation performed in cases of suspected perforation. The patient needs to be well enough to sit upright for at least 10 minutes.
- A normal erect chest X-ray does not exclude a perforation.
- There should be a low threshold for senior review and proceeding to CT scanning to confirm the diagnosis.

CASE 2.15

A 45-year-old man presents with thoracic back discomfort and shortness of breath. As part of his assessment, you request a chest X-ray.

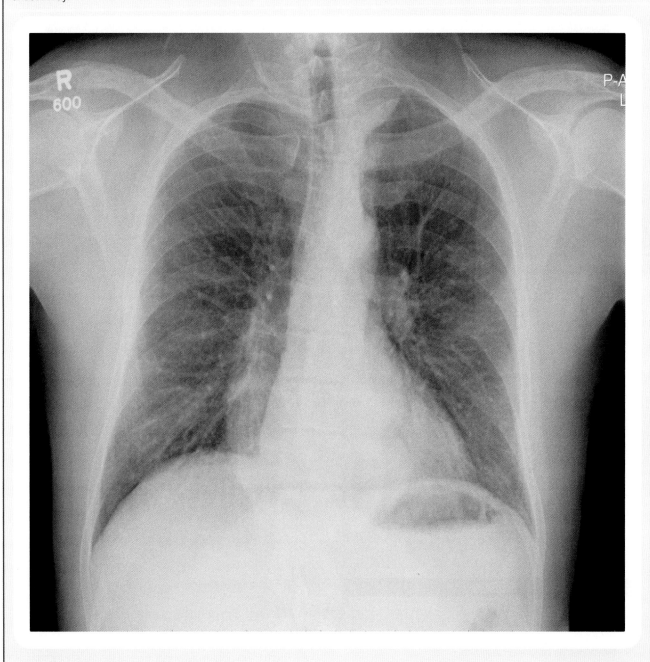

Continue

CASE **2.15**   *Contd.*

ANNOTATED X-RAY

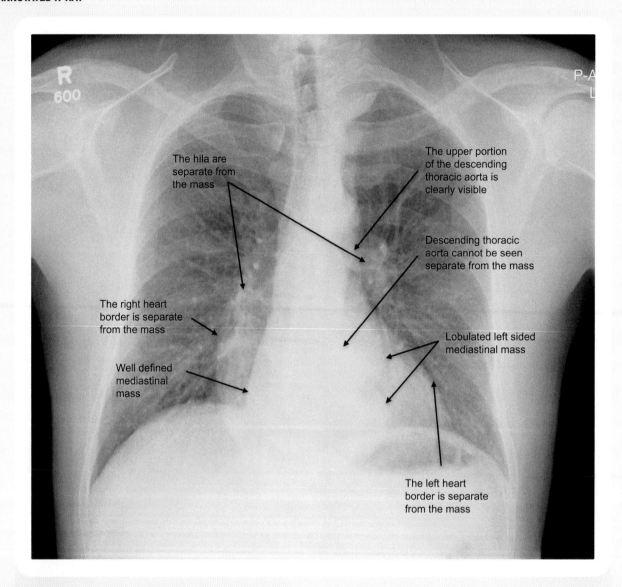

The hila are separate from the mass

The upper portion of the descending thoracic aorta is clearly visible

Descending thoracic aorta cannot be seen separate from the mass

The right heart border is separate from the mass

Well defined mediastinal mass

Lobulated left sided mediastinal mass

The left heart border is separate from the mass

🔍 PRESENT YOUR FINDINGS

- This is a PA chest X-ray of an adult.
- It has been anonymised, and the date of the examination has been removed. I would like to confirm these details before proceeding.
- The patient is slightly rotated, but there is good inspiratory achievement, and the X-ray is sufficiently penetrated.
- The striking abnormality is a smooth-contoured right-sided mediastinal soft tissue mass. The right heart border is seen separate from the mass. On inspection of the retrocardiac area, there is also a lobulated soft tissue density in the left paravertebral region. This is separate from the left cardiac silhouette, but the descending thoracic aorta cannot be seen separate from the mass. There is no definite continuation of the soft tissue masses below the diaphragm.

- The trachea is central (allowing for the patient's rotation).
- The lungs and pleural spaces are clear.
- Both hila are visible and appear normal.
- There is no free subdiaphragmatic gas.
- There is no abnormality in the visualised bony thorax.

IN SUMMARY – This chest X-ray demonstrates bilateral mediastinal masses. The hila and the heart borders are seen separate from the masses. The upper portion of the descending thoracic aorta is visible, but the rest of it cannot be seen separate from the mass. This is thus likely to represent a posterior mediastinal mass. The differential for mediastinal masses includes lymphadenopathy, neurofibroma, schwannoma, extramedullary haematopoiesis and a descending thoracic aortic aneurysm. I would like to review any previous X-rays to assess for change. CT is warranted.

QUESTIONS

1. Regarding the normal mediastinum, which of the following is/are correct?
   A) The anterior border of the anterior mediastinum is the sternum, and the posterior border is the pericardium, aorta and brachiocephalic vessels
   B) The aortopulmonary window should have a convex border
   C) The anterior border of the middle mediastinum is the anterior pericardium, and the posterior border is the posterior pericardium and posterior tracheal wall
   D) The right paratracheal line should be greater than 5 mm in width
   E) The posterior mediastinum is bordered posteriorly by the vertebral column

2. Regarding mediastinal masses, which of the following statements is/are true?
   A) The presence of air bronchograms within a mass abutting the mediastinum suggests lung rather than mediastinal pathology
   B) A posterior mediastinal mass makes an obtuse angle with the mediastinal surface
   C) Fascial tissues planes separate the mediastinal compartments
   D) Pathology may affect multiple mediastinal compartments
   E) A normal mediastinum on a chest X-ray excludes mediastinal pathology

3. Which of the following is/are features of an anterior mediastinal mass on chest X-ray?
   A) The right heart border is confluent with the mass (the silhouette sign)
   B) The proximal pulmonary arteries are demonstrated separate from the mass (the hilum overlay sign)
   C) The mass extends superiorly above the clavicle (the cervicothoracic sign)
   D) The mass obliterates the retrosternal space on lateral chest X-ray
   E) The mass obliterates the anterior junctional line

4. Which of the following is/are in the differential diagnose for an anterior mediastinal mass in a 65-year-old patient?
   A) Thyroid goitre
   B) Thymus
   C) Teratoma
   D) Thymoma
   E) Lymphoma

5. Regarding middle mediastinal masses, which of the following is/are true?
   A) Normal variant anatomy can mimic a middle mediastinal mass
   B) New unilateral elevated hemidiaphragm may result from a middle mediastinal mass
   C) In patients presenting with a hoarse voice, the aorto-pulmonary window should be scrutinised
   D) A sliding hiatus hernia can appear as a middle mediastinal mass
   E) Enlarged proximal pulmonary arteries can mimic middle mediastinal lymphadenopathy

Continue

CASE 2.15 *Contd.*

ANSWERS TO QUESTIONS

1. Regarding the normal mediastinum, which of the following is/are correct?

   The correct answers are **A) The anterior border of the anterior mediastinum is the sternum, and the posterior border is the pericardium, aorta and brachiocephalic vessels, C) The anterior border of the middle mediastinum is the anterior pericardium, and the posterior border is the posterior pericardium and posterior tracheal wall and E) The posterior mediastinum is bordered posteriorly by the vertebral column**.

   Knowledge of the mediastinal compartments is important to direct the differential diagnosis of mediastinal pathology. The mediastinum is commonly divided into three compartments: anterior, middle and posterior.

   A) The anterior border of the anterior mediastinum is the sternum, and the posterior border is the pericardium, aorta and brachiocephalic vessels – Correct. The anterior mediastinum is everything between the sternum and the heart and great vessels (i.e. anterior to the pericardium). Its contents include the thymus (which involutes in adulthood), lymph nodes and some blood vessels.

   B) The aortopulmonary window should have a convex border – Incorrect. Between the aortic knuckle and left main pulmonary artery, there should be a concave region of soft tissue, known as the aortopulmonary window. This is visible on frontal chest X-rays. If the aortopulmonary window is convex, pathology, such as lymph node enlargement, needs excluding.

   C) The anterior border of the middle mediastinum is the anterior pericardium, and the posterior border is the posterior pericardium and posterior tracheal wall – Correct. The middle mediastinum consists of the pericardium and its contents (the heart and great vessels), the pulmonary trunk and the trachea/main bronchi. Its posterior boundary is the posterior pericardium and the posterior tracheal wall.

   D) The right paratracheal line should be greater than 5 mm in width – Incorrect. The right paratracheal line is seen through the superior vena cava. It is formed by the right lateral wall of the trachea and the medial border of the right lung. If visible, it should be of uniform thickness, and less than 5 mm wide (it is only visible on 50%–60% of chest X-rays). If it measures more than 5 mm in width, lymphadenopathy should be suspected.

   E) The posterior mediastinum is bordered posteriorly by the vertebral column – Correct. The posterior mediastinum is the area posterior to the pericardium. Its posterior border is formed by the vertebral column. Its contents include the oesophagus, the descending thoracic aorta, azygous and hemiazygous veins, vagus nerve and the thoracic duct.

❶ KEY POINT

The mediastinum is divided into three compartments. Knowledge of their boundaries helps in formulating a differential diagnosis for lesions in each compartment by allowing you to think of the normal anatomical structures within the compartment, and then think of pathology affecting those structures.

2. Regarding mediastinal masses, which of the following statements is/are true?

   The correct answers are **A) The presence of air bronchograms within a mass abutting the mediastinum suggests lung rather than mediastinal pathology, B) A posterior mediastinal mass makes an obtuse angle with the mediastinal surface and D) Pathology may affect multiple mediastinal compartments**.

   A) The presence of air bronchograms within a mass abutting the mediastinum suggests lung rather than mediastinal pathology – Correct. Sometimes it can be difficult to distinguish a lung mass from a mediastinal mass, particularly if the lung mass abuts the mediastinal surface. The presence of air bronchograms within a mass confirms that it is related to lung parenchyma.

   B) A posterior mediastinal mass forms an obtuse angle with the mediastinal surface – Correct. This can help distinguish among lung masses outside the mediastinum (but next to it), which can form acute angles with the mediastinal surfaces.

   C) Fascial tissue planes separate the mediastinal compartments – Incorrect. The divisions of the mediastinum into anterior, middle and posterior are essentially arbitrary. There are no anatomical fascial planes which separate the mediastinal compartments.

   D) Pathology may affect multiple mediastinal compartments – Correct. As there are no anatomical boundaries among the mediastinal compartments, pathology may affect multiple compartments. This can occur in mediastinitis, mediastinal haematoma, bronchogenic malignancy and lymphadenopathy.

   E) A normal mediastinum on a chest X-ray excludes mediastinal pathology – Incorrect. Chest X-ray provides a limited assessment of the mediastinum, as there are multiple structures overlapping one another. If there is ongoing concern, further investigation with CT is usually the next investigative step.

❶ KEY POINTS

1. When faced with a potential mediastinal mass on a chest X-ray, the first step is to confirm that it represents a mediastinal mass, rather than a lung mass abutting the mediastinum.

2. Remember that certain pathologies can affect multiple mediastinal compartments.

3. Which of the following is/are features of an anterior mediastinal mass on chest X-ray?

   The correct answers are **A) The right heart border is confluent with the mass (the silhouette sign), B) The proximal pulmonary arteries are demonstrated separate from the mass (the hilum overlay sign), D) The mass obliterates the retrosternal space on lateral chest X-ray and E) The mass obliterates the anterior junctional line**.

   Localising a mass to a particular mediastinal compartment can be difficult on chest X-ray. There are several radiographic signs that, if present, can help with this process.

   A) The right heart border is confluent with the mass (the silhouette sign) – Correct. The reason why we see the heart shadow clearly on a chest X-ray is because it is surrounded by aerated lung, which is of different radiographic density from that of the heart. When a soft tissue mass touches the border of the heart, the clarity of the heart border is obliterated, because the aerated lung is displaced and replaced by an entity of similar radiographic density. Likewise, if the border of the heart is preserved, then a mass cannot be abutting that surface. The silhouette sign actually refers to loss of part of the silhouette of the structure in question. Loss of the right heart border could potentially localise a mass to the anterior or middle mediastinum, or the adjacent lung.

   B) The proximal pulmonary arteries are demonstrated separate from the mass (the hilum overlay sign) – Correct. The pulmonary arteries and other hilar structures are part of the middle mediastinum. If the mass seen is separate from normally positioned pulmonary arteries, then the mass cannot be in the middle mediastinum. A middle mediastinal mass would either display the silhouette sign with the abutting pulmonary vessels or displace them laterally. The hilum overlay sign therefore localises the mass to either the anterior or posterior mediastinum.

   C) The mass extends superiorly above the clavicle (the cervicothoracic sign) – Incorrect. The anterior mediastinum stops at the level of the clavicle. Therefore, if a mediastinal mass extends above the clavicle, it must either represent a posterior mediastinal mass or it is located in the neck. This is termed the cervicothoracic sign and therefore is not a sign of an anterior mediastinal mass. Remember that an enlarged thyroid goitre, which is a neck mass, can extend retrosternally into the anterior mediastinum.

   D) The mass obliterates the retrosternal space on lateral chest X-ray – Correct. Lateral X-rays are rarely performed in the UK these days. There should be aerated lung visible anterior to the cardiac shadow and posterior to the sternum on a lateral X-ray. An anterior mediastinal mass may obliterate the retrosternal space on lateral chest X-ray.

   E) The mass obliterates the anterior junctional line – Correct. The anterior junctional line is formed by the anterior apposition of the lungs behind the upper two-thirds of the sternum. Loss of this line suggests that there is pathology within the anterior mediastinum which is displacing the two lung edges.

❶ KEY POINTS

1. The silhouette sign, hilum overlay sign and cervicothoracic sign are useful to help confirm on chest X-ray in which mediastinal compartment a lesion is located.
2. CT provides a more comprehensive assessment of the mediastinum and allows pathology to be located accurately.

4. Which of the following is/are in the differential diagnoses for an anterior mediastinal mass in a 65-year-old patient?

   The correct answers are **A) Thyroid goitre, C) Teratoma, D) Thymoma and E) Lymphoma**.

   All of the listed options are potential causes of anterior mediastinal masses. In this question, the age of the patient is the discriminator.

   A) Thyroid goitre – Correct. The thyroid gland can enlarge retrosternally and manifest as an anterior mediastinal mass (although technically it is a neck mass).

   B) Thymus – Incorrect. Whilst the thymus is a normal anterior mediastinal mass, it undergoes atrophy during childhood and adolescence and therefore should not be in the differential diagnosis for a patient of this age. Abnormalities arising from the remnants of the thymus gland, on the other hand, are a possible differential (see D).

   C) Teratoma – Correct. Teratoma is a germ cell tumour; a potential cause of an anterior mediastinal mass.

   D) Thymoma – Correct. Although normal thymic tissue should not be part of the differential of an anterior mediastinal mass in adults, abnormal thymic tissue should be included. Thymoma is the most common pathology (thymic carcinoma is much rarer) and should be sought in patients with new-onset myasthenia gravis, as there is an association between these two diseases.

   E) Lymphoma – Correct. Lymphoma is a potential cause of an anterior mediastinal mass.

❶ KEY POINT

The differential for anterior mediastinal masses can be remembered as the four Ts: Thyroid, Thymic, Teratoma and Terrible lymphoma.

5. Regarding middle mediastinal masses, which of the following is/are true?

   The correct answers are **A) Normal variant anatomy can mimic a middle mediastinal mass, B) New unilateral elevated hemidiaphragm may result from a middle mediastinal mass, C) In patients presenting with a hoarse voice, the aortopulmonary window should be scrutinised**

Continue

CASE 2.15 *Contd.*

and E) Enlarged proximal pulmonary arteries can mimic middle mediastinal lymphadenopathy.

This question tests your knowledge of the contents of the middle mediastinum, which includes the heart, pericardium, ascending aorta and aortic arch, superior vena cava, inferior vena cava, brachiocephalic vessels, pulmonary arteries, trachea, main bronchi, lymph nodes and nerves (phrenic, vagus and left recurrent laryngeal).

A) Normal variant anatomy can mimic a middle mediastinal mass – Correct. In particular, a right-sided aortic arch could be seen as a right superior middle mediastinal mass. Other normal variants which can mimic middle mediastinal pathology include a left-sided superior vena cava and prominent azygous vein (near to the right paratracheal strip) due to azygous continuation of the inferior vena cava.

B) New-onset unilateral elevated hemidiaphragm may result from a middle mediastinal mass – Correct. A phrenic nerve palsy can result in a unilateral elevated hemidiaphragm. Pathology can result in neural damage, as it courses through the middle mediastinum.

C) In patients presenting with a hoarse voice, the aortopulmonary window should be scrutinised – Correct. The left recurrent laryngeal nerve descends into the middle mediastinum and loops around the arch of the aorta before ascending superiorly again. Look carefully for a left hilar or aortopulmonary window mass causing left recurrent laryngeal nerve palsy in patients having a chest X-ray for a hoarse voice. In contrast, the right recurrent laryngeal nerve has a much shorter intrathoracic course, passing around the right subclavian artery. It is thus less likely to be affected by mediastinal pathology.

D) A sliding hiatus hernia can appear as a middle mediastinal mass – Incorrect. The oesophagus is a posterior mediastinal structure. A sliding hiatus hernia can often be observed on chest X-ray, but usually as a distinct soft tissue entity from the heart shadow.

E) Enlarged proximal pulmonary arteries can mimic middle mediastinal lymphadenopathy – Correct. Remember that not all hilar soft tissue masses will represent lymphadenopathy. The proximal pulmonary arteries themselves can enlarge, e.g. in pulmonary artery hypertension or in the presence of a longstanding uncorrected atrial septal defect. It is often difficult to differentiate this from lymph node enlargement on the chest X-ray, and a CT scan may be required for further assessment.

TABLE C2.15.1 Differential Diagnosis of Mediastinal Masses by Their Location

ANTERIOR MEDIASTINUM	MIDDLE MEDIASTINUM	POSTERIOR MEDIASTINUM
Thyroid mass (although this is technically a neck mass)	Lymphadenopathy	Lymphadenopathy
Thymus/thymic mass	Central bronchogenic tumours	Nerve sheath tumours (neurofibroma, schwannoma)
Teratoma	Foregut duplication cysts	Sympathetic ganglion (neuroblastoma)
Lymphoma		Paraspinal abscess
		Extramedullary haematopoiesis
		Descending thoracic aortic aneurysm

❗ **KEY POINTS**

1. Most middle mediastinal masses consist of bronchogenic malignancy or lymphadenopathy (Table C1.15.1). Other causes include foregut duplication cysts (e.g. oesophageal or bronchogenic).
2. Remember that any anatomical structure in the middle mediastinum can be affected by pathology.
3. The clinical information (e.g. hoarse voice) or other chest X-ray findings (e.g. elevated hemidiaphragm) should prompt you to scrutinise the middle mediastinum for pathology.

IMPORTANT LEARNING POINTS

- The first step in assessing mediastinal masses on the chest X-ray is to confirm that the mass is mediastinal, and not a lung mass abutting the mediastinum – look for air bronchograms within the mass and assess the angle the mass makes with the mediastinal surface.
- Then attempt to localise the mass to the anterior, middle or posterior mediastinum. Use hilum overlay and cervicothoracic signs to help. In addition, scrutinising the right paratracheal strip, the anterior junctional line and aortopulmonary window can help. This helps narrow your differential diagnosis.
- The clinical context may help target your concentration, e.g. left hilum and aortopulmonary window in a patient with hoarse voice.
- Remember that pathology may affect multiple mediastinal compartments.
- CT is commonly performed to help assess mediastinal masses further.

CASE **2.16**

An unkempt 40-year-old woman presents to A&E with a worsening cough and foul-smelling, blood-stained sputum. She is feverish and breathless. She has a background of type II diabetes and was recently diagnosed with pneumonia. She says she did not take her antibiotics as they 'didn't agree with her' and she failed to attend her GP follow-up appointments. Below is her chest X-ray.

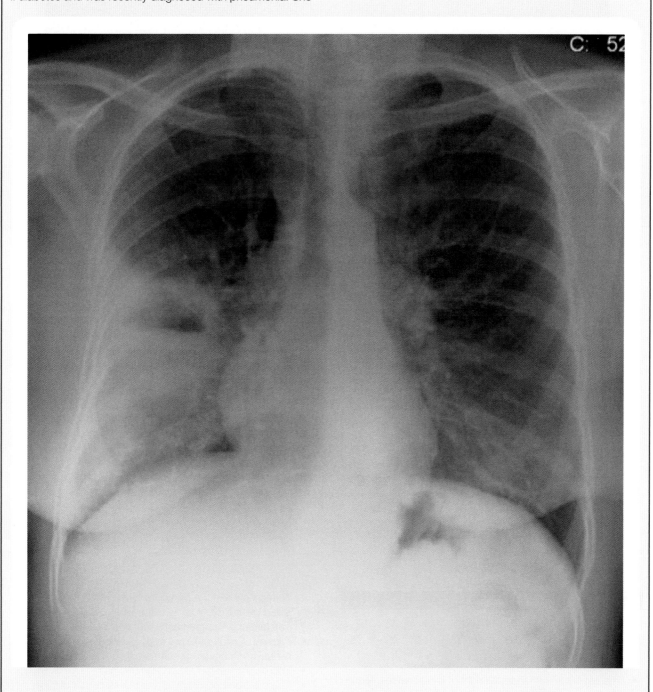

Continue

CASE **2.16**   *Contd.*

ANNOTATED X-RAY

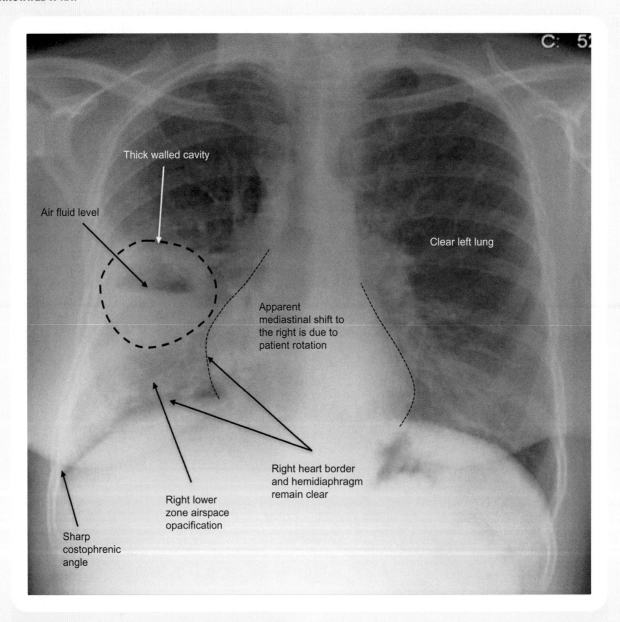

Thick walled cavity

Air fluid level

Clear left lung

Apparent mediastinal shift to the right is due to patient rotation

Right heart border and hemidiaphragm remain clear

Right lower zone airspace opacification

Sharp costophrenic angle

C: 5

🔍 **PRESENT YOUR FINDINGS**

- This is a PA chest X-ray of an adult.
- There are no patient identifiers on the X-ray. I would like to ensure that this is the correct patient, and to check the date and time when the X-ray was taken.
- The patient is rotated to the right. It is otherwise a technically adequate X-ray, with suitable penetration and good inspiratory achievement. There are no important areas cut off at the edges of the film.
- The most striking abnormality is the thick-walled cavity within the right midzone. This contains an air-fluid level.
- There is surrounding airspace opacification in the right lower zone, in keeping with consolidation. Both the right hemidiaphragm and heart border are clearly defined. Therefore it is not possible to localise the

consolidation into a particular lobe. There is no right-sided pleural effusion.
- The left lung and pleural space are clear.
- Allowing for the patient's rotation, the heart and mediastinal contours are unremarkable.
- There is no free subdiaphragmatic gas.
- There is no abnormality of the bones or soft tissues.

IN SUMMARY – This X-ray shows a cavity in the right lung, with an air-fluid level and surrounding consolidation. Given the clinical history, the findings are in keeping with a lung abscess and pneumonia. There is no evidence of associated empyema.

QUESTIONS

1. The differential diagnosis of a cavitating lung lesion includes which of the following?
   A) Lung abscess
   B) Cavitating tumour
   C) Granulomatosis with polyangiitis
   D) Pulmonary infarction
   E) Influenza pneumonia

2. Which of the following is/are risk factors for developing a lung abscess?
   A) Emphysema
   B) Immunocompetence
   C) Alcoholism
   D) Poor dental hygiene
   E) Penetrating pulmonary trauma

3. Which of the following is/are correct regarding the aetiology of lung abscesses?
   A) Most lung abscesses are caused by aerobic bacteria
   B) Lung abscesses are almost always caused by a single microorganism
   C) Lung abscesses can complicate pyogenic pneumonia
   D) Fungi are more likely to cause lung abscesses in immunocompromised patients
   E) An abscess can develop in a preexisting lung cyst

4. Which of the following imaging modalities provides the best assessment of a lung abscess?
   A) PA chest X-ray
   B) PA and lateral chest X-rays
   C) Unenhanced CT
   D) CT with IV contrast
   E) Ultrasound

5. Regarding the treatment of a lung abscess, which of the following is/are correct?
   A) Oxygen is contraindicated if the causative organism is an aerobic bacterium
   B) Postural draining may be helpful
   C) Antibiotics should be continued until the patient's temperature has normalised
   D) The patient should have regular follow-up
   E) Surgery is indicated for lung abscesses which have not resolved within 2 weeks of antibiotics

Continue

CASE **2.16** *Contd.*

ANSWERS TO QUESTIONS

1. The differential diagnosis of a cavitating lung lesion includes which of the following?
   The correct answers are **A) Lung abscess, B) Cavitating tumour, C) Granulomatosis with polyangiitis and D) Pulmonary infarction**.
   A lung cavity can be described as a gas-filled area within pulmonary consolidation, a nodule or a mass. They are usually thick-walled and can be filled with fluid and/or air. If both air and fluid are present, a fluid level can usually be seen. Lung cavities have a variety of causes. Differentiating among the causes involves clinical assessment, blood tests, microbiology tests, imaging features and, sometimes, biopsy.
   A) Lung abscess – Correct. Lung abscesses are collections of pus, debris and fluid within lung cavities. They can occur as a result of necrotising pneumonia (primary abscess), or following the infection of a preexisting lung abnormality such as a bulla, or due to proximal bronchial obstruction (secondary abscess). Risk factors include immunosuppression, alcoholism, underlying lung disease (e.g. cystic fibrosis) and factors that increase the risk of aspiration (e.g. cerebral palsy, stroke).
   B) Cavitating tumour – Correct. Some tumours, such as squamous cell carcinoma, are known to cavitate. Sarcoma, lymphoma and transitional cell carcinoma are also recognised causes of a cavitating tumour. Other features on the imaging, such as malignant disease elsewhere, may suggest an underlying tumour; however, often a biopsy, either via bronchoscopy or under CT guidance, is required to confirm the diagnosis.
   C) Granulomatosis with polyangiitis – Correct. Granulomatosis with polyangiitis was previously known as Wegener granulomatosis. It is a vasculitis of small- and medium-sized arteries which usually affects the upper airways, lungs and kidneys. Within the lungs, it results in multiple nodules, half of which cavitate. The presence of antineutrophil cytoplasmic antibodies (ANCA) supports the diagnosis; however, biopsy is required for confirmation.
   D) Pulmonary infarction – Correct. Pulmonary infarction can result in necrosis of the lung and thus lead to cavity formation. Infarction of the lung is most commonly due to thromboembolic disease, but can also be caused by septic emboli and sickle cell disease.
   E) Influenza pneumonia – Incorrect. Influenza is very infectious and usually occurs in epidemics. Whilst it affects lots of people, it very rarely results in pneumonia. Influenza pneumonia is not a recognised cause of necrotising pneumonia and therefore will not cause lung cavities/abscesses.

❶ KEY POINT

CAVITY is a mnemonic for the causes of lung cavities. It stands for:
- Cancer (e.g. squamous cell carcinoma)
- Autoimmune (e.g. Granulomatosis with polyangiitis)
- Vascular (e.g. thrombotic and septic emboli)
- Infection (e.g. lung abscess)
- Trauma (e.g. pneumatocoele)
- Youth (congenital abnormalities such as sequestration and congenital cystic adenoid malformation (CCAM))

2. Which of the following is/are risk factors for developing a lung abscess?
   The correct answer is **A) Emphysema, C) Alcoholism, D) Poor dental hygiene and E) Penetrating pulmonary trauma**.
   Lung abscesses can either be primary, which occur in normal lung, or secondary infection of an existing lung abnormality. There are a variety of risk factors for developing lung abscesses.
   A) Emphysema – Correct. Infection of an emphysematous bulla can result in a secondary lung abscess. Other lung cavities which can become infected include pneumatocoeles, Langerhans cell histiocytosis and neurofibromatosis type 1. Bulla and other lung cavities, such as TB cavities, can also be infected with Aspergillus, leading to an aspergilloma. An obstructing bronchial tumour is another risk factor for secondary lung abscess formation.
   B) Immunocompetence – Incorrect. Immunosuppression NOT immunocompetence is a risk factor for infection and lung abscesses. This is associated with diabetes mellitus, chemotherapy and other medications such as steroids. Be careful reading the question and answers in examinations – the answer given here is immunocompetence, which can easily be misread!
   C) Alcoholism – Correct. Primary abscesses are most commonly due to necrotising pneumonia resulting from aspiration of oral bacteria. Any condition which increases the chance of aspiration and is associated with poor oral hygiene will increase the risk of lung abscesses. Alcoholism is associated with both of these. In addition, alcoholics often have a degree of immunosuppression, which adds to the risk. Other conditions which increase the risk of aspiration include strokes, cerebral palsy, other central nervous system disorders and achalasia (a condition in which the lower oesophageal sphincter fails to relax. This leads to impaired passage of oesophageal contents into the stomach with accumulation of fluid in the oesophagus and overspill into the trachea and lungs).
   D) Poor dental hygiene – Correct. As discussed in C, poor oral hygiene is a risk factor. Patient groups at highest risk of this include alcoholics, drug users and the homeless.
   E) Penetrating pulmonary trauma – Correct. Penetrating pulmonary trauma increases the risk of lung abscess formation.

3. Which of the following is/are correct regarding the aetiology of lung abscesses?
   The correct answers are **C) Lung abscesses can complicate pyogenic pneumonia, D) Fungi are more likely to cause lung abscesses in**

immunocompromised patients and E) An abscess can develop in a preexisting lung cyst.

Lung abscesses can be caused by bacterial (aerobic or anaerobic) or fungal infection. The exact organism responsible for the abscess can be difficult to isolate in cultures due to contamination with the normal upper airway flora.

A) Most lung abscesses are caused by aerobic bacteria – Incorrect. Most lung abscesses are the result of anaerobic bacteria or mixed aerobic and anaerobic infections.

B) Lung abscesses are almost always caused by a single microorganism – Incorrect. Whilst lung abscesses can be caused by a single organism, they are often the result of a mixed bacterial infection.

C) Lung abscesses can complicate pyogenic pneumonia – Correct. Pyogenic pneumonia, such as *S. aureus*, *Klebsiella pneumoniae* and *Streptococcus*, can result in a necrotising pneumonia, lung necrosis and abscess formation. TB is another common bacterial cause of lung abscesses.

D) Fungi are more likely to cause lung abscesses in immunocompromised patients – Correct. Fungi such as *Aspergillus*, *Coccidioidomycosis* and *Cryptococcus* are more commonly associated with lung abscesses in the immunocompromised, compared to immunocompetent patients. Atypical bacterial infections, such as nocardia and mycobacterium, are also more frequent in immunocompromised patients.

E) An abscess can develop in a preexisting lung cyst – Correct. As already discussed, abscesses can form within pre-existing cavities. Such abscesses are known as secondary abscesses. Emphysematous bullae, traumatic pneumatocoeles and sarcoid-related cavities are examples of potential sites for secondary abscesses.

4. Which of the following imaging modalities provides the best assessment of a lung abscess?

The correct answer is **D) CT with IV contrast**.

Imaging has a role in diagnosing a lung abscess and monitoring its response to treatment.

A) PA chest X-ray – Incorrect. Lung abscesses typically appear as a thick-walled cavity with an air-fluid level. As they are frequently due to aspiration, they are most commonly found in the lower lobes, or the posterior segments of the upper lobes. As the infection resolves, the cavity wall becomes thin and well defined. Chest X-ray also allows the identification of pleural fluid, which may represent a coexisting empyema. Chest X-ray is, however, inferior to CT for assessing a lung abscess.

B) PA and lateral chest X-rays – Incorrect. Whilst the lateral view will help to localise the abscess more accurately, this imaging combination is still inferior to CT.

C) Unenhanced CT – Incorrect. See D.

D) CT with IV contrast – Correct. CT provides the most accurate assessment of the lungs. It can show the size, shape and location of an abscess, as well as any associated features, such as coexistent consolidation or pleural fluid, or underlying lung disease, such as

emphysema. IV contrast permits the edge of the abscess to be seen clearly as the margins can blur into any surrounding consolidation. CT will also help differentiate a lung abscess from other causes of a lung cavitation.

E) Ultrasound – Incorrect. Ultrasound can be used to identify and characterise pleural fluid accurately. It is often used to guide pleural aspiration or drainage. However, as the ultrasound beams are scattered by gas, it is not possible to assess the lung accurately. Peripheral abscesses that are close to or in contact with the pleural cavity can often be seen as hypoechoic, round structures.

> ⊕ KEY POINT
>
> Contrast-enhanced CT is the most accurate method for assessing lung abscesses.

5. Regarding the treatment of a lung abscess, which of the following is/are correct?

The correct answer is **B) Postural draining may be helpful and D) The patient should be regularly followed up**.

As with most lung infections, the management of lung abscesses is centred around antibiotics.

A) Oxygen is contraindicated if the causative organism is an aerobic bacterium – Incorrect. The patient should be given supplementary oxygen if their oxygen levels are low. The presence of aerobic bacteria is not a contraindication to this.

B) Postural draining may be helpful – Correct. Postural drainage with chest physiotherapy is aimed at allowing as much of the pus as possible to drain from the abscess via the bronchial tree. Postural drainage is one of the main therapeutic measures for lung abscesses.

C) Antibiotics should be continued until the patient's temperature has normalised – Incorrect. The mainstay of treatment is appropriate antimicrobial agents (usually antibiotics, but antifungals may be needed if there is an underlying fungal infection). Patients with lung abscesses usually need prolonged courses of antimicrobials. Most patients are treated for 4 to 6 weeks. The choice of antimicrobial should be tailored to the patient, any isolated organism and local sensitivities.

D) The patient should be regularly followed up – Correct. It is important that these patients are followed up clinically and radiologically (often with chest X-ray). Reasons for a poor response to antimicrobial therapy include a resistant infection, the wrong choice of antimicrobial and bronchial obstruction (either by a foreign body or a tumour). Identifying a poor response to treatment early will allow appropriate alternative management to be instigated.

E) Surgery is indicated for lung abscesses which have not resolved within 2 weeks of antibiotics – Incorrect. Lung abscesses often take several weeks to respond,

Continue

CASE 2.16   *Contd.*

and patients are usually treated with antibiotics for at least 4 weeks. Surgery usually consists of lobectomy or pneumonectomy, but this is associated with a number of complications, including empyema formation and a bronchopleural fistula; it is therefore reserved for patients not responding to conventional treatment. Percutaneous drainage of the abscess under CT guidance is an alternative treatment option.

❗ KEY POINT

Lung abscesses are usually treated with prolonged antimicrobials and postural drainage.

 IMPORTANT LEARNING POINTS

- There are several potential causes for a lung cavity, including lung abscess and malignancy. The clinical findings and results of investigations will help determine the cause.
- Conditions which lead to immunosuppression, increase the risk of aspiration or are associated with poor oral hygiene increase the chance of lung abscesses.
- Lung abscesses are most accurately imaged using contrast-enhanced CT.
- Prolonged antimicrobials and postural drainage are the mainstay of treatment, with invasive options, such as CT-guided drainage and surgery, reserved for patients who fail to respond.

CASE 2.17

A 70-year-old female smoker presents with a 3-week history of cough, haemoptysis and breathlessness. She has lost some weight over the last 2 months. A chest X-ray has been performed for further assessment.

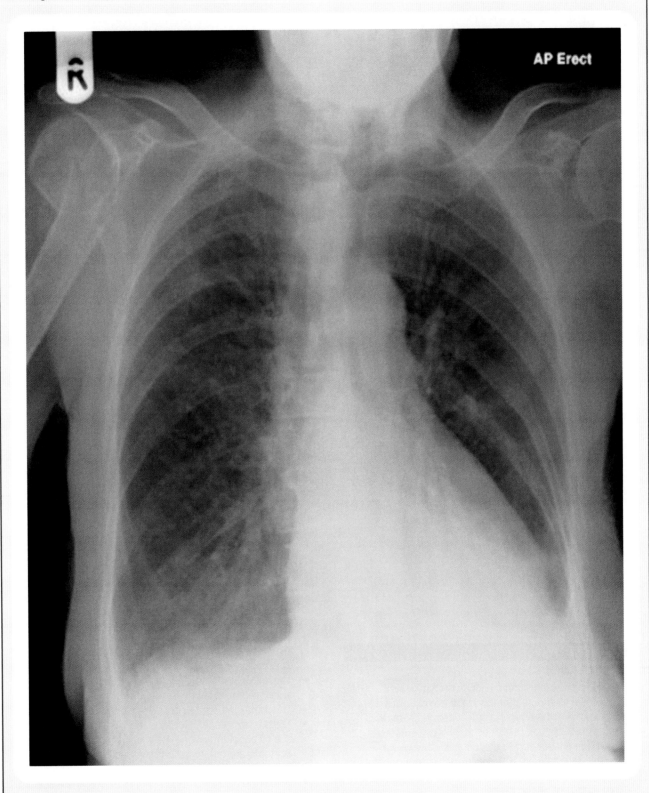

Continue

CASE 2.17 *Contd.*

ANNOTATED X-RAY

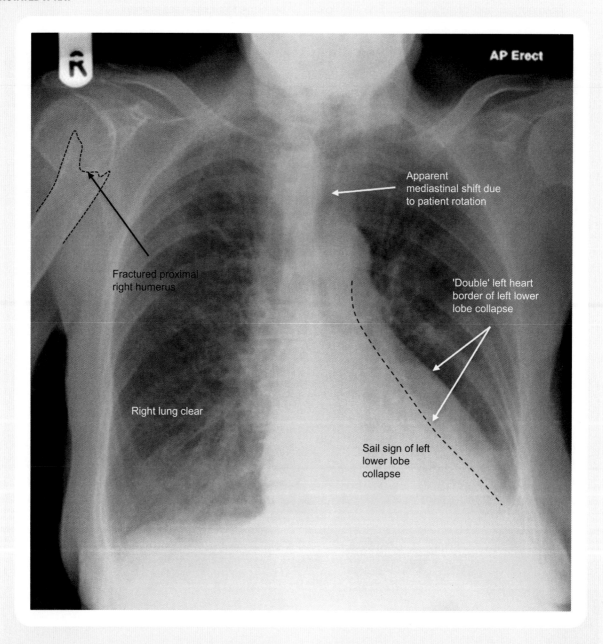

🔍 PRESENT YOUR FINDINGS

- This is an AP chest X-ray of an adult.
- There are no identifying markings on the X-ray. I would like to ensure that this is the correct patient, and to check the time and date when the X-ray was taken.
- The patient is rotated to the left. It is otherwise a technically adequate X-ray, with satisfactory penetration and inspiratory achievement. There are no important areas cut off the X-ray.
- There is increased left-sided retrocardiac density, the appearance of a double left heart border and loss of clarity of the left hemidiaphragm. These findings

are in keeping with the sail sign of left lower lobe collapse.
- The left costophrenic angle is blunted, in keeping with a small pleural effusion.
- The remaining right lung and left lung are clear.
- There is apparent shift of the mediastinum to the left due to patient rotation. The mediastinal and cardiac contours are otherwise unremarkable.
- There is no free subdiaphragmatic gas.
- Within the partially imaged right humerus, there is a displaced fracture through the surgical neck. It is difficult to assess the bone texture at this site. The bone texture elsewhere appears normal.

IN SUMMARY – This chest X-ray shows a left lower lobe collapse. The cause of this is not visible on the X-ray; however, given the clinical history, I am concerned that there is an underlying malignancy. Additionally, there is a displaced fracture through the surgical neck of the right humerus. Whilst the bone texture at this site appears relatively normal, given the lung findings, we must consider a pathological fracture from a metastasis.

QUESTIONS

1. Which of the following malignancies could cause the chest X-ray appearances in this patient?
   A) Primary bronchogenic carcinoma
   B) Breast cancer
   C) Thyroid cancer
   D) Colon cancer
   E) Prostate cancer
2. Which of the following is/are causes of a left lower lobe collapse?
   A) Lymph node enlargement
   B) Endoluminal bronchial mass
   C) Inhaled foreign body
   D) Mucous plug
   E) Pancoast tumour
3. Which of the following is/are malignant causes of a pathological fracture?
   A) Multiple myeloma
   B) Unicameral bone cyst
   C) Paget disease
   D) Chondromyxoid fibroma
   E) Osteosarcoma
4. The following tests should be considered to investigate this patient further:
   A) Lateral chest X-ray
   B) CT scan
   C) Bronchoscopy
   D) MRCP scan
   E) X-rays of the right shoulder and humerus
5. The patient has undergone further tests which confirm a lung tumour at the left hilum, a pathological fracture of the right proximal humerus and several liver metastases. Which of the following is/are possible treatment options?
   A) Chemotherapy
   B) Radiotherapy
   C) Antibiotics to treat the lobar collapse
   D) Surgical resection of the primary lung tumour
   E) Surgical fixation of the humeral fracture

Continue

CASE 2.17   *Contd.*

ANSWERS TO QUESTIONS

1. Which of the following malignancies could cause the chest X-ray appearances in this patient?

The correct answers are **A) Primary bronchogenic carcinoma, B) Breast cancer, C) Thyroid cancer and D) Colon cancer**.

Lobar collapse has a variety of causes, but with the clinical history available and the findings of a probably pathological fracture, we must consider malignancy as the top differential. There are various tumours which can result in these X-ray appearances.

A) Primary bronchogenic carcinoma – Correct. A primary bronchogenic carcinoma can occur in the bronchial tree or the lung parenchyma. When large enough, these tumours can obstruct the lumen of that bronchus (either directly or by extrinsic compression), leading to reduced airflow distally and collapse of the affected pulmonary lobe/segment. The presence of malignancy often also leads to an impaired immune system, and patients may then develop a secondary respiratory tract infection. Bone metastases from lung cancer can result in pathological fractures. Lung cancer classically causes lytic bone metastases, but about 15% can be mixed lytic and sclerotic metastases.

B) Breast cancer – Correct. Breast cancer can metastasise to any part of the body, and when it affects the lung, it may involve the bronchus with an endoluminal deposit, leading to lobar collapse. Another possible mechanism of lobar collapse is extrinsic compression of a bronchus by enlarged lymph nodes. Bone metastases from breast cancer are typically lytic, but 25% are mixed lytic and sclerotic.

C) Thyroid cancer – Correct. There are four histological types of thyroid cancer – papillary, follicular, medullary and anaplastic. Similar to breast cancer, thyroid malignancy can metastasise and form endobronchial deposits, leading to lobar collapse. Bone metastases from thyroid cancer are usually mixed lytic and sclerotic.

D) Colon cancer – Correct. Colon cancer often metastasises to the liver and lungs. It rarely metastasises to bone, but if it does occur, then it usually leads to lytic metastases which can result in a pathological fracture.

E) Prostate cancer – Incorrect. Prostate cancer typically causes sclerotic bone metastases.

❗ KEY POINT

It is easy to not assess the X-ray fully once you have identified an abnormality you think is responsible for the clinical findings. This phenomenon is known as 'satisfaction of search'. It is important, however, to review the X-ray comprehensively, as there may be other significant pathologies.

2. Which of the following is/are causes of a left lower lobe collapse?

The correct answers are **A) Lymph node enlargement, B) Endoluminal bronchial mass, C) Inhaled foreign body and D) Mucous plug**.

A bronchus or bronchiole can be occluded by three methods – extrinsic pathology compressing the tube walls from the outside; pathology in the tube wall becoming large enough to push into the lumen, causing occlusion; and a lesion within the lumen causing blockage. Blockage of a bronchus or bronchiole can result in distal collapse. This occurs because that lobe or segment of lung cannot be ventilated, and as the gas within the distal bronchial tree is resorbed, the area of lung will collapse. The causes of lobar collapse include malignancy and nonmalignant causes.

A) Lymph node enlargement – Correct. Lymph nodes are parts of the immune system which 'filter' the blood. They can become enlarged due to infection, inflammatory conditions (such as sarcoidosis) or malignancy. At the lung hilum, the bronchi are surrounded by lymph nodes. If the lymphadenopathy is large enough, it can encircle the bronchus and lead to extrinsic compression with lobar collapse.

B) Endoluminal bronchial mass – Correct. If a tumour arises intraluminally within the bronchus, then it may grow large enough to obstruct the lumen of that tube. Squamous cell carcinoma is the commonest malignant tumour to arise in the airways. Papillomas and hamartomas are benign tumours of the airways. Thyroid, oesophageal and lung cancer can all spread directly into the airways by local extension.

C) Inhaled foreign body – Correct. A foreign body, such as a peanut, can sometimes be inhaled into the lower respiratory tract and become lodged within a bronchi, occluding its lumen and leading to distal collapse. Foreign bodies are rarely visible on chest X-ray. If suspected, bronchoscopy may be required to confirm the diagnosis and remove the foreign body. The right lower lobe is the bronchus most likely to be affected by an inhaled foreign body due to its straight course and wider diameter.

D) Mucous plug – Correct. Mucous plugs can result in endoluminal obstruction of a bronchus/bronchiole with distal collapse. Patients with cystic fibrosis or bronchiectasis who get viscid secretions can also present in a similar way. They can also occur postoperatively if the patient is unable to cough effectively due to pain. Treatment involves chest physiotherapy to dislodge the mucous plug.

E) Pancoast tumour – Incorrect. A Pancoast tumour affects the apex of the upper lobes of the lungs. They can lead to rib bony erosion and may infiltrate the nearby brachial plexus, but due to their location, it will not directly cause lower lobe collapse.

❶ KEY POINT

The treatment of a lobar collapse is directed at the cause – chest physiotherapy for a mucous plug, bronchoscopic removal for a foreign body and treatment of any underlying malignancy.

3. Which of the following is/are malignant causes of a pathological fracture?
   The correct answers are **A) Multiple myeloma and E) Osteosarcoma**.
   A pathological fracture is a fracture occurring in abnormal bone. Because the bone is abnormal and weakened, pathological fractures can occur with significantly less force. Pathological fractures occurring within normal bone most commonly affect the vertebrae, hip and wrist. The causes of pathological fractures can be benign or malignant and involve focal or diffuse processes. Osteoporosis is the commonest cause of pathological fractures.
   A) Multiple myeloma – Correct. Multiple myeloma is a malignant cancer of plasma cells. The abnormal cells collect in the bone marrow, where they interfere with the normal production of blood cells, as well as structurally weakening the bone. Multiple myeloma can result in bone pain and pathological fractures, anaemia, renal failure and neurological symptoms.
   B) Unicameral bone cyst – Incorrect. Unicameral bone cysts are also known as simple bone cysts. They are fluid-filled areas within bone which often present as a pathological fracture. They are benign lesions.
   C) Paget disease – Incorrect. Paget disease is a benign abnormality of bone turnover (osteoblasts and osteoclasts). It often results in increased bone deposition, with thickened cortices affecting the pelvis and femurs. Pathological fractures can occur and usually involve the vertebrae. Malignant degeneration of Paget disease does occur, but it is very rare (<1%).
   D) Chondromyxoid fibroma – Incorrect. Chondromyxoid fibromas are rare bone tumours which have abnormal fibrous deposition within areas of bone. They can result in pathological fractures but are benign tumours.
   E) Osteosarcoma – Correct. Osteosarcoma is a primary malignant bone tumour after multiple myeloma. It typically affects adolescents and young adults and usually occurs around the knee. It has an aggressive appearance, with bone destruction and periosteal reaction, and can result in pathological fractures.

❶ KEY POINT

Osteoporosis is the commonest cause of a pathological fracture. Remember that osteoporosis is a diagnosis made by dual-energy X-ray absorptiometry (DEXA) scanning; it is not possible to diagnose on X-rays. If the cortices appear thin on an X-ray, you can thus state there is osteopaenia, but you cannot tell if there is osteoporosis.

4. The following tests should be considered to investigate this lady further:
   The correct answers are **B) CT scan, C) Bronchoscopy and E) X-rays of the right shoulder and humerus**.
   This patient needs further investigation to determine the cause of the lobar collapse and identify whether the fracture is pathological.
   A) Lateral chest X-ray – Incorrect. Whilst a lateral chest X-ray would confirm the lobar collapse, it is unlikely to identify the cause. Further imaging with CT will still be required, and thus a lateral X-ray will give the patient an additional, albeit relatively small, radiation dose without taking us any further.
   B) CT scan – Correct. The chest X-ray combined with the clinical history raises concern about an underlying malignant process. CT of the chest, abdomen and pelvis will help confirm this and allow other involved areas, such as the liver or adrenals, to be identified. This staging process helps to determine suitability of treatment options, and gives clinicians an idea of prognosis.
   C) Bronchoscopy – Correct. A bronchoscopy would be ideal, as it will allow direct visualisation of the pathology causing the left lower lobe collapse, and therefore differentiation between a tumour and a mucous plug. Additionally, it would permit a biopsy of any tumour to be obtained, which would help guide further treatment. A bronchoscopy is undertaken by an experienced thoracic physician after considering the benefits and risks of the procedure dependent on patient co-morbidities and frailty.
   D) MRCP scan – Incorrect. Magnetic resonance cholangiopancreatography is an MRI scan of the gallbladder and biliary system. It is, in simple terms, the MRI version of an ERCP. It uses a heavily T2-weighted MRI protocol, in which fluid (including bile) is bright and gallstones are dark, to get clear images of the biliary system in patients with gallstones and suspected obstructive jaundice. This test is not needed here, as there is no mention of biliary dysfunction.
   E) X-rays of the right shoulder and humerus – Correct. The chest X-ray has only partially imaged the right shoulder fracture. Further dedicated views are required to assess the type of fracture (simple or comminuted) and any displacement. It will also allow an assessment of the underlying bone to see if there is a lytic lesion at the fracture site. Images of the entire humerus are important to exclude any other pathological lesions in the shaft of the humerus.

5. The patient has undergone further tests, which confirm a lung tumour at the left hilum, a pathological fracture of the right proximal humerus and several liver metastases. Which of the following is/are possible treatment options?
   The correct answers are **A) Chemotherapy, B) Radiotherapy and E) Surgical fixation of the humeral fracture**.
   The treatment of cancer depends on its type, including histology, spread (staging), the co-morbidities of the

Continue

CASE **2.17**   *Contd.*

patient and the patient's wishes. In this case, we must also think about the appropriate management for the humeral fracture. The specific details of these treatments are beyond the expected knowledge of a medical student/junior doctor, but a rough idea is helpful.

A) Chemotherapy – Correct. Chemotherapy is a systemic treatment using cytotoxic antineoplastic drugs. The chemotherapy agent/agents (often given in combinations) is/are usually delivered via the peripheral venous system. Chemotherapy can have a detrimental effect on normal tissues, leading to side effects. The choice of chemotherapeutic agent is determined by the type of cancer and its histology. Sometimes chemotherapy is used in isolation, and sometimes in combination with radiotherapy and surgery.

B) Radiotherapy – Correct. Some histological types of cancer are radiosensitive. In this case, radiotherapy may be useful to deliver to the humeral metastasis; if not, then an orthopaedic technique such as internal fixation may be required.

C) Antibiotics to treat the lobar collapse – Incorrect. The lobar collapse is caused by mechanical obstruction of the bronchus by the tumour. This does increase the risk of distal infection; however, unless there is evidence of additional infection, antibiotics are not required.

D) Surgical resection of the primary lung tumour – Incorrect. Surgical resection of a lung tumour is a procedure usually with curative intent. In this case, the patient has liver and bone metastases. Surgery is therefore not indicated in this case.

E) Surgical fixation of the humeral fracture – Correct. Proximal humeral fractures can be treated surgically or nonsurgically, depending on the type of fracture, the degree of displacement and the comorbidities of the patient. Pathological fractures are often fixed surgically to ensure that they heal.

❶ KEY POINT

The management of patients with lung cancer is often complicated, and treatment decisions are usually made in a MDT meeting, in which physicians, including oncologists, thoracic surgeons, radiologists, pathologists and other healthcare professionals can discuss each case.

IMPORTANT LEARNING POINTS

- Always look carefully at the entire X-ray, even if you have found an abnormality which would account for the patient's clinical findings.
- Lobar collapses can be due to malignant and nonmalignant processes, and the treatment is determined by the underlying cause.
- Pathological fractures can also be due to malignant and nonmalignant causes, with the commonest being osteoporosis.
- The management of cancer patients is often complex, and treatment decisions are usually made at MDT meetings.

CASE 2.18

A 70-year-old female with a background of breast cancer, for which she received chemotherapy, has been admitted to intensive care with increasing shortness of breath. A chest X-ray has been performed to assess the position of the lines which have been placed.

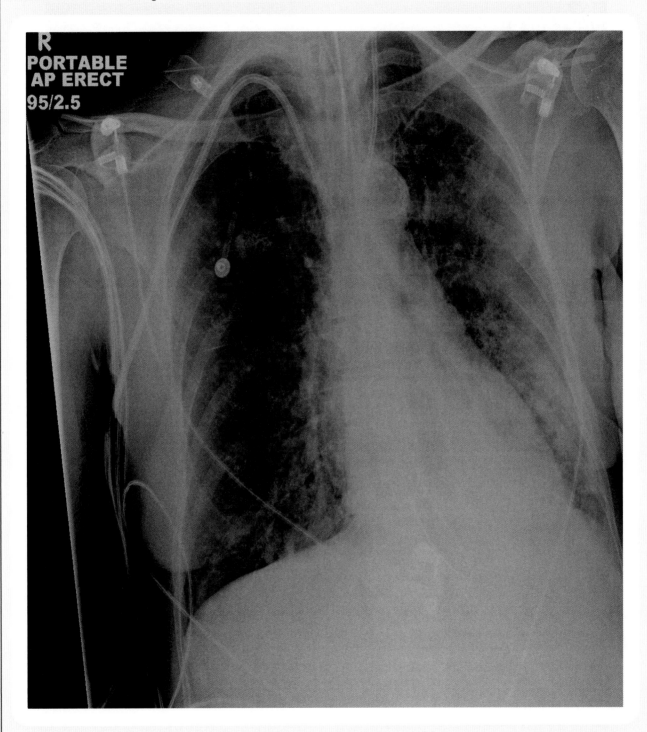

Continue

CASE **2.18** *Contd.*

ANNOTATED X-RAY

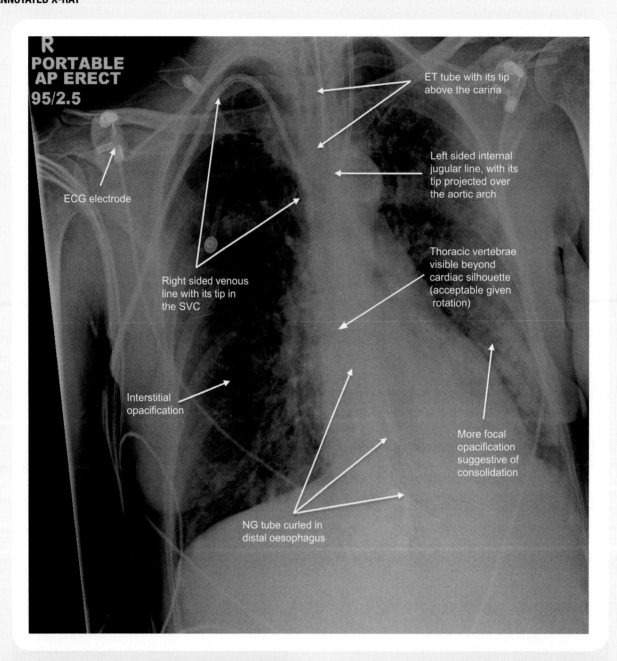

R
PORTABLE
AP ERECT
95/2.5

ET tube with its tip above the carina

Left sided internal jugular line, with its tip projected over the aortic arch

ECG electrode

Thoracic vertebrae visible beyond cardiac silhouette (acceptable given rotation)

Right sided venous line with its tip in the SVC

Interstitial opacification

More focal opacification suggestive of consolidation

NG tube curled in distal oesophagus

🔍 **PRESENT YOUR FINDINGS**

- This is a portable AP erect chest X-ray of an adult patient.
- There are no patient identifiers on the X-ray. I would like to confirm the patient's details and the time and date when the X-ray was taken.
- Apart from slight patient rotation, it is a technically adequate X-ray.
- There is a left-sided internal jugular line in situ. Its tip is projected over the aortic arch. This could be due to patient rotation; however, it may be due to misplacement into a central artery.
- The NG tube is coiled in the distal oesophagus and needs resiting.

- There is a tunnelled right-sided central line (Hickmann line) with its tip projected over the superior vena cava.
- The tip of the ET tube is above the carina.
- There is extensive bilateral interstitial opacification, in keeping with pulmonary oedema. There is more focal consolidation in the left lower zone, which may indicate pneumonia.
- No pneumothorax.
- The cardiac and mediastinal contours are unremarkable given the patient rotation.
- There is no free subdiaphragmatic gas.
- There is no abnormality of the bones or soft tissues.

IN SUMMARY – This chest X-ray shows that the NG tube is coiled in the distal oesophagus and needs to be removed. The left internal jugular line is projected over the aortic arch. This may be due to patient rotation; however, a repeat, nonrotated X-ray is needed to help exclude misplacement in a central artery. The other lines are in satisfactory positions. Additionally, there is pulmonary oedema and left lower zone consolidation.

QUESTIONS

1. An NG tube has been passed for feeding in a patient with dysphagia due to a distal oesophageal stricture. Which of the following is/are correct?
   A) It is safe to use for feeding as long as it was passed easily and the patient is not coughing
   B) It is safe to use if the pH of the aspirate is less than 7 (i.e. acidic)
   C) A chest X-ray is always required to confirm position
   D) As well as after insertion, the position of the NG tube should be confirmed before each feed, or anytime it has been dislodged
   E) If it is difficult to pass the NG tube on the ward, then this can be performed using fluoroscopic guidance in the radiology department

2. Which of the following corresponds to a correctly positioned NG tube on a chest X-ray?
   A) Coiled in the oropharynx
   B) Tip projected over the lower mediastinum
   C) NG tube projected over the mediastinum, with the tip below the left hemidiaphragm over the gastric bubble
   D) Projected over the right lung
   E) Tip projected just below the left hemidiaphragm

3. When intubating a patient with an endotracheal tube, which of the following is/are correct?
   A) Ideally, a trained anaesthetist should perform the procedure, using a laryngoscope
   B) There is one size of tube available for an adult and one size for a child

C) The size of the endotracheal tube refers to the internal diameter of the tube
D) The correct position for the tube tip in an adult is about 5 cm above the carina, or midway between the clavicles and the carina
E) It is most often malpositioned in the right main bronchus

4. Which of the following is/are true regarding central venous lines?
   A) They can be inserted via a subclavian or internal jugular vein approach
   B) Ultrasound can be used to visualise placement of the needle directly, as part of the Seldinger technique
   C) The correct position of the tube tip is within the right atrium
   D) A recognised complication of insertion is pneumothorax
   E) Central venous lines should always be used for taking blood, as this prevents the need for peripheral venepuncture, with its associated pain/discomfort

5. Reviewing the postinsertion chest X-ray, you think that the central venous line may have been mistakenly placed into an artery. What is the most appropriate initial step?
   A) As long as it bleeds and flushes, it is safe to use
   B) Immediately remove and resite
   C) Analyse a sample taken from the line on an arterial blood gas machine to confirm whether venous or arterial
   D) Request an urgent CT for confirmation of the line position
   E) Request a linogram (contrast is injected into the line and X-rays taken) to confirm line position

Continue

CASE 2.18 *Contd.*

ANSWERS TO QUESTIONS

1. An NG tube has been passed for feeding in a patient with dysphagia due to a distal oesophageal stricture. Which of the following is/are correct?

   The correct answers are **D) As well as after insertion, the position of the NG tube should be confirmed before each feed, or any time it has been dislodged and E) If it is difficult to pass the NG tube on the ward, then this can be performed using fluoroscopic guidance in the radiology department**.

   Feeding via a misplaced NG tube can have potentially fatal consequences if feed enters the lung and results in a pneumonia/pneumonitis. Such events should not happen, and, as such, they are referred to as 'never events'. Knowledge of how to confirm the correct placement of an NG tube is therefore vital.

   A) It is safe to use for feeding as long as it was passed easily and the patient is not coughing – Incorrect. As NG tubes are inserted blindly on the wards, there is no way of confirming their position clinically. An NG tube which is misplaced into the trachea and bronchial tree can be passed easily. It may cause coughing during the placement, but this may settle. Additionally, the syringe test or whoosh test, which involves injecting a syringe full of air into the NG tube and auscultating over the stomach, should not be used to confirm position.

   B) It is safe to use if pH of the aspirate is less than 7 (i.e. acidic) – Incorrect. The pH of NG tube aspirates can be used; however, the pH must be less than 5.5 to ensure correct placement. Medications such as proton pump inhibitors can alter the pH and make this method of assessment difficult.

   C) A chest X-ray is always required to confirm position – Incorrect. The position of most NG tubes can be confirmed using the pH test. If the pH is >5.5, or there is no aspirate, a chest X-ray should be performed. Chest X-ray confirmation of NG tube position should also be routinely performed in intensive care patients, those with swallowing problems and confused patients.

   D) As well as after insertion, the position of the NG tube should be confirmed before each feed or any time it has been dislodged – Correct. It is important to ensure the NG tube is correctly positioned after insertion, before each feed, and following any episode in which the tube may have been dislodged (e.g. vomiting).

   E) If it is difficult to pass the NG tube on the ward, then this can be performed using fluoroscopic guidance in the radiology department – Correct. Most NG tubes can be easily passed blindly on the ward. However, it may be difficult to do so, particularly in patients with oesophageal strictures. In such cases, the NG tube can be inserted in the radiology department using fluoroscopic screening. This uses continuous or intermittent X-rays to image the NG tube as it is being inserted. It helps the operator negotiate any strictures and allows confirmation of the tube position at the end of the procedure. Occasionally, in particularly difficult cases, a slippery flexible guidewire may be inserted across the stricture initially, with the NG tube passed over this.

❗ KEY POINT

It is important you are aware of how the position of an NG tube can be confirmed. In most patients, this can be done on the ward by confirming an acidic aspirate (pH <5.5). If there is any doubt, a chest X-ray can be performed.

2. Which of the following corresponds to a correctly positioned NG tube on a chest X-ray?

   The correct answer is **C) NG tube projected over the mediastinum, with the tip below the left hemidiaphragm over the gastric bubble**.

   In 2012, nearly 10% of the incidents reported to the National Patient Safety Agency related to NG tube placement. As discussed in question 1, the chest X-ray is used in cases in which the position of the NG tube cannot be confirmed on pH testing or where there is ongoing doubt. It is therefore important to know what a correctly positioned NG tube should look like on a chest X-ray, and what the common appearances for misplaced tubes are.

   A) Coiled in the oropharynx – Incorrect. The NG tube can be coiled in the oropharynx. This is usually evident clinically, as the patient will be coughing and the tube is usually visible. However, in patients who are unconscious or have lost their gag reflex, this may not be so obvious. If the NG is coiled in the oropharynx, it should be removed and resited. On a chest X-ray, the tube will be projected over the upper central part of the chest. It may not actually be included on the chest X-ray if it is coiled too high up.

   B) Tip projected over the lower mediastinum – Incorrect. This finding is in keeping with the tip of the NG tube being within the distal oesophagus. If used to feed in this position, there is a risk that the feed will be aspirated, especially if the patient is supine. If the NG tube is required to decompress the stomach and small bowel, it will not be able to achieve this, as its tip is not beyond the gastro-oesophageal junction. It needs to be advanced so that its tip will be well beyond the gastro-oesophageal junction.

   C) NG tube projected over the mediastinum, with the tip below the left hemidiaphragm over the gastric bubble – Correct. This is the appearance of a correctly positioned NG tube. The tip should be well below the left hemidiaphragm. It should also clearly bisect the carina and cross the diaphragm in the midline.

   D) Projected over the right lung – Incorrect. This indicates that the NG tube has been misplaced into the trachea and through the right main bronchus into the lung (NG tubes are more likely to pass down the right main bronchus than the left, as it is wider and more vertically orientated). This is a potentially fatal situation, as instilling feed in this position can result in pneumonia and pneumonitis. The tube needs to be removed and resited immediately.

Often, misplaced NG tubes like this will be detected by the radiographer performing the X-ray, who can then remove the tube whilst the patient is in the radiology department. However, you should not assume this to be the case.

E) Tip projected just below the left hemidiaphragm – Incorrect. On first inspection, you may think that this is a correctly positioned NG tube. However, you must remember that the diaphragm curves front to back, as well as medial to lateral. The gastro-oesophageal junction is therefore actually a few centimetres below the top of the left hemidiaphragm, as seen on a frontal chest X-ray. This NG tube should be advanced 5 to 10 cm, and a repeat X-ray should be considered if there is still doubt about position.

! KEY POINTS

1. It is vital that you be sure that an NG tube is correctly sited, particularly if it is to be used for feeding. If you are in doubt, do not use the tube until a senior or a radiologist has reviewed the X-ray.
2. Other rare complications of NG tube placement include placement through a base of skull fracture (a possibility in a patient experiencing trauma) into the brain, and through an oesophageal perforation into the posterior mediastinum. These are very rare but have serious consequences.

3. When intubating a patient with an endotracheal tube, which of the following is/are correct?
   The correct answers are **A) Ideally, a trained anaesthetist should perform the procedure using a laryngoscope, C) The size of the endotracheal tube refers to the internal diameter of the tube, D) The correct position for the tube tip in an adult is about 5 cm above the carina, or midway between the clavicles and the carina and E) It is most often malpositioned in the right main bronchus**.
   Intubation is a difficult skill which should only be performed by trained practitioners. It is useful to have some knowledge of this procedure and potential complications.

   A) Ideally, a trained anaesthetist should perform the procedure using a laryngoscope – Correct. A trained anaesthetist should perform the procedure of endotracheal intubation because it is a complex procedure with many possible complications – these include breaking/chipping teeth with the laryngoscope, perforating the upper oropharynx and intubating the oesophagus.
   B) There is one size of tube available for an adult and one size for a child – Incorrect. There are many different tube sizes for adult and paediatric patients. It is important to use a correctly sized tube to ensure a good seal with the trachea.
   C) The size of the endotracheal tube refers to the internal diameter of the tube – Correct. A size '5' tube thus

refers to an endotracheal tube with an internal diameter of 5 mm.

D) The correct position for the tube tip in an adult is about 5 cm above the carina, or midway between the clavicles and the carina – Correct. The tube tip should be above the carina and at sufficient distance to allow movements in the tube position when the patient flexes/extends their neck.

E) It is most often malpositioned in the right main bronchus – Correct. This is the most common position for a misplaced endotracheal tube and is due to the right main bronchus being straighter and at a less acute angle relative to the trachea than the left main bronchus. The left lung will not be ventilated if the right main bronchus has been intubated. This results in collapse of the entire left lung.

4. Which of the following is/are true regarding central venous lines?
   The correct answers are **A) They can be inserted via a subclavian or internal jugular vein approach, B) Ultrasound can be used to visualise placement of the needle directly, as part of the Seldinger technique and D) A recognised complication of insertion is pneumothorax**.
   A central venous line is a catheter which has its tip in one of the central veins (superior or inferior vena cava). This can be used to provide venous access in patients who require frequent blood sampling, access to large central veins for administration of IV fluids and medications, and central venous pressure monitoring. A postinsertion chest X-ray should be performed to assess the position of the line and detect any other complications, such as a pneumothorax.

   A) They can be inserted via a subclavian or internal jugular vein approach – Correct. The internal jugular veins are most frequently used, as they have the lowest risk of complications. If these are not suitable, due to thrombosis for example, a subclavian vein may be used. A PICC is a type of central line which, as the name suggests, is inserted through a peripheral vein – usually the basilic vein in the arm. It is then positioned so that its tip is in a central vein. Umbilical vein catheters are a type of central venous catheter which can be used in neonates.
   Most central lines are temporary and have to be removed or changed within 7 days due to the risk of infection. Longer-lasting central venous catheters can be inserted in patients requiring prolonged central venous access, often for total parenteral nutrition or certain types of chemotherapy. Such lines are tunnelled under the skin before entering the venous system, which helps prevent infection from entering the venous system.
   B) Ultrasound can be used to visualise placement of the needle directly, as part of the Seldinger technique – Correct. Ultrasound provides direct visualisation of the vein and helps reduce complications when inserting central lines. It also allows the veins to be assessed prior to cannulation, to identify any potential

Continue

CASE **2.18**   *Contd.*

problems, such as thrombosis. In the Seldinger technique, a needle is initially placed in the vein. A guidewire is then passed through the needle into the vein, and the needle is then removed. The catheter can then be fed over the guide directly into the vein.

C) The correct position of the tube tip is within the right atrium – Incorrect. The tips of central lines should be in the mid or lower superior vena cava. This lies on the right side of the mediastinum, just above the right atrium. If the line lies within the right atrium, it can touch the sinoatrial node or bundle of His, resulting in arrhythmias. The exception to the rule is umbilical vein catheters (in neonates), which should be positioned in the upper inferior vena cava.

D) A recognised complication of insertion is pneumothorax – Correct. This is a common complication, particularly with subclavian venous catheters, and should be actively looked for in the follow-up chest X-ray.

E) Central venous lines should always be used for taking blood, as this prevents the need for peripheral venepuncture, with its associated pain/discomfort – Incorrect. Some central lines have multiple lumens. In these cases, venepuncture can usually be performed using the designated lumen. If there is only a single lumen, it is usually best not to use it for venepuncture, as this can cause the line to become blocked, preventing it from being used for IV fluids/medications.

5. Reviewing the postinsertion chest X-ray, you think that the central venous line may have been mistakenly placed into an artery. What is the most appropriate initial step? The correct answer is **C) Analyse a sample taken from the line on an arterial blood gas machine to confirm whether venous or arterial**.

Accidental placement within a central artery, such as the common carotid artery at the neck or the subclavian artery, is a potential complication of central venous catheters. Instilling IV medication, such as total parenteral nutrition, into an arterial line has serious consequences, including stroke. Knowledge of the normal venous and arterial anatomy on chest X-ray is thus needed to determine if a venous catheter is misplaced line.

Right-sided internal jugular or subclavian vein lines should traverse the right brachiocephalic vein, which forms the superior right border of the mediastinum, directly down into the superior vena cava. If a right-sided central line crosses the midline of the mediastinum, you must consider whether it is within an artery (subclavian or common carotid) and is passing into the aortic arch. See p. 11 for an example X-ray of correctly positioned right- and left-sided central venous lines.

Left-sided internal jugular or subclavian vein lines need to run through the left brachiocephalic vein before entering the superior vena cava. The left brachiocephalic vein runs diagonally down the upper mediastinum from the

patient's left to right. Therefore if the catheter does not cross the midline of the mediastinum, you must consider whether it may be arterial and in the aorta.

A) As long as it bleeds and flushes it is safe to use – Incorrect. Arterially placed lines will bleed and flush, so this does not tell you whether the line is venous or arterial.

B) Immediately remove and resite – Incorrect. If the line is arterial, it will need removal and resiting. However, you may not be able to compress the puncture site in the artery adequately, as it may be within the mediastinum or under the clavicle, therefore raising the potential for significant haemorrhage. If the line is arterial, you should discuss the situation with a senior clinician and potentially the cardiothoracic surgeons before removing it.

C) Analyse a sample taken from the line on an arterial blood gas machine to confirm whether venous or arterial – Correct. The position of a central catheter is not always clear cut on a chest X-ray. Analysing a sample of blood from the catheter for oxygen saturations and $PaO_2/PaCO_2$ is a quick, simple method for helping to determine where the line is within an artery or vein.

D) Request an urgent CT for confirmation of the line position – Incorrect. There is usually enough information from the chest X-ray and blood gas analysis to determine whether the line is within an artery or vein. CT will allow further evaluation of the position of the line, if this is required.

E) Request a linogram (contrast is injected into the line and X-rays taken) to confirm line position – Incorrect. Again, this is not the most appropriate next step. Linograms are primarily used to check the patency of a previously inserted central venous catheter, and to look for other complications, such as fibrin sheath formation or fracture of the line.

IMPORTANT LEARNING POINTS

- The complications from misplaced lines can be serious.
- The position of most NG tubes can be confirmed using the pH test, but if there is doubt, a chest X-ray should be performed.
- The main complication of endotracheal tube insertion to be aware of is insertion too far, resulting in intubation of the right main bronchus.
- Central lines should have their tip in the mid or lower superior vena cava.
- If you think a central line may be arterial, assess a sample of blood using a blood gas machine and discuss urgently with your seniors.
- If you are in doubt about the position of any line, then you should discuss with your seniors or radiology.

CASE 2.19

A 45-year-old female presents to A&E with chest pain and light-headedness. Pulmonary embolism is suspected, and a chest X-ray is performed.

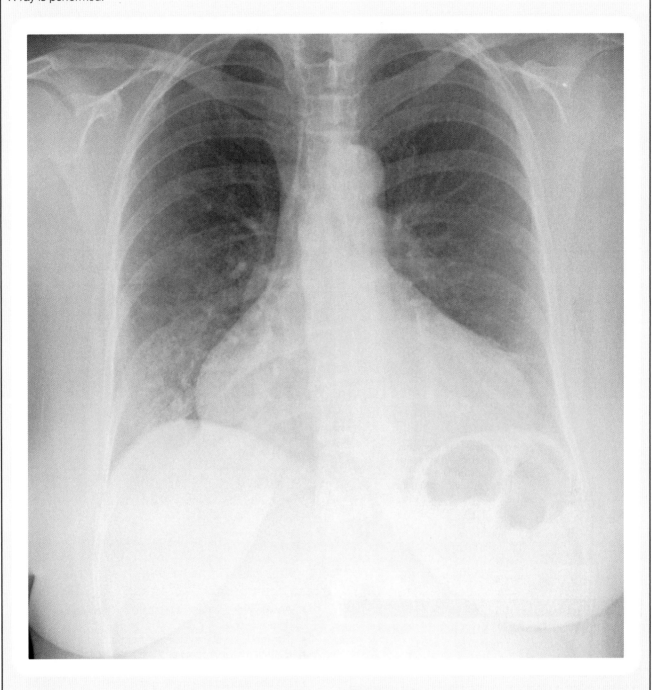

Continue

CASE **2.19** *Contd.*

ANNOTATED X-RAY

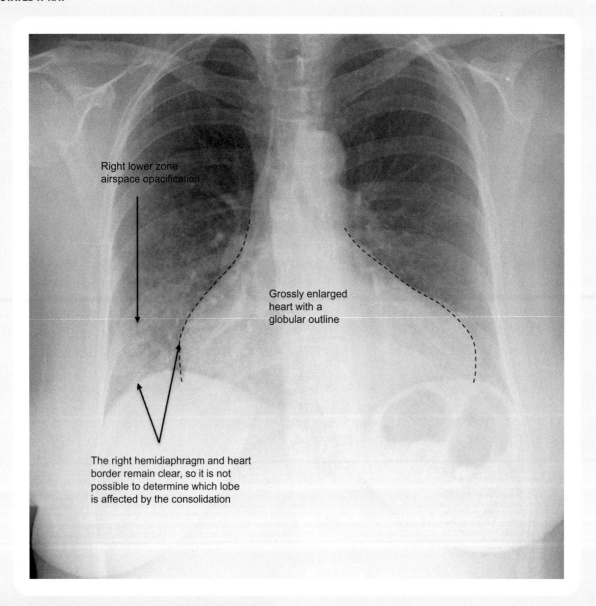

Right lower zone
airspace opacification

Grossly enlarged
heart with a
globular outline

The right hemidiaphragm and heart
border remain clear, so it is not
possible to determine which lobe
is affected by the consolidation

PRESENT YOUR FINDINGS

- This is a PA chest X-ray of an adult.
- There are no identifying markings. I would like to ensure this is the correct patient and check the date and time when the X-ray was taken.
- The patient is slightly rotated to the right. It is otherwise a technically adequate X-ray, with suitable penetration and a good inspiratory effort. The apex of the left lung is cut off.
- The most striking abnormality is the enlarged heart. In addition, it has a globular appearance, which is suggestive of a pericardial effusion.
- There is airspace opacification in the right lower zone in keeping with consolidation. Both the right hemidiaphragm and right heart border are clear, so it is not possible to locate this consolidation more accurately to a lobe. The lungs are otherwise clear.

- Allowing for the patient rotation, the trachea is unremarkable.
- The mediastinal contours are normal.
- Both hemidiaphragms and the costophrenic angles are clearly demarcated.
- No free subdiaphragmatic gas is seen.
- There is no abnormality of the imaged soft tissues or skeleton.

IN SUMMARY – This chest X-ray shows an enlarged, globular heart in keeping with a pericardial effusion. In addition, there is right lower zone consolidation. Both of these pathologies may be contributing to the patient's clinical condition. I would like to assess the patient for signs of haemodynamic instability and review any previous imaging to see if the pericardial effusion is new.

QUESTIONS

1. Which of the following regarding a pericardial effusion is correct?
   A) It is due to fluid accumulating in the myocardium
   B) The fluid accumulates outside of the parietal pericardium
   C) The fluid accumulates between the endocardium and myocardium
   D) The fluid accumulates between the visceral and parietal pericardium
   E) The fluid accumulates within the pericardial fat

2. The causes of a pericardial effusion include which of the following?
   A) Renal failure
   B) Postmyocardial infarction
   C) Malignancy
   D) Hypothyroidism
   E) Viral infection such as Coxsackie virus

3. Which of the following clinical signs is/are in keeping with a pericardial effusion?
   A) Muffled heart sounds
   B) Hypotension
   C) Reduced jugular venous pulse
   D) Pericardial friction rub
   E) Rise in blood pressure on inspiration

4. Which of the following appearances on chest X-ray is consistent with a pericardial effusion?
   A) 'Egg on a string'–shaped heart
   B) Globular-shaped heart with a blurred right heart border and a sharp left heart border
   C) Snowman sign heart
   D) Globular heart with a sharp right heart border and a sharp left heart border
   E) Boot-shaped heart

5. Which of the following is/are correct regarding the treatment of a pericardial effusion?
   A) Not all pericardial effusions need active treatment
   B) Pericardial effusions are life-threatening and require urgent pericardiocentesis
   C) Aspirin and colchicine may be used
   D) Steroids are contraindicated
   E) Antibiotics can be used

Continue

CASE 2.19 *Contd.*

ANSWERS TO QUESTIONS

1. Which of the following regarding a pericardial effusion is correct?

   The correct answer is **D) The fluid accumulates between the visceral and parietal pericardium**.

   Normally, there is a small amount of fluid within the pericardial cavity. This is the area enclosed between the visceral pericardium (attached to the heart) and the parietal pericardium. A pericardial effusion is an abnormal collection of fluid within the pericardial cavity. As with other fluid collections, the constituents may be blood (red cells), pus (white cells), serum (no cells) or malignancy (cancer cells).

2. The causes of a pericardial effusion include which of the following?

   The correct answers are **A) Renal failure, B) Postmyocardial infarction, C) Malignancy, D) Hypothyroidism and E) Viral infection such as Coxsackie virus**.

   There are many different causes of a pericardial effusion. Other causes not mentioned in the question include idiopathic, trauma, postcardiac surgery, postradiotherapy, autoimmune disease such as rheumatoid arthritis and systemic lupus erythematosus, and medications such as hydralazine.

   A) Renal failure – Correct. Renal failure leads to fluid retention in the body, with an increase in the intravascular hydrostatic pressure. Hence fluid accumulates within the pericardial sac, as well as in other body compartments such as the pleural and abdominal cavities. A similar picture may be seen with cardiac failure (raised intravascular hydrostatic pressure) and liver failure (reduced plasma oncotic pressure, secondary to reduced albumin synthesis).

   B) Postmyocardial infarction – Correct. This may occur due to rupture of a wall, or secondary to immunologically mediated pericarditis. The latter is known as Dressler syndrome, and the classic presentation is with a triad of pericardial effusion, fever and pleuritic pain.

   C) Malignancy – Correct. Malignancy can result in a pericardial effusion via direct tumour extension, retrograde extension via the lymphatics or due to haematological seeding. Lung and breast cancer, as well as leukaemia and lymphoma, are the commonest malignant causes of a pericardial effusion.

   D) Hypothyroidism – Correct. This is a recognised cause. In hypothyroidism, there is albumin leak into interstitial and extracellular spaces due to capillary dysfunction, accompanied by poor lymphatic clearance due to poor lymphatic tone. The hypothyroid infiltrates that accumulate in the pericardial sac are rarely of a large enough volume to cause cardiac tamponade.

   E) Viral infection such as Coxsackie virus – Correct. Viral infections are the commonest cause of infectious pericarditis/pericardial effusions. Other infectious causes include bacterial (pneumococcal, staphylococcal, streptococcal), TB and fungal infections.

3. Which of the following clinical signs is/are in keeping with a pericardial effusion?

   The correct answers are **A) Muffled heart sounds, B) Hypotension and D) Pericardial friction rub**.

   The clinical signs associated with a pericardial effusion are related to its size and underlying cause. Small pericardial effusions will be difficult or impossible to detect on clinical examination, whereas large effusions can result in cardiac tamponade and cardiac arrest.

   A) Muffled heart sounds – Correct. This is one of the triad of classic findings of pericardial tamponade. In the same way a pleural effusion will reduce the breath sounds heard when auscultating the chest, a pericardial effusion will result in muffled heart sounds.

   B) Hypotension – Correct. This is another part of the classic triad of clinical findings. As the effusion enlarges, it compromises cardiac output (reduced stroke volume, as the heart is not able to contract efficiently). This results in hypotension. There will be a reflex tachycardia as the body attempts to increase the cardiac output.

   C) Reduced jugular venous pulse – Incorrect. Cardiac tamponade causes an elevated jugular venous pulse – this is the third part of the classic triad. The increased pressure from the fluid in the pericardium impairs venous return to the heart, resulting in a raised jugular venous pulse. This helps distinguish cardiac tamponade as the cause of shock (hypotension/tachycardia) from hypovolaemia, which will have a reduced jugular venous pulse.

   D) Pericardial friction rub – Correct. This is found in pericarditis, which often results in a pericardial effusion.

   E) Rise in blood pressure on inspiration – Incorrect. Normally, there is a small drop in systolic blood pressure during inspiration. This is due to the effects of the relative negative intrathoracic pressure (during inspiration) on venous return to the right side of the heart and on the pulmonary circulation. Cardiac tamponade can result in a larger than normal drop in blood pressure during inspiration (>10 mmHg). This is due to the detrimental effects of the tamponade on stroke volume and left ventricular filling. This phenomenon is known as pulsus paradoxus. It can also be seen in asthma, obstructive sleep apnoea and croup.

🛈 KEY POINTS

1. Pericardial effusion may be asymptomatic. If large enough, it can result in cardiac tamponade.

2. The classic triad of cardiac tamponade is known as Beck's Triad and consists of muffled heart sounds, hypotension and a raised jugular venous pulse. Pulsus paradoxus is also a feature.

4. Which of the following appearances on chest X-ray is consistent with a pericardial effusion?

   The correct answer is **D) Globular heart with a sharp right heart border and a sharp left heart border**.

A pericardial effusion can be detected on chest X-ray due to its effects on heart shape. Echocardiogram, CT and MRI are all more sensitive than plain X-rays for identifying pericardial effusions.

A) 'Egg on a string'–shaped heart – Incorrect. This is the classic finding in transposition of the great vessels, a type of congenital heart disease.

B) Globular-shaped heart with a blurred right heart border and a sharp left heart border – Incorrect. Pericardial effusions do result in a globular heart, but the heart borders are typically sharp. See D for more details.

C) Snowman sign heart – Incorrect. This rare appearance of the heart is due to total anomalous pulmonary venous return.

D) Globular heart with a sharp right heart border and a sharp left heart border – Correct. The fluid in the pericardial space leads to an enlarged cardiac silhouette, classically with a globular shape. This globular shape of the cardiac silhouette is often described as the 'water bottle sign'. It is also said to reduce the cardiac pulsation, leading to reduced movement and a sharp cardiac outline on chest X-rays. Remember that there needs to be approximately 300 mL of pericardial fluid before there will be detectable changes on a chest X-ray.

E) Boot-shaped heart – Incorrect. The boot-shaped heart is typically seen with tetralogy of Fallot.

❶ KEY POINTS

1. A globular heart with clear margins is the classic chest X-ray finding in pericardial effusion; however, other modalities, such as echocardiogram and CT, are more sensitive for detecting pericardial fluid.
2. A diagnostic pericardiocentesis may be performed to establish the aetiology of the pericardial effusion.

5. Which of the following is/are correct regarding the treatment of a pericardial effusion?
The correct answer is **A) Not all pericardial effusions need active treatment, C) Aspirin and colchicine may be used and E) Antibiotics can be used**.
The treatment of pericardial effusions depends on their size, the symptoms they are causing and the underlying cause.

A) Not all pericardial effusions need active treatment – Correct. If the pericardial effusion is small, the patient asymptomatic and there is no haemodynamic compromise, the patient may be treated conservatively with regular clinical and echocardiogram follow-up.

B) Pericardial effusions are life-threatening and require urgent pericardiocentesis – Incorrect. Whilst large pericardial effusions can result in cardiac tamponade necessitating urgent pericardiocentesis, this is not usually the case. If required, pericardiocentesis should ideally be performed under echocardiogram guidance. Patients with chronic large pericardial effusions may require repeated pericardiocentesis. If this is unsuccessful, a surgical option, such as a pleuropericardial window, may be required.

C) Aspirin and colchicine may be used – Correct. The medical management of pericardial effusions depends on the underlying cause. Most pericardial effusions are either virally induced or idiopathic. Such patients may be treated with aspirin or another nonsteroidal antiinflammatory drug if there is no haemodynamic compromise. Colchicine can be used in combination with aspirin, or as an alternative.

D) Steroids are contraindicated – Incorrect. Steroids can be used to treat patients with recurrent pericardial effusions which are unresponsive to aspirin or colchicine. They are also indicated in cases of pericardial effusion due to an underlying inflammatory or autoimmune cause.

E) Antibiotics can be used – Correct. IV antibiotics, combined with pericardial drainage, are indicated in patients with purulent pericardial effusions. TB pericardial effusions will require prolonged courses of anti-TB antibiotics.

❶ KEY POINTS

1. The treatment of pericardial effusions depends on their size and the underlying aetiology.
2. Patients who are haemodynamically compromised should be considered for urgent pericardiocentesis.

IMPORTANT LEARNING POINTS

- There are a variety of causes of pericardial effusions; however, viral infection and idiopathic are the most common types.
- Diagnosis is often made by the clinical findings and the finding of an enlarged, globular heart on chest X-ray.
- ECHO and CT provide a more accurate assessment for pericardial fluid.
- Treatment depends on the size and cause of the pericardial effusion. Large effusions causing haemodynamic compromise need to be treated urgently, often with pericardiocentesis.

CASE 2.20

A 70-year-old man presents with a cough and shortness of breath. A chest X-ray has been performed.

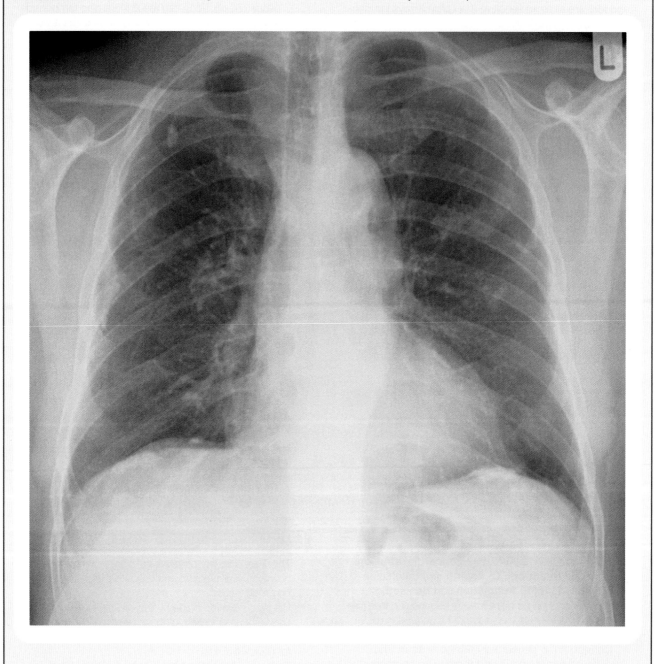

ANNOTATED X-RAY

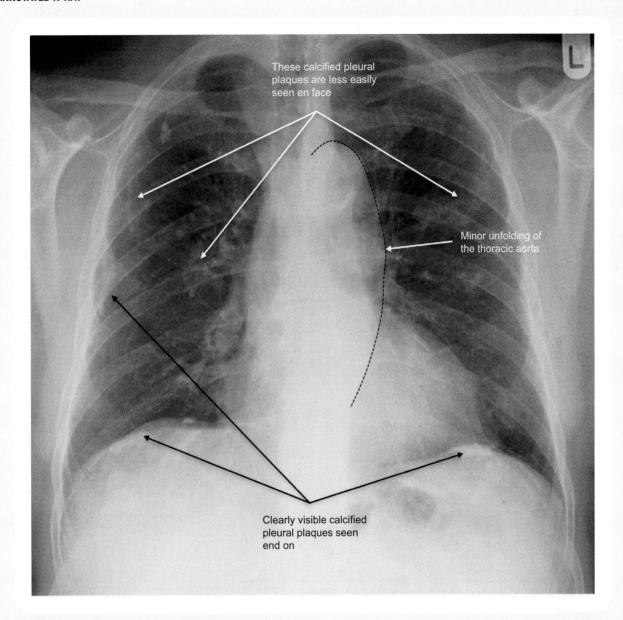

These calcified pleural plaques are less easily seen en face

Minor unfolding of the thoracic aorta

Clearly visible calcified pleural plaques seen end on

🔍 PRESENT YOUR FINDINGS

- This is a PA chest X-ray of an adult.
- There are no identifying markings. I would like to ensure that this is the correct patient, and to check the date and time when the X-ray was taken.
- The patient is slightly rotated to the right. It is otherwise a technically adequate X-ray, with adequate penetration and a good inspiratory effort. There are no important areas cut off at the edges of the X-ray.
- The most striking abnormalities are the areas of calcification on the hemidiaphragms and the right lateral chest wall, which are in keeping with calcified pleural plaques. There are further pleural plaques projected over the lungs.
- The lungs are otherwise clear, and there is no evidence of pleural effusions.

- Allowing for the minor patient rotation, the trachea is unremarkable.
- There is minor unfolding of the thoracic aorta.
- The heart is not enlarged, and the cardiac contours are normal.
- No free subdiaphragmatic gas is seen.
- There is no abnormality of the imaged soft tissues or skeleton.

IN SUMMARY – This chest X-ray shows bilateral calcified pleural plaques suggestive of previous asbestos exposure. No cause for the patient's breathlessness is identified.

Continue

CASE **2.20**   *Contd.*

QUESTIONS

1. Which of the following are causes of pleural calcification?
   A) Previous empyema
   B) Previous simple pleural effusion
   C) Previous radiotherapy
   D) Asbestos-related pleural disease
   E) Previous haemothorax

2. What is the commonest symptom relating to pleural plaques?
   A) Asymptomatic
   B) Haemoptysis
   C) Breathlessness
   D) Chest pain
   E) Weight loss

3. Which of the following is/are correct regarding the imaging of pleural plaques?
   A) Most pleural plaques are calcified
   B) They tend to spare the lung apices
   C) Chest X-ray will detect >75% of pleural plaques
   D) CT is more sensitive than chest X-ray for detecting pleural plaques
   E) The parietal pleura is most commonly involved

4. Which of the following can occur secondary to asbestos exposure?
   A) Mesothelioma
   B) Laryngeal carcinoma
   C) Round atelectasis
   D) Pulmonary fibrosis
   E) Emphysema

5. Which of the following cause calcification on a chest X-ray?
   A) Emphysema
   B) Previous varicella pneumonia
   C) Silicosis
   D) Mitral valve disease
   E) Early pulmonary artery hypertension

ANSWERS TO QUESTIONS

1. Which of the following are causes of pleural calcification?
   The correct answers are **A) Previous empyema, C) Previous radiotherapy, D) Asbestos-related pleural disease and E) Previous haemothorax**.
   Calcification on a chest X-ray may originate from the lung parenchyma, pleural space, mediastinal structures or overlying bone/soft tissues. Pleural calcification is most easily seen at the lateral chest wall and the diaphragms, as the pleural space is adjacent to lung in these locations and therefore any calcification will be easily detectable due to its contrast with the adjacent aerated lung. At other sites, the lung is overlying the pleural surface, and pleural calcification can be more difficult to detect on chest X-ray.
   A) Previous empyema – Correct. Previous infection in the pleural space leads to inflammation and scarring, which can result in pleural calcification. It is most commonly seen with previous TB.
   B) Previous simple pleural effusion – Incorrect. A simple pleural effusion will not cause scarring or pleural calcification.
   C) Previous radiotherapy – Correct. Radiotherapy leads to inflammation, and the end result of this is scarring with calcification. Radiotherapy also produces scarring in the lung that is included in the radiotherapy field.
   D) Asbestos-related pleural disease – Correct. Pleural plaques are the commonest manifestation of asbestos-related diseases. Approximately 10% of pleural plaques calcify. Asbestos fibres get deposited in the pleural space and result in a chronic inflammatory process, which leads to plaque formation.
   E) Previous haemothorax – Correct. A haemothorax may be traumatic or iatrogenic in nature. As with other causes of pleural inflammation, a haemothorax can result in pleural calcification.

❗ KEY POINT

Whilst there are several causes for calcification in the pleural space, calcified and noncalcified pleural plaques are almost pathognomonic of previous asbestos exposure.

2. What is the commonest symptom relating to pleural plaques?
   The correct answer is **A) Asymptomatic**.
   Pleural plaques are focal areas of pleural thickening. They are the most common form of asbestos-related disease and have no functional significance. In contrast, diffuse pleural thickening, which is also associated with asbestos exposure but is much less common than pleural plaques, can result in lung symptoms due to reduced lung function.
   A) Asymptomatic – Correct. Pleural plaques are considered a benign pathology, although they usually signify previous asbestos exposure. They cause no

symptoms and are found incidentally on chest X-ray or CT. They do not require any treatment.
   B) Haemoptysis – Incorrect. Pleural plaques are not associated with haemoptysis.
   C) Breathlessness – Incorrect. Pleural plaques do not cause breathlessness or reduce lung function.
   D) Chest pain – Incorrect. If a patient with pleural plaques has chest pain, an alternative diagnosis, such as mesothelioma, must be considered.
   E) Weight loss – Incorrect. Again, pleural plaques themselves do not cause chest pain. If a patient with known pleural plaques has weight loss, an alternative diagnosis, such as mesothelioma, must be considered.

❗ KEY POINT

Whilst pleural plaques are considered benign, their significance is that they imply previous asbestos exposure, which can result in other more serious complications (see question 4).

3. Which of the following is/are correct regarding the imaging of pleural plaques?
   The correct answers are **B) They tend to spare the lung apices, D) CT is more sensitive than chest X-ray for detecting pleural plaques and E) The parietal pleura is most commonly involved**.
   Pleural plaques are not uncommonly identified on chest X-ray. They are often an incidental finding and can result in a bizarre appearance due to their size, shape and calcification. Some knowledge of the imaging features of pleural plaques is therefore useful.
   A) Most pleural plaques are calcified – Incorrect. Calcified pleural plaques are more easily detected on chest X-ray, but only approximately 10% of pleural plaques are calcified.
   B) They tend to spare the lung apices – Correct. Pleural plaques predominantly affect the parietal pleura of the mid and lower zones, with sparing of the lung apices and costophrenic angles. The mediastinal pleura can also be involved, although the visceral pleura is commonly spared. Unless extensive, pleural plaques do not cause any impairment in lung function.
   C) Chest X-ray will detect >75% of pleural plaques – Incorrect. Calcified pleural plaques are much more easily seen on chest X-ray than noncalcified plaques. As we have already discussed, almost 90% of pleural plaques are noncalcified. Chest X-rays thus detect only about 10% to 20% of pleural plaques.
   D) CT is more sensitive than chest X-ray for detecting pleural plaques – Correct. CT allows cross-sectional imaging of the chest. This permits a much more accurate assessment of the lung and pleura, particularly as the levels of contrast on CT (the 'windows') can be adjusted. CT is therefore much better at demonstrating pleural plaques, including noncalcified plaques, than chest X-ray. It can also show other

Continue

CASE 2.20   *Contd.*

complications of asbestos exposure, such as malignancy and pulmonary fibrosis.

E) The parietal pleura is most commonly involved – Correct. See B.

4. Which of the following can occur secondary to asbestos exposure?

The correct answers are **A) Mesothelioma, B) Laryngeal carcinoma, C) Round atelectasis and D) Pulmonary fibrosis**.

Asbestos exposure can cause diseases of the lung, pleural and airways. It can also cause malignancies of the lung, pleura and the gastrointestinal tract. There is a long lag period between exposure to asbestos and the occurrence of asbestos-related disease. Amosite and crocidolite are the most harmful type of asbestos fibres. Pleural plaques and simple pleural effusions are the most common manifestations.

A) Mesothelioma – Correct. Mesothelioma is a rare cancer which develops in the mesothelial cells, most commonly in the pleura. It can also arise in the peritoneum and pericardium. Asbestos exposure increases the chance of developing malignant mesothelioma as 90% of mesothelioma cases are associated with asbestos exposure. Unlike pleural plaques, malignant mesothelioma can cause a variety of symptoms, including chest wall pain, shortness of breath, haemoptysis and weight loss. It usually presents in combination with a pleural effusion and typically results in contraction of the involved hemithorax. It also often metastasises through haematogenous spread. The diagnosis is confirmed by pleural fluid cytology or pleural biopsy. The prognosis remains poor.

B) Laryngeal carcinoma – Correct. There is a recognised association between asbestos exposure and laryngeal carcinoma.

C) Round atelectasis – Correct. As the name suggests, round atelectasis describes an area of collapsed lung which has a round configuration. It is not specific to asbestos-related lung disease; however, when it occurs in patients with previous asbestos exposure, it is located adjacent to an area of pleural thickening. Other features which suggest the diagnosis include the comet tail sign (vessels and bronchi curve in towards the mass), and the fact the mass is not completely surrounded by lung.

D) Pulmonary fibrosis – Correct. Asbestos-induced pulmonary fibrosis is known as asbestosis. Like other forms of fibrosis, there is an increase in the interstitial lung markings, which progresses to 'honeycombing' later. It typically affects the lung periphery (just under the pleural surface) and progresses from the lung bases upwards.

E) Emphysema – Incorrect. There is no association between asbestos exposure and emphysema. Emphysema may coexist with asbestos-related diseases, and smoking increases the risk of asbestos-related malignancies.

❗ KEY POINT

Asbestos-related diseases usually affect the lung, but other structures, such as the peritoneum and larynx, can be involved.

5. Which of the following cause calcification on a chest X-ray?

The correct answers are **B) Previous varicella pneumonia, C) Silicosis and D) Mitral valve disease**.

As mentioned earlier, calcification on a chest X-ray can arise from a number of different structures. The causes of pleural calcification have been discussed earlier in the question.

A) Emphysema – Incorrect. Emphysema results in destruction of the lung parenchyma, and in bullae formation. It does not cause pulmonary calcification.

B) Previous varicella pneumonia – Correct. Old chicken pox (varicella pneumonia) is a classic cause for multiple calcified pulmonary nodules. Other infectious causes of calcified nodules include TB, histoplasmosis and schistosomiasis.

C) Silicosis – Correct. Silicosis is an inhalational lung disease caused by inhaled silicon dioxide. It can result in various radiological findings, including a reticular pattern of interstitial lung markings, calcified lung nodules and hilar lymph node enlargement. Coal workers' pneumoconiosis is another occupational lung disease in which you may see calcified pulmonary nodules.

D) Mitral valve disease – Correct. The mitral and aortic valves are most commonly affected in valvular heart disease. Valvular heart disease can result in calcification of the valves and surrounding tissues, as well as enlargement of cardiac chambers and abnormal pulmonary vascularity.

E) Early pulmonary artery hypertension – Incorrect. Whilst calcified pulmonary arteries are pathognomonic of pulmonary artery hypertension, this is a rare finding that only occurs in advanced disease. Other features include enlarged pulmonary arteries and rapid tapering of the pulmonary arteries.

👥 IMPORTANT LEARNING POINTS

- There are many causes of calcification on a chest X-ray.
- Pleural plaques are asymptomatic and benign but indicate previous asbestos exposure.
- They are best identified on CT.
- Complications of asbestos exposure include malignancy, such as mesothelioma, bronchogenic cancer and laryngeal carcinoma, as well as pulmonary fibrosis and round atelectasis.

Abdominal X-rays

Cindy Chew and Zeshan Qureshi

3

Chapter Outline

This introduction to the chapter is aimed at providing a systematic framework for approaching abdominal X-rays (AXRs). Further details and examples of the specific X-rays findings discussed next are covered more extensively in the example cases later in the chapter and in the bonus X-ray chapter.

> **❶ KEY POINT**
>
> Systematic approach to abdominal X-rays
> 1. Projection
> 2. Patient details
> 3. Technical adequacy
> 4. Obvious abnormalities
> 5. Systematic review of the X-ray
> 6. Summary

PROJECTION

- The standard abdominal X-ray is an AP X-ray with the patient in the supine position. You can assume this is the case unless told otherwise.
- Sometimes, a lateral decubitus (the patient is rolled onto their left side and the X-ray taken in an AP direction) or a lateral shoot through (the patient is supine but a lateral X-ray is taken) abdominal X-ray is performed. Such X-rays should be clearly labelled. They are most frequently undertaken in neonates to confirm or exclude a pneumoperitoneum.

PATIENT DETAILS

- It is important to check you are looking at the correct X-ray from the correct patient.

- The patient details should be listed on the film.
- State the name, age (or date of birth) and the date on which the film was taken.

TECHNICAL ADEQUACY

- The entire abdomen should be included in the X-ray.
- Check the X-ray includes the hemidiaphragms down to the symphysis pubis and hernial orifices.
- If the entire abdomen has not been included, you need to decide whether a repeat/additional X-ray is required.

OBVIOUS ABNORMALITIES

- If there is an obvious abnormality, such as small bowel dilatation, comment on this before conducting your systematic review of the film.

SYSTEMATIC REVIEW OF THE FILM

ASSESS THE BOWEL (SEE FIG. 3.1)

When looking at the bowel try to identify:
- Large and small bowel
- Diameter of the bowel
- Bowel wall thickness

LARGE BOWEL

- The large bowel is normally the easiest to identify as it typically runs around the outside of the abdomen.
- Apart from its position, the large bowel can also be identified by the presence of haustra (horizontal lines that only partially cross the width of the large bowel).

- The large bowel should be no wider than 7 cm, except the caecum, which can be up to 10 cm.
- Identify the rectum within the pelvis – it usually contains air.
- Follow this around to the sigmoid colon and up the descending colon, which lies on the right side of the X-ray.

- Follow the transverse colon (often this hangs down through the middle of the film before rising again to the hepatic flexure).
- Follow the ascending colon from the hepatic flexure down to the caecum.

  If you can follow the entire large bowel around, then identifying the small bowel is easy as it is the remaining part of the intestine.

SMALL BOWEL

- The small bowel normally lies more centrally and should be no more than 3 cm in diameter.
- The small bowel can also be identified by the valvulae conniventes, which are lines that traverse the full width of the small bowel.

> **! KEY POINT**
>
> Remember, in a 'normal' abdominal X-ray, the large and small bowel can be difficult to see clearly. The small and large bowel become much easier to recognise when there is bowel dilatation, which may be functional or due to mechanical obstruction.

BOWEL OBSTRUCTION (SEE FIG. 3.2)

- The most common finding on an abdominal X-ray in an exam is bowel obstruction. The first thing to do is identify the level of the bowel obstruction. Then try to determine the cause of obstruction, although this is often not possible on an abdominal X-ray.

  If there is large bowel obstruction:
- The level of obstruction is usually visible on the X-ray.
- Malignancy commonly causes large bowel obstruction. This may be visible on the X-ray as a cut-off

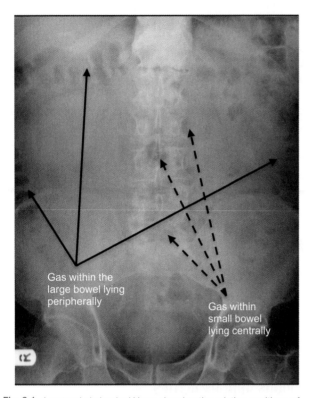

Fig. 3.1 A normal abdominal X-ray showing the relative positions of small and large bowel.

Gas within the large bowel lying peripherally

Gas within small bowel lying centrally

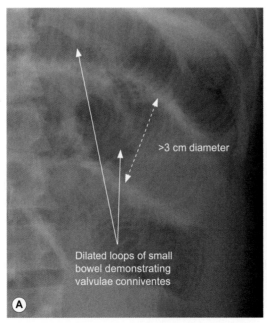

>3 cm diameter

Dilated loops of small bowel demonstrating valvulae conniventes

(A)

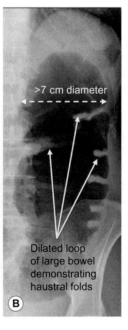

>7 cm diameter

Dilated loop of large bowel demonstrating haustral folds

(B)

Fig. 3.2 **(A)** Dilated small bowel. **(B)** Dilated large bowel.

point but the patient will require further imaging for confirmation.

- The other cause not to be missed on the abdominal X-ray is a sigmoid volvulus.
- If the ileocaecal valve is competent (or the patient is X-rayed early during the obstruction), then the bowel dilatation will be confined to the large bowel. On the other hand, if the ileocaecal valve is incompetent, the backpressure from large bowel obstruction can result in additional dilatation of the small bowel. This is beneficial in the short term as it reduces the pressure within the large bowel, reducing the risk of perforation.
  If the small bowel is dilated alone:
- The cause is most likely either adhesions or a hernia.
- Evidence of previous surgery, such as surgical clips, may suggest adhesions.
- Looking at the region of the inguinal canal is essential for identifying inguinal hernias.

EXTRALUMINAL GAS (PNEUMOPERITONEUM)

- There are a variety of features visible on an abdominal X-ray to suggest extraluminal gas (pneumoperitoneum).
- The features of pneumoperitoneum on abdominal X-rays include:
  - Rigler's sign (see Fig. 3.3B): Normally, only the inner wall of the bowel is visible, due to the contrast of the inner wall against air present inside of the bowel. In a pneumoperitoneum, air is also present outside the bowel. This can make both sides of the bowel wall clearly visible. Such an appearance is known as Rigler's sign.
  - Free subdiaphragmatic gas (see Fig. 3.3A): As in an erect chest X-ray, free intraperitoneal gas can outline the hemidiaphragms. This is known as the crescent sign.
  - The 'continuous diaphragm sign' may also be present. Normally, the central portion of the diaphragm is not discretely seen (since it merges with the cardiac silhouette). If the diaphragm can be seen continuously across the midline (see Fig. 3.3B), then this is highly suggestive of gas within an abnormal space (i.e. the mediastinum, pericardium or the peritoneal cavity).
  - Visualisation of the falciform ligament (see Fig. 3.3B): Free intraperitoneal gas can outline the falciform ligament, which appears as a vertical line in the right upper quadrant extending towards the umbilicus.
  - Triangular lucencies: Free gas between bowel loops can often result in triangular lucent areas.
  - Hyperlucency of the liver (see Fig. 3.3B): Free abdominal gas overlying the liver can cause the liver to appear more lucent than usual.

- Football sign: A round area of air, usually towards the top of the film, mainly found in neonates.

> ❶ KEY POINT
>
> Pneumoperitoneum is usually more easily detected on an erect chest X-ray, so make sure you request and scrutinise the erect chest X-ray in patients with possible pneumoperitoneum, even if there are no suggestive features on the abdominal X-ray.

THUMBPRINTING OF THE BOWEL WALL

- Thumbprinting is thickening of the bowel wall caused by oedema, haemorrhage or tumour (Fig. 3.4). It is so named because it looks like someone has pushed their thumb into it in several places, resulting in a wavy pattern. There are a variety of causes, but the most common are inflammatory bowel disease and ischaemic colitis.
- If you see an enlarged colon with thumbprinting, you should always question whether this is inflammatory-bowel-disease-related toxic megacolon.

LIVER, SPLEEN, GALLBLADDER, KIDNEYS AND PANCREAS

- The abdominal X-ray provides a limited assessment of the solid abdominal organs (liver, spleen, kidneys) and gallbladder (ultrasound is much better for imaging these structures) (Fig. 3.5).
- Look at the size of the liver and spleen; hepato- or splenomegaly can sometimes be visible as an enlarged soft tissue density arising from the right or left upper quadrants, respectively. There may be indirect evidence of their enlargement due to displacement of the bowel.
- Gas within the portal system or biliary tree may sometimes be visible as lucent lines projected over the liver, and suggest bowel ischaemia or biliary pathology, respectively. Portal vein gas extends to the periphery of the liver whilst biliary tree gas is centred around the porta hepatis. It is useful to look for these findings although X-ray is less accurate compared with ultrasound or CT.
- Look for gallstones within the gallbladder. However, remember that the majority of gallstones are radiolucent and will not be seen on X-ray.
- Look for calcification along the renal tract; with practice, the kidneys can be visualised on most AXRs (T12–L2) and the ureters run vertically over the transverse processes of the lumbar spine.
- Calcifications may represent renal calculi or calcification within the renal parenchyma (medullary or cortical calcification).

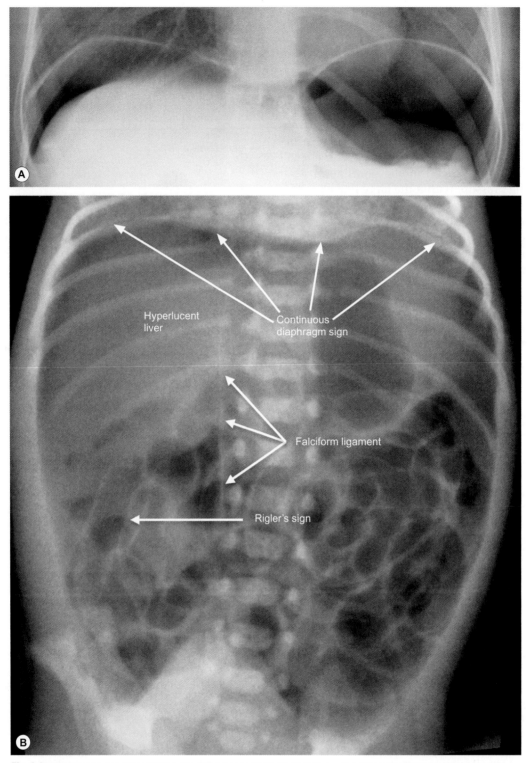

Fig. 3.3 (A) Free air under the diaphragm. **(B)** A neonatal abdominal X-ray showing several signs of pneumoperitoneum; hyperlucency of the liver, subdiaphragmatic gas creating a continuous diaphragm sign, visualisation of the falciform ligament and Rigler's sign.

- There may be calculi within the bladder itself.
- Beware of phleboliths (calcified pelvic vessels), which are common. If you do not look at their position carefully, you may mistake them for renal or bladder calculi.
- Assess for calcification in the distribution of the pancreas, which is suggestive of chronic pancreatitis.

ABDOMINAL AORTA

- Always look for the aorta and iliac vessels (Fig. 3.6).
- With increasing age, the aortic wall is increasingly calcified, so the two walls can be seen and measured; an aorta larger than 3 cm in diameter suggests an aneurysm and requires further investigation and possible surgery.

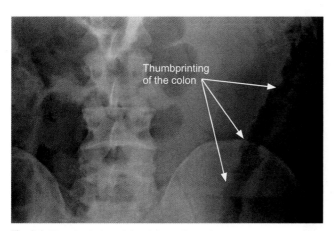

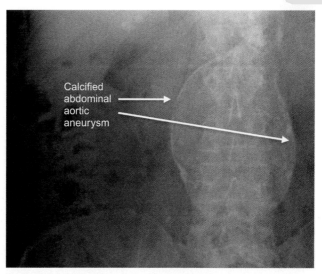

Fig. 3.4 Thumbprinting of the descending colon.

Fig. 3.6 A calcified abdominal aortic aneurysm.

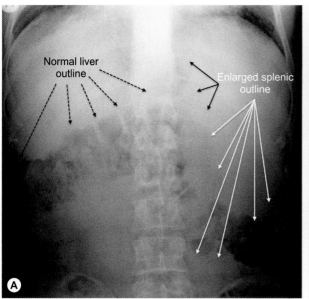

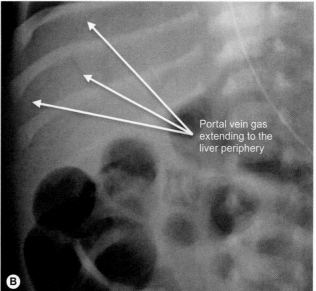

Fig. 3.5 Normal liver outline and an enlarged spleen **(A)**; branching linear lucencies extending to the liver periphery **(B)** in keeping with portal vein gas.

BONES

- Assess all of the imaged bones, looking for alterations in density, such as osteoporosis, lucent areas and sclerosis (Fig. 3.7).
- Look for pelvic and hip fractures.
- Look specifically at the spine – often, osteoporotic fractures can be seen, as well as scoliosis and metastatic deposits.

> ⓘ KEY POINT
>
> Abdominal X-rays provide limited assessment of the aorta and cannot exclude significant pathology; ultrasound and CT are much more accurate for assessing the aorta and other abdominal blood vessels.

FOREIGN BODIES

- Mention clips from previous surgery and any indwelling lines, such as umbilical catheters in neonates, ureteric drains (Fig. 3.7) or surgical drains. Sterilisation clips can commonly be seen.

SUMMARY

- State your key findings (either as a description or a diagnosis), put forward a differential diagnosis and suggest any further relevant imaging and an appropriate initial management plan.

You can use the checklist presented in Table 3.1 to assess the abdominal X-rays shown in this chapter. Example cases follow (Cases 3.1–3.20).

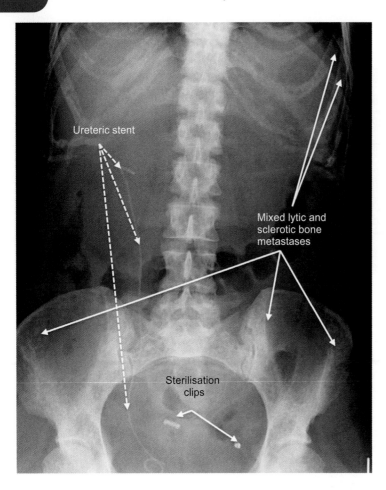

Fig. 3.7 Right-sided ureteric stent and sterilisation clips. Diffusely abnormal bones in keeping with mixed and sclerotic bone metastases.

TABLE 3.1	**Abdominal X-ray Checklist**	
Technical Aspects		
Checks patient details (name, date of birth, hospital number)		✓
Checks the date of the X-ray		✓
Identifies the projection of the X-ray		✓
Assesses technical quality of X-ray		✓
Obvious Abnormalities		
Describes any obvious abnormality		✓
Systematic Review of the X-ray		
Assesses the large bowel (diameter, wall thickening)		✓
Assesses small bowel (diameter, wall thickening)		✓
Comments on evidence of extraluminal gas (pneumoperitoneum)		✓
Comments on any obvious abnormality of the liver, gallbladder or spleen (e.g. radio-opaque gallstones)		✓
Assesses the urinary tract (kidney, ureters and bladder) e.g. calculi		✓
Comments on any abnormality of the major vascular structures (aorta and iliac vessels) e.g. vascular calcification, aneurysm		✓
Assesses the imaged skeleton		✓
Comments on iatrogenic abnormalities (surgical clips, stents, etc.)		✓
Summary		
Presents findings		✓
Reviews relevant previous imaging if appropriate		✓
Provides a differential diagnosis where appropriate		✓
Suggests appropriate further imaging/investigations if relevant		✓

CASE EXAMPLES

CASE 3.1

A 56-year-old woman has presented to A&E with a 4-day history of colicky lower abdominal pain, nausea and vomiting. She has not moved her bowels for 4 days. On examination, her abdomen is generally tender but not peritonitic. As part of her investigations, you request an abdominal X-ray to exclude bowel obstruction.

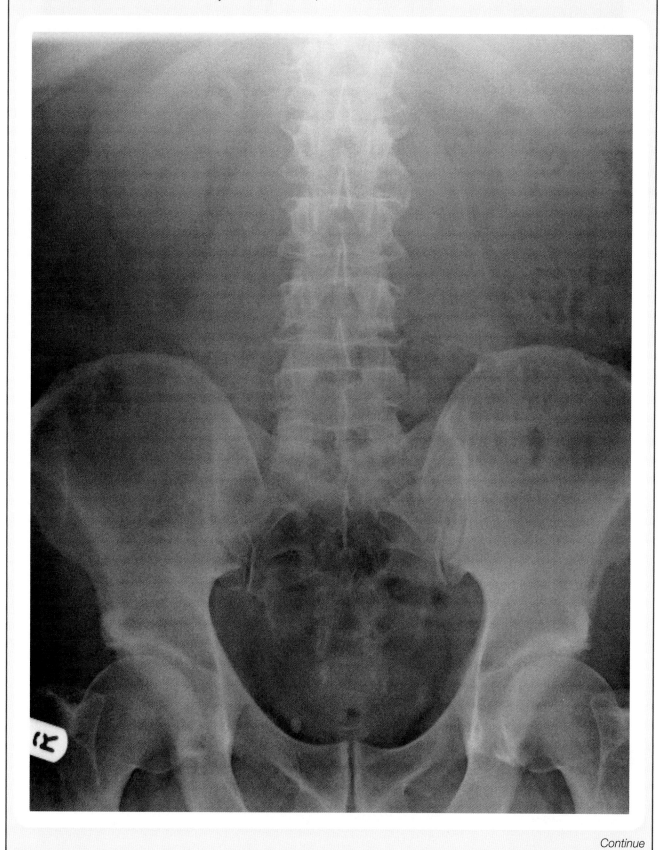

Continue

ANNOTATED X-RAY

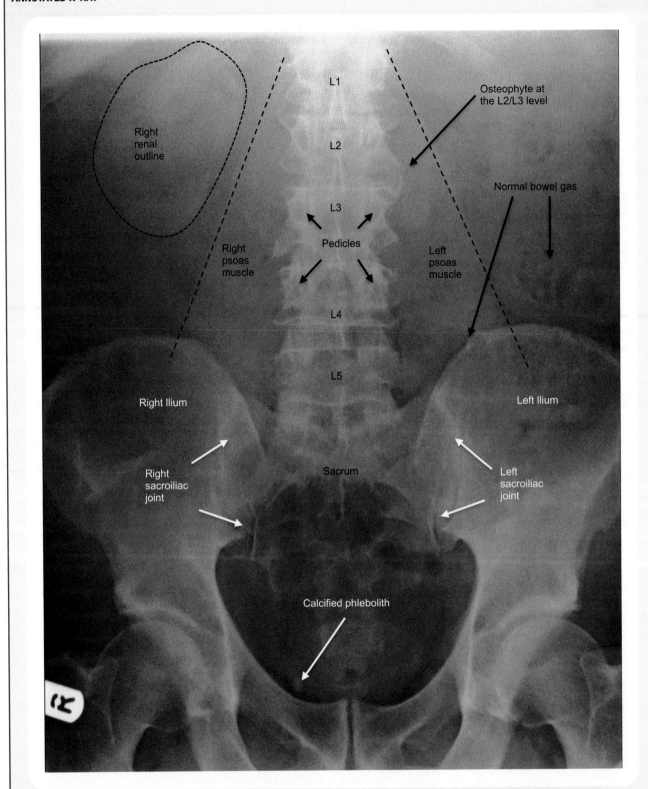

Right renal outline

L1

L2

L3

Pedicles

Right psoas muscle

Left psoas muscle

Osteophyte at the L2/L3 level

Normal bowel gas

L4

L5

Right Ilium

Left Ilium

Right sacroiliac joint

Sacrum

Left sacroiliac joint

Calcified phlebolith

🔍 PRESENT YOUR FINDINGS

- This is a supine anteroposterior (AP) X-ray of the abdomen.
- It has been anonymised and the timing of the examination is not available. I would like to confirm the patient's details and timing of the examination before I make any further assessment.
- The hemidiaphragms have not been included in the study; therefore, the entire abdomen has not been imaged, making this is a technically inadequate film.
- The bowel gas pattern is normal.

- There is no evidence of bowel obstruction, perforation or mucosal oedema.
- There is a small rounded area of calcification projected over the right side of the pelvis in keeping with a calcified phlebolith.
- There is no obvious abnormality of the visible solid abdominal organs.
- There is a left-sided osteophyte at the L2/L3 level. The imaged skeleton is otherwise normal.

IN SUMMARY – Apart from some minor degenerative changes in the spine, this is a normal abdominal X-ray.

QUESTIONS

1. Which of the following is/are appropriate indications for an abdominal X-ray?
   A) Acute abdominal pain
   B) Acute gastrointestinal bleed
   C) Altered bowel habit
   D) Acute exacerbation of inflammatory bowel disease
   E) First-line investigation for suspected migrated intra-uterine contraceptive device (IUCD)

2. Which of the following statements about the radiation dose associated with abdominal X-rays is correct?
   A) Abdominal X-rays do not involve the use of ionising radiation
   B) Abdominal X-rays do involve the use of ionising radiation but the dose is negligible (significantly less than a chest X-ray)
   C) Abdominal X-rays do involve the use of ionising radiation and the dose is similar to a chest X-ray
   D) Abdominal X-rays do involve the use of ionising radiation and the dose is significantly higher than a chest X-ray
   E) Abdominal X-rays do involve the use of ionising radiation and the dose is similar to a computed tomography (CT) scan of the abdomen

3. How can you differentiate small from large bowel on an abdominal X-ray?
   A) Small bowel usually lies centrally and has haustra
   B) Small bowel usually lies peripherally and has valvulae conniventes
   C) Large bowel usually lies centrally and has valvulae conniventes
   D) Large bowel usually lies peripherally and has haustra
   E) There is no reliable method for differentiating small from large bowel on an abdominal X-ray

4. What is the upper limit of normal for the diameter of the small and large bowel?
   A) Small bowel 1 cm, large bowel 3 cm
   B) Small bowel 3 cm, large bowel 7 cm
   C) Small bowel 6 cm, large bowel 9 cm
   D) Small and large bowel 6 cm
   E) Small and large bowel 3 cm

5. Regarding the visible skeleton on an abdominal X-ray, which of the following is/are true?
   A) The pedicles of the imaged vertebrae should be visible
   B) Both sacroiliac (SI) joints should be visible
   C) A normal appearance of the bones excludes bone metastases
   D) Due to the technique used, fractures are unlikely to be visible
   E) An accurate assessment of the vertebral alignment can be made

Continue

CASE 3.1   *Contd.*

ANSWERS TO QUESTIONS

1. Which of the following is/are appropriate indications for an abdominal X-ray?
   The correct answers are **A) Acute abdominal pain and D) Acute exacerbation of inflammatory bowel disease**.
   Abdominal X-rays are associated with a relatively high dose of ionising radiation and have limited indications. 'Making the best use of clinical radiology services' is the Royal College of Radiologists' guidelines for requesting imaging investigations. These guidelines describe the appropriate imaging for various different pathologies. They are now available as a smartphone/tablet app (iRefer).
   A) Acute abdominal pain – Correct. An abdominal X-ray is an appropriate investigation in acute abdominal pain if there is concern regarding bowel obstruction or perforation. An erect chest X-ray should also be performed to help diagnose a pneumoperitoneum (see Chapter 2 for further details). Patients presenting with abdominal pain who are not suspected of having bowel obstruction or perforation should not routinely have an abdominal X-ray performed unless another indication is present.
   B) Acute gastrointestinal bleed – Incorrect. Abdominal X-rays are of no use in patients with acute gastrointestinal bleeds. Such patients are usually investigated with endoscopy or occasionally with CT and conventional angiography.
   C) Altered bowel habit – Incorrect. Abdominal X-rays are of limited use in patients with altered bowel habit. In particular, they should not be routinely requested to exclude faecal loading or constipation. (Abdominal X-rays may be indicated in certain geriatric and psychiatric patients to show the extent of faecal impaction, or to investigate altered bowel habit.) CT colonography or colonoscopy are more appropriate and useful investigations in patients with altered bowel habit (where the most significant concern is possible colon cancer).
   D) Acute exacerbation of inflammatory bowel disease – Correct. Abdominal X-rays are useful to identify mucosal oedema in acute exacerbations of inflammatory bowel disease and to monitor for the development of toxic dilatation of the colon, which is a medical emergency.
   E) First-line investigation for suspected migrated IUCD – Incorrect. The first-line investigation for suspected missing/migrated IUCD is ultrasound. Ultrasound does not involve ionising radiation and can identify IUCDs which may not be evident on clinical examination. If the IUCD is not visible on ultrasound, then an abdominal X-ray is used to check for extrauterine migration.

① KEY POINT

Abdominal X-rays are associated with a relatively high radiation dose and have limited indications. The following are the main indications suspected:
- Small or large bowel obstruction
- Perforated viscus (although an erect chest X-ray is more sensitive for identifying a pneumoperitoneum)
- Acute exacerbation of inflammatory bowel disease of the colon
- Constipation is an indication for abdominal X-rays only in specific circumstances.

2. Which of the following statements about the radiation dose associated with abdominal X-rays is correct?
   The correct answer is **D) Abdominal X-rays do involve the use of ionising radiation and the dose is significantly higher than a chest X-ray.**
   X-rays are a form of ionising radiation and have the potential to damage tissues. It is therefore necessary for medical staff requesting X-rays to have an understanding of the relative dose of an X-ray examination and the potential hazards for the patient.
   An abdominal X-ray uses 30 to 50 times the dose of a chest X-ray. This is because the chest is largely composed of gas-filled alveoli which absorb relatively few X-rays, whereas a higher dose is needed to penetrate through the many layers of soft tissues in the abdominal cavity. CT examinations use hundreds of X-rays to produce images. Therefore, the dose associated with a CT is significantly higher than an abdominal X-ray.

① KEY POINTS

1. To put the dose of X-ray examinations into perspective, it is useful to remember that a chest X-ray gives the equivalent dose of roughly 3 days background radiation or a 6-hour flight. Therefore, an abdominal X-ray, which uses 30 to 50 times more radiation than a chest X-ray, equates to approximately 3 months background radiation and a CT anywhere between 6 and 18 months.
2. Under UK IRMER legislation, any investigation exposing a patient to ionising radiation must be justified. When making a request for an X-ray, CT, nuclear medicine examination or fluoroscopy, the referrer must provide enough clinical information for the examination to be justified. Examinations associated with a low dose of radiation, such as extremity X-rays, are easier to justify than high-dose examinations such as CT.
3. The biological effects of X-rays and other forms of ionising radiation can be generally divided into two categories:
   - Deterministic effects include skin erythema, hair loss and cataracts and do not occur below a threshold dose.
   - Stochastic effects occur by chance but are more likely to occur with increasing doses of radiation. Carcinogenesis is the most concerning stochastic effect of radiation.

3. How can you differentiate small from large bowel on an abdominal X-ray?
   The correct answer is **D) Large bowel usually lies peripherally and has haustra.**
   Being able to confidently distinguish small and large bowel is important in the assessment of X-rays with dilated bowel, as the causes and management of small and large bowel obstruction differ (Table C3.1.1).
   Small bowel usually lies centrally and contains valvulae conniventes. These are lines which traverse the full

width of the bowel loop. In contrast, the large bowel usually lies peripherally and contains haustra, which are horizontal lines that only partially cross the bowel loop. Large bowel often contains faecal material which can be visible on X-ray.

Table C3.1.1 The Differences Between Small and Large Bowel on Abdominal X-ray

SMALL BOWEL	LARGE BOWEL
Central location	Peripheral location
Valvulae conniventes (traverse the entire width of bowel)	Haustral folds (partially cross the bowel loops)
	Contains faecal material

❗ KEY POINT

The ascending and descending colon and rectum are retroperitoneal structures which consequently usually have a relatively constant position. The transverse and sigmoid colon have a mobile mesentery and can have variable positions.

4. What is the upper limit of normal for the diameter of the small and large bowel?
    The correct answer is **B) Small bowel 3 cm, large bowel 7 cm.**
    Due to the divergent nature of the X-ray beam, an abdominal X-ray results in some magnification of the bowel loops. However, as a rule of thumb the diameter of small bowel loops should be no larger than 3 cm and that of the large bowel should be less than 7 cm. The caecum can have a diameter of up to 10 cm.

❗ KEY POINTS

1. The upper limit of normal bowel diameter on an abdominal X-ray can be remembered by the 3/7/10 rule. The small bowel should be less than 3 cm, the large bowel 7 cm and the caecum 10 cm.
2. The normal range for bowel diameter given earlier is slightly arbitrary. Therefore, if there is a clinical diagnosis of bowel obstruction and associated prominent but not technically dilated bowel loops on the abdominal X-ray, the patient should be treated accordingly even though the bowel loop diameter is still within the 'normal range'.

5. Regarding the visible skeleton on an abdominal X-ray, which of the following is/are true?
    The correct answers are **A) The pedicles of the imaged vertebrae should be visible and B) Both SI joints should be visible**.
    It is important to assess all the structures included in the X-ray. Skeletal pathology identified on abdominal X-rays

may be the cause of the patient's symptoms, a consequence of relevant pathology or an incidental finding.

A) The pedicles of the imaged vertebrae should be visible – Correct. The pedicles of the lower thoracic and lumbar spine should be visible 'end on'. It is important to ensure both pedicles are visible. Loss of one or both pedicles suggests the presence of a destructive mass, such as a bone metastasis, affecting that vertebra.

B) Both SI joints should be visible – Correct. Both SI joints should be visible. Symmetrical bilateral fused SI joints are seen in ankylosing spondylitis, inflammatory bowel disease and hyperparathyroidism. Reiter syndrome and psoriatic arthritis can cause asymmetrical bilateral fusion of the SI joints. Infection and degenerative disease usually cause unilateral fusion.

C) A normal appearance of the bones excludes bone metastases – Incorrect. Bone metastases can be sclerotic, lytic or mixed. X-rays are an insensitive test for excluding bone metastases as approximately 50% of the bone must be eroded for a lytic deposit to be identifiable on X-ray. CT, MRI and bone scans have a higher sensitivity for identifying bony metastatic disease compared to X-rays.

D) Due to the technique used, fractures are unlikely to be visible – Incorrect. Fractures may be visible. In particular, fractures of the femoral neck or pubic rami may present with abdominal pain. It is therefore important to assess the imaged skeleton for the presence of fractures.

E) An accurate assessment of the vertebral alignment can be made – Incorrect. An abdominal X-ray allows assessment of the AP alignment of the vertebral column. A scoliosis of the lumbar spine, for example, will be visible. However, no comment can be made regarding the lateral vertebral alignment. Therefore a kyphosis or spondylolisthesis (anterior or posterior displacement of a vertebra in relation to the vertebra below) will not be visible; specific lateral views are required to assess for these.

📖 IMPORTANT LEARNING POINTS

-   There are only a few indications for an abdominal X-ray, such as bowel obstruction, perforation and exclusion of toxic megacolon.
-   Abdominal X-rays use a relatively large dose of radiation compared to chest X-rays.
-   Small bowel tends to lie centrally and contains valvulae conniventes, whereas large bowel is usually peripheral with incomplete haustral folds. The upper limit of normal for bowel diameter is 3 cm for small bowel, 7 cm for large bowel and 10 cm for the caecum.
-   It is important to assess all the structures on an abdominal X-ray, including the bones.

CASE 3.2

A 35-year-old nonbinary person is recovering on the surgical ward following a laparoscopic appendicectomy yesterday. The operative findings described a localised perforation of the appendix. You are called to review the patient as they are complaining of abdominal distension, nausea and vomiting. An abdominal X-ray has been performed.

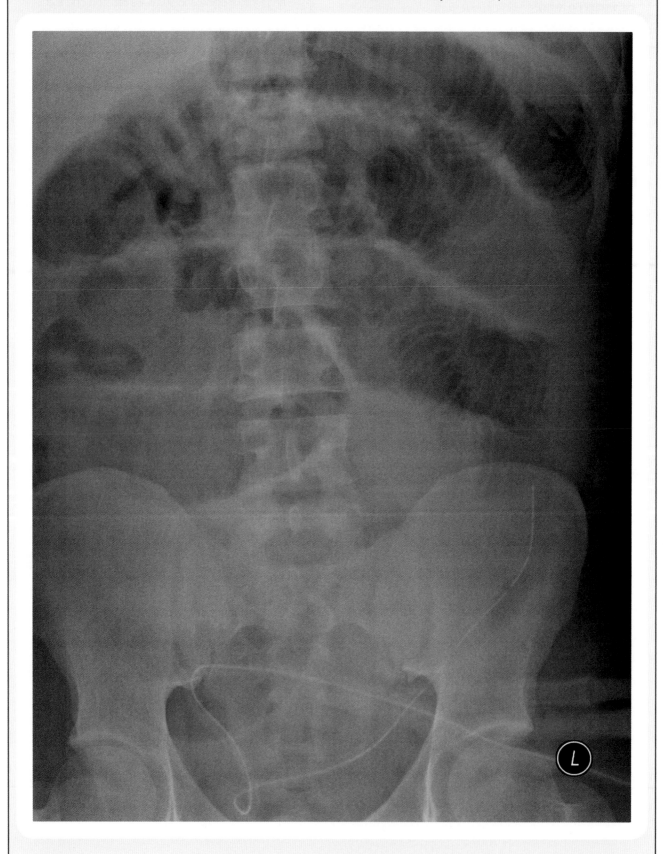

ANNOTATED X-RAY

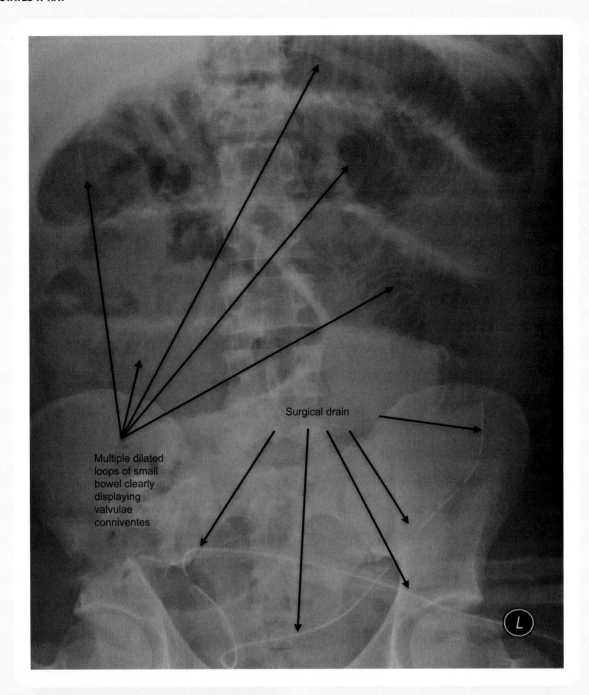

Multiple dilated
loops of small
bowel clearly
displaying
valvulae
conniventes

Surgical drain

L

🔍 PRESENT YOUR FINDINGS

- This is a supine AP abdominal X-ray.
- There are no patient identifiable data on the X-ray.
  I would like to confirm the patient's name, date of
  birth and date and time that the X-ray was performed
  before making any further assessment.
- The diaphragms and hernial orifices are not visualised –
  the entire abdomen has therefore not been imaged and
  the film is technically inadequate. I would check to see if
  the film has been repeated.
- The most striking abnormality is multiple loops of
  dilated bowel within the central and epigastric regions
  of the abdomen. Mucosal markings are discernible running across the entire diameter of the bowel consistent
  with valvulae conniventes in keeping with dilated small
  bowel.
- There is no evidence of pneumoperitoneum, nor any
  dilatation of the large bowel. There is some gas evident
  in the sigmoid colon in the left iliac fossa.
- A surgical drain is present in the left iliac fossa.
- There is no obvious abnormality of the visible solid
  abdominal organs.
- No skeletal abnormality.

Continue

CASE 3.2   *Contd.*

IN SUMMARY – This abdominal X-ray demonstrates small bowel obstruction. Given the presence of an abdominal drain, there has likely been recent abdominal surgery, which is confirmed in the clinical history. The most likely aetiology in this scenario is therefore a small bowel ileus. There is some gas in the large bowel, mitigating against complete small bowel obstruction. However, I would examine the patient carefully for the presence of a hernia as the hernial orifices have been incompletely imaged.

QUESTIONS

1. Which feature on AXR favours small bowel obstruction over large bowel obstruction?
   A) Mucosal markings that only extend partially across the bowel loops
   B) Centrally located loops of bowel
   C) Bowel diameter of 5 cm
   D) Extensive faecal shadowing within the lumen of the bowel loops
   E) Pneumoperitoneum
2. Which of the following favours a functional ileus over mechanical small bowel obstruction?
   A) Marked crampy abdominal pain with distension
   B) Bilious vomiting
   C) History of several previous abdominal operations
   D) Peritonism
   E) Absent bowel sounds
3. What is the most common aetiology of mechanical small bowel obstruction in adults in the UK?
   A) Adhesions
   B) Intussusception
   C) Crohn's disease
   D) Gallstone ileus
   E) Inguinal hernia
4. Which of the following is/are part of the management of an adult patient with small bowel obstruction?
   A) Measure the patient's urea and electrolytes
   B) Place an NG tube
   C) Monitor fluid balance
   D) Consider a CT scan
   E) Encourage the patient to drink plenty of fluids to compensate for their increased fluid losses
5. What is the diagnostic investigation of choice in a neonate with bilious vomiting and suspected proximal small bowel obstruction?
   A) Ultrasound
   B) CT scan of the abdomen
   C) Barium meal
   D) MR scan of the abdomen
   E) Diagnostic laparoscopy

ANSWERS TO QUESTIONS

1. Which feature on AXR favours small bowel obstruction over large bowel obstruction?
   The correct answer is **B) Centrally located loops of bowel**.
   When assessing bowel loops on plain film, the first step is to decide if the loops represent small or large bowel. The position (peripheral versus central), the bowel markings (haustra versus valvulae conniventes) and the size of the bowel loops can help distinguish large from small bowel.
   A) Mucosal markings that only extend partially across the bowel loops – Incorrect. Mucosal markings that extend only partially across the bowel loops represent haustra, which are found in the large bowel. Markings which go completely across the bowel are valvulae conniventes which are found in the small bowel. Beware that occasionally haustral markings can cross the entire bowel when seen en face.
   B) Centrally located loops of bowel – Correct. The position of the dilated loops of bowel can help differentiate between large and small bowel. Generally, small bowel loops are centrally placed in the abdomen and large bowel loops are around the periphery. This normal pattern may not be present if there has been previous surgery, such as a hemicolectomy or if there is congenital malrotation of the bowel.
   C) Bowel diameter of 5 cm – Incorrect. The diameter of bowel can be useful in certain circumstances. Normal small bowel should be less than 3 cm in diameter and normal large bowel less than 7 cm – the caecum can measure up to 10 cm. Dilated small bowel and normal calibre large bowel could both measure 5 cm in diameter so this will not help distinguish between the two. However, if the loops of bowel are markedly distended, e.g. >10 cm in diameter, this is likely to represent large bowel because small bowel is unlikely to be able to dilate to this degree without perforating.
   D) Extensive faecal shadowing within the lumen of the bowel loops – Incorrect. In general, the large bowel lumen can contain faecal shadowing, gas and fluid whereas the small bowel contains gas and fluid. The 'small bowel faeces' sign consists of apparent faeculent material within the lumen of the small bowel and is postulated to be a marker of small bowel obstruction but is more commonly seen and described on CT than X-ray.
   E) Pneumoperitoneum – Incorrect. Perforation can complicate both small bowel and large bowel obstruction. Therefore, evidence of pneumoperitoneum does not help distinguish between the two pathologies.

❶ KEY POINT

It can be difficult to distinguish dilated small bowel from dilated large bowel on the abdominal X-ray. Use the features in Table C3.2.1 to help differentiate the two. However remember: Small and large bowel dilatation are not mutually exclusive and they may exist concomitantly.

Table C3.2.1 Differentiating Small and Large Bowel

SMALL BOWEL	LARGE BOWEL
Central location	Peripheral location
Valvulae conniventes (traverse the entire width of bowel)	Haustral folds (partially cross the bowel loops)
> 3 cm in diameter, but usually not larger than 6 cm	> 6 cm in diameter
	Contains faecal material

2. Which of the following favours a functional ileus over mechanical small bowel obstruction?
   The correct answer is **E) Absent bowel sounds**.
   Distinguishing between functional and mechanical obstruction is important because functional ileus is treated conservatively whereas mechanical obstruction might require an operation.
   A) Marked crampy abdominal pain with distension – Incorrect. An ileus can result in abdominal distension and discomfort but does not usually result in marked crampy abdominal pain, in contrast to mechanical small bowel obstruction.
   B) Bilious vomiting – Incorrect. Bilious vomiting occurs in both functional and mechanical small bowel obstruction so will not favour one diagnosis over the other.
   C) History of several previous abdominal operations – Incorrect. The history of previous surgical operations favours the possibility of adhesional (i.e. mechanical) small bowel obstruction.
   D) Peritonism – Incorrect. The presence of peritonism is a concerning sign which may imply perforation, uncommon in simple functional ileus.
   E) Absent bowel sounds – Correct. Ileus is due to paralysis of peristalsis. Classically, the bowel sounds are absent. In comparison, in mechanical obstruction, the bowel sounds may be high-pitched and tinkling.

❶ KEY POINTS

1. The history is key in determining whether dilated bowel loops on an abdominal X-ray likely represent a functional ileus or a mechanical obstruction. The quality of bowel sounds may also be a useful clinical sign. Distinguishing ileus from obstruction is difficult from X-ray alone.
2. Causes of an ileus include recent surgery, intraabdominal infection, pancreatitis, trauma (e.g. head or spinal injury), metabolic upset (e.g. hyponatraemia, hypokalaemia, hypoxia, hypothermia and diabetic ketoacidosis) and medications (e.g. general anaesthesia, tricyclic antidepressants).
3. A water-soluble contrast follow-through examination can help distinguish between functional and mechanical small bowel obstruction. The patient drinks contrast material and the bowel is imaged with X-rays to see how long it takes for the contrast material to reach the colon. If it takes more than 4 hours, it implies a mechanical small bowel obstruction is present.

Continue

3. What is the most common aetiology of mechanical small bowel obstruction in adults in the UK?
   The correct answer is **A) Adhesions**.
   Knowledge of the common causes of small bowel obstruction is vital. Occasionally, the answer will be on the film, e.g. bowel gas seen below the inguinal ligament (identified as an imaginary line drawn between the anterior superior iliac spine and the pubic symphysis) to suggest an inguinal hernia as the cause.
   A) Adhesions – Correct. Postoperative adhesions are the most common cause of small bowel obstruction overall. However, there usually needs to have been a preceding history of abdominal surgery and this should be asked specifically if not volunteered by the patient. If the patient has never had an operation which breeches the peritoneum before, then an alternative cause must be considered.
   B) Intussusception – Incorrect. Intussusception can cause small bowel obstruction but is relatively rare in the adult population. In these rare cases, there is often a pathological lead point such as a polyp or tumour. In comparison, intussusception is a more common cause of small bowel obstruction in children. In this age group it usually occurs in the context of a recent viral illness, with enlarged Peyer's patches (lymphoid tissue in the small bowel) postulated to act as the lead point.
   C) Crohn's disease – Incorrect. Crohn's disease can involve the small bowel. Both acute inflammation and its subsequent sequelae, such as stricture formation or fistulation, can result in upstream small bowel obstruction, but it is not the most common cause of small bowel obstruction in adults.
   D) Gallstone ileus – Incorrect. Gallstone ileus is a rare cause of small bowel obstruction, favoured by examiners historically. It occurs when a large gallstone erodes through the gallbladder wall into the small bowel (usually the adjacent duodenum) and then travels through the small bowel before becoming impacted, usually at the ileocaecal valve and resulting in proximal obstruction. The pathognomonic findings on abdominal X-ray are dilated loops of small bowel, pneumobilia (air in the biliary tree) and a calcific entity in the vicinity of the ileocaecal valve. Interestingly, gallstone ileus is a misnomer as the gallstone results in mechanical obstruction rather than an ileus.
   E) Inguinal hernia – Incorrect. Inguinal hernias can contain small bowel and result in small bowel obstruction. However, overall, this aetiology is not as common as adhesional small bowel obstruction.

❗ KEY POINTS

1. Overall, functional ileus is the most common cause of dilated loops of small bowel. However, adhesions and hernias are the most common mechanical causes. Consequently, it is imperative to enquire about previous abdominal surgical operations and to carefully examine the groins for the presence of an inguinal or femoral hernia.

2. Potential causes of small bowel obstruction could be related to the lumen (gallstones, foreign bodies, bezoars), bowel wall/mucosa (inflammatory strictures; e.g. Crohn's, ulcerative colitis, necrotising enterocolitis, malignancy strictures, congenital atresia, e.g. duodenal atresia) or from extrinsic compression (adhesions, hernias, volvulus, intussusception).

4. Which of the following is/are part of the management of an adult patient with small bowel obstruction?
   The correct answers are **A) Measure the patient's urea and electrolytes, B) Place an NG tube, C) Monitor fluid balance and D) Consider a CT scan**.
   Knowledge of the initial steps in the management of small bowel obstruction is important so that once the diagnosis is identified on the abdominal film these steps can be instigated.
   A) Measure the patient's urea and electrolytes – Correct. It is important to identify any biochemical derangement that may be contributing to a functional ileus or that may result from loss of potassium-rich fluid into the bowel lumen. Correct hypokalaemia in a safe manner. Additionally, metabolic derangement may be the underlying cause of a functional small bowel obstruction (ileus).
   B) Place an NG tube – Correct. Placing an NG tube can help provide relief to the patient from nausea and vomiting by decompressing the stomach. It also helps with monitoring fluid balance as the output from the NG tube can be easily and accurately recorded.
   C) Monitor fluid balance – Correct. Patients with small bowel obstruction can lose a significant volume of fluid into the bowel lumen. It is important that urine output is documented to help calculate replacement fluid requirements.
   D) Consider a CT scan – Correct. Adhesional small bowel obstruction is often managed conservatively initially. However, if the patient fails to improve or there are concerning signs, such as peritonism, hypotension, tachycardia or lactic acidosis, an urgent CT scan should be considered to determine the aetiology of the obstruction and assess for evidence of bowel ischaemia or perforation.
   E) Encourage the patient to drink plenty of fluids to compensate for their increased fluid losses – Incorrect. Whilst it is imperative to replace the fluid loss of a patient with small bowel obstruction, the enteral route should not be used for two reasons. Firstly, the patient will be vomiting and unable to absorb significant volumes of oral fluid intake. Secondly, the patient should be placed nil by mouth in case surgical intervention is required. Intravenous fluid replacement with appropriate electrolyte supplements is vital.

❗ KEY POINT

Small bowel obstruction is usually managed conservatively in the initial period. Adhesional and functional small bowel obstructions usually respond to such measures. Other causes may require definitive treatment, such as surgery in the case of a strangulated hernia, or an air enema in a child with intussusception.

5. What is the diagnostic investigation of choice in a neonate with bilious vomiting and suspected proximal small bowel obstruction?

The correct answer is **C) Barium meal**.

In this scenario, midgut volvulus secondary to malrotation requires exclusion. In malrotation, the small bowel has an unusually narrow peritoneal attachment, with the ligament of Treitz (the duodenojejunal junction) displaced inferiorly and towards the right of the midline. The narrow peritoneal attachment of the small bowel makes it prone to volvulus.

A) Ultrasound – Incorrect. Ultrasound is readily available and does not involve ionising radiation. It is sometimes possible to demonstrate that the third part of the duodenum lies in a retroperitoneal position by passing posterior to the superior mesenteric artery, with ultrasound. In addition, the normal relation of the superior mesenteric artery to the superior mesenteric vein (SMA on the left and SMV on the right) demonstrated by ultrasound makes malrotation unlikely. However, bowel gas may obscure these findings and it is not considered the gold standard diagnostic investigation in this scenario.

B) CT scan of the abdomen – Incorrect. Whilst a CT could, in theory, demonstrate a malrotation abnormality, the associated radiation dose cannot be justified in the paediatric population for routine use.

C) Barium meal – Correct. A fluoroscopic study can be performed. Demonstrating a normally sited duodenojejunal flexure (to the left of the vertebral column at the level of L1) excludes malrotation. The corkscrew sign (spiral appearance of the distal duodenum and proximal jejunum) is suggestive of midgut volvulus. It is the diagnostic investigation of choice in this situation.

D) MR scan of the abdomen – Incorrect. MR is currently a limited resource. It is time consuming and requires careful logistical planning and often needs to be performed under general anaesthesia to obtain diagnostic images in a neonate. It is not feasible to use MR to exclude the diagnosis of malrotation in the emergency setting.

E) Diagnostic laparoscopy – Incorrect. If small bowel obstruction secondary to malrotation is confirmed, the neonate will undergo a laparotomy. Diagnostic laparoscopy is not the investigation of choice in this scenario; it is unnecessary when good noninvasive diagnostic tests are available.

🛈 KEY POINT

Midgut volvulus secondary to malrotation is a potentially life-threatening surgical emergency. Prompt diagnosis with barium meal and early discussion with the regional paediatric surgery service is required.

IMPORTANT LEARNING POINTS

- Distinguishing between small and large bowel dilatation on abdominal X-ray can be challenging. Centrally placed loops of bowel with mucosal markings traversing the entire bowel, and a dilatation not in excess of 6 to 7 cm in diameter favour small bowel over large bowel.
- There are a variety of causes of small bowel obstruction which can be categorised into functional and mechanical (luminal, mucosal and extrinsic) causes. The age of the patient influences the most likely aetiology.
- Small bowel obstruction management is often conservative initially but the patients should be reviewed regularly. CT may be required to identify adult patients who will require surgical intervention.

CASE **3.3**

A 65-year-old man presents with absolute constipation (i.e. no bowel motions or flatus passed), nausea and faeculent vomiting. There is a preceding history of increasing constipation over the last month with blood mixed in with the stool. There has been 3 kg unintentional weight loss over the preceding 2 months. An abdominal X-ray has been performed.

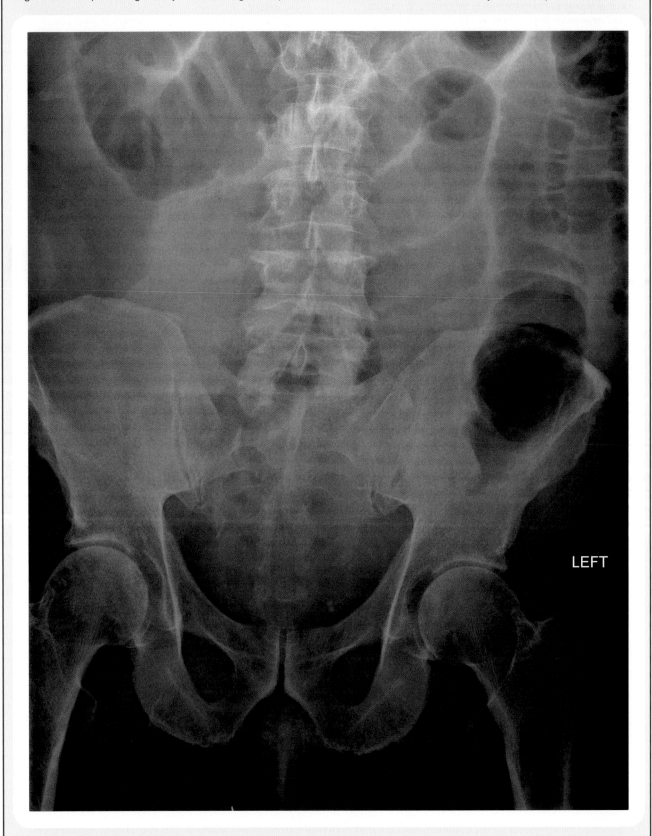

LEFT

ANNOTATED X-RAY

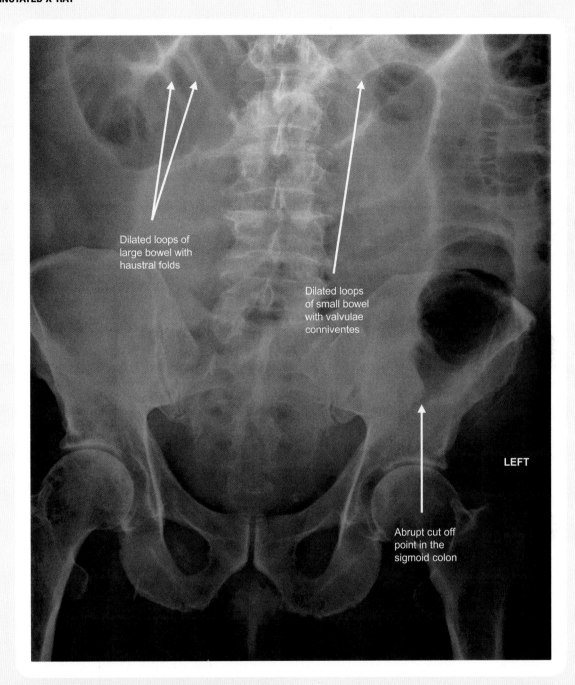

PRESENT YOUR FINDINGS

- This is a supine AP abdominal X-ray.
- There are no patient identifiable data on the X-ray but I would like to confirm the patient's name, date of birth and date and time that the X-ray was performed before assessing the X-ray further.
- The hernial orifices are demonstrated but the diaphragmatic contours have not been included. Consequently, this is technically inadequate as the entire abdomen has not been adequately visualised.
- The most striking abnormality is dilated gas-filled loops of bowel around the periphery of the

abdomen. Haustral folds are noted consistent with dilated large bowel. There is an abrupt cut-off point in the sigmoid colon in the left iliac fossa. No gas is demonstrated in the rectum. The prominent loops of gas-filled bowel within the central abdomen demonstrate valvulae conniventes and are consistent with dilated small bowel.
- There is no evidence of pneumoperitoneum or mucosal oedema.
- There is no obvious abnormality of the visible solid abdominal organs.
- No skeletal abnormality.

Continue

CASE **3.3** *Contd.*

IN SUMMARY – This abdominal X-ray demonstrates small and large bowel dilatation with a calibre change in the sigmoid colon, in keeping with mechanical large bowel obstruction due to sigmoid colon pathology. There is secondary small bowel dilatation due to backpressure and an incompetent ileocaecal valve. Given the history, I am concerned that the sigmoid pathology represents colorectal malignancy. I would ask for urgent surgical assessment, request an erect chest X-ray to look for evidence of pneumoperitoneum and consider the requirement for a CT scan.

QUESTIONS

1. Which of the following support/supports the diagnosis of mechanical large bowel obstruction over functional large bowel obstruction (pseudo-obstruction)?
   A) An abrupt change in calibre of the dilated large bowel
   B) Lack of gas within the distal large bowel
   C) Preceding history of unintentional weight loss and per rectum (PR) bleeding
   D) Radiological or clinical evidence of bowel ischaemia
   E) Recent (<24 hours) laparotomy
2. Which of the following is the commonest cause of large bowel obstruction?
   A) Adhesions
   B) Inguinal hernia
   C) Adenocarcinoma
   D) Diverticular disease
   E) Volvulus
3. A stricture within the large bowel may result in obstruction. Which of the following is/are causes of large bowel stricture formation?
   A) Diverticular disease
   B) Necrotising enterocolitis
   C) Bowel ischaemia
   D) Classic Hirschsprung disease
   E) Inflammatory bowel disease
4. Which of the following is the diagnostic investigation of choice for a patient with suspected colorectal cancer?
   A) Abdominal X-ray
   B) Colonoscopy
   C) Barium enema
   D) Virtual CT colonoscopy
   E) Ultrasound of the abdomen
5. Which of the following is/are potentially part of the initial management of a patient with mechanical large bowel obstruction secondary to colorectal malignancy?
   A) Laparotomy and Hartmann's procedure
   B) Laparoscopic colonic resection with primary anastomosis
   C) Neoadjuvant chemotherapy
   D) Stent placement
   E) Neoadjuvant radiotherapy

ANSWERS TO QUESTIONS

1. Which of the following support/supports the diagnosis of mechanical large bowel obstruction over functional large bowel obstruction (pseudo-obstruction)?

The correct answers are **A) An abrupt change in calibre of the dilated large bowel, B) Lack of gas within the distal large bowel, C) Preceding history of unintentional weight loss and PR bleeding and D) Radiological or clinical evidence of bowel ischaemia**.

It is important to realise that dilated large bowel can be due to a mechanical or functional cause.

A) An abrupt change in calibre of the dilated large bowel – Correct. The presence of an abrupt change in calibre of the dilated large bowel implies there is mechanical obstruction at the point of calibre transition.

B) Lack of gas within the distal large bowel – Correct. In cases of complete mechanical obstruction, there is collapse of the bowel distal to the point of obstruction. Therefore, the presence of gas throughout dilated loops of large bowel favours a functional rather than a mechanical aetiology. However, it is important to realise that there may be gas in the distal bowel if there is partial mechanical obstruction.

C) Preceding history of unintentional weight loss and PR bleeding – Correct. The presence of dilated large bowel with this clinical history is highly concerning for mechanical large bowel obstruction secondary to colorectal cancer.

D) Radiological or clinical evidence of bowel ischaemia – Correct. If severe enough and present for sufficient time, mechanical bowel obstruction can result in bowel ischaemia. Ischaemia should not result from simple functional bowel dilatation.

E) Recent (<24 hours) laparotomy – Incorrect. In the immediate postoperative period (<24 hours post laparotomy), the most common cause of dilated loops of large bowel will be a functional pseudo-obstruction. All types of surgery which breech the abdominal parietal peritoneum can cause pseudo-obstruction but the risk is greater with open procedures in comparison to laparoscopic techniques. Ensuring the patient is adequately hydrated and correcting biochemical abnormalities are both important. A repeat abdominal X-ray can be useful. Persistent bowel distension which does not improve with conservative measures warrants further assessment either with CT or occasionally with water-soluble enema in the case of recent large bowel surgery to exclude an anastomotic leak or intraabdominal collection as the cause.

❗ KEY POINT

The aetiology of large bowel obstruction is divided into functional and mechanical. It is important to interpret the radiological findings in the clinical context. If a presumed functional obstruction fails to improve, further investigation is warranted.

2. Which of the following is the commonest cause of large bowel obstruction?

The correct answer is **C) Adenocarcinoma**.

There are several causes of large bowel obstruction, some of which can be diagnosed by an abdominal X-ray. However, it is often necessary to resort to CT imaging to identify the aetiology and determine the anatomical cut-off point in the presence of mechanical obstruction.

A) Adhesions – Incorrect. Adhesions are the most common cause of small bowel obstruction. In the vast majority of cases, adhesions are secondary to scarring from previous abdominal surgery but can also occur following inflammatory bowel disease or diverticular disease and localised perforation. Adhesional large bowel obstruction is possible but rare.

B) Inguinal hernia – Incorrect. Bowel can pass into an inguinal hernia. If the bowel becomes irreducible, bowel obstruction can occur as a result. This usually affects small bowel more frequently and is only rarely described in the context of large bowel obstruction.

C) Adenocarcinoma – Correct. Adenocarcinoma of the large bowel is the most common cause of large bowel obstruction. The majority of large bowel adenocarcinomas occur in the rectum and sigmoid region. There are multiple risk factors for the development of adenocarcinoma of the large bowel including male sex, increasing age, family history, history of inflammatory bowel disease and a low-fibre high-fat diet (perhaps the most relevant).

D) Diverticular disease – Incorrect. Diverticular disease can cause large bowel obstruction but it is not the most common cause. Diverticula are herniations of mucosa through the circular muscles of the large bowel. Diverticular disease is most commonly found in the sigmoid colon and has been associated with lack of dietary fibre. The diverticula can become acutely inflamed and result in diverticulitis. This can result in rectal bleeding, bowel perforation and the formation of fistulas or strictures that can subsequently cause bowel obstruction. It can sometimes be difficult to exclude a diagnosis of adenocarcinoma in an area of active diverticulitis during the acute presentation. Follow-up imaging or direct visualisation is important in these cases.

E) Volvulus – Incorrect. Volvulus can cause large bowel obstruction but it is not the most common cause. Volvulus most commonly affects the sigmoid colon and the caecum. Sigmoid volvulus often occurs in constipated elderly patients. The bowel twists on its long mesentery and causes a closed-loop obstruction. Deflation of the bowel with a rigid sigmoidoscopy is often effective in relieving the obstruction.

Continue

CASE 3.3   *Contd.*

❶ KEY POINTS

1. Always consider malignancy as a cause of large bowel obstruction. As the majority of large bowel malignant tumours occur in the rectum or sigmoid colon, constipation often occurs earlier than vomiting in such patients as the site of mechanical obstruction is relatively low. Malignant large bowel obstruction can result in bowel or tumour perforation and subsequent faecal peritonitis. Due to the high mortality associated with these potential complications, patients with suspected malignant large bowel obstruction need prompt surgical review and treatment.

2. Other common causes of large bowel obstruction include sigmoid volvulus, inflammatory and ischaemic strictures, marked constipation and extrinsic bowel compression by a tumour.

---

3. A stricture within the large bowel may result in obstruction. Which of the following is/are causes of large bowel stricture formation?
   The correct answers are **A) Diverticular disease, B) Necrotising enterocolitis, C) Bowel ischaemia and E) Inflammatory bowel disease**.
   Strictures are a well-recognised cause of mechanical large bowel obstruction. They can result from a variety of different pathologies, but are usually neoplastic, inflammatory or ischaemic in nature.
   A) Diverticular disease – Correct. Long-standing diverticular disease can result in localised smooth muscle hypertrophy and stricture formation.
   B) Necrotising enterocolitis – Correct. Necrotising enterocolitis is a disease of the large bowel in premature neonates. If the neonate survives the initial insult, subsequent stricture formation is a recognised complication.
   C) Bowel ischaemia – Correct. A stricture can arise in the segment of previously ischaemic bowel.
   D) Classic Hirschsprung disease – Incorrect. Hirschsprung disease usually presents in childhood. It results in the absence of ganglion cells in Auerbach's and Meissner's plexuses (involved in the innervations of the bowel to enable coordinated peristalsis) in the rectum. Classically, the disease manifests with gross distension of the sigmoid colon proximal to the aganglionic segment of rectum. However, stricture formation is not usually a feature.
   E) Inflammatory bowel disease – Correct. Stricture formation is a feature of inflammatory bowel disease. It most commonly affects the small bowel in Crohn's disease.

❶ KEY POINTS

1. Contrast enemas (barium or water soluble) and CT can identify and help characterise a stricture. Most benign strictures tend to have smooth contours on imaging, whereas malignant strictures are often irregular.

2. Direct visualisation using colonoscopy or sigmoidoscopy has the advantage over other imaging techniques of allowing biopsies of the stricture to be taken to confirm the underlying aetiology.

---

4. Which of the following is the diagnostic investigation of choice for a patient with suspected colorectal cancer? The correct answer is **B) Colonoscopy**.
   A) Abdominal X-ray – Incorrect. Abdominal X-rays are often the initial investigation performed in patients presenting with an acute abdomen. Although they may demonstrate dilated loops of large bowel with a cut-off point, it is not possible to infer the aetiology of the change in calibre. For example, diverticular disease, previous bowel ischaemia and inflammatory bowel disease can all cause strictures and will be indistinguishable from a malignant stricture on abdominal X-ray.
   B) Colonoscopy – Correct. Direct visualisation with colonoscopy is the diagnostic investigation of choice for suspected colorectal cancer as it always allows the area of concern to be biopsied, thus enabling histological diagnosis. The patient must be fit enough to undergo purgative bowel preparation in order to allow the colonoscope to pass to the caecum. Colorectal malignancy often affects the elderly, some of whom are too frail to tolerate this preparation, which is why alternative investigations are sometimes performed to exclude gross colonic pathology.
   C) Barium enema – Incorrect. Barium enema used to be a common investigation for suspected large bowel pathology. It is no longer a recommended examination of the large bowel in the UK. CT or CT colonography provides superior diagnostic information with similar radiation penalty and should be performed instead.
   D) Virtual CT colonoscopy – Incorrect. A degree of bowel preparation is still required and the patient must be able to tolerate rolling on their side as well as insufflation of the colon with a considerable volume of carbon dioxide gas. As the entire abdomen and pelvis is imaged, further information regarding potential metastatic disease can be gained at the same time. However, the lack of ability to acquire a tissue diagnosis means that colonoscopy still remains the gold standard diagnostic investigation.
   E) Ultrasound of the abdomen – Incorrect. Ultrasound is a useful tool for assessing the solid viscera of the abdomen. The presence of gas within the bowel often precludes sonographic assessment of these structures and therefore is not used to interrogate the bowel in cases of suspected colorectal malignancy.

❶ KEY POINT

Once a malignant tumour is identified, the patient will require staging investigations, which will guide management and provide an indication of prognosis. CT of the chest, abdomen and pelvis is usually performed to assess the spread of the tumour. Additionally, MRI of the rectum is used in the local staging of patients with rectal cancers.

5. Which of the following is/are potentially part of the initial management of a patient with mechanical large bowel obstruction secondary to colorectal malignancy?

The correct answers are **A) Laparotomy and Hartmann's procedure, B) Laparoscopic colonic resection with primary anastomosis and D) Stent placement**.

The definitive treatment of colorectal malignancy is surgical resection. However, the treatment is dependent on many factors including the stage of the disease (e.g. distant metastases) at presentation as well as comorbidities. Those presenting with mechanical large bowel obstruction usually undergo a procedure to alleviate the obstruction, even if the cancer is incurable.

A) Laparotomy and Hartmann's procedure – Correct. In the case of malignant distal large bowel obstruction complicated by perforation and faeculent peritonitis, a Hartmann's procedure may be performed. This is an emergency operation which involves resection of the affected sigmoid colon, over-sewing of the distal rectal stump and bringing out a proximal end colostomy or ileostomy.

B) Laparoscopic colonic resection with primary anastomosis – Correct. Provided there is no high-grade proximal obstruction and depending on the local surgical expertise, resection of the colorectal tumour may be tackled by the less invasive laparoscopic approach with primary anastomosis in certain cases.

C) Neoadjuvant chemotherapy – Incorrect. Depending on the staging, there is a role of neoadjuvant chemoradiotherapy in rectal cancer to shrink the tumour and increase the chance of subsequent complete surgical excision with clear margins. However, this is not likely to be an initial option if the patient presents with complete obstruction.

D) Stent placement – Correct. Attempting definitive surgical excision in the presence of high-grade obstruction in the emergency setting can be difficult and can result in faecal contamination of the peritoneal cavity. Placing a stent with the aid of fluoroscopic monitoring, across the stricturing lesion can relieve the obstruction. The tumour and stent can then be excised in an urgent elective setting with the hope of a better surgical outcome for the patient. It can also be used as a palliative treatment.

E) Neoadjuvant radiotherapy – Incorrect. There is no role for neoadjuvant radiotherapy in the initial management of colorectal adenocarcinoma (see answer 5C).

❗ KEY POINT

Although surgical excision is the definitive treatment for colorectal malignancy, the appropriate initial management should be tailored to the patient. Some of the available options are previously described. Occasionally, a palliative defunctioning ileostomy (a loop of ileum upstream of the mechanical obstruction is brought out as a stoma, allowing the luminal contents to be diverted into the stoma bag) will be performed to relieve obstruction in a patient not fit for radical resection.

IMPORTANT LEARNING POINTS

- When presented with X-ray evidence of large bowel obstruction, the first diagnostic decision to be made is whether the dilatation is functional or mechanical in aetiology. In the case of the latter, malignancy must be excluded.
- There are a variety of investigations available for suspected colorectal malignancy. The burden of the preparation and demands of each investigation should be considered for each patient.
- Management of large bowel obstruction depends on the presentation (emergency with perforation or obstruction versus elective with weight loss, altered bowel habit, etc.), the comorbid conditions of the patient and the stage of their disease.

CASE 3.4

An 85-year-old woman presents with abdominal pain, distension and absolute constipation. She has had a previous stroke and is a nursing home resident. There has been a preceding history of constipation. An abdominal X-ray is performed.

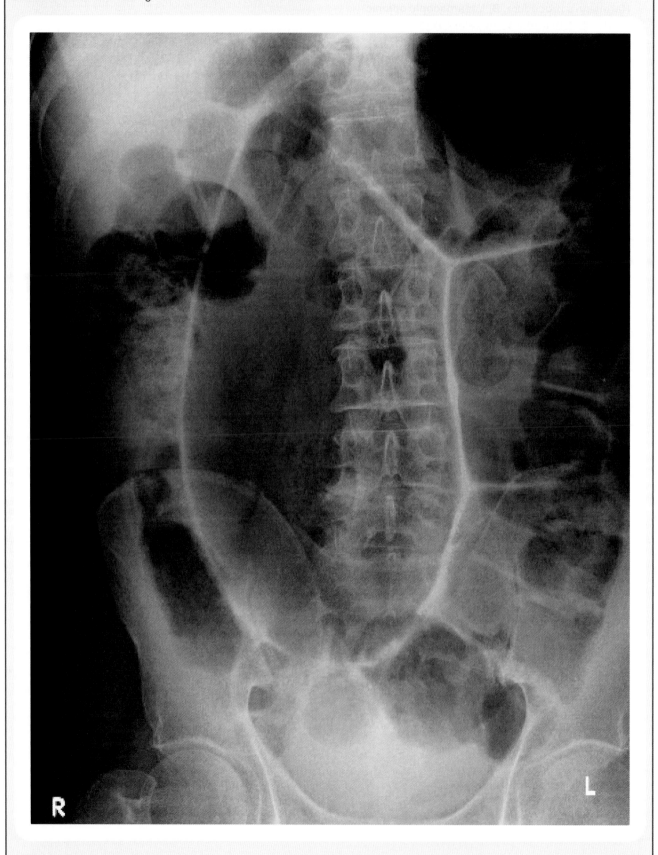

ANNOTATED X-RAY

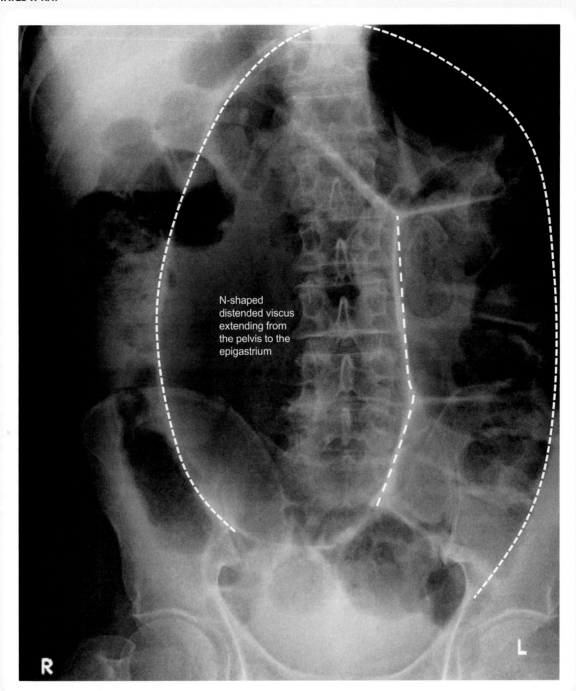

N-shaped distended viscus extending from the pelvis to the epigastrium

R

L

🔍 PRESENT YOUR FINDINGS

- This is a supine AP abdominal X-ray.
- There are no patient identifiable data on the X-ray but I would like to confirm the patient's name, date of birth and date and time that the X-ray was performed before making further assessment.
- The hernial orifices, diaphragmatic contours and left flank have not been included. Consequently, this is technically inadequate as the entire abdomen has not been adequately visualised.
- The most striking abnormality is a grossly distended loop of bowel extending from the pelvis towards the

epigastrium. This has a 'N-shaped' configuration and is devoid of haustra. The findings are consistent with a sigmoid volvulus.
- The remainder of the bowel is unremarkable.
- No evidence of pneumoperitoneum or mucosal oedema.
- There is no obvious abnormality of the visible solid abdominal organs.
- No skeletal abnormality.

IN SUMMARY – This abdominal X-ray demonstrates a large sigmoid volvulus. I would arrange urgent surgical review of the patient.

Continue

CASE 3.4 *Contd.*

QUESTIONS

1. Which of the following structures can undergo volvulus?
   A) Oesophagus
   B) Stomach
   C) Duodenum
   D) Caecum
   E) Sigmoid colon
2. Which patient demographic is most at risk of sigmoid volvulus?
   A) Infants
   B) Adolescents
   C) Pregnant women
   D) Middle-aged men
   E) The elderly
3. Regarding caecal volvulus, which of the following is correct?
   A) Caecal volvulus is the most common cause of volvulus
   B) Everyone is at risk of caecal volvulus
   C) Caecal volvulus generally affects older patients than sigmoid volvulus
   D) All forms of caecal volvulus involve torsion
   E) The 'swirl' sign is a useful CT sign of volvulus

4. Which of the following is/are radiological signs of sigmoid volvulus on the abdominal X-ray?
   A) Convergence of the lower margins of the distended loops in the left iliac fossa
   B) A dilated loop of bowel extending from the left iliac fossa to the liver or above it
   C) A dilated loop of bowel extending from the left iliac fossa to the left flank overlying the descending colon
   D) Thickened bowel wall with thumbprinting
   E) The coffee bean sign
5. Which of the following is/are potentially part of the initial management of suspected sigmoid volvulus?
   A) Water-soluble enema
   B) CT scan
   C) Rigid sigmoidoscopy
   D) Urgent laparotomy and sigmoid colectomy
   E) Percutaneous endoscopic colostomy

ANSWERS TO QUESTIONS

1. Which of the following structures can undergo volvulus?
   The correct answers are **B) Stomach, C) Duodenum, D) Caecum and E) Sigmoid colon**.
   Volvulus can affect any part of the intraabdominal gastrointestinal tract and consists of twisting of the segment around its mesentery.
   A) Oesophagus – Incorrect. The oesophagus does not have a mesentery and therefore volvulus does not affect this part of the gastrointestinal tract.
   B) Stomach – Correct. The stomach can twist along its long axis from cardia to pylorus and the greater curvature comes to lie to the right of the lesser curvature. The twisted stomach is at risk of resultant vascular compromise.
   C) Duodenum – Correct. Volvulus involving the small bowel is a complication of malrotated bowel. The vast majority of cases occur within the first year of life.
   D) Caecum – Correct. Volvulus of the caecum accounts for approximately 11% of all intestinal volvulus.
   E) Sigmoid colon – Correct. Sigmoid volvulus is the most common intestinal volvulus.

❗ KEY POINT

Any part of the intraabdominal gastrointestinal tract can twist on its mesentery. Sigmoid volvulus is the most common type of volvulus.

2. Which patient demographic is most at risk of sigmoid volvulus?
   The correct answer is **E) The elderly**.
   A) Infants – Incorrect. Midgut volvulus secondary to malrotation and intussusception are the most common causes of intestinal obstruction in the infant.
   B) Adolescents – Incorrect. Involvement of the small bowel by Crohn's disease and complicated acute appendicitis are probably the most likely causes of bowel obstruction in this age group.
   C) Pregnant women – Incorrect. Chronically constipated patients are at increased risk of sigmoid volvulus. Pregnancy can result in constipation but sigmoid volvulus is not a recognised feature in this demographic cohort.
   D) Middle-aged men – Incorrect. The risk of sigmoid volvulus increases with age but middle-aged men are not most at risk.
   E) The elderly – Correct. The elderly are most at risk of sigmoid volvulus.

❗ KEY POINT

In addition to age, a tortuous sigmoid colon on a long mesentery and chronic constipation are other risk factors for the development of sigmoid volvulus.

3. Regarding caecal volvulus, which of the following is/are correct?
   The correct answer is **E) The 'swirl' sign is a useful CT sign of volvulus**.
   A) Caecal volvulus is the most common cause of volvulus – Incorrect. Sigmoid volvulus is the most common type of volvulus, not caecal volvulus.

B) Everyone is at risk of caecal volvulus – Incorrect. A normally sited caecum with normal peritoneal fixation cannot undergo volvulus. Approximately 11% to 25% of the population has deficient peritoneal fixation and are at risk of caecal volvulus.
   C) Caecal volvulus generally affects older patients than sigmoid volvulus – Incorrect. Caecal volvulus generally affects a younger age group than sigmoid volvulus, usually between the ages of 20 and 40 years.
   D) All forms of caecal volvulus involve torsion – Incorrect. Caecal bascule is a variant of caecal volvulus where the caecum folds anteriorly but without any associated torsion.
   E) The 'swirl' sign is a useful CT sign of volvulus – Correct. The 'swirl' sign refers to twisting of the mesenteric vessels on CT at the point within the mesentery about which the bowel has rotated. All forms of volvulus may demonstrate this sign.

❗ KEY POINT

Only patients with deficient retroperitoneal fixation of the caecum are at risk of caecal volvulus.

4. Which of the following is/are radiological signs of sigmoid volvulus on the abdominal X-ray?
   The correct answers are **A) Convergence of the lower margins of the distended loops in the left iliac fossa, B) A dilated loop of bowel extending from the left iliac fossa to the liver or above it, C) A dilated loop of bowel extending from the left iliac fossa to the left flank overlying the descending colon and E) The coffee bean sign**.
   There are a variety of features on abdominal X-rays which can be used to identify a sigmoid volvulus.
   A) Convergence of the lower margins of the distended loops in the left iliac fossa – Correct. The sigmoid colon usually lies in the left iliac fossa. Once a sigmoid volvulus has formed, the closed-loop obstructed bowel dilates into the abdomen from the left iliac fossa.
   B) A dilated loop of bowel extending from the left iliac fossa to the liver or above it – Correct. This finding is termed the 'liver overlap sign'. It is a marker of the degree of distension.
   C) A dilated loop of bowel extending from the left iliac fossa to the left flank overlying the descending colon – Correct. This description refers to the 'left flank overlap sign'. Similarly to the liver overlap sign, it is a marker of degree of distension.
   D) Thickened bowel wall with thumbprinting – Incorrect. This describes mucosal oedema, which is a feature of inflammatory bowel disease, not sigmoid volvulus.
   E) The coffee bean sign – Correct. As the sigmoid colon twists on its mesentery, the compression together of the two medial walls produces a 'Y'-shaped shadow at the centre of the dilated bowel loop. This is said to resemble a coffee bean in appearance with its central indentation.

Continue

CASE **3.4**   *Contd.*

KEY POINTS

1. Other features that can occur in sigmoid volvulus include loss of the haustra markings due to the degree of distension. Another measure of severity is if the apex of the dilated bowel extends above the 10th vertebral body.
2. Always look for evidence of pneumoperitoneum in the presence of a sigmoid volvulus.
3. Water-soluble contrast enema and CT can help confirm the presence of a sigmoid volvulus (Table C3.4.1).

Table C3.4.1   Differentiating Sigmoid and Caecal Volvulus on Abdominal X-ray

SIGMOID VOLVULUS	CAECAL VOLVULUS
Arises from left lower quadrant	Arises from right lower quadrant
Extends towards the epigastrium – may overlap the liver (liver overlap sign) and may project above the transverse colon (Northern exposure sign)	Extends towards the left upper quadrant
Devoid of haustra	Haustra usually maintained
Coffee bean or 'n' shaped	Soft tissue indentation of the ileocolic valve
Often associated with proximal large bowel obstruction	Often associated with small bowel obstruction; however, the distal large bowel may be collapsed
Contrast enema will confirm the obstruction in the sigmoid colon. The volvulus appears like a bird's beak	Contrast enema will demonstrate a nondilated distal colon with the obstruction in the caecum

5. Which of the following is/are potentially part of the initial management of suspected sigmoid volvulus?
The correct answers are **A) Water-soluble enema, B) CT scan, C) Rigid sigmoidoscopy and D) Urgent laparotomy and sigmoid colectomy**.

A) Water-soluble enema – Correct. In situations where the diagnosis of sigmoid volvulus is not clear, an enema with water-soluble contrast medium can be performed. The contrast is run into the colon in a retrograde manner from a rectal catheter whilst screening with fluoroscopy. A twisted beak-like sign at the point of convergence in the sigmoid colon confirms the diagnosis.

B) CT scan – Correct. CT can be performed to confirm the diagnosis of sigmoid volvulus in atypical cases and to look for potential complications such as evidence of bowel ischaemia or perforation.

C) Rigid sigmoidoscopy – Correct. Most cases of sigmoid volvulus can initially be managed nonoperatively. Performing a rigid sigmoidoscopy can look for an obstructing lesion causing the large bowel dilatation but it also provides therapeutic decompression by passing a rectal tube into the proximal sigmoid colon.

D) Urgent laparotomy and sigmoid colectomy – Correct. Sigmoid volvulus can be complicated by bowel ischaemia and/or perforation. In these cases, urgent laparotomy and colectomy is required.

E) Percutaneous endoscopic colostomy – Incorrect. This involves creating a colostomy to allow alternative outflow tracts, relieving pressure and stopping the sigmoid colon over extending. Percutaneous endoscopic colostomy is a method of treating patients with recurrent sigmoid volvulus who are not fit for elective laparotomy and sigmoid colectomy. It is not usually performed for the first presentation of acute sigmoid volvulus.

KEY POINT

Once the diagnosis of sigmoid volvulus has been made either by abdominal X-ray, contrast enema or CT, then therapeutic decompression should be performed. The patient should then be placed on laxatives and elective sigmoid colectomy considered to prevent recurrence.

IMPORTANT LEARNING POINTS

- Sigmoid volvulus is the most common cause of volvulus. Caecal, midgut (associated with malrotation) and gastric volvulus are all much rarer.
- Sigmoid volvulus can be diagnosed by plain film and initially managed conservatively in most cases.
- Look for evidence of complications of volvulus, such as perforation, which will require urgent surgical intervention.

CASE **3.5**

A 40-year-old man with known ulcerative colitis presents with severe abdominal pain worse with movement. There has been a preceding history of increasing frequency of bloody diarrhoea and pyrexia. An abdominal X-ray has been performed.

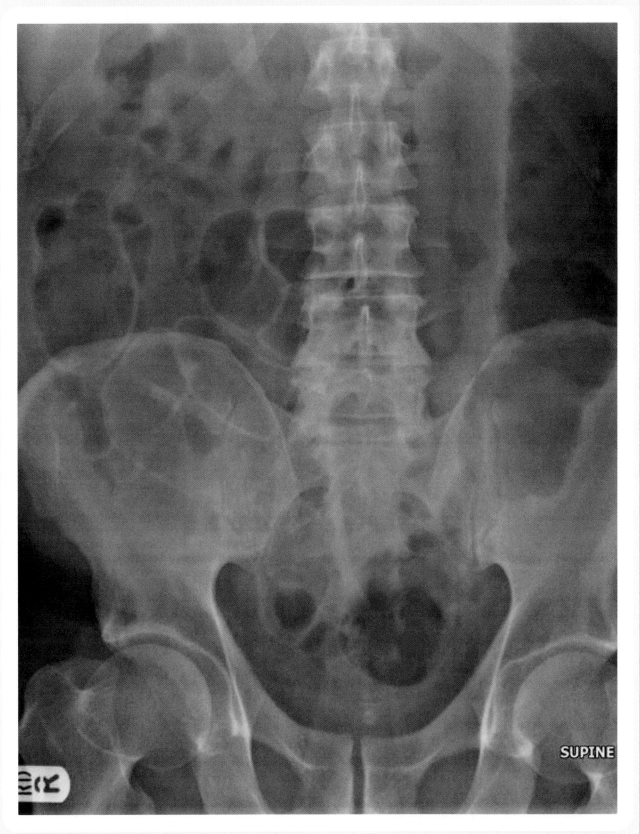

Continue

CASE **3.5**   *Contd.*

ANNOTATED X-RAY

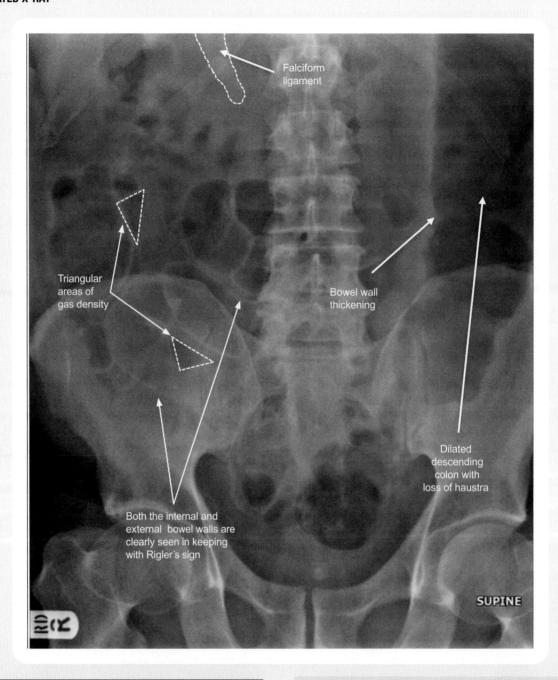

Falciform ligament

Triangular areas of gas density

Bowel wall thickening

Dilated descending colon with loss of haustra

Both the internal and external bowel walls are clearly seen in keeping with Rigler's sign

SUPINE

R

🔍 **PRESENT YOUR FINDINGS**

- This is a supine AP abdominal X-ray.
- There are no patient identifiable data on the X-ray. I would like to confirm the patient's name, date of birth and date and time that the X-ray was performed before making further assessment.
- The hernial orifices are demonstrated but the dia-phragmatic contours have not been included. The transverse colon is not clearly seen. Consequently, this is technically inadequate as the entire abdomen has not been adequately visualised.
- The most striking abnormality is the clearly defined walls of several loops of small bowel

within the right flank, consistent with Rigler's sign. Furthermore, there are several triangular pockets of gas density and the falciform ligament is clearly visible. These findings are indicative of extraluminal gas.
- There is dilatation of the descending colon, which has lost its haustral markings and demonstrates a thickened wall, suggestive of mucosal oedema. The transverse colon has not been included on the X-ray.
- There is no obvious abnormality of the visible solid abdominal organs.
- No skeletal abnormality.

IN SUMMARY – This abdominal X-ray demonstrates a pneumoperitoneum. Given the history and appearance of the descending colon, perforation of toxic megacolon due to acute exacerbation of the known ulcerative colitis is the most likely aetiology. I would arrange an urgent surgical review.

QUESTIONS

1. Which of the following is/are recognised causes of pneumoperitoneum?
   A) Perforated duodenal ulcer
   B) Diverticulitis
   C) Recent laparotomy
   D) Intraabdominal infection with a gas-forming organism
   E) Cholecystitis

2. Which of the following is/are X-ray signs of free intraperitoneal gas?
   A) A convex pocket of gas under the left hemidiaphragm with air–fluid level on erect chest X-ray
   B) Well-defined wall of small bowel loops on abdominal X-ray
   C) Visualisation of the falciform ligament on abdominal X-ray
   D) Triangular-shaped areas of gas density on abdominal X-ray
   E) Well-defined contours of the intraabdominal organs

3. Which of the following statements regarding imaging in suspected pneumoperitoneum is true?
   A) Gas in the right upper quadrant between the liver and the diaphragm on a chest X-ray always represents a pneumoperitoneum
   B) Prior to performing an erect chest X-ray the patient should be sat up for 1 minute
   C) Lack of subdiaphragmatic gas on erect chest X-ray excludes a pneumoperitoneum
   D) Performing an abdominal X-ray with the patient lying on their side is an alternative to performing an erect chest X-ray
   E) No further imaging is required once a pneumoperitoneum is demonstrated on erect chest or abdominal X-ray

4. Which of the following is/are potentially part of the initial management of a patient with pneumoperitoneum diagnosed on abdominal X-ray?
   A) Urgent laparotomy
   B) Urgent CT scan
   C) Intravenous broad-spectrum antibiotics
   D) Endoscopy
   E) Urgent anaesthetic review

5. With regard to the CT appearances in perforation, which of the following is true?
   A) Free fluid in the abdominal cavity is pathognomonic of a lower GI perforation
   B) Gas in the anterior portion of the abdomen only occurs in upper GI perforation
   C) The presence of diverticula indicates a lower GI site of perforation
   D) Oedema of the duodenal wall and localised stranding favours an upper GI site of perforation
   E) It is always possible to determine the precise origin of perforation on CT

Continue

CASE 3.5 *Contd.*

ANSWERS TO QUESTIONS

1. Which of the following is/are recognised causes of pneumoperitoneum?

The correct answers are **A) Perforated duodenal ulcer, B) Diverticulitis, C) Recent laparotomy and D) Intraabdominal infection with a gas-forming organism**.

Free gas within the abdominal cavity can irritate the parietal peritoneum and result in peritonism on clinical examination. Pneumoperitoneum is often, incorrectly, thought to be synonymous with bowel perforation. However, there are a variety of other causes.

A) Perforated duodenal ulcer – Correct. Duodenal ulcers could also affect the posterior wall of the first part of the duodenum and result in retroperitoneal free gas if they perforate. The gastroduodenal artery runs in this region and the patient may experience haematemesis. Duodenal ulcers are often benign and *Helicobacter pylori* infection is implicated in the aetiology of 90% of cases. Other risk factors for peptic ulcers include NSAID use and smoking.

B) Diverticulitis – Correct. Diverticulitis refers to active inflammation of diverticula, which are mucosal herniations through the circular muscles of the bowel. They occur most commonly in the sigmoid colon. Active inflammation can result in perforation of the bowel wall. This may seal off, resulting in a contained perforation, in which case flecks of extraluminal gas may only be discernible locally on CT. However, if the perforation is not sealed off, a pneumoperitoneum will result.

C) Recent laparotomy – Correct. An iatrogenic pneumoperitoneum is to be expected following recent abdominal surgery, particularly laparoscopic surgery where the abdominal cavity is insufflated with carbon dioxide during the procedure. Free gas related to surgery is usually reabsorbed within 7 days.

D) Intraabdominal infection with a gas-forming organism – Correct. Intraabdominal infection with a gas-forming organism can result in gas within the abdominal cavity.

E) Cholecystitis – Incorrect. Cholecystitis is inflammation of the gallbladder. It is most frequently related to gallstone disease. There is usually right upper quadrant pain. Murphy's sign may be positive. To elicit this sign, the right upper quadrant is palpated as the patient breathes in. If the patient stops breathing in and winces as the gallbladder is palpated, then Murphy's sign is present (though remember for Murphy's sign to be positive, the same action on the left must NOT result in the patient stopping breathing in). There may be pericholecystic fluid due to the localised inflammation but pneumoperitoneum is not recognised in uncomplicated cases of cholecystitis. Even if the gallbladder perforates there will not be a pneumoperitoneum, because unlike the gastrointestinal tract, the biliary system and gallbladder contain bile and not air/gas.

❗ KEY POINT

There are a variety of causes of pneumoperitoneum other than a perforated hollow viscus. The clinical scenario helps determine the aetiology.

2. Which of the following is/are X-ray signs of free intraperitoneal gas?

The correct answers are **B) Well-defined wall of small bowel loops on abdominal X-ray, C) Visualisation of the falciform ligament on abdominal X-ray, D) Triangular-shaped areas of gas density on abdominal X-ray and E) Well-defined contours of the intraabdominal organs**.

A pneumoperitoneum is usually identified first on plain X-rays, such as an erect chest X-ray, supine or lateral decubitus abdominal X-rays. Therefore it is important to understand and recognise the signs of pneumoperitoneum on these imaging modalities.

A) A convex pocket of gas under the left hemidiaphragm with air-fluid level on erect chest X-ray – Incorrect. This description refers to the normal gastric bubble, which should not be mistaken for a pneumoperitoneum on the erect chest X-ray. In the case of pneumoperitoneum, there is only a thin layer of soft tissue superior to the gas collection (usually 1–2 mm thick), which represents the diaphragm. In comparison, gas in the stomach has a thicker layer of superior soft tissue consisting of stomach wall in addition to the diaphragm.

B) Well-defined wall of small bowel loops on abdominal X-ray – Correct. This description refers to Rigler's sign. The appearance of the soft tissue density of the bowel walls is exaggerated on abdominal X-ray in pneumoperitoneum as there is radiolucent gas on both sides of the bowel wall (within the bowel lumen and on the outside of the bowel). Usually, there is only gas within the lumen so the outer aspect of the bowel wall is less well defined.

C) Visualisation of the falciform ligament on abdominal X-ray – Correct. Usually the falciform ligament lies in contact with the liver. As both structures are of similar soft tissue density, it is not normally discernible. On a supine X-ray, free intraperitoneal gas may rise anteriorly and lift the falciform ligament away from the liver and surround it with radiolucent gas. In this scenario, a linear soft tissue density will be demonstrated in the right upper quadrant running obliquely.

D) Triangular-shaped areas of gas density on abdominal X-ray – Correct. Intraluminal gas conforms to the smooth contoured shape of the bowel. Presence of triangular bubbles implies there is free gas between loops of bowel.

E) Well-defined contours of the intraabdominal organs – Correct. Similar in principle to why the bowel wall is particularly well defined in Rigler's sign, abdominal organs may also be outlined by free gas and therefore clearly seen in pneumoperitoneum. Retroperitoneal perforation may also exaggerate the outline of the psoas major muscles.

❗ KEY POINTS

1. Diagnosing pneumoperitoneum on an abdominal X-ray alone is difficult. There will usually be an accompanying erect chest X-ray to help.
2. There are several possible mimics of free intraperitoneal gas to be aware of:
   - The gastric bubble can be confused with free sub-diaphragmatic gas. Remember: the gastric bubble has a relatively thick superior wall and there is often an air-fluid level present.
   - A loop of bowel can be interposed between the right hemidiaphragm and the liver, which results in a pseudocrescent sign. This is known as Chilaiditi's phenomenon. Look for a relatively thick diaphragmatic contour (composed of bowel wall and diaphragm) and the presence of a bowel loop (usually haustra will be visible).
   - A false Rigler's sign occurs when there are two adjacent gas-filled loops of bowel. The intraluminal gas within each bowel loop outlines both internal bowel walls, which mimics the Rigler's sign.

   In such cases, the clinical condition of the patient will often not be consistent with a pneumoperitoneum. However, if you are in doubt, ask a radiologist to review the X-ray.

3. Which of the following statements regarding imaging in suspected pneumoperitoneum is true?
   The correct answer is **D) Performing an abdominal X-ray with the patient lying on their side is an alternative to performing an erect chest X-ray**.
   An erect chest X-ray is often the first investigation performed in a patient with suspected pneumoperitoneum as it is quick, can be performed portably and does not expose the patient to a significant amount of ionising radiation. However, it is important to be aware of some of the limitations of the erect chest X-ray in patients with suspected pneumoperitoneum, which are discussed later.
   A) Gas in the right upper quadrant between the liver and the diaphragm on a chest X-ray always represents a pneumoperitoneum – Incorrect. Chilaiditi syndrome is when a loop of transverse colon interposes itself between the liver and right hemidiaphragm. It is a rare phenomenon but a favourite topic for questioning medical students and junior doctors by consultant surgeons! The appearance may mimic perforation. Look for haustral folds to mitigate against pneumoperitoneum. Furthermore, the clinical condition of the patient is important – it is usually an incidental diagnosis made on a chest X-ray performed for suspected chest pathology. It may not always be possible to differentiate between Chilaiditi syndrome and pneumoperitoneum on a chest X-ray – in such cases, further imaging, such as a lateral decubitus abdominal X-ray or more likely a CT scan, can be considered.

   B) Prior to performing an erect chest X-ray, the patient should be sat up for 1 minute – Incorrect. To improve the sensitivity of an erect chest X-ray, the patient should sit in the erect position for 10 to 20 minutes prior to performing the investigation to allow free gas to collect beneath the diaphragm.
   C) Lack of subdiaphragmatic gas on erect chest X-ray excludes a pneumoperitoneum – Incorrect. The erect chest X-ray is not 100% sensitive for detecting free intraperitoneal gas. Consequently, a normal erect chest X-ray cannot fully exclude pneumoperitoneum. In particular, sealed perforations are unlikely to be demonstrated (see explanation for question 1 option B). If there is ongoing clinical concern, further imaging with CT is warranted.
   D) Performing an abdominal X-ray with the patient lying on their side is an alternative to performing an erect chest X-ray – Correct. A lateral decubitus abdominal X-ray can be performed as described. This only requires the patient to lie on their side, which may be better tolerated than attempting to sit an ill patient upright for an erect chest X-ray. Usually, the patient lies with their left hand side down and right side up. Free gas can then be identified. Lateral decubitus X-rays are more frequently used in the paediatric population than adults. This is because infants and children are more sensitive to the detrimental effects of ionising radiation compared to adults, and a lateral decubitus X-ray has a significantly lower dose of ionising radiation compared with a CT. On the other hand, CT provides a more comprehensive and accurate assessment of the abdomen and pelvis.
   E) No further imaging is required once a pneumoperitoneum is demonstrated on erect chest or abdominal X-ray – Incorrect. Nowadays, most surgeons request a CT scan in patients with pneumoperitoneum prior to laparotomy. Modern CT scanners are readily available and the study can be performed in seconds. It will help identify the aetiology and may be able to distinguish between upper GI and lower GI perforation. This, in turn, may dictate the surgical approach for the operation.

❗ KEY POINT

No imaging modality is 100% sensitive, so pathology can never be definitively excluded. If there is clinical suspicion of perforation but no evidence of pneumoperitoneum on erect chest X-ray or abdominal X-ray, the patient should proceed to CT, which has a much higher sensitivity.

4. Which of the following is/are potentially part of the initial management of a patient with pneumoperitoneum diagnosed on abdominal X-ray?
   The correct answers are **A) Urgent laparotomy, B) Urgent CT scan, C) Intravenous broad-spectrum antibiotics and E) Urgent anaesthetic review**.

Continue

CASE **3.5**   *Contd.*

Patients with a pneumoperitoneum are usually acutely unwell. Management is aimed at stabilising the patient, identifying the underlying cause and instigating definitive management.

A) Urgent laparotomy – Correct. Most cases of pneumoperitoneum are the result of bowel perforation. Laparotomy usually enables definitive treatment.

B) Urgent CT scan – Correct. Most patients with evidence of pneumoperitoneum will go on to have a CT scan to help determine the aetiology of the free gas and attempt to localise the site of perforation to guide the surgeon.

C) Intravenous broad-spectrum antibiotics – Correct. A patient with perforated small or large bowel may benefit from administration of antibiotics. It is important to commence appropriate antibiotic therapy prior to surgery. This is particularly relevant if the site of perforation is the lower GI tract and there is resultant faeculent contamination of the peritoneal cavity.

D) Endoscopy – Incorrect. Perforation is a recognised risk of endoscopy. It is not used in the initial management of a patient with pneumoperitoneum. A patient with haematemesis from suspected gastric or duodenal ulcer will undergo oesophagogastroduodenoscopy in an attempt to stop the bleeding. However, if the ulcer perforates, management will be surgical.

E) Urgent anaesthetic review – Correct. Early anaesthetic review is vital in patients with perforation. Some patients may be too high risk for an anaesthetic (e.g. a very frail elderly patient) and early review enables prompt palliative care involvement. Alerting the on-call anaesthetist will highlight the situation to the emergency theatres to ensure a space is free on the emergency list for the patient if appropriate.

❗ KEY POINT

Patients with pneumoperitoneum should be discussed early with radiology, surgery and anaesthetics to ensure optimal diagnostic and therapeutic management.

5. With regard to the CT appearances in perforation, which of the following is true?
   The correct answer is **D) Oedema of the duodenal wall and localised stranding favours an upper GI site of perforation**.
   The wide availability, accuracy and rapid speed of CT scanning make it the most attractive imaging modality in patients with a pneumoperitoneum or acute abdomen. CT is used to try to identify the underlying pathology whilst permitting accurate assessment of the rest of the abdominal and pelvic cavities.

   A) Free fluid in the abdominal cavity is pathognomonic of a lower GI perforation – Incorrect. Free fluid is a nonspecific sign, which can occur in both upper and lower GI perforation, as well as many other abdominal and pelvic pathologies. Occasionally, there may be evidence of faeces in the peritoneal cavity. This clearly implicates the large bowel.

B) Gas in the anterior portion of the abdomen only occurs in upper GI perforation – Incorrect. Free gas localised to the upper abdomen or retroperitoneum can favour an upper GI perforation. However, as patients are scanned in the supine position, the anterior abdomen is where most free gas will collect, so this does not help distinguish between upper and lower GI sites of perforation.

C) The presence of diverticula indicates a lower GI site of perforation – Incorrect. Diverticula are extremely common. Their presence alone does not implicate the large bowel in cases of pneumoperitoneum. There must be other supporting evidence to imply active inflammation, such as surrounding flecks of extraluminal gas, reactive lymphadenopathy or pericolic abscess formation.

D) Oedema of the duodenal wall and localised stranding favours an upper GI site of perforation – Correct. Sometimes CT can demonstrate the defect in the bowel wall at the site of perforation. However, as omentum attempts to wall off perforations, this is not always discernible. Wall oedema and local stranding are secondary signs which support the notion of active inflammation in the vicinity. If this occurs in the duodenum, it suggests that it might be the site of perforation (i.e. an upper GI source).

E) It is always possible to determine the precise origin of perforation on CT – Incorrect. CT can often only suggest the site of perforation by evidence of secondary inflammatory change. As the physical defect in the bowel is not always seen and because several of the CT signs are nonspecific, it is not always possible to predict the exact origin of the perforation. Even with the use of enteral contrast (oral or rectal), it may not be possible to identify the site of perforation as the surrounding omentum will often seal off the perforation by the time the scan is performed.

❗ KEY POINT

CT provides detailed information regarding the intraabdominal situation. However, clinicians should be aware that it is not 100% specific for identifying the site of perforation.

👥 IMPORTANT LEARNING POINTS

- There are various causes of a pneumoperitoneum including perforated viscus, recent laparotomy/laparoscopy and rarely a gas-forming intraperitoneal infection.
- The signs of pneumoperitoneum on abdominal X-ray can be subtle. Always look for an accompanying erect chest X-ray to help make the diagnosis.
- CT is commonly used to confirm the pneumoperitoneum and assess the underlying cause.
- Be aware of the limitations in sensitivity and specificity of the common imaging modalities.
- Involve radiology, surgery and anaesthetics early in the management of patients with suspected perforation.

CASE 3.6

A 42-year-old man who has known ulcerative colitis presented with abdominal pain, diarrhoea and rectal bleeding.

He is febrile and has raised inflammatory markers. He undergoes an abdominal X-ray.

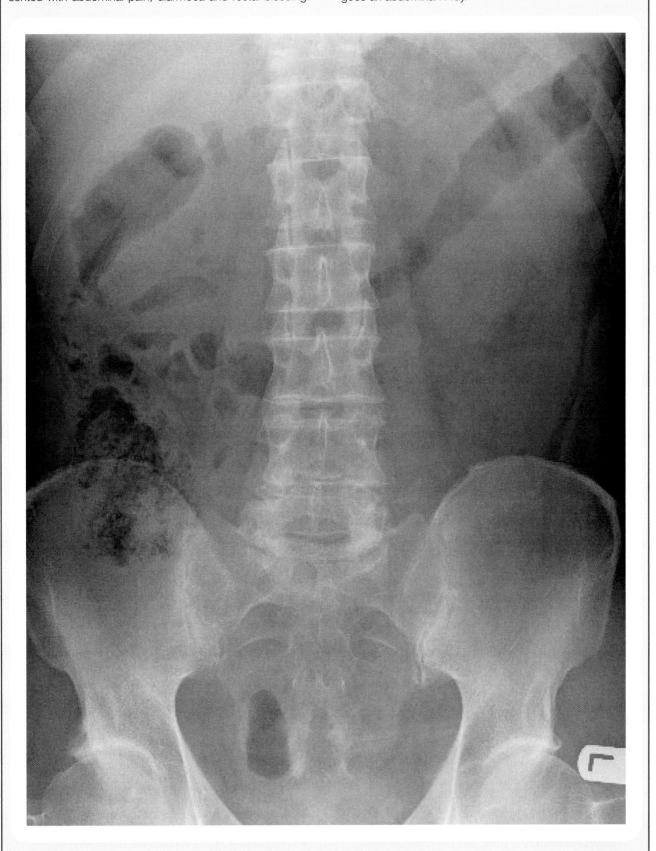

Continue

CASE **3.6**   *Contd.*

ANNOTATED X-RAY

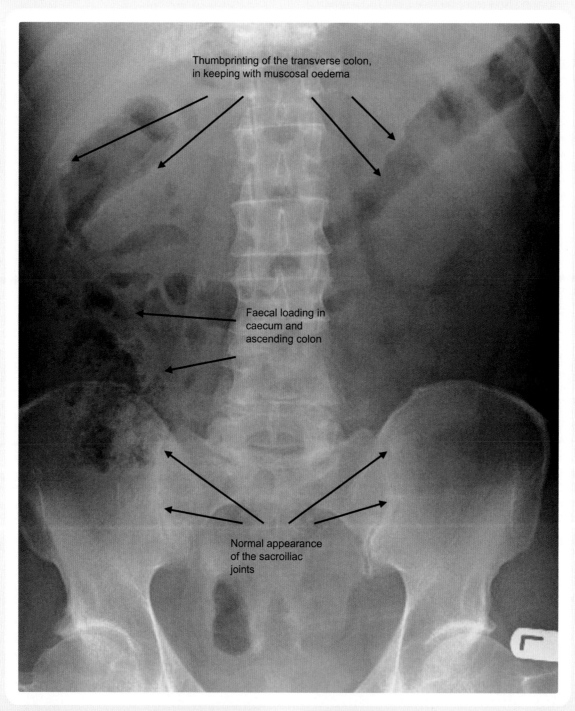

Thumbprinting of the transverse colon, in keeping with muscosal oedema

Faecal loading in caecum and ascending colon

Normal appearance of the sacroiliac joints

🔍 PRESENT YOUR FINDINGS

- This is a supine AP abdominal X-ray.
- There are no patient identifiable data on the X-ray. I would ordinarily confirm the patient's name, date of birth and date and time that the X-ray was performed before making further assessment.
- The hernial orifices and diaphragmatic contours have not been included. Consequently, this is a technically inadequate film as the entire abdomen has not been adequately visualised.

- The most striking abnormality is the appearance of the transverse colon, which has thumbprinting of its walls. This is consistent with mucosal oedema.
- There is faecal loading within the caecum and proximal ascending colon. The descending and sigmoid colon are difficult to identify.
- No evidence of bowel dilatation or perforation.
- No obvious abnormality of the visible solid abdominal organs.
- The sacroiliac joints appear normal. No skeletal abnormality.

IN SUMMARY – This abdominal X-ray shows mucosal oedema within the transverse colon and the hepatic and splenic flexures. Given the patient's past medical history, the findings are most likely due to a flare of ulcerative colitis, although other forms of colitis are a possibility.

QUESTIONS

1. Which of the following is the **least** likely to cause colitis?
   A) *Clostridium difficile* infection
   B) *Staphylococcus* infection
   C) Cytomegalovirus infection
   D) Neutropenia
   E) Inflammatory bowel disease

2. Which of the following is/are useful in the initial assessment of a patient with bloody diarrhoea?
   A) Accurate history and examination
   B) Bloods including full blood count, U&Es, CRP and blood cultures
   C) Stool cultures
   D) Urgent MRI
   E) Urgent CT abdomen and pelvis

3. Which of the following is more commonly found in Crohn's disease rather than ulcerative colitis?
   A) Involvement of only the superficial layers of the mucosa
   B) Continuous involvement from the rectum moving proximally
   C) Fistula formation
   D) Colorectal cancer
   E) Primary sclerosing cholangitis

4. In patients with a severe flare of ulcerative colitis, which potentially life-threatening complication is usually assessed for with serial abdominal X-rays?
   A) Pericolonic abscess
   B) Fistulation
   C) Stricture formation
   D) Toxic megacolon
   E) Colorectal cancer

5. Which of the following is/are part of the initial management of a severe flare of ulcerative colitis?
   A) IV fluid resuscitation
   B) IV corticosteroids
   C) Nutritional support
   D) Venous thromboembolism prophylaxis
   E) Urgent colectomy

Continue

CASE **3.6**   *Contd.*

ANSWERS TO QUESTIONS

1. Which of the following is the **least** likely to cause colitis? The correct answer is **B)** *Staphylococcus* **infection**. Colitis can be ischaemic, infective or inflammatory in nature and results in bowel wall thickening/ mucosal oedema and in some cases haemorrhage. Thumbprinting is a term used to describe thickened bowel wall on an abdominal X-ray, with the appearance of bowel wall indentations the size of a thumb. It can be caused by oedema (infective or inflammatory aetiology), tumour (lymphoma or leukaemia) or haemorrhage (ischaemia, coagulopathy, Henoch–Schönlein disease, disseminated intravascular coagulopathy) within the bowel wall.

A) *C. difficile* infection – Incorrect. *C. difficile* infection is a common cause of infective colitis particularly in hospitalised patients. Risk factors for its development include increasing age, prolonged hospital admission, recent antibiotics (any antibiotics can be a cause, with clindamycin, broad-spectrum penicillins and cephalosporins being most frequently implicated) and proton pump inhibitors. *C. difficile* is the commonest cause of pseudomembranous colitis due to the production of toxins A and B.

B) *Staphylococcus* infection – Correct. *Staphylococcus* is a very uncommon cause of colitis. It is, however, often implicated in colitis as many of the antibiotics used to treat staphylococcal infections are strongly associated with *C. difficile* infection.

C) Cytomegalovirus infection – Incorrect. Cytomegalovirus is a recognised cause of colitis. It usually affects immunocompromised patients. It can cause superficial or deep ulceration and localised or diffuse colitis. Often it is difficult to distinguish from pseudomembranous colitis on X-ray.

D) Neutropenia – Incorrect. Acute necrotising colitis occurs in patients who are immunocompromised and neutropenic. Classically, it is seen in young patients being treated for leukaemia and affects the right side of the colon. It is also known as typhlitis or neutropenic colitis.

E) Inflammatory bowel disease – Incorrect. Inflammatory bowel disease (ulcerative colitis and Crohn's disease) is a common cause of colitis, particularly in younger patients.

❶ KEY POINTS

1. Other causes of infective colitis include *Salmonella, Shigella, Campylobacter* and *Yersinia* infections.
2. Radiotherapy, chemotherapy and ischaemia are other noninfective causes of colitis.
3. The distribution of colitis, the degree of wall thickening and other findings in the abdomen and pelvis on CT can help differentiate the causes of colitis. However, the history, examination and other investigations such as stool cultures are often more helpful.

2. Which of the following is/are useful in the initial assessment of a patient with bloody diarrhoea?

The correct answers are **A) Accurate history and examination, B) Bloods including full blood count, U&Es, CRP and blood cultures and C) Stool cultures**. As alluded to in question 1, there are several different causes of bloody diarrhoea and colitis. Initial investigations are aimed at identifying the underlying aetiology and assessing for potential complications.

A) Accurate history and examination – Correct. Accurate clinical assessment helps to determine the underlying aetiology. For example, a recent hospital admission or treatment with high-risk antibiotics would increase the likelihood of *C. difficile* infection, whereas a history of food poisoning raises the possibility of another type of infective colitis, such as *Salmonella*. There may be extraintestinal signs, such as erythema nodosum and iritis, which will point to an inflammatory aetiology. Ischaemic colitis should be considered in patients with significant vascular disease or a history of atrial fibrillation/atrial myxoma. History and examination also play an important role in assessing the patient's clinical status and the severity of the colitis.

B) Bloods including full blood count, U&Es, CRP and blood cultures – Correct. Routine blood tests are essential to assess for anaemia and dehydration. Inflammatory markers are useful for assessing severity and response to treatment. Lactate is a useful test in patients suspected to have ischaemic colitis (infarcted tissue results in raised lactate). Blood cultures should be considered in all patients.

C) Stool cultures – Correct. An infectious cause is one of the commonest causes of bloody diarrhoea. Therefore, stool cultures are essential in the initial assessment of any patient presenting with bloody diarrhoea. However, the results will not be available for a few days.

D) Urgent MRI – Incorrect. MRI allows accurate assessment of the gastrointestinal tract, particularly the small bowel. It is also very useful for assessing pelvic and perineal disease, such as fistulae. However, it is not suitable for acutely unwell patients, due to the relatively long imaging times. It is mainly used to assess disease burden and response to therapy in relatively quiescent Crohn's disease. It is not necessary in the investigation or management of the majority of other forms of colitis.

E) Urgent CT abdomen and pelvis – Incorrect. Contrast-enhanced CT can be useful in patients with colitis. However, CT is not part of the initial management of patients with bloody diarrhoea – most of these patients can be managed without cross sectional imaging, with CT being reserved for a few cases. The pattern of bowel involvement identified on CT can help distinguish different types of colitis. For example, pseudomembranous colitis often involves the rectum and extends proximally to a variable extent. The bowel wall is usually very thickened (>15 mm) and there might be pericolonic fat changes and ascites. In contrast, ischaemic colitis typically occurs in a vascular territory or a watershed area, usually the splenic flexure or descending colon. It is less frequently associated with ascites. There may be evidence of vascular disease, thrombus within one of the mesenteric vessels or bowel wall ischaemia. CT is also very useful for identifying complications such as perforation or abscess formation.

> **❗ KEY POINT**
>
> It is important to identify the underlying cause as this will guide management. Antibiotics, for example, may be considered if there is an infective aetiology, anticoagulation can be used in certain types of ischaemic colitis and antiinflammatory medications can be used in inflammatory bowel disease.

Table C3.5.1 Differences Between Crohn's Disease and Ulcerative Colitis

	CROHN'S DISEASE	ULCERATIVE COLITIS
Part of GI tract involved	Any part, especially the terminal ileum	Colon only (can involve terminal ileum = backwash ileitis)
	Discontinuous (skip lesion)	Continuous, starting in the rectum and extending proximally
Continuity of involvement	Oral and perianal disease common	Oral and perianal areas spared
Depth of inflammation	Transmural deep fissures and fistulae common	Mucosal superficial ulcers. Fistulation is rare
Common complications	Perianal and intraabdominal abscess, fistula formation	Toxic megacolon
Risk of colorectal cancer	Increased risk of colorectal cancer (if colon affected)	High risk of colorectal cancer
Other associated conditions	Gallstones, sacroiliitis	Primary sclerosing cholangitis, cholangiocarcinoma

3. Which of the following is more commonly found in Crohn's disease rather than ulcerative colitis (Table C3.5.1)?
   The correct answer is **C) Fistula formation**.
   Crohn's disease and ulcerative colitis can present similarly, with diarrhoea, abdominal pain and rectal bleeding. However, their underlying pathologies are very different. Crohn's disease results in transmural inflammation (involvement of the whole thickness of the bowel wall) and is therefore more commonly

associated with the formation of fistulae and fissures, particularly in the perianal region. It tends to involve the small bowel, particularly the terminal ileum with skip lesions (normal areas of bowel interspersed between diseases areas). On the other hand, ulcerative colitis causes superficial mucosal inflammation and thus fistulation is rare. The disease typically starts at the rectum and extends proximally in a continuous fashion (no skip lesions). The perianal area is usually spared. The terminal ileum can be involved (backwash ileitis). Ulcerative colitis is also associated with a significantly higher risk for the development of colorectal cancer. Additionally, primary sclerosing cholangitis is much more frequent in patients with ulcerative colitis compared to those with Crohn's disease and the general population.

4. In patients with a severe flare of ulcerative colitis, which potentially life-threatening complication is usually assessed for with serial abdominal X-rays? The correct answer is **D) Toxic megacolon**.
   Patients with a severe flare of ulcerative colitis, as with any colitis, can be very unwell. They are at risk of developing toxic megacolon which can result in bowel perforation and is associated with increased mortality.
   A) Pericolonic abscess – Incorrect. Ulcerative colitis results in inflammation within the superficial mucosa, whereas Crohn's disease causes transmural inflammation. Therefore, pericolic abscess formation is much more common with Crohn's disease. Additionally, contrast-enhanced CT, not serial abdominal X-rays, would be the investigation of choice in patients suspected to have an intraabdominal abscess.
   B) Fistulation – Incorrect. Again, fistulation is uncommon in ulcerative colitis as the inflammation is not transmural. In Crohn's disease fistula formation is much more common. However, abdominal X-rays are not useful diagnostically. MRI is more useful.
   C) Stricture formation – Incorrect. Stricture formation is a recognised complication of both ulcerative colitis and Crohn's disease but is unlikely to occur in the acute setting. Again, abdominal X-rays are not useful in the identification of strictures unless there is resultant bowel obstruction. Water-soluble or barium contrast examinations, CT and MRI are more useful.
   D) Toxic megacolon – Correct. Toxic megacolon is an acute form of colonic dilatation, which occurs most commonly in ulcerative colitis or pseudomembranous colitis. It can also complicate Crohn's disease and other forms of colitis, albeit more rarely. Toxic megacolon can lead to perforation, sepsis and shock. Serial abdominal X-rays can be used to detect the development of toxic megacolon; the X-ray features are a dilated, ahaustral colon (>7 cm). Treatment can be conservative (e.g. steroids for ulcerative colitis) or more radical (e.g. colectomy) if the patient does not improve.

Continue

CASE **3.6**   *Contd.*

E) Colorectal cancer – Incorrect. Ulcerative colitis significantly increases the risk of colorectal cancer. For this reason, patients will often undergo an elective total colectomy. However, colorectal cancer is not a complication which develops in the acute setting. Furthermore, serial abdominal X-rays would be an insensitive method of screening for colorectal cancer.

❗ KEY POINT

The severity of an acute flare of ulcerative colitis can be estimated using clinical parameters.
   Factors suggestive of a severe flare include:
- More than six episodes of bloody diarrhoea per day
- Temperature >37.5°C
- Pulse >90 beats per minute
- Haemoglobin <100 g/L
- Erythrocyte sedimentation rate (ESR) >30 mm/h
- Serum albumin <30 g/L
- Dilated bowel on abdominal X-ray.

5. Which of the following is/are part of the initial management of a severe flare of ulcerative colitis?
   The correct answers are **A) IV fluid resuscitation, B) IV corticosteroids, C) Nutritional support and D) Venous thromboembolism prophylaxis**.
   A severe flare of ulcerative colitis is associated with high morbidity and mortality and should be managed in hospital by a gastroenterologist with regular surgical input. The initial management is medical.
   A) IV fluid resuscitation – Correct. These patients are likely to be dehydrated due to diarrhoea and increased insensible losses from pyrexia. They should receive IV fluids to replace fluid and electrolyte losses.
   B) IV corticosteroids – Correct. Intravenous methylprednisolone or hydrocortisone is used to dampen down the inflammatory response. Topical steroids may also be used. If, however, the patient fails to respond, other antiinflammatory drugs, such as ciclosporin (immunosuppressant) or infliximab (monoclonal antibody against tumour necrosis factor alpha), should be considered.
   C) Nutritional support – Correct. Nutritional support, preferably enteral, is used in malnourished patients.

D) Venous thromboembolism prophylaxis – Correct. Patients with an acute flare of inflammatory bowel disease are at risk of developing deep vein thrombosis. Therefore, even in the presence of bloody diarrhoea, the patients should receive appropriate venous thromboembolism prophylaxis.
E) Urgent colectomy – Incorrect. The initial management is medical with IV steroids +/– ciclosporin/infliximab. However, if the patient fails to improve after optimal medical therapy or if they develop toxic megacolon, an urgent colectomy should be considered.

❗ KEY POINT

The patient's response to treatment should be monitored:
- Clinically
  - Abdominal pain
  - Pulse rate
  - Stool frequency/amount of blood
  - Temperature
- Biochemically
  - Haemoglobin
  - ESR and CRP
  - Albumin
  - U&Es
- Radiologically
  Serial abdominal X-rays assessing for the development of toxic megacolon. The frequency of these X-rays is determined by the clinical condition of the patient. They are usually initially performed daily.

 IMPORTANT LEARNING POINTS

- Thumbprinting is an X-ray sign of bowel wall oedema, haemorrhage or tumour infiltration.
- Colitis is a common cause of mucosal oedema and can be infective, inflammatory or ischaemic in nature.
- Clinical, biochemical and radiological assessments are all important in investigating patients with colitis/bloody diarrhoea.
- Toxic megacolon is a serious complication of colitis. It is most commonly associated with ulcerative colitis and pseudomembranous colitis. Serial abdominal X-rays are used to screen for its development.

CASE **3.7**

An 85-year-old man presents to hospital as an emergency in an ambulance with severe abdominal pain and distension. He is hypotensive and tachycardic and is in new-onset atrial fibrillation. As he is being resuscitated in the emergency department, an abdominal X-ray is performed.

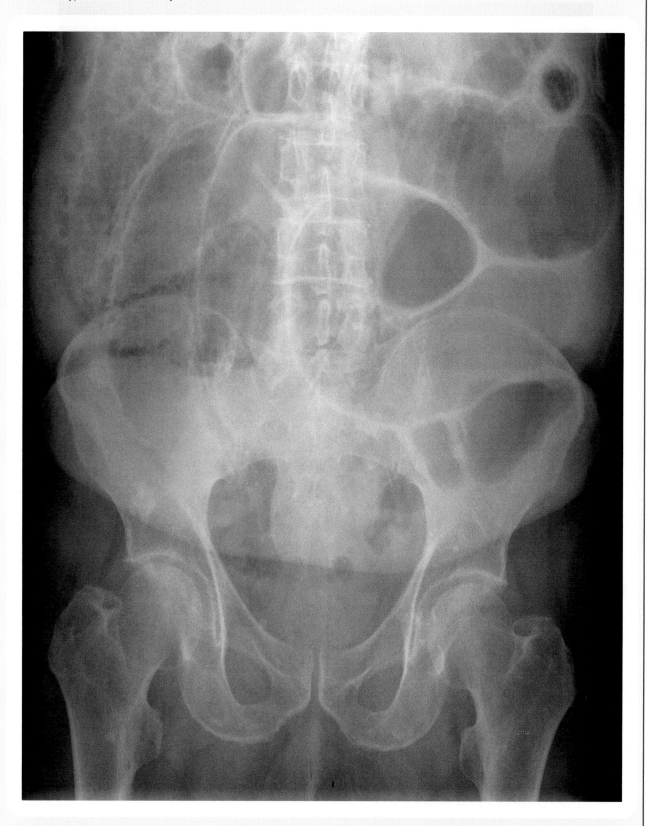

Continue

CASE **3.7** *Contd.*

ANNOTATED X-RAY

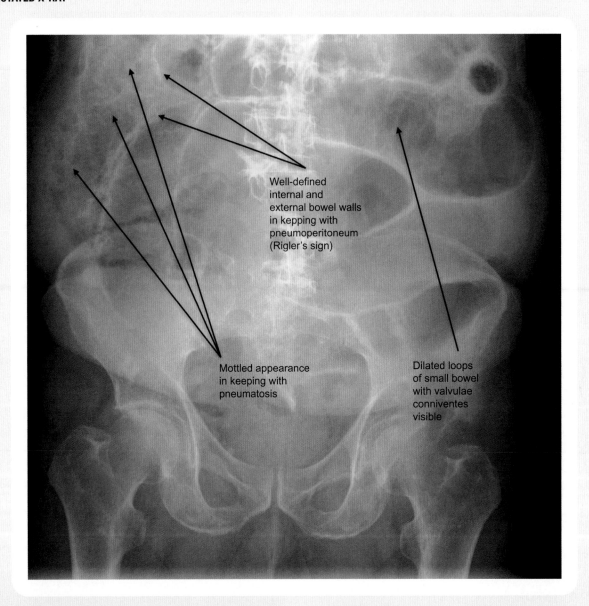

Well-defined internal and external bowel walls in kepping with pneumoperitoneum (Rigler's sign)

Mottled appearance in keeping with pneumatosis

Dilated loops of small bowel with valvulae conniventes visible

PRESENT YOUR FINDINGS

- This is a supine AP abdominal X-ray.
- There are no patient identifiable data on the X-ray. I would like to confirm the patient's name, date of birth and date and time that the X-ray was performed before making further assessment.
- The hernial orifices are demonstrated but the diaphragmatic contours have not been included. Consequently, this is technically inadequate as the entire abdomen has not been adequately visualised.
- The most striking abnormality is the multiple foci of gas density in the right upper quadrant, which appear to outline the bowel wall, suspicious for gas within the bowel wall (pneumatosis intestinalis). This is concerning for bowel ischaemia. It is not possible to determine whether there is any associated portal venous gas, due to overlying bowel loops.
- In addition, there are multiple loops of distended bowel, predominantly in the upper central abdomen. Some of the loops have markings across their diameter suggestive of valvulae conniventes, favouring small bowel over large bowel.
- The walls of several of the bowel loops in the right flank are well-defined suggestive of Rigler's sign (clear demonstration of the bowel wall due to adjacent intra- and extraluminal gas – suggestive of associated free intraabdominal gas).
- There is no obvious abnormality of the visible abdominal organs.
- No skeletal abnormality.

IN SUMMARY – This abdominal X-ray demonstrates dilated loops of bowel, likely small bowel, with evidence of gas within the bowel wall and possibly a pneumoperitoneum. Given the history, I am concerned that the patient has bowel ischaemia. A thrombotic event related to the new-onset atrial fibrillation may be implicated. I would arrange urgent surgical review. An erect chest X-ray may help confirm the presence of a pneumoperitoneum. A CT scan is likely to be required.

QUESTIONS

1. Which of the following is/are part of the differential diagnosis for gas in the bowel wall (pneumatosis intestinalis)?
   A) Idiopathic
   B) Obstructive airways disease
   C) Recent barium swallow
   D) Trauma
   E) Intestinal ischaemia

2. Which of the following is/are potentially part of the management of a patient with suspected acute bowel ischaemia?
   A) Erect chest X-ray and abdominal X-ray
   B) Perform a CT scan
   C) Consider the role of interventional radiology
   D) Consider vasopressin to maintain blood pressure in hypovolaemic patients
   E) Emergency laparotomy and resection of the ischaemic bowel

3. Which of the following is/are radiological features of acute bowel ischaemia?
   A) Lack of mucosal enhancement in a segment of bowel on contrast-enhanced CT
   B) Dilatation of multiple bowel loops
   C) Pneumatosis intestinalis
   D) Branching pattern of gas within the central liver that does not reach the periphery
   E) Filling defect in the superior mesenteric artery on contrast-enhanced CT

4. Regarding CT imaging in suspected acute bowel ischaemia, which of the following is/are true?
   A) Oral contrast medium should be given to help visualise the bowel
   B) A CT of the abdomen and pelvis without IV contrast may be performed
   C) A CT of the abdomen and pelvis with arterial phase contrast may be performed
   D) A CT of the abdomen and pelvis with portal venous phase contrast may be performed
   E) The patient should have an appropriate medical escort to and from the CT scanner

5. Bowel ischaemia can be acute or chronic. Which feature is least specific to chronic bowel ischaemia?
   A) Postprandial abdominal pain
   B) Malabsorption
   C) Weight loss
   D) Rectal bleeding
   E) The presence of cardiovascular risk factors

Continue

CASE **3.7** *Contd.*

ANSWERS TO QUESTIONS

1. Which of the following is/are part of the differential diagnosis for gas in the bowel wall (pneumatosis intestinalis)?

   The correct answers are **A) Idiopathic, B) Obstructive airways disease, D) Trauma and E) Intestinal ischaemia**.

   There are numerous causes of gas in the bowel wall. They include a variety of benign aetiologies as well as some life-threatening causes. The accompanying clinical history may help differentiate.

   A) Idiopathic – Correct. In up to 15% of cases, no cause is identified. This condition is termed pneumatosis cystoides intestinalis and usually affects the colon.

   B) Obstructive airways disease – Correct. Both chronic obstructive pulmonary disease and asthma can be implicated in pneumatosis intestinalis. It is also associated with cystic fibrosis and ventilator support using positive end-expiratory pressure.

   C) Recent barium swallow – Incorrect. There are a variety of iatrogenic causes of pneumatosis intestinalis including recent barium enema, CT colonoscopy or conventional colonoscopy. However, a recent barium swallow is not a cause of pneumatosis intestinalis.

   D) Trauma – Correct. Pneumatosis intestinalis secondary to trauma is a recognised phenomenon.

   E) Intestinal ischaemia – Correct. Pneumatosis intestinalis is a sign of bowel ischaemia. The arterial blood supply may be directly compromised in thromboembolic events or perfusion pressure may be limited in states of either hypovolaemia or reduced cardiac output. It should be remembered that mechanical bowel obstruction, if present for sufficient time, can also result in compromise of the vascular blood supply to the mucosa and cause venous stasis and venous infarction.

   ❗ KEY POINT

   Bowel ischaemia should always be considered the cause of pneumatosis intestinalis until proven otherwise.

2. Which of the following is/are potentially part of the management of a patient with suspected acute bowel ischaemia?

   The correct answers are **A) Erect chest X-ray and abdominal X-ray, B) Perform a CT scan, C) Consider the role of interventional radiology and E) Emergency laparotomy and resection of the ischaemic bowel**.

   Acute bowel ischaemia is a surgical emergency and warrants urgent surgical review whenever this diagnosis is entertained. A CT scan is often performed in patients with suspected bowel ischaemia but remember a normal CT cannot exclude early bowel ischaemia.

   A) Erect chest X-ray and abdominal X-ray – Correct. An erect chest X-ray and abdominal X-ray are readily available and are important initial investigations which can be performed as the patient is resuscitated. The chest X-ray is used to identify a pneumoperitoneum, as well as any chest pathology which may be relevant. The abdominal X-ray may show features of pneumatosis intestinalis as in this case, as well as bowel obstruction, perforation or mucosal thickening.

   B) Perform a CT scan – Correct. CT is more sensitive for diagnosing bowel ischaemia than plain films. It can also help determine the aetiology of the ischaemia.

   C) Consider the role of interventional radiology – Correct. If there is a thrombus in a mesenteric artery causing the ischaemia, management may involve attempts at revascularisation with intraarterial thrombolysis or thrombectomy via an endovascular route.

   D) Consider vasopressin to maintain blood pressure in hypovolaemic patients – Incorrect. Vasopressin may be used in patients with active variceal bleeding to help stop bleeding and maintain blood pressure. However, as it causes splanchnic vasoconstriction, it will exacerbate the bowel ischaemia and is contraindicated in this situation.

   E) Emergency laparotomy and resection of the ischaemic bowel – Correct. The surgical team should always be involved early in the management of any patient with suspected bowel ischaemia. Irreversible bowel ischaemia requires resection, ideally before it perforates.

   ❗ KEY POINTS

   1. X-rays are usually the first investigations to be performed. However, contrast-enhanced CT is much more sensitive and specific for detecting bowel ischaemia.
   2. If acute bowel ischaemia is not diagnosed and treated promptly, the prognosis is extremely poor.

3. Which of the following is/are radiological features of acute bowel ischaemia?

   The correct answer is **A) Lack of mucosal enhancement in a segment of bowel on contrast-enhanced CT, B) Dilatation of multiple bowel loops, C) Pneumatosis intestinalis and E) Filling defect in the superior mesenteric artery on contrast-enhanced CT**.

   Imaging plays a key role in confirming the diagnosis and excluding differentials.

   A) Lack of mucosal enhancement in a segment of bowel on contrast-enhanced CT – Correct. In cases of bowel ischaemia secondary to compromise of the arterial blood supply, the segment of the affected bowel may fail to enhance following intravenous contrast administration on CT imaging.

   B) Dilatation of multiple bowel loops – Correct. Dilatation of the bowel is a sign of bowel ischaemia but if it occurs early in the process, with no other accompanying signs, it can be nonspecific.

   C) Pneumatosis intestinalis – Correct. Bowel ischaemia is one of the life-threatening causes of pneumatosis intestinalis.

D) Branching pattern of gas within the central liver that does not reach the periphery – Incorrect. This description refers to gas in the biliary tree (aerobilia), which most commonly occurs after ERCP (endoscopic retrograde cholangiopancreatography) and sphincterotomy. Portal venous gas typically extends from the central part (large main portal vein) to the periphery (smaller portal vein branches) of the liver. Gas in the bile ducts is typically seen more centrally in the liver, within the common hepatic and bile ducts.

E) Filling defect in the superior mesenteric artery on contrast-enhanced CT – Correct. There may be evidence of a filling defect due to thrombus in one of the mesenteric arteries on CT in a patient with bowel ischaemia.

> **❗ KEY POINT**
>
> CT is more sensitive than abdominal film at detecting the presence of pneumatosis intestinalis. The signs of established bowel ischaemia are usually readily discernible. However, early bowel ischaemia is more difficult to diagnose because the earliest imaging manifestations are nonspecific. Correlation with the clinical picture (history, examination and blood results, such as serum lactate) is therefore of paramount importance.

4. Regarding CT imaging in suspected acute bowel ischaemia, which of the following is/are true?
   The correct answers are **B) A CT of the abdomen and pelvis without IV contrast may be performed, C) A CT of the abdomen and pelvis with arterial phase contrast may be performed, D) A CT of the abdomen and pelvis with portal venous phase contrast may be performed and E) The patient should have an appropriate medical escort to and from the CT scanner**.
   Oral contrast is often administered to patients with suspected bowel pathology before a CT of the abdomen/pelvis, depending on the local protocols. However, in suspected acute bowel ischaemia, this should not be administered because it takes time for the contrast to pass to the bowel and time is of the essence. It can also affect the interpretation of the scan.
   A) Oral contrast medium should be given to help visualise the bowel – Incorrect. If bowel ischaemia is suspected, the patient should not be given oral contrast medium prior to the CT scan. This prevents assessment of mucosal enhancement. It is the radiologist's job to protocol the scan appropriately (i.e. decide what type of contrast, if any, is required); however, it is an important point for junior doctors and nursing staff on the wards to appreciate.
   B) A CT of the abdomen and pelvis without IV contrast may be performed – Correct. A comprehensive CT study for the investigation of suspected bowel ischaemia may involve scanning the abdomen three times – once without contrast, once when the intravenous contrast is within the arterial system (arterial phase) and finally when the contrast is in the portal venous system (portal venous phase). It can therefore result in a significant radiation dose to the patient. The rationale behind the initial unenhanced scan is to look for the presence of calcified atherosclerotic plaque in the mesenteric arteries which may not be discernible on the postcontrast images.
   C) A CT of the abdomen and pelvis with arterial phase contrast may be performed – Correct. See B for further details. The rationale behind the arterial phase scan is to look for filling defects in the mesenteric arteries, particularly the superior mesenteric artery, which may be the cause of the ischaemic event.
   D) A CT of the abdomen and pelvis with portal venous phase contrast may be performed – Correct. See B for further details. The rationale behind the portal venous phase study is that this is the phase at which bowel mucosa normally enhances maximally. It provides an opportunity to assess for lack of mucosal perfusion.
   E) The patient should have an appropriate medical escort to and from the CT scanner – Correct. Patients with suspected acute bowel ischaemia are very unwell. They should be accompanied to and from the radiology department with a medical escort and the surgical team should be involved with the patient's care early so that the results of the CT can be acted on immediately if required.

> **❗ KEY POINTS**
>
> 1. A CT scan is often performed in patients with suspected bowel ischaemia. The supervising radiologist should emphasise the importance not to administer oral contrast to these patients. All doctors managing these patients should be aware that a comprehensive CT study in such cases is potentially high dose and requires IV contrast medium.
> 2. Contrast-induced nephropathy is a risk of IV contrast administration and is more common in patients with underlying renal disease or acute renal failure. However, the benefits of administering IV contrast to make the correct diagnosis may outweigh the risks of inducing renal failure (the patient may need to undergo temporary renal replacement therapy if this occurs). Such decisions should be made by senior clinicians on a patient-by-patient basis.

5. Bowel ischaemia can be acute or chronic. Which feature is least specific to chronic bowel ischaemia?
   The correct answer is **D) Rectal bleeding**.
   A) Postprandial abdominal pain – Incorrect. Abdominal pain following eating is a classical symptom of chronic mesenteric insufficiency. It is also known as 'abdominal angina'. Due to the excellent collateral supply of the bowel, marked stenosis of the coeliac axis, superior mesenteric artery or inferior mesenteric artery are usually required to cause the classic symptoms of mesenteric angina (pain after eating).

Continue

B) Malabsorption – Incorrect. Malabsorption is a feature of chronic bowel ischaemia.

C) Weight loss – Incorrect. Patients with chronic bowel ischaemia have often lost a significant amount of weight because eating is painful and due to the resultant malabsorption.

D) Rectal bleeding – Correct. Rectal bleeding can occur in both conditions and therefore does not help distinguish between the two entities clinically without any other supporting symptoms.

E) The presence of cardiovascular risk factors – Incorrect. The most common cause of chronic mesenteric ischaemia is atherosclerosis. Patients with evidence of ischaemic heart disease, peripheral vascular disease or cardiovascular risk factors (smoking history, diabetes mellitus, hypertension, hyperlipidaemia, etc.) are at risk of chronic bowel ischaemia. Acute bowel ischaemia is usually a thromboembolic event. It may also occur in patients with cardiovascular risk factors, particularly those with atrial fibrillation.

IMPORTANT LEARNING POINTS

- Although there are a variety of causes for pneumatosis intestinalis, bowel ischaemia should always be considered, as it is a life-threatening condition.
- In patients with suspected acute bowel ischaemia, early diagnosis and treatment is vital.
- Plain X-rays are the initial imaging modalities; however, CT is usually required to confirm the diagnosis.
- Patients undergoing CT for the investigation of ischaemic bowel should not receive oral contrast medium. However they will require intravenous contrast.
- Chronic bowel ischaemia can present like malignancy (weight loss and loss of appetite); however, there is typically abdominal pain following eating and a significant cardiovascular history. CT can distinguish between these conditions.

CASE **3.8**

A 35-year-old man, who is currently an inpatient on a psychiatric ward, presents with no bowel motions for the past 5 days. He has a background medical history of depression and is currently taking a tricyclic antidepressant. An abdominal X-ray is performed as part of his assessment.

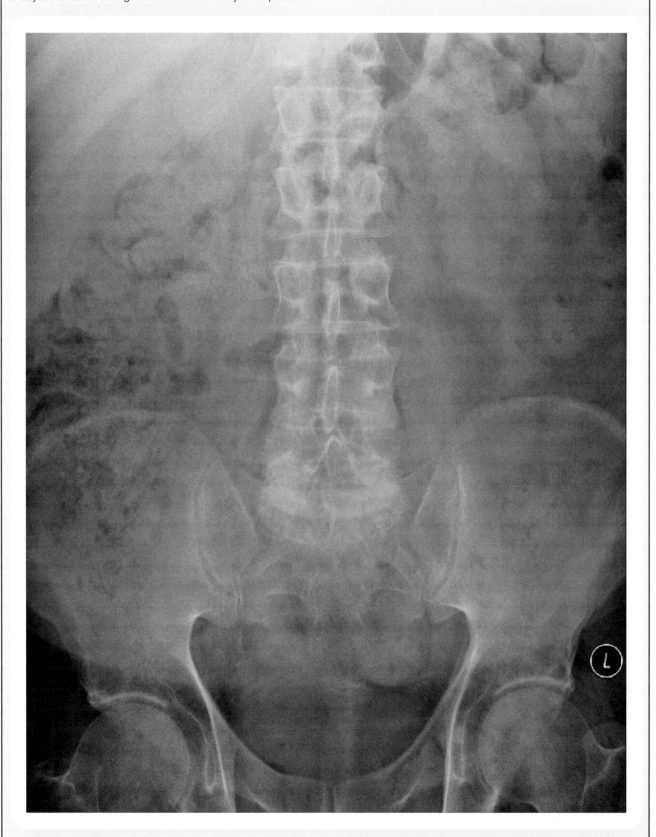

Continue

CASE **3.8**   *Contd.*

ANNOTATED X-RAY

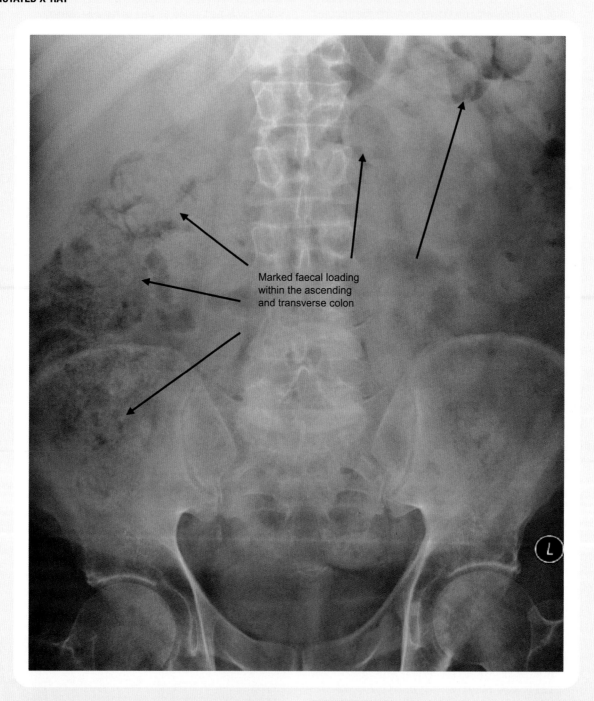

Marked faecal loading within the ascending and transverse colon

PRESENT YOUR FINDINGS

- This is a supine AP abdominal X-ray.
- The patient details and date of the investigation are not present on the film. I would ensure this relates to the correct patient before making any further assessment.
- The entire abdomen has not been completely imaged as the diaphragms, pubic symphysis and lateral aspects of the flanks are not completely imaged.
- There are no dilated loops of bowel to suggest the presence of large or small bowel obstruction.
- There is no plain film evidence of perforation or mucosal oedema.

- There is no obvious abnormality of the visible solid abdominal organs.
- The visualised skeleton is unremarkable.

IN SUMMARY – This abdominal X-ray demonstrates faeces evident within the colon. Antimuscarinic side effects from the patient's tricyclic antidepressant may be implicated. There is no evidence of bowel obstruction. In this case, a trial of laxative and consideration of using an antidepressant less likely to cause constipation could be potential initial management options.

QUESTIONS

1. Which of the following is a red flag symptom in a patient presenting with constipation?
   A) Opening bowels <3 per week
   B) Passing hard stool
   C) Tenesmus
   D) Straining to pass stool
   E) Nausea

2. Which of the following is/are recognised causes of constipation?
   A) Lack of dietary fibre
   B) Opioid medication
   C) Hypercalcaemia
   D) Hyperthyroidism
   E) Anal fissure

3. Which of the following is/are medical options for the management of constipation?
   A) Lactulose
   B) Loperamide
   C) Senna
   D) Docusate sodium
   E) Glycerol suppositories

4. Which of the following is/are correct regarding imaging in constipation?
   A) Abdominal X-ray is indicated in all patients with suspected constipation
   B) A transit study is useful to diagnose slow transit
   C) A gastrografin follow-through study may have a therapeutic effect
   D) A barium swallow can cause constipation
   E) Fluoroscopic studies can assess the mechanism of defaecation

5. Which of the following is/are potential complications of chronic constipation?
   A) Haemorrhoids
   B) Rectal prolapse
   C) Faecal incontinence
   D) Perforation
   E) Colorectal malignancy

Continue

CASE 3.8   *Contd.*

ANSWERS TO QUESTIONS

1. Which of the following is a red flag symptom in a patient presenting with constipation?
   The correct answer is **C) Tenesmus**.
   Constipation is a common symptom. However, occasionally it can herald a serious underlying pathology, such as colorectal malignancy. It is important to screen for the presence of any red flag symptoms (see key points for a list of red flag symptoms in constipation) which may herald a serious underlying pathology.
   A) Opening bowels <3 per week – Incorrect. Infrequent bowel movement is part of the definition of constipation, and in itself does not signify sinister underlying pathology. Although fewer than three motions per week is stated as a marker of constipation, any reduction in frequency of defaecation from the patient's usual bowel habit is a more important factor.
   B) Passing hard stool – Incorrect. The sensation of passing hard stool is part of the definition of constipation. Again, this does not indicate serious underlying pathology on its own. The Bristol Stool Chart is a method of quantifying stool character.
   C) Tenesmus – Correct. Tenesmus is the sensation of incomplete rectal emptying. It is considered a red flag symptom as the sensation may be due to a mass lesion in the rectum. There are a variety of other potential causes of tenesmus, including inflammatory or infective colitis as well as haemorrhoids.
   D) Straining to pass stool – Incorrect. Difficulty defaecating is part of the definition of constipation.
   E) Nausea – Incorrect. Nausea is not a red flag symptom in a patient with constipation.

❶ KEY POINTS

1. In addition to tenesmus, other red flag symptoms include new-onset constipation in an elderly patient, unexplained iron-deficiency anaemia, rectal bleeding (particularly when mixed in with the stool), a positive faecal occult blood test, family history of colorectal cancer or inflammatory bowel disease and recent unintentional weight loss.
2. The further management of a patient with red flags will vary slightly depending on the clinical context; however, direct visualisation of the colon, using colonoscopy, is often indicated.

2. Which of the following is/are recognised causes of constipation?
   The correct answers are **A) Lack of dietary fibre, B) Opioid medication, C) Hypercalcaemia and E) Anal fissure**.
   There are a variety of causes of constipation, many of which are readily correctable.
   A) Lack of dietary fibre – Correct. Dietary factors including lack of fibre and poor fluid intake can cause constipation.

B) Opioid medication – Correct. Many medications can result in constipation as a side effect. Opioid analgesia has a particularly potent constipating effect and the concomitant prescription of a laxative should be considered.
C) Hypercalcaemia – Correct. Hypercalcaemia can result in constipation. Patients with hypercalcaemia may also be dehydrated which may exacerbate the problem.
D) Hyperthyroidism – Incorrect. Hypothyroidism is a metabolic disorder which can result in constipation. Hyperthyroidism may cause diarrhoea.
E) Anal fissure – Correct. Anal fissures can make defaecation painful and constipation may result, particularly amongst children.

❶ KEY POINT

Clinical assessment should be aimed at identifying potentially reversible causes of constipation.

3. Which of the following is/are medical options for the management of constipation?
   The correct answers are **A) Lactulose, C) Senna, D) Docusate sodium and E) Glycerol suppositories**.
   Constipation is usually managed conservatively. Treatment is aimed at increasing fluid and fibre intake, treating any reversible causes and the use of laxatives.
   A) Lactulose – Correct. Lactulose is an example of an osmotic laxative. It works by drawing water into the lumen of the bowel to make the stool less viscous and therefore easier to pass.
   B) Loperamide – Incorrect. Loperamide is an opioid receptor agonist which acts in the large bowel. It is used in the treatment of diarrhoea and works by prolonging the transit time of the colon, allowing more water from the faeces to be reabsorbed. In contrast to opioid analgesics, loperamide does not act on the central nervous system.
   C) Senna – Correct. Senna is a stimulant laxative. Senna is broken down in the gastrointestinal tract and its components stimulate the Auerbach's plexus in the bowel and cause increased peristalsis.
   D) Docusate sodium – Correct. Docusate sodium has stimulant and softening actions. This is a surface-active compound and produces softer stool by reducing surface tension in a similar manner to detergent. It also has weak stimulant effects.
   E) Glycerol suppositories – Correct. Glycerol suppositories act as a rectal stimulant and alter the consistency of the stool, making it easier to pass.

❶ KEY POINT

Different laxatives work by different pharmacological methods such as stimulant action, stool softening or osmotic effect. Combining laxatives with different actions may be beneficial to manage constipation.

4. Which of the following is/are correct regarding imaging in constipation?
The correct answers are **B) A transit study is useful to diagnose slow transit, C) A gastrografin follow-through study may have a therapeutic effect, D) A barium swallow can cause constipation and E) Fluoroscopic studies can assess the mechanism of defaecation**.
There are a variety of radiological investigations which can be of use in patients with constipation.

A) Abdominal X-ray is indicated in all patients with suspected constipation – Incorrect. According to the Royal College of Radiologists making best use of clinical radiology services guidelines, an abdominal X-ray should not be performed to diagnose constipation and is only indicated in selected cases, such as to show the extent of faecal impaction in the elderly or psychiatric patients.

B) A transit study is useful to diagnose slow transit – Correct. A transit study involves the patient swallowing special capsules. One is swallowed each day for 6 days. Each capsule contains different shaped radio-opaque markers. On the 7th day, an abdominal X-ray is performed. The transit time can be determined by assessing the shapes and numbers of the visible radio-opaque markers discernible within the gastrointestinal tract. Transit studies can also be performed using ingested radionuclide rather than radio-opaque markers. Transit studies are a specialised investigation that are only occasionally required in the investigation of constipation. They should not be routinely requested.

C) A gastrografin follow-through study may have a therapeutic effect – Correct. Gastrografin is a contrast medium which also has an osmotic laxative effect. It is sometimes used following gastrointestinal surgery to exclude mechanical obstruction (these patients are prone to paralytic ileus) and promote resumption of normal bowel function.

D) A barium swallow can cause constipation – Correct. Barium contrast medium can cause constipation. Patients should be advised to stay hydrated following barium investigations to prevent this from occurring. Their stools may also be coloured white by the barium for a short period of time following the examination.

E) Fluoroscopic studies can assess the mechanism of defaecation – Correct. A defaecating proctogram is a specialised examination performed under fluoroscopic imaging to assess the mechanism of defaecation. This involves inserting contrast medium into the rectum and then screening as the patient empties their bowels. Dynamic MRI can also be used to assess the mechanism of defaecation.

> ❗ KEY POINT
>
> Most patients with constipation do not require any imaging. Abdominal X-rays should be reserved for selected cases.

5. Which of the following is/are potential complications of chronic constipation?
The correct answers are **A) Haemorrhoids, B) Rectal prolapse, C) Faecal incontinence and D) Perforation**.
Constipation is often a straightforward condition to manage. However, it can be associated with a variety of complications.

A) Haemorrhoids – Correct. Excessive straining can result in haemorrhoids.

B) Rectal prolapse – Correct. Rectal prolapse may result from chronic constipation.

C) Faecal incontinence – Correct. Overflow diarrhoea can occur in patients with constipation and result in faecal incontinence.

D) Perforation – Correct. A faecaloma from chronic constipation can rarely result in colonic perforation. This is known as stercoral perforation.

E) Colorectal malignancy – Incorrect. Chronic constipation is not known to cause colorectal malignancy. However, a change in bowel habit may be the presenting symptom for colorectal malignancy.

> ❗ KEY POINT
>
> It is important to manage patients with constipation well to avoid some of the potentially serious complications of chronic constipation.

👥 IMPORTANT LEARNING POINTS

- Constipation is a common symptom but it is important to assess for red flag symptoms which may herald a sinister aetiology.
- The abdominal X-ray should not be routinely used to diagnose constipation.
- Constipation should be managed appropriately with treatment of reversible causes, advice to increase fluid and fibre intake and combinations of complimentary laxatives if required to prevent the risk of any complications of chronic constipation.

CASE **3.9**

A 45-year-old woman presented with left upper quadrant pain and discomfort. Clinical examination raised the possibility of a fullness in the left upper quadrant. Full blood count revealed pancytopaenia. An abdominal X-ray was performed as part of her assessment to exclude bowel obstruction.

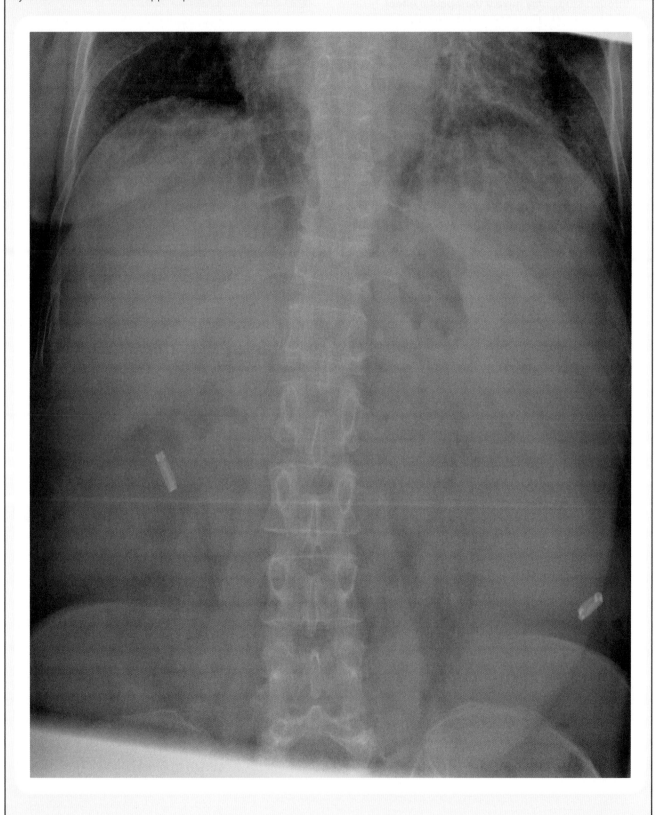

ANNOTATED X-RAY

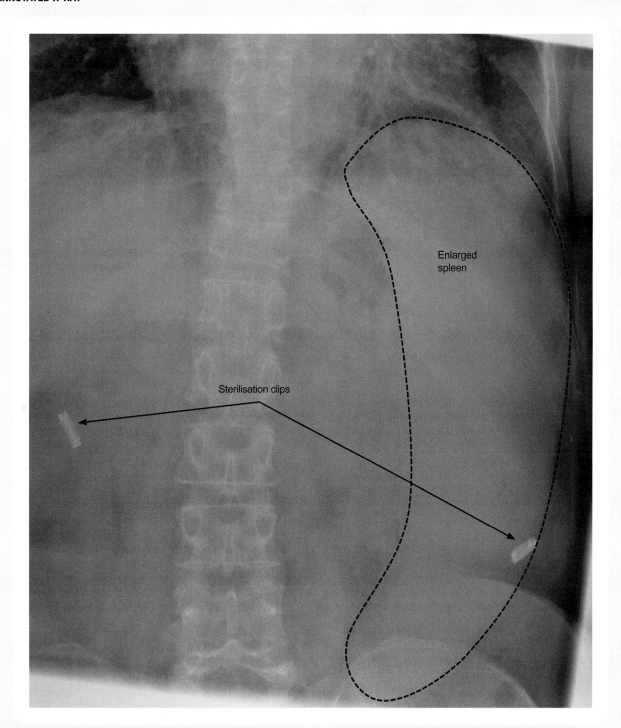

Enlarged
spleen

Sterilisation clips

🔍 PRESENT YOUR FINDINGS

- This is a supine AP abdominal X-ray.
- There are no patient identifiable markings nor a time and date stamp. I would ensure this investigation relates to the correct patient before proceeding further.
- This is an inadequate X-ray as the pelvis and hernial orifices are not visible.
- The most striking abnormality is a large curved soft tissue density arising in the left upper quadrant and extending inferiorly. It is consistent with an enlarged spleen.
- The liver outline does not appear enlarged.
- There is a paucity of bowel gas, but no evidence of obstruction, perforation or mucosal oedema.
- Two metallic density clips are noted in the flanks and presumably represent displaced sterilisation clips.
- There is no other significant abnormality of the visible abdominal organs.
- No skeletal abnormality.

Continue

CASE **3.9**   *Contd.*

IN SUMMARY – This abdominal X-ray demonstrates likely splenomegaly. In addition, incidental note is made of displaced sterilisation clips. I would like to confirm my suspicions with clinical examination of the patient's abdomen and abdominal ultrasound. The full blood count findings suggest there is associated hypersplenism.

QUESTIONS

1. Which of the following features is/are consistent with splenomegaly during clinical examination of the abdomen?
   A) A mass extending from the left costal margin towards the umbilicus
   B) A mass which moves down with inspiration
   C) A mass with a palpable notch on the medial aspect
   D) Inability to palpate deep to the mass
   E) A mass which is dull to percussion

2. Regarding the spleen, which of the following statements is/are correct?
   A) It may be congenitally absent
   B) Splenosis is a normal variant
   C) It can measure up to 12 cm in normal adults
   D) It has a role in maintaining normal circulating erythrocytes
   E) It has a role in cell-mediated immunity

3. Which of the following is/are causes of massive splenomegaly?
   A) Chronic myeloid leukaemia
   B) Myelofibrosis
   C) Malaria
   D) Sickle cell anaemia
   E) Primary lymphoma of the spleen

4. Which of the following is/are indications for splenectomy?
   A) Hereditary spherocytosis complicated with pigmented gallstones
   B) Idiopathic thombocytopaenic purpura not responsive to steroid therapy
   C) Non-Hodgkin lymphoma confined to the spleen
   D) Gastric variceal bleeding due to portal hypertension resulting from splenic vein thrombosis
   E) Small, peripheral, single traumatic splenic laceration

5. Regarding management of splenectomy patients, which of the following is/are true?
   A) In the postoperative period, heparin should be avoided due to increased bleeding tendency
   B) Prophylactic oral penicillin V should be considered
   C) Patients should receive pneumococcal, meningococcal and haemophilus influenza vaccines 2 to 3 weeks before elective surgery for splenectomy or at the time of emergency surgery
   D) Travel to malaria endemic regions should be avoided
   E) The patient should carry a medical alert card

ANSWERS TO QUESTIONS

1. Which of the following features is/are consistent with splenomegaly during clinical examination of the abdomen?

   The correct answers are **A) A mass extending from the left costal margin towards the umbilicus, B) A mass which moves down with inspiration, C) A mass with a palpable notch on the medial aspect and E) A mass which is dull to percussion**.

   A mass arising from the left upper quadrant may be splenic or renal in origin. Certain features on clinical examination can help differentiate the two.

   A) A mass extending from the left costal margin towards the umbilicus – Correct. This is a feature of splenomegaly.

   B) A mass which moves down with inspiration – Correct. This is a feature of splenomegaly.

   C) A mass with a palpable notch on the medial aspect – Correct. This is a feature of splenomegaly.

   D) Inability to palpate deep to the mass – Incorrect. It should be possible to palpate deep to an enlarged spleen. In comparison, it is not possible to palpate deep to a left renal mass.

   E) A mass which is dull to percussion – Correct. This is a feature of splenomegaly.

❗ KEY POINTS

1. When a mass is palpated in the left upper quadrant/left flank, it is important to try and distinguish an enlarged spleen from left renal pathology. The key differentiating factors include the fact that renal masses may move deeply and vertically on inspiration in comparison to superficially and diagonally in splenomegaly. There is a palpable notch with splenomegaly. The percussion note may be resonant overlying the left kidney due to interposed bowel and there may be bilateral renal masses, depending on the pathology – e.g. polycystic kidneys.

2. Ultrasound can be used as the first-line investigation for differentiating a splenic and left renal mass, and provides an assessment of splenic size and appearance.

2. Regarding the spleen, which of the following statements is/are correct?

   The correct answers are **A) It may be congenitally absent, C) It can measure up to 12 cm in normal adults, D) It has a role in maintaining normal circulating erythrocytes and E) It has a role in cell-mediate immunity**.

   A) It may be congenitally absent – Correct. Congenital asplenia may occur in isolation or in conjunction with other congenital anomalies.

   B) Splenosis is a normal variant – Incorrect. Splenosis is a rare acquired condition of ectopic splenic tissue due to autotransplantation of splenic fragments following splenic trauma. Splenic foci can occur throughout the abdominal cavity, and the thorax if the diaphragm was also breached at the time of the trauma. It should not be confused with a splenunculus (also known as accessory or supernumerary spleen), a normal variant which is an area of splenic tissue adjacent to the spleen which failed to fuse during embryological development. It is of no clinical relevance, other than the fact it may mimic pathology, e.g. lymphadenopathy.

   C) It can measure up to 12 cm in normal adults – Correct. The upper limit of normal is considered 12 cm for most adults. A spleen that measures 12 to 20 cm is enlarged. The term massive splenomegaly refers to a spleen in excess of 20 cm.

   D) It has a role in maintaining normal circulating erythrocytes – Correct. The red pulp area of the spleen filters erythrocytes and removes abnormal cells from the circulation. The spleen also acts as a reservoir of erythrocytes.

   E) It has a role in cell-mediated immunity – Correct. The white pulp area of the spleen produces both B- and T-lymphocytes so is involved in both humoral and cell-mediated immunity.

❗ KEY POINT

The spleen has multiple important functions. Normal splenic variants, such as splenunculi, can mimic pathology.

3. Which of the following is/are causes of massive splenomegaly?

   The correct answers are **A) Chronic myeloid leukaemia, B) Myelofibrosis, C) Malaria and E) Primary lymphoma of the spleen**.

   The spleen normally measures up to approximately 12 cm in adults. There are many causes of splenomegaly. They can be divided into splenomegaly (12–20 cm) and massive splenomegaly (in excess of 20 cm) (Table C3.9.1).

   A) Chronic myeloid leukaemia – Correct. This is a cause of massive splenomegaly.

   B) Myelofibrosis – Correct. This is a cause of massive splenomegaly.

Table C3.9.1   Causes of Splenomegaly

SPLENOMEGALY (12–20 CM)	MASSIVE SPLENOMEGALY (>20 CM)
Portal hypertension (See abdominal X-ray Case 3.14 for further details)	Myelofibrosis
Haemoglobinopathies (Thalassaemia, spherocytosis, early sickle cell anaemia[a])	Chronic myeloid leukaemia
Infection (mononucleosis, AIDS, bacterial endocarditis, splenic abscess, histoplasmosis)	Primary lymphoma of the spleen
Autoimmune disorders (rheumatoid arthritis, SLE, sarcoidosis)	Malaria
Metabolic disorders (amyloidosis, Gaucher disease, Niemann–Pick disease)	Leishmaniasis

[a]Later sickle cell anaemia results in a small spleen due to repeated infarcts (autosplenectomy).

Continue

CASE **3.9** *Contd.*

C) Malaria – Correct. This is a cause of massive splenomegaly.
D) Sickle cell anaemia – Incorrect. Sickle cell anaemia can affect the spleen but is does not result in massive splenomegaly. Most patients with sickle cell anaemia have undergone an autosplenectomy before the end of childhood secondary to multiple splenic infarcts due to the number of impacted abnormal erythrocytes. A splenic sequestration crisis causes acute and painful splenic enlargement (but not massive enlargement) due to trapped erythrocytes, which can lead to hypovolaemic shock and marked anaemia.
E) Primary lymphoma of the spleen – Correct. This is a cause of massive splenomegaly.

! KEY POINT

Splenomegaly refers to an increase in splenic size, whereas hypersplenism is the overactivity of the spleen. The two are separate conditions but may coexist.

4. Which of the following is/are indications for splenectomy?
The correct answers are **A) Hereditary spherocytosis complicated with pigmented gallstones, B) Idiopathic thombocytopaenic purpura not responsive to steroid therapy, C) Non-Hodgkin lymphoma confined to the spleen and D) Variceal bleeding due to portal hypertension resulting from splenic vein thrombosis.**
A) Hereditary spherocytosis complicated with pigmented gallstones – Correct. Hereditary spherocytosis is an autosomal dominant condition which results in spherical-shaped erythrocytes which are fragile and prone to destruction in the spleen. In addition to resultant gallbladder disease, splenectomy is indicated when severe haemolytic crises have occurred or when health is impaired.
B) Idiopathic thombocytopaenic purpura not responsive to steroid therapy – Correct. Splenectomy is indicated in idiopathic thrombocytopaenic purpura if the acute phase cannot be controlled with steroids or if a patient has two relapses whilst on steroids.
C) Non-Hodgkin lymphoma confined to the spleen – Correct. This is an indication for splenectomy but it is rare for non-Hodgkin lymphoma to only affect the spleen.
D) Variceal bleeding due to portal hypertension resulting from splenic vein thrombosis – Correct. Splenectomy can be curative in this specific case of portal hypertension.
E) Small, peripheral, single traumatic splenic laceration – Incorrect. Splenectomy would not be performed after a single traumatic laceration in a patient who is haemodynamically stable. Patients are being increasingly managed conservatively and when surgery is performed, spleen-saving procedures such as local suturing and partial splenectomy are being attempted.

! KEY POINT

The majority of indications for splenectomy are related to haematological conditions that cannot be managed adequately with medication. The role of splenectomy in trauma is in decline. It is important to realise that enlarged spleens are at greater risk of traumatic rupture as they are less protected by the ribs. Patients with splenic trauma should be closely observed because there can be delayed rupture to the spleen after a period of apparent stability.

5. Regarding management of splenectomy patients, which of the following is/are true?
The correct answers are **B) Prophylactic oral penicillin V should be considered, C) Patients should receive pneumococcal, meningococcal and haemophilus influenza vaccines 2 to 3 weeks before elective surgery for splenectomy or at the time of emergency surgery, D) Travel to malaria endemic regions should be avoided and E) The patient should carry a medical alert card.**
A) In the postoperative period, heparin should be avoided due to increased bleeding tendency – Incorrect. Postsplenectomy, there is a transient increase in platelets and white cell count. Low-dose heparin is advised in all patients as venous thromboembolism prophylaxis.
B) Prophylactic oral penicillin V should be considered – Correct. Prophylactic antibiotics should be considered in splenectomy patients. The highest risk groups are those aged <16 years and >50 years. The 2-year period immediately postoperatively poses the highest risk, although the risk remains elevated throughout life
C) Patients should receive pneumococcal, meningococcal and haemophilus influenza vaccines 2 to 3 weeks before elective surgery for splenectomy or at the time of emergency surgery – Correct.
D) Travel to malaria endemic regions should be avoided – Correct.
E) The patient should carry a medical alert card – Correct.

! KEY POINT

Postsplenectomy patients are at risk of life-threatening sepsis. This should be managed with appropriate vaccination prior to splenectomy and prophylactic antibiotic therapy as appropriate.

IMPORTANT LEARNING POINTS

- A palpable spleen always indicates splenomegaly, as the spleen has to increase in size by three times before it can be palpated.
- There are multiple causes of splenomegaly, but only a few conditions result in massive splenomegaly.
- Ultrasound is the first-line investigation for assessing splenic size.
- Enlarged spleens are more prone to traumatic injury.
- Postsplenectomy patients are at increased risk of infection.

CASE 3.10

A 77-year-old woman presents with colicky upper abdominal pain, nausea and vomiting. As part of her workup, she undergoes an abdominal X-ray to exclude obstruction.

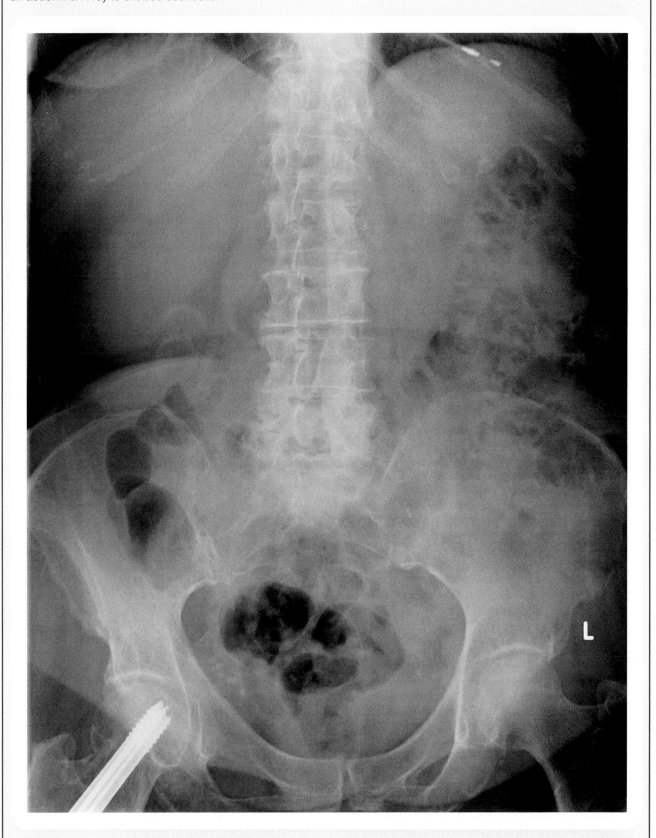

Continue

CASE 3.10   *Contd.*

ANNOTATED X-RAY

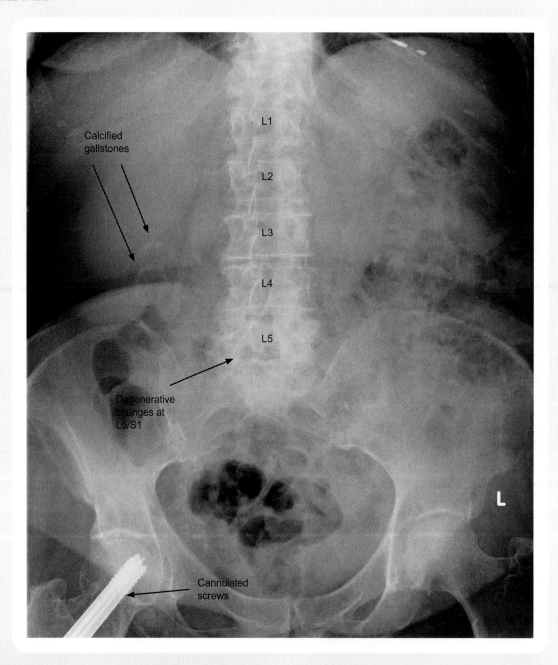

Calcified
gallstones

L1

L2

L3

L4

L5

Degenerative
changes at
L5/S1

Cannulated
screws

L

🔍 **PRESENT YOUR FINDINGS**

- This is a supine AP X-ray of the abdomen.
- It has been anonymised and the timing of the examination is not available. I would like to check this is the correct patient, as well as the time and date of the examination.
- The lateral aspects of the abdomen have not been fully included in the film. It is otherwise technically adequate.
- No evidence of bowel obstruction, perforation or mucosal oedema.
- There are two round areas of calcification projected over the right side of the abdomen at the level of L3/4. Given their position and appearance, they may represent calcified gallstones. Alternatively, they could be calcified lymph nodes.

- There is no pneumobilia (air in the biliary tree) visible.
- There is no obvious abnormality of the visible solid abdominal organs.
- Cannulated screws within the right femoral neck are visible. There are also degenerative changes within the spine, most marked at the L5/S1 level. Otherwise, no significant abnormality of the imaged skeleton can be seen.

IN SUMMARY – This abdominal X-ray shows two calcified areas within the right side of the abdomen, which may represent gallstones. Abdominal ultrasound would be useful to confirm this finding and assess for possible complications. There is no bowel obstruction.

QUESTIONS

1. Which of the following is/are risk factors for developing gallstones?
   A) Obesity
   B) Crohn's disease
   C) Increasing age
   D) Male sex
   E) Haemolytic anaemia

2. Gallstones can present in which of the following ways?
   A) Incidental finding
   B) Biliary colic
   C) Acute hepatitis
   D) Acute cholecystitis
   E) Obstructive jaundice

3. What is the most appropriate first-line investigation for a patient suspected of having gallstones?
   A) Abdominal X-ray
   B) CT
   C) Magnetic resonance cholangio-pancreatography (MRCP)
   D) Endoscopic retrograde cholangio-pancreatography (ERCP)
   E) Ultrasound

4. What is the imaging modality of choice for diagnosing a common bile duct stone?
   A) Ultrasound
   B) MRCP
   C) CT
   D) ERCP
   E) Abdominal X-ray

5. What is the most appropriate management of a patient diagnosed with gallstone-induced acute cholecystitis?
   A) Analgesia, IV fluids, antibiotics and cholecystectomy
   B) Analgesia and discharge with outpatient follow-up
   C) Urgent ERCP
   D) Percutaneous drainage of the gallbladder
   E) Gallstone lithotripsy

Continue

CASE **3.10** *Contd.*

ANSWERS TO QUESTIONS

1. Which of the following is/are risk factors for developing gallstones?
   The correct answers are **A) Obesity, B) Crohn's disease, C) Increasing age and E) Haemolytic anaemia**.
   Gallstones form from constituents of bile. There are three main types. Approximately 20% are cholesterol stones, which form in bile containing high levels of cholesterol or low levels of bile salts. Five to ten per-cent are pigmented stones, which form in patients with increased levels of bile pigment. Most gallstones (75%) are a mixture of the two.
   A) Obesity – Correct. Obesity and a high cholesterol diet are recognised risk factors for developing gallstones, particularly the cholesterol type, due to super-satura-tion of bile with cholesterol.
   B) Crohn's disease – Correct. Crohn's disease, particu-larly when it affects the terminal ileum, predisposes patients to gallstones. The diseased small bowel cannot effectively reabsorb bile acids, interrupting the enterohepatic circulation of bile. Bile salts help keep cholesterol in suspension and prevent its precipita-tion. Reduced levels of these salts predisposes to cholesterol stones. Other conditions which affect the terminal ileum and surgical resection of the terminal ileum can also predispose to gallstones.
   C) Increasing age – Correct. Gallstones increase in prev-alence with age.
   D) Male sex – Incorrect. Gallstones are two to three times more common in women than men.
   E) Haemolytic anaemia – Correct. Haemolytic anaemias, such as thalassaemia and sickle cell disease, cause an increase in bilirubin as a by-product of red cell breakdown, which can cause pigmented gallstones.

> **KEY POINT**
> Gallstones can occur in any patient but people at increased risk include those who are middle aged, obese and female.

2. Gallstones can present in which of the following ways?
   The correct answers are **A) Incidental finding, B) Biliary colic, D) Acute cholecystitis and E) Obstructive jaundice**.
   Gallstones can present in a variety of different ways. In addition to the options listed in the question, other pre-sentations include acute pancreatitis, chronic cholecys-titis and gallstone ileus.
   A) Incidental finding – Correct. Most patients with gall-stones are asymptomatic, with the stones being diag-nosed incidentally when they undergo imaging, such as ultrasound or CT, for another reason.
   B) Biliary colic – Correct. Biliary colic is a classic pre-sentation of gallstones. It is caused by transient obstruction of the cystic duct or gallbladder outlet by a gallstone. The pain is typically severe, located in the epigastrium and right upper quadrant and waxes and wanes in intensity. It often occurs after meals. The episode ends when the stone falls back into the

gallbladder or into the common bile duct. Patients can commonly suffer from recurrent attacks of biliary colic. Differential diagnoses include renal colic, bowel obstruction and angina.
   C) Acute hepatitis – Incorrect. Acute hepatitis is usually the result of alcohol excess or viral infection of the liver and not associated with gallstones.
   D) Acute cholecystitis – Correct. Acute cholecystitis is inflammation of the gallbladder. It is almost always caused by gallstones (90%–95% of cases). Patients usually have an episode of biliary colic, but the pain is very severe. There is often evidence of localised peritonism (tenderness, rigidity and Murphy's sign). Inflammatory markers tend to be elevated. The diag-nosis can be made clinically in patients with known gallstones. However, ultrasound can be used to iden-tify features of gallbladder inflammation. It may prog-ress to empyema or emphysema (from gas-producing bacteria) of the gallbladder, particularly in the elderly and in diabetic patients.
   E) Obstructive jaundice – Correct. Gallstones lodged in the common bile duct can cause obstructive jaun-dice. In contrast to malignant causes of obstructive jaundice, common bile duct stones usually result in an acute onset of jaundice associated with pain. Rarely, a gallstone impacted in the gallbladder neck or cystic duct can cause extrinsic compression of the common bile duct. This is known as Mirizzi syndrome.

> **KEY POINT**
> Gallstones can present in a variety of ways – incidental findings, biliary colic, cholecystitis, biliary obstruction, acute pancreatitis and, rarely, gallstone ileus.

3. What is the most appropriate first-line investigation for a patient suspected of having gallstones?
   The correct answer is **E) Ultrasound**.
   Gallstone disease is a common differential diagnosis for patients presenting with abdominal pain. Understanding the appropriate imaging investigations is therefore important.
   A) Abdominal X-ray – Incorrect. Abdominal X-rays are not sensitive for detecting gallstones as only approxi-mately 15% of gallstones contain enough calcium to be visible. Abdominal X-rays can be used to exclude differential diagnoses for the clinical findings, such as bowel obstruction. Additionally, abdominal X-rays may provide limited assessment of the potential complica-tions of gallstones such as pneumobilia (air within the biliary system), suggesting the presence of a choledo-choenteric fistula or gallbladder wall calcification from chronic cholecystitis).
   B) CT – Incorrect. Whilst CT provides detailed images of the abdominal organs, including the gallbladder and biliary tree, it is less sensitive than ultrasound for detecting gallstones. In addition, CT uses a significant amount of ionising radiation. Therefore, it is not used routinely for diagnosing gallstones. It is useful for

excluding the differential diagnoses of cholecystitis, such as appendicitis and diverticulitis.

C) MRCP – Incorrect. MRCP is a type of MRI examination. It can provide an accurate, noninvasive assessment of the gallbladder and bile ducts without the use of ionising radiation. Gallstones are usually seen as filling defects. However, gallbladder polyps and tumours can be indistinguishable from gallstones on MRCP. Additionally, MRI is expensive, not readily available and requires the patient to lie very still, which may be difficult if the patient is in severe pain. For these reasons, it is not used as a first-line imaging modality in the assessment of gallstone disease. The main indication is the investigation of obstructive jaundice, which may be caused by an intraductal calculi, cholangiocarcinoma or extrinsic compression by a pancreatic mass or enlarged lymph nodes.

D) ERCP – Incorrect. ERCP is an endoscopic procedure that involves cannulating the common bile duct via its ampulla in the duodenum. X-ray contrast can then be injected into the extrahepatic bile ducts and calculi appear as filling defects. It provides better assessment of the bile ducts than the gallbladder. ERCP is an invasive procedure with a risk of inducing acute pancreatitis. It is therefore not used as a diagnostic test.

E) Ultrasound – Correct. Ultrasound is a cheap, readily available investigation which is quick to perform and highly sensitive for diagnosing gallstones. Patients should be fasted for at least 6 hours prior to scanning (clear fluids are permitted). This allows the gallbladder to distend with bile (remember: the gallbladder contracts and empties in response to eating) and improves the diagnostic accuracy of the scan. Ultrasound has higher specificity compared with MRCP as it is able to distinguish between gallstones (echogenic masses within the gallbladder which are mobile and cast an acoustic shadow) and gallbladder polyps/tumours (gallbladder wall thickening, nonmobile and no acoustic shadow). Additionally, ultrasound is useful for identifying complications of gallstones, such as cholecystitis (gallbladder wall thickening and surrounding pericholecystic fluid), biliary dilatation and pneumobilia (air within the bile ducts).

❶ KEY POINT

Ultrasound is the first-line investigation for suspected gallstone disease. Patients should be fasted for the scan.

4. What is the imaging modality of choice for diagnosing a common bile duct stone?
The correct answer is **B) MRCP**.
Biliary obstruction can result in deranged liver function tests with jaundice, biliary sepsis and acute pancreatitis. Bile duct stones are one cause of biliary obstruction. Others include bile duct strictures, bile duct malignancy (cholangiocarcinoma) and extrinsic compression, such as masses in the pancreatic head.

A) Ultrasound – Incorrect. Ultrasound can diagnose biliary dilatation as it is able to assess the intrahepatic bile ducts as well as the proximal common bile duct (CBD). However, it is often difficult to image the entire length of the CBD due to overlying bowel gas. Therefore, the cause of biliary obstruction, such as an obstructing common bile duct stone, is often not visible on ultrasound, particularly if it is located distally in the CBD.

B) MRCP – Correct. MRCP provides an accurate assessment of the entire bile duct system, including the distal CBD. An obstructive CBD stone will be shown as a rounded filling defect within the CBD, with dilatation of the proximal ductal system. MRCP is noninvasive and does not use ionising radiation. It is the imaging modality of choice for diagnosing CBD stones.

C) CT – Incorrect. CT can identify biliary dilatation and if the calculi are radio-opaque a CBD stone may be seen. However, not all gallstones are visible on CT. CT is more useful in the investigation of patient with obstructive jaundice in whom a pancreatic mass is suspected.

D) ERCP – Incorrect. As described in question 3, ERCP will allow the diagnosis of intraductal stones. However, because it is an invasive test with significant associated complications, such as pancreatitis, it has been superseded by MRCP for diagnosing CBD stones. Its role is limited to treatment of bile duct obstructions (stones can be removed, and a sphincterotomy performed to encourage any further CBD stones to pass into the duodenum, whilst strictures can be stented).

E) Abdominal X-ray – Incorrect. As discussed in question 3, abdominal X-rays have limited ability to diagnose gallstones and their complications.

❶ KEY POINT

Biliary obstruction can be caused by a variety of pathologies, including gallstones. Ultrasound is usually the first-line investigation in a patient with suspected biliary obstruction, as it can quickly and accurately identify biliary dilatation and guide further investigations. MRCP is the preferred imaging modality for diagnosing CBD stones, whilst CT is preferred if there is suspicion of a pancreatic mass/tumour causing biliary obstruction.

5. What is the most appropriate management of a patient diagnosed with gallstone-induced acute cholecystitis?
The correct answer is **A) Analgesia, IV fluids, antibiotics and cholecystectomy**.
Acute cholecystitis is a common surgical problem and knowledge of its management is important. However, not all patients with gallstones need surgical treatment; those with asymptomatic gallstones or infrequent biliary colic are usually managed conservatively (avoid fatty foods, analgesia). Patients with biliary obstruction, acute pancreatitis or cholangitis due to a CBD stone often need ERCP to remove the stone and a cholecystectomy.

Continue

CASE 3.10   *Contd.*

A) Analgesia, IV fluids, antibiotics and cholecystectomy – Correct. Basic management of patients with acute cholecystitis includes appropriate analgesia, IV fluid resuscitation, keeping the patient nil by mouth, inserting an NG tube if the patient is vomiting and commencing broad-spectrum IV antibiotics. Cholecystectomy, preferably laparoscopic, is usually performed within a few days of admission, although it can be delayed for 6 weeks and performed on a semielective basis. Early cholecystectomy is often preferred as it is associated with lower risk of complications compared to the delayed surgery. It also prevents any further episodes of acute cholecystitis during the waiting period.

B) Analgesia and discharge with outpatient follow-up – Incorrect. As mentioned earlier – cholecystectomy is required to prevent recurrent attacks and reduce the risk of complications, such as gallbladder perforation.

C) Urgent ERCP – Incorrect. ERCP is used to treat CBD obstructions, such as CBD stones.

D) Percutaneous drainage of the gallbladder – Incorrect. Percutaneous cholecystostomy is an ultrasound-guided drainage procedure of the gallbladder. It is used as an intermediate intervention in critically unwell patients with gallstone-induced acute cholecystitis who are not fit for cholecystectomy. Once the patient has recovered sufficiently, they will need to undergo cholecystectomy. Percutaneous cholecystostomy can also be employed in patients with acalculous cholecystitis.

E) Gallstone lithotripsy – Incorrect. Nonsurgical treatments of gallstones, such as lithotripsy, have limited success rates (much lower than lithotripsy for renal calculi) and have largely been replaced by laparoscopic cholecystectomy.

IMPORTANT LEARNING POINTS

- Gallstones are common. Risk factors include obesity, increasing age and female sex.
- They are often asymptomatic but can cause a variety of symptoms and complications including biliary colic, cholecystitis, biliary obstruction and pancreatitis.
- First-line imaging for suspected gallstones is ultrasound. MRCP is used to identify CBD stones.
- Treatment depends on the presentation. Acute cholecystitis is usually managed surgically.

CASE **3.11**

A 38-year-old man presents to A&E with acute left-sided loin pain, urinary frequency and haematuria. As part of his workup, an abdominal X-ray is performed.

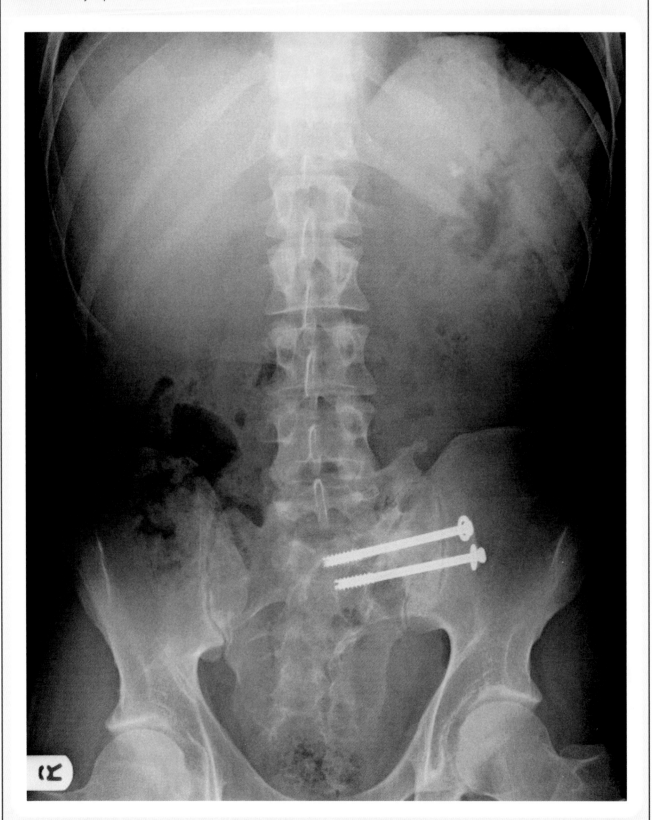

Continue

CASE **3.11**   *Contd.*

ANNOTATED X-RAY

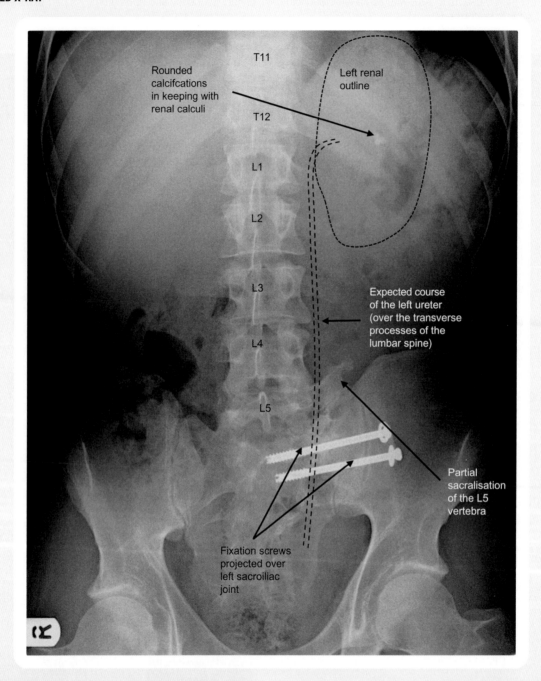

T11

Rounded
calcifcations
in keeping with
renal calculi

Left renal
outline

T12

L1

L2

L3

Expected course
of the left ureter
(over the transverse
processes of the
lumbar spine)

L4

L5

Partial
sacralisation
of the L5
vertebra

Fixation screws
projected over
left sacroiliac
joint

🔍 PRESENT YOUR FINDINGS

- This is a supine AP X-ray of the abdomen.
- It has been anonymised and the timing of the examination is not available. I would like to check the name and date of birth, as well as the time and date of the examination.
- The hernial orifices and right hemidiaphragm have not been included on the image; therefore, this is a technically inadequate X-ray.
- The most pertinent abnormality is the rounded areas of calcification projected over the left upper quadrant at the level of T12/L1. Given their position (overlying the left renal outline) and appearance, they are most in keeping with small renal calculi.

- There is no evidence of urinary calculi in the expected distribution of the left ureter, nor are there any visible right-sided urinary tract calculi.
- The bowel gas pattern is normal. No plain film evidence of bowel obstruction, perforation or mucosal oedema.
- Fixation screws are projected over the left sacroiliac joint. There is an abnormal area of bone on the left side of the L5 vertebral body which is in keeping with partial sacralisation of the L5 vertebra (a congenital anomaly, which is usually of no clinical significance, where the transverse process of the L5 vertebral body fuses onto the sacrum). Otherwise, there is no significant abnormality of the imaged skeleton.

IN SUMMARY – This abdominal X-ray shows multiple small left-sided renal calculi.

QUESTIONS

1. Which of the following is/are risk factors for developing renal calculi?
   A) Hypercalcaemia
   B) Renal tubular acidosis
   C) Overhydration
   D) Inflammatory bowel disease
   E) Recurrent urinary tract infections

2. Which of the following are symptoms associated with renal calculi?
   A) Pain
   B) Nausea and vomiting
   C) Dysuria
   D) Haematuria
   E) All of the above

3. Which type of renal stone is **least** likely to be visible on an X-ray?
   A) Uric acid
   B) Calcium oxalate
   C) Calcium phosphate
   D) Struvite
   E) Cysteine

4. What is the diagnostic modality of choice for identifying renal calculi?
   A) Abdominal X-ray/KUB
   B) Intravenous urogram
   C) Ultrasound
   D) Noncontrast CT KUB
   E) Contrast-enhanced CT of the abdomen and pelvis

5. What is the most appropriate initial management of a well patient with renal colic and a small (<5 mm) left-sided calculus at the left vesicoureteric junction identified on CT KUB?
   A) Urgent ureteroscopy and stone retrieval
   B) Urgent ESWL
   C) Urgent percutaneous nephrostomy
   D) Conservative approach (supportive treatment with analgesia and antiemetics and follow-up with X-ray KUBs (if the stone is visible on X-ray) until the stone has passed)
   E) Percutaneous nephrolithotomy

Continue

CASE **3.11** *Contd.*

ANSWERS TO QUESTIONS

1. Which of the following is/are risk factors for developing renal calculi?

The correct answers are **A) Hypercalcaemia, B) Renal tubular acidosis, D) Inflammatory bowel disease and E) Recurrent urinary tract infections**.

Renal calculi are common, occurring in 5% to 10% of the population. They typically occur in middle age (30–60 years) and affect men more commonly than women. There are several risk factors for developing renal calculi.

A) Hypercalcaemia – Correct. Calcium is a component of most renal calculi, in the form of calcium oxalate or calcium phosphate. There is increased risk of developing calcium containing renal calculi with conditions that cause hypercalcaemia, such as primary hyperparathyroidism, malignancy, sarcoidosis, Addison disease and medications (thiazides, vitamin D analogues, lithium).

B) Renal tubular acidosis – Correct. There is an increased risk of developing calcium renal stones in type 1 renal tubular acidosis. This is due to alkaline urine, hypercalciuria and low citrate which are associated with this condition.

C) Overhydration – Incorrect. Renal calculi are more common in hot climates due to dehydration. Dehydration results in concentrated urine, which can become supersaturated with substances that result in stone formation.

D) Inflammatory bowel disease – Correct. Calcium oxalate stones are more common in patients with Crohn's disease or those who have had a previous small bowel resection. Normally, calcium within the lumen of the GI tract binds to oxalate and the resultant calcium oxalate is poorly absorbed from the GI tract. Fat malabsorption occurs in patients who have had small bowel resections or Crohn's disease (due to the disruption of the enterohepatic circulation of bile acids). Unabsorbed fats preferentially bind with luminal calcium. This results in oxalate binding with sodium in the GI tract. Sodium oxalate is absorbed in the colon and results in high serum oxalate levels, increasing the risk of calcium oxalate stone formation.

E) Recurrent urinary tract infections – Correct. Struvite stones (magnesium ammonium phosphate) form in alkaline urine which contains ammonia. These conditions can occur in the presence of urease-producing bacteria, such as *Proteus*, *Klebsiella* and *Enterobacter* (urease metabolises urea into ammonia and carbon dioxide). Struvite stones typically occur in patients who have had multiple urinary tract infections such as those with vesicoureteric reflux, neurogenic bladder and obstructive uropathies.

2. Which of the following are symptoms associated with renal calculi?

The correct answer is **E) All of the above**.

Many patients with renal calculi are asymptomatic; however, renal calculi can cause a variety of symptoms.

A) Pain – Incorrect. Renal colic is the classic symptom associated with urinary tract calculi. It is caused by a calculus becoming lodged in a ureter, with resultant hyperperistalsis of the ureter in an attempt to overcome the blockage. The three anatomical sites at which calculi typically become obstructed are a) the pelvi-ureteric junction, b) where the ureter crosses over the iliac vessels and c) at the vesico-ureteric junction. Additionally, any pathological narrowing, such as a stricture, can cause stone impaction. The pain usually starts acutely, spreads from the loin to groin and comes in waves. In contrast to peritonitis, patients with renal colic usually writhe around the bed in agony.

B) Nausea and vomiting – Incorrect. Nausea and vomiting is common. It is mediated via an autonomic response to the pain. The ganglion which receives pain signals from the kidneys also supplies the stomach.

C) Dysuria – Incorrect. Dysuria can occur with urinary tract calculi. It is also commonly seen in cystitis (bladder inflammation, which is often secondary to infection).

D) Haematuria – Incorrect. Haematuria is another classic clinical finding in patients with renal calculi. It is often microscopic and is related to inflammation and trauma caused by the calculus. However, the absence of haematuria on urinalysis does not exclude renal calculi.

E) All of the above – Correct. As the previous answers suggest, renal calculi can cause a variety of symptoms. They can also cause fever and rigors if there is superimposed infection, acute kidney injury secondary to ureteral obstruction, or be asymptomatic.

> ❗ KEY POINT
>
> Dissecting or leaking abdominal aortic aneurysms can cause loin pain similar in nature to renal colic. In addition, if the aneurysm is adjacent to a ureter, there may be haematuria. Therefore, it is important to consider this serious differential diagnosis particularly in patients aged over 65 years presenting with renal colic for the first time.

3. Which type of renal stone is **least** likely to be visible on an X-ray?

The correct answer is **A) Uric acid**.

Different types of renal calculi have varying X-ray density. Overall, approximately 75% to 90% of renal calculi are radio-opaque (i.e. visible) on plain X-rays, and almost all stones are radio-opaque on CT. The exception is calculi that form in patients with HIV being treated with the protease inhibitor indinavir; these stones are classically radiolucent even on CT.

A) Uric acid – Correct. Uric acid stones are the least radio-opaque stones out of the listed options. They are typically radiolucent on X-ray but usually visible on CT. They form in patients with increased levels of uric acid, such as those with gout or who are being treated for myeloproliferative disorders. They account for approximately 10% of renal calculi. Xanthine stones are also typically radiolucent but are a rare cause of renal calculi.

B) Calcium oxalate – Incorrect. Calcium containing renal calculi are the most common type of stone, accounting for approximately 75%. They are the most radio-opaque renal calculi.

C) Calcium phosphate – Incorrect. See answer B.

D) Struvite – Incorrect. Struvite calculi form in the presence of urease-producing bacteria (see question 1) and account for approximately 15% of renal stones. They are generally radio-opaque, and are the second densest type of renal calculi. Most staghorn calculi are composed of struvite.

E) Cysteine – Incorrect. Cysteine stones are rare. They occur in patients with cystinuria, an uncommon autosomal recessive condition. Cysteine stones are usually radio-opaque on plain X-ray but less dense than calcium containing or struvite stones.

> ❗ KEY POINT
>
> Not all renal calculi are radio-opaque on X-ray. Therefore, a normal abdominal/KUB X-ray does not exclude renal calculi. CT is much more sensitive for identifying renal calculi.

4. What is the diagnostic modality of choice for identifying renal calculi?

The correct answer is **D) Noncontrast CT KUB**.

Imaging is used to confirm the diagnosis of renal/urinary tract calculi, exclude differential diagnoses, such as appendicitis and diverticulitis, and identify any complications, such as hydronephrosis. All the options listed can help diagnose urinary tract calculi.

A) Abdominal X-ray/KUB – Incorrect. Whilst 75% to 90% of renal calculi are radio-opaque, they can be difficult to identify on abdominal X-ray if they are small. Additionally, it can be difficult to differentiate urinary tract calculi from other causes of renal, abdominal or pelvic calcification such as nephrocalcinosis and calcified phleboliths. An abdominal/KUB X-ray should be performed if a calculus is identified on CT; X-rays can be used to monitor its response to treatment if the calculus is radio-opaque and visible on the X-ray. Additionally, if a patient is known to have radio-opaque calculi, plain X-rays can be used if they re-present with acute pain to assess any change in position of the known calculi.

B) Intravenous urogram – Incorrect. In the past, IVUs were the diagnostic test of choice for urinary tract calculi. However, they have now been superseded by CT. IVUs involve intravenous administration of contrast followed by plain X-rays of the kidneys, ureter and bladder (KUB) once the contrast is within the urinary collecting system. Urinary calculi, including radiolucent calculi, will show as filling defects within the urinary tract. Additionally, urinary tract obstruction (hydronephrosis) secondary to the urinary tract calculus can be diagnosed.

C) Ultrasound – Incorrect. Ultrasound can occasionally identify renal calculi. However, this modality is not as sensitive as CT. Additionally, it is usually impossible to image the entire ureter due to overlying bowel gas. Therefore, ultrasound has a low sensitivity for detecting urinary tract calculi. Ultrasound is good at identifying urinary tract obstruction which may be caused by calculi. Furthermore, it can identify other causes of loin pain and haematuria such as renal tumours, as well as gynaecological pathology, such as ovarian cysts, which can present in a similar manner.

D) Noncontrast CT KUB – Correct. Noncontrast CT KUB is the imaging modality of choice. It is a low-dose noncontrast CT which has a sensitivity of 95% to 100% and a higher specificity than IVU. It is readily available and quick to perform. As it is a noncontrast examination, it can be safely performed in patients with renal impairment (which may be secondary to urinary tract calculi). As well as identifying calculi, CT KUB can assess for complications (e.g. urinary tract obstruction causing hydronephrosis). Additionally, it permits an assessment of the other abdominal and pelvic organs, helping to identify or exclude other differential diagnoses, such as appendicitis and diverticulitis (although the accuracy for this is limited by the low-dose nature of the examination and the lack of intravenous contrast). As discussed in question 3, a small proportion of urinary tract calculi are not visible on CT; however, there may still be secondary signs of urinary tract calculi, such as perinephric and periureteral stranding.

E) Contrast-enhanced CT of the abdomen and pelvis – Incorrect. Standard contrast-enhanced CT can identify urinary tract calculi, but it uses a higher dose of radiation than CT KUB and requires intravenous contrast. Therefore, noncontrast scans are preferred. It does, however, provide a better assessment of the abdominal and pelvic organs. Additionally, a delayed phase scan, where the patient is imaged when the contrast is being excreted into the urinary tract (CT urogram), would help identify non-radio-opaque calculi as these would appear as filling defects in the urinary tracts.

5. What is the most appropriate initial management of a well patient with renal colic and a small (<5 mm) left-sided calculus at the left vesicoureteric junction identified on CT KUB?

The correct answer is **D) Conservative approach (supportive treatment with analgesia and antiemetics and follow-up with X-ray KUBs (if the stone is visible on X-ray) until the stone has passed)**.

The management of urinary tract calculi depends on the size and site of the stone and whether there is evidence of associated infection.

A) Urgent ureteroscopy and stone retrieval – Incorrect. Ureteroscopy is an invasive procedure reserved for patients with larger stones, persistent pain or those who fail to respond to conservative therapy. A ureteroscope is inserted via the urethra, through the bladder and into the appropriate ureter. Most ureteric calculi are accessible. However, results are best for those calculi located in the distal ureters.

B) Urgent ESWL – Incorrect. ESWL is another treatment modality reserved for patients who fail conservative management or have large stones. An external energy

Continue

CASE **3.11** *Contd.*

source causes shock waves which are targeted towards the stone. The aim is to fragment stones to allow them to pass through the ureters. The fragments can cause renal colic and ESWL may fail in large and hard stones.

C) Urgent percutaneous nephrostomy – Incorrect. Urgent percutaneous nephrostomy is needed in patients with an obstructed kidney and superimposed infection. It is usually performed under sedation with antibiotic coverage to reduce the risk of septicaemia. Once the collecting system has been suitably drained and the infection treated, the access gained via the nephrostomy can be used for nephrolithotomy (procedure to remove the stone) if required. An alternative approach to draining an infected, obstructed collecting system is from below (in a retrograde fashion) with an endoscopically placed ureteric stent extending from the bladder, up the ureter and into the renal pelvis.

D) Conservative approach (supportive treatment with analgesia and anti-emetics and follow-up with X-ray KUBs (if the stone is visible on X-ray) until the stone has passed) – Correct. Most small (<5 mm) stones in the ureter pass spontaneously, particularly if they are located distally. Patients can therefore be treated conservatively if there is no evidence of an infected, obstructed collecting system (see earlier). The mainstay of treatment is analgesia (NSAIDs such as diclofenac are used as first line), anti-emetics and IV

fluids if dehydrated. Medications such as tamsulosin (an alpha-blocker) or nifedipine (a calcium channel blocker) can be used to facilitate the passage of the stone. If visible on X-rays, the progress of such stones can be monitored by serial X-ray KUBs. If the stone fails to pass after 4 to 6 weeks, the pain becomes intolerable or if the patient develops an infected, obstructed collecting system, an alternative treatment option is required (see earlier).

E) Percutaneous nephrolithotomy – Incorrect. Percutaneous nephrolithotomy is used to fragment large renal calculi. It is usually reserved for large or complex stones or patients in which ESWL and ureteroscopy have failed. ESWL may fail in very large or hard stones.

IMPORTANT LEARNING POINTS

- Renal calculi are common and can cause a variety of symptoms; however, most stones are asymptomatic.
- Seventy-five to ninety percent of stones are visible on X-rays, whilst almost all are visible on CT.
- Noncontrast low-dose CT KUB is the imaging modality of choice, with X-ray KUBs reserved for follow-up of radio-opaque stones.
- Treatment depends on the size and site of the stone and the presence of infection or urinary tract obstruction.

CASE 3.12

A 52-year-old man presents with central abdominal pain, nausea and vomiting. He has not opened his bowels for several days. He has had similar episodes in the past. As part of your assessment, you request an abdominal X-ray.

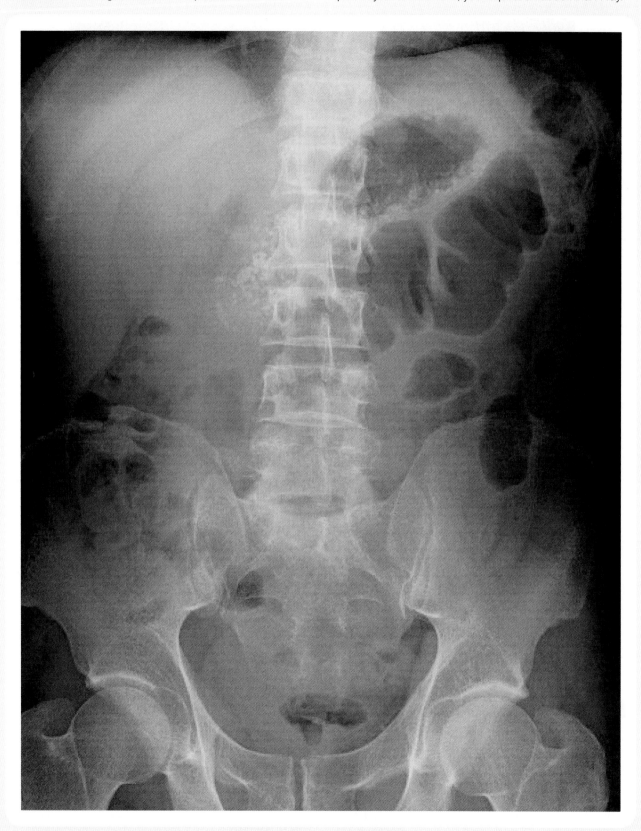

Continue

CASE **3.12**   *Contd.*

ANNOTATED X-RAY

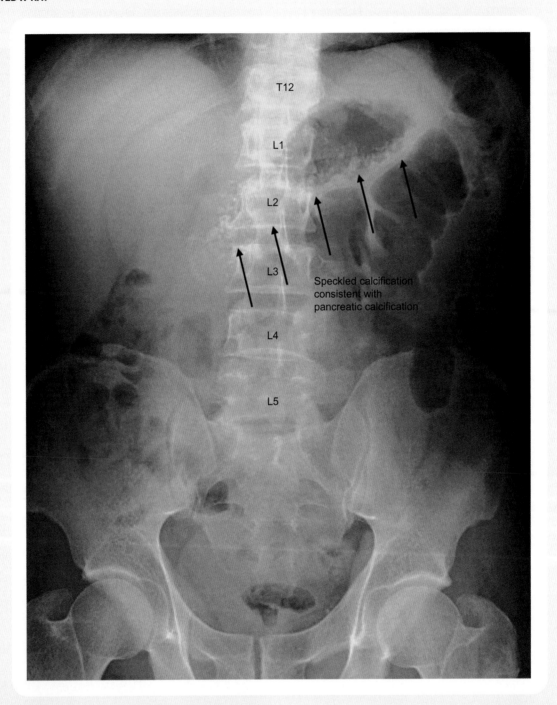

T12

L1

L2

L3

L4

L5

Speckled calcification
consistent with
pancreatic calcification

🔍 PRESENT YOUR FINDINGS

- This is a supine AP X-ray of the abdomen.
- There are no identifying marks on the X-ray but I would check this was the correct patient, date and time.
- It is a technically adequate X-ray.
- The most obvious abnormality is an area of speckled calcification centrally within the abdomen, projected over the L2 vertebral body, and extending into the left upper quadrant. Given its location, it is most in keeping with pancreatic calcification, secondary to chronic pancreatitis.

- The bowel gas pattern is normal. No plain film evidence of bowel obstruction, perforation or mucosal oedema.
- There is no obvious abnormality of the visible solid abdominal organs.
- No skeletal abnormality.

IN SUMMARY – This X-ray shows pancreatic calcification, in keeping with chronic pancreatitis.

QUESTIONS

1. Which of the following is the commonest cause of **chronic** pancreatitis?
   A) Hyperparathyroidism
   B) Hyperlipidaemia
   C) Alcohol
   D) Hereditary
   E) Gallstones

2. Which of the following is/are causes for **acute** pancreatitis?
   A) Gallstones
   B) ERCP
   C) Alcohol
   D) Renal calculi
   E) Idiopathic

3. In patients presenting with acute pancreatitis, which of the following is most correct?
   A) An abdominal X-ray can reliably exclude acute pancreatitis
   B) An urgent CT is required to confirm the diagnosis
   C) Elevated serum amylase is a specific marker of pancreatitis
   D) An MRCP should be requested to assess for gallstones
   E) An ultrasound should be requested to assess for gallstones

4. The initial management of acute pancreatitis includes which of the following?
   A) Discharge the patient, as pancreatitis is a self-limiting condition
   B) Analgesia, treatment of shock with IV fluids, consideration of urinary catheterisation to measure urine output and NG tube if the patient is vomiting
   C) Discharge the patient with strong analgesia and arrange follow-up in the general surgical clinic for the following week
   D) Urgent laparotomy
   E) Urgent MIRP

5. With regard to the complications of acute pancreatitis, which of the following is/are correct?
   A) All patients with acute pancreatitis will require a CT to identify potential complications
   B) Noncontrast CT is the preferred imaging modality for detecting complications
   C) CT can reliably diagnose a pancreatic pseudocyst within the first week
   D) A pancreatic abscess is a recognised complication and often requires drainage (either surgically, endoscopically or percutaneously)
   E) Pancreatic necrosis has a good prognosis

Continue

CASE **3.12**   *Contd.*

ANSWERS TO QUESTIONS

1. Which of the following is the commonest cause of **chronic** pancreatitis?

    The correct answer is **C) Alcohol**.

    Chronic pancreatitis is caused by repeated and prolonged episodes of pancreatic inflammation, which results in stricture formation within the pancreatic ducts and fibrous replacement of the pancreatic parenchyma. Typically, patients complain of severe epigastric pain radiating through to their back. This is because the pancreas is a retroperitoneal structure and inflammation compresses somatic nerves on the posterior abdominal wall. Over time, there can be loss of endocrine and exocrine pancreatic function, leading to diabetes mellitus and malabsorption/steatorrhoea, respectively. Weight loss is a common finding, due to exocrine dysfunction, as the pancreas is not able to produce enzymes required for digestion of ingested food.

    A) Hyperparathyroidism – Incorrect. Hyperparathyroidism is a rare cause of chronic pancreatitis. High levels of serum calcium can result in repeated episodes of inflammation in the pancreas. Hypercalcaemia can also cause inflammation of the gastric mucosa, resulting in peptic ulceration.

    B) Hyperlipidaemia – Incorrect. Significantly elevated levels of triglycerides, usually as a result of genetic defects rather than dietary factors, is a rare cause of chronic pancreatitis. Hypercholesterolaemia is not associated with pancreatitis.

    C) Alcohol – Correct. Alcohol is by far the commonest cause of chronic pancreatitis, accounting for 80% of the cases. Whilst most of these patients drink excessively, chronic pancreatitis can occur in patients drinking within the advised alcohol limits, suggesting there are other factors that act in conjunction with alcohol to predispose to the development of pancreatitis.

    D) Hereditary – Incorrect. Hereditary pancreatitis is a rare autosomal dominant condition caused by abnormalities in the trypsinogen gene. Episodes of pancreatitis usually start to present in childhood. It is associated with a significantly increased risk of pancreatic cancer.

    E) Gallstones – Incorrect. Gallstones and biliary tract disease can obstruct the pancreatic duct, leading to the premature activation of digestive pancreatic enzymes within the pancreatic ducts. However, patients who have an episode of acute pancreatitis due to gallstones usually undergo ERCP and cholecystectomy to prevent further episodes of pancreatitis.

2. Which of the following is/are causes for **acute** pancreatitis?

    The correct answers are **A) Gallstones, B) ERCP, C) Alcohol and E) Idiopathic**.

    There are several causes of acute pancreatitis, many of which overlap with the causes of chronic pancreatitis (see question 1).

    A) Gallstones – Correct. Along with alcohol, gallstones and biliary disease are the commonest cause of acute pancreatitis. It is believed that obstruction at the ampulla of Vater can cause reflux of bile into the pancreatic duct, resulting in premature activation of the digestive pancreatic enzymes.

    B) ERCP – Correct. Acute pancreatitis is an infrequent but well-recognised complication of ERCP. The pathogenesis is unclear but may be related to mechanical trauma, hydrostatic pressure from contrast injection, chemical injury or infection.

    C) Alcohol – Correct. Alcohol is one of the commonest causes of acute pancreatitis, accounting for approximately 40% of cases.

    D) Renal calculi – Incorrect. Renal calculi do not cause pancreatitis per se; however, hypercalcaemia, which is a risk factor for renal calculi, can cause acute pancreatitis.

    E) Idiopathic – Correct. Twenty percent of cases of acute pancreatitis are classed as idiopathic. A proportion of these cases may be caused by biliary sludge and microcrystals.

> ❶ KEY POINT

'I GET SMASHED' is a useful mnemonic for the causes of acute pancreatitis. It stands for: Idiopathic, Gallstones, Ethanol, Trauma, Steroids, Mumps, Autoimmune and inherited (e.g. polyarteritis nodosa), Scorpion stings, Hyperlipidaemia/hypercalcaemia, ERCP/surgery, Drugs (such as thiazides and azathioprine).

3. In patients presenting with acute pancreatitis, which of the following is most correct?

    The correct answer is **E) An ultrasound should be requested to assess for gallstones**.

    The diagnosis of acute pancreatitis is usually clinical and biochemical, with severe abdominal pain, often with vomiting, and a raised serum amylase highly suggestive. Imaging is used to exclude other differential diagnoses, such as a perforated viscus or bowel obstruction, etc., to help identify the underlying cause and to detect complications.

    A) An abdominal X-ray can reliably exclude acute pancreatitis – Incorrect. Acute pancreatitis cannot be diagnosed by abdominal X-ray. The role of the abdominal and erect chest X-rays is to help exclude other differential diagnoses, such as a perforated viscus and bowel obstruction. As in this case, calcification within the pancreas as a result of chronic pancreatitis can sometimes be seen. However, its absence does not exclude the diagnosis of chronic pancreatitis.

    B) An urgent CT is required to confirm the diagnosis – Incorrect. The diagnosis of acute pancreatitis is usually biochemical. CT is occasionally used for diagnosis if the biochemical and clinical findings are equivocal. However, the main role of CT in acute pancreatitis is to identify complications, such as pancreatic necrosis, abscesses and peripancreatic fluid collections.

    C) Elevated serum amylase is a specific marker of pancreatitis – Incorrect. Elevated amylase is a sensitive but nonspecific marker of pancreatic inflammation. Other causes of elevated amylase include perforated duodenal ulcer, acute cholecystitis, mesenteric ischaemia, ruptured or dissected aortic aneurysm and ruptured ectopic pregnancy. However, such conditions usually result in a mildly elevated amylase <1000 IU, whereas acute pancreatitis often causes the amylase to be very high (>1000 IU).

D) An MRCP should be requested to assess for gallstones – Incorrect. MRCP is a noninvasive technique for assessing the bile and pancreatic ducts (ERCP is an invasive technique, which permits assessment as well as allowing treatment). MRCP does not use ionising radiation. It is less accurate than ultrasound at detecting gallstones.

E) An ultrasound should be requested to assess for gallstones – Correct. Gallstones are one of the commonest causes of acute pancreatitis and they should be excluded in acute pancreatitis. Ultrasound is a sensitive and specific technique for identifying gallstones. It is cheap, readily available and does not involve ionising radiation. Patients should be fasted for at least 6 hours prior to scanning to allow the gallbladder to distend with bile, thus improving the accuracy. If there is biliary dilation, suggesting bile duct stone, MRCP should be performed to guide decision regarding stone extraction with ERCP.

❶ KEY POINT

The amylase rise in acute pancreatitis is transient. Therefore, if a patient presents several days after the onset of acute pancreatitis, the amylase may be normal. Serum amylase is less useful in chronic pancreatitis as there is often not enough functioning pancreatic parenchyma to cause a rise in amylase.

4. The initial management of acute pancreatitis includes which of the following?
The correct answer is **B) Analgesia, treatment of shock with IV fluids, consideration of urinary catheterisation to measure urine output and NG tube if the patient is vomiting**.
Treatment of acute pancreatitis is usually supportive; there is no specific initial management.

A) Discharge the patient, as pancreatitis is a self-limiting condition – Incorrect. Acute pancreatitis is usually a self-limiting condition. However, patients can become very unwell. They need to be admitted for analgesia, fluid resuscitation, investigation of the underlying cause (e.g. gallstones) and management of potential complications.

B) Analgesia, treatment of shock with IV fluids, consideration of urinary catheterisation to measure urine output and NG tube if the patient is vomiting – Correct. All these options should be considered. Antibiotics should be reserved for specific infections. Further management will depend on the severity of the pancreatitis and development of complications.

C) Discharge the patient with strong analgesia and arrange follow-up in the general surgical clinic for the following week – Incorrect. See entry for answer A. The patient may need to be followed up in the outpatient clinic once discharged.

D) Urgent laparotomy – Incorrect. The initial treatment is supportive. Even in cases of gallstone pancreatitis, cholecystectomy is deferred to a later date.

E) Urgent MIRP – Incorrect. MIRP can be used to treat pancreatic necrosis, a complication associated with acute pancreatitis. However, this is not part of the initial management.

❶ KEY POINTS

1. The severity of acute pancreatitis can be estimated using various scoring systems, such as the Modified Glasgow prognostic score.
2. The Modified Glasgow prognostic score can be remembered by the mnemonic 'PANCREAS'
P = PaO$_2$ <8 kPa on air
A = Age >55
N = Neutrophils (white cell count) >15 × 10^9/L
C = Calcium <2 mmol/L
R = Raised urea >16 mmol/L
E = Elevated enzymes (LDH >600 units/L, ALT >100 units/L)
A = Albumin <32 g/L
S = Sugar (glucose) >10 mmol/L (in the absence of diabetes)
If three or more criteria are present, then the attack of acute pancreatitis is severe.
3. Patients with mild pancreatitis can usually be managed on a surgical ward. Those with severe pancreatitis are more prone to developing complications, have a worse prognosis and should be managed in high dependency or intensive care units.

5. With regard to the complications of acute pancreatitis, which of the following is/are correct?
The correct answer is **D) A pancreatic abscess is a recognised complication and often requires drainage (either surgically, endoscopically or percutaneously)**.
Complications are more common in patients with severe episodes of acute pancreatitis. Complications include pancreatic necrosis, acute fluid collection, pseudocysts, pancreatic abscesses, infected pancreatic necrosis, haemorrhage and pseudoaneurysm formation of the splenic or gastroduodenal arteries.

A) All patients with acute pancreatitis will require a CT to identify potential complications – Incorrect. CT is the main imaging technique for identifying complications of acute pancreatitis, commonly being performed after 48 hours from the onset. However, it is usually reserved for patients with severe pancreatitis. Those with mild episodes do not routinely require a CT.

B) Noncontrast CT is the preferred imaging modality for detecting complications – Incorrect. CT with IV contrast is required to accurately assess for complications. In particular, contrast enhancement permits assessment for pancreatic necrosis. It also improves assessment of the other abdominal organs. Contraindications to IV contrast include previous

Continue

CASE **3.12** *Contd.*

contrast allergic reactions. Caution is required with IV contrast in patients taking metformin and those with renal impairment.

C) CT can reliably diagnose a pancreatic pseudocyst within the first week – Incorrect. Peripancreatic fluid collections identified in the acute setting are termed 'acute fluid collections'. They contain enzyme-rich fluid, allowing them to dissect into other body compartments, such as the mediastinum or adjacent organs, but they do not have a fibrous capsule. Fifty percent of acute fluid collections resolve. Those that persist for more than 4 to 6 weeks are termed pseudocysts (therefore, pseudocysts cannot be detected at 1 week, since they are defined as only existing from 4 weeks onwards). Pseudocysts are so called because of the presence of a fibrous capsule (true cysts have epithelial lined capsule). Most pseudocysts resolve spontaneously, especially if they are small (<4 cm). Complications from pseudocysts are infrequent and include: haemorrhage, obstruction of the bile ducts or small bowel, infection or rupture leading to peritonitis.

D) A pancreatic abscess is a recognised complication and often requires drainage (either surgically, endoscopically or percutaneously) – Correct. A fluid collection in or around the pancreas that becomes infected and contains pus is termed a pancreatic abscess. The patient is usually very unwell. These typically form after 4 weeks from the onset of acute pancreatitis. CT may show gas within a peri/intrapancreatic fluid collection. Treatment is often with percutaneous drainage (either CT or ultrasound guided). Endoscopic and surgical drainage may be required.

E) Pancreatic necrosis has a good prognosis – Incorrect. Pancreatic necrosis has a poor prognosis. The prognosis deteriorates with increasing amounts of necrotic pancreas (30% necrosis = 10% mortality, 90% necrosis = 50% mortality). Superimposed infection worsens the prognosis and requires surgery.

IMPORTANT LEARNING POINTS

- Pancreatic calcification is associated with chronic pancreatitis; however, the abdominal X-ray cannot reliably diagnose or exclude pancreatitis – acute or chronic.
- Ultrasound is often the first line to identify gallstone as a cause of pancreatitis. CT is reserved for imaging complications of pancreatitis, or to exclude mimics such as hollow organ perforation.
- Treatment of acute pancreatitis is usually supportive. However, complications may require specific management, such as percutaneous drainage.

A 55-year-old female presented with a palpable pelvic mass. There was a history of menorrhagia and lower abdominal pain. An abdominal X-ray was performed.

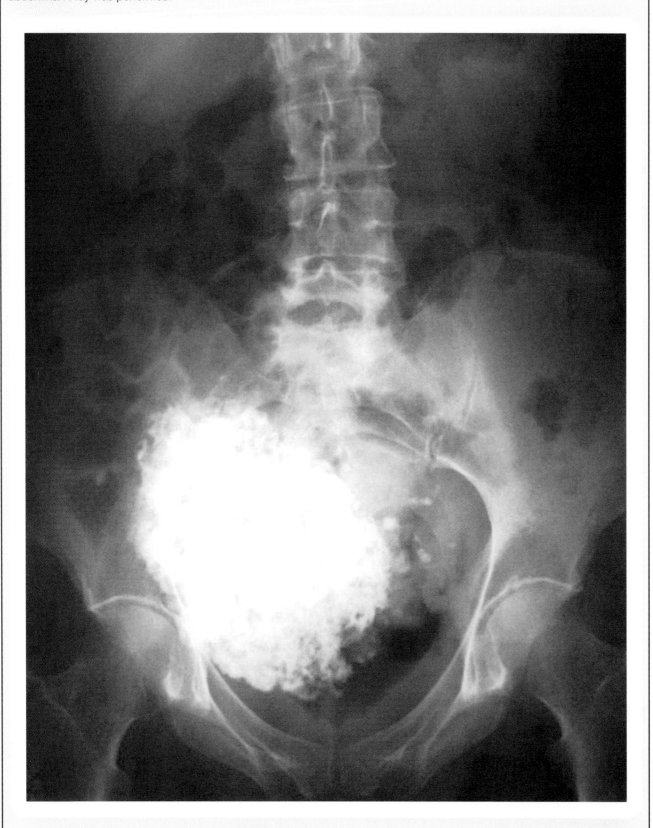

Continue

CASE **3.13** *Contd.*

ANNOTATED X-RAY

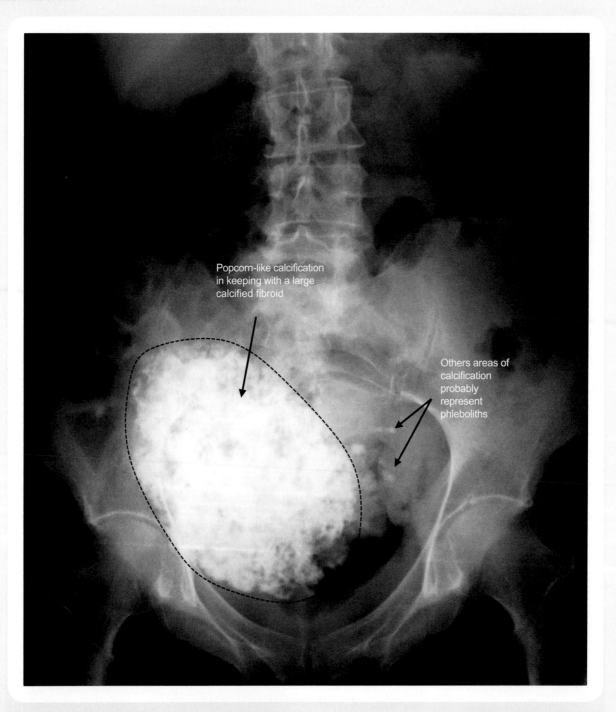

Popcorn-like calcification in keeping with a large calcified fibroid

Others areas of calcification probably represent phleboliths

🔍 PRESENT YOUR FINDINGS

- This is a supine AP abdominal X-ray.
- There are no patient identifiable data, nor a time or date stamp on the X-ray. I would confirm this relates to the correct patient before proceeding with interpretation.
- The upper aspect of the abdomen has not been included; therefore, the X-ray is technically inadequate.
- The most obvious abnormality is a large area of 'popcorn'-like calcification projected over the right

hemipelvis. The findings are suggestive of a large calcified uterine fibroid.
- The further distinct small areas of calcification projected over the pelvis likely represent calcified phleboliths.
- The bowel gas pattern is normal, with no evidence of obstruction, perforation or mucosal oedema.
- No significant abnormality of the other visible abdominal organs.
- The visualised skeleton is unremarkable.

IN SUMMARY – This abdominal X-ray demonstrates a large area of calcification in the pelvis which is consistent with a large calcified uterine fibroid. This could be confirmed with ultrasound. I would refer to any previous imaging, if available, to assess for any change in size and seek gynaecological input into the management of the patient's symptoms.

QUESTIONS

1. Which of the following is/are common symptoms of uterine fibroids?
   A) Asymptomatic
   B) Menorrhagia
   C) Urinary frequency
   D) Dysmenorrhoea
   E) Postcoital bleeding
2. Which of the following is the most common location for uterine fibroids?
   A) Subserosal
   B) Intramural
   C) Submucosal
   D) Pedunculated submucosal
   E) Pedunculated subserosal
3. Which of the following imaging techniques provides the most comprehensive assessment of uterine fibroids?
   A) X-ray
   B) Hysterosalpingogram
   C) Transabdominal ultrasound
   D) CT of the abdomen and pelvis
   E) MRI of the pelvis
4. Which of the following is/are potential medical management options for uterine fibroids and their associated symptoms?
   A) Levonorgestrel IUCD
   B) Tranexamic acid
   C) Gonadotropin-releasing hormone analogues
   D) Hormone replacement therapy
   E) Danazol
5. Which of the following is/are potential interventional management options for uterine fibroids?
   A) Radiotherapy
   B) Uterine artery embolisation
   C) Hysterectomy
   D) Myomectomy
   E) MR-guided focused ultrasound

Continue

CASE 3.13 *Contd.*

ANSWERS TO QUESTIONS

1. Which of the following is/are common symptoms of uterine fibroids?

   The correct answers are **A) Asymptomatic, B) Menorrhagia, C) Urinary frequency and D) Dysmenorrhoea**.

   Uterine fibroids are a benign tumour arising from smooth muscle (myometrium) of the uterus. They are a common pathology and can result in a variety of disabling symptoms for many women. Being hormone dependent, fibroids are most common in premenopausal women, can grow during pregnancy and usually involute after menopause.

   A) Asymptomatic – Correct. Some patients may have fibroids but never experience any symptoms related to them.

   B) Menorrhagia – Correct. Heavy and prolonged menstrual bleeding is a common symptom related to uterine fibroids.

   C) Urinary frequency – Correct. Anterior uterine fibroids may exert local pressure effects on the urinary bladder, resulting in urinary frequency. They may also cause difficulty in emptying the bladder (urinary retention) and therefore predispose the patient to urinary tract infections.

   D) Dysmenorrhoea – Correct. Lower abdominal pain related to menstruation is a recognised feature of uterine fibroids.

   E) Postcoital bleeding – Incorrect. Fibroids can result in dyspareunia (pain during intercourse); however, bleeding following intercourse is not a common finding. Postcoital bleeding should raise the possibility of cervical pathology. Genitourinary infection and local vaginal pathology may also present in this manner.

❗ KEY POINTS

1. The size, position and number of uterine fibroids may relate to the symptoms experienced by the patient.
2. Other clinical features which may occur with fibroids include infertility, miscarriage, premature labour and abnormal foetal positioning. Pedunculated fibroids, rarely, may twist on their pedicles, resulting in torsion. Very rarely, fibroids can undergo malignant (sarcomatous) degeneration.
3. Pregnancy, including an ectopic pregnancy, is another important differential diagnosis in any woman of childbearing age with abdominal pain. The β-hCG (human chorionic gonadotropin) should be measured. It is especially important to exclude pregnancy before exposing the patient to X-rays due to the potential teratogenic effects of ionising radiation.

2. Which of the following is the most common location for uterine fibroids?

   The correct answer is **B) Intramural**.

   From interior to exterior, the layers of the uterus are the uterine cavity, endometrium, mucosa, submucosa, myometrium and serosa.

   A) Subserosal – Incorrect. Subserosal fibroids are located just under the visceral peritoneal covering of the uterus. They are not the most common location for fibroids.

   B) Intramural – Correct. Fibroids within the myometrium (intramural) are the most common subtype.

   C) Submucosal – Incorrect. These fibroids grow inwards and can distort the endometrial cavity. However, they are not the most common location for fibroids.

   D) Pedunculated submucosal – Incorrect. Submucosal fibroids may protrude sufficiently into the endometrial cavity to develop a stalk. This is termed a pedunculated fibroid. They are not the most common location for fibroids.

   E) Pedunculated subserosal – Incorrect. Pedunculated subserosal fibroids pose the rare risk of detaching from the uterus and seeding elsewhere in the abdomen. They are uncommon.

❗ KEY POINTS

1. Intramural fibroids are the commonest location for uterine fibroids. In addition to the locations mentioned earlier, other rare locations for fibroids include the cervix and uterine supporting structures.
2. Submucosal fibroids are less common than intramural ones but are more likely to produce symptoms.
3. The location of the fibroid(s) guides which treatment options are suitable. For example, pedunculated subserosal fibroids are a relative contraindication for uterine embolisation due to the risk of fibroid separation and resultant serious complications.

3. Which of the following imaging techniques provides the most comprehensive assessment of uterine fibroids?

   The correct answer is **E) MRI of the pelvis**.

   Imaging is used to confirm the diagnosis, and identify the number and location of the fibroids. There are a variety of different imaging options.

   A) X-ray – Incorrect. Uterine fibroids will only be readily discernible on a X-ray if they are calcified and this is often not the case.

   B) Hysterosalpingogram – Incorrect. Hysterosalpingogram is performed to confirm patency of the fallopian tubes in patients with fertility issues. Whilst the associated mass effect of a uterine fibroid may be discernible with this imaging technique, it is not commonly used to assess the fibroid uterus as fibroids which do not indent/distort the uterine cavity are unlikely to be detected.

   C) Transabdominal ultrasound – Incorrect. Ultrasound is good at identifying and assessing uterine fibroids. Transvaginal ultrasound in particular generates excellent images of the uterus.

   D) CT of the abdomen and pelvis – Incorrect. Fibroids are soft tissue masses which have a similar appearance on CT to the surrounding myometrium. CT scanning is not as good at characterising such soft

tissue entities as MR. Additionally, CT involves a significant dose of ionising radiation to the pelvis and reproductive organs of these young patients. For these reasons, it is not routinely performed in the workup of patients with suspected uterine fibroids.
E) MRI of the pelvis – Correct. MRI provides the best soft tissue contrast and is performed when deciding treatment options for symptomatic patients. Compared with ultrasound, MRI allows a better assessment of the relationship of the fibroids to other pelvic structures. It does not involve any ionising radiation. On the down side, MRI is much less readily available than ultrasound.

> **❗ KEY POINT**
>
> Ultrasound and MR imaging are the mainstay techniques in diagnostic imaging of uterine fibroids, neither of which use ionising radiation.

4. Which of the following is/are potential medical management options for uterine fibroids and their associated symptoms?
   The correct answers are **A) Levonorgestrel IUCD, B) Tranexamic acid, C) Gonadotropin-releasing hormone analogues and E) Danazol**.
   Most fibroids do not need treatment as they are asymptomatic. Medical therapies are aimed at either reducing the symptoms, such as menorrhagia, or shrinking the fibroid.
   A) Levonorgestrel IUCD – Correct. The Mirena coil is an effective way to deliver progesterone locally to the uterus. It can help with the symptom of menorrhagia and may result in amenorrhoea. It may be of limited use in patients with large fibroids which deform the uterine cavity, precluding insertion of the device or promoting rapid expulsion once placed.
   B) Tranexamic acid – Correct. Tranexamic acid is an antifibrinolytic agent which prevents the breakdown of clots and can be used in patients with menorrhagia.
   C) Gonadotropin-releasing hormone analogues – Correct. These agents can cause shrinkage of uterine fibroids by reducing circulating oestrogen levels. Prolonged use is limited by side effects of postmenopausal symptoms and osteoporosis. They may be used as a neoadjuvant approach prior to surgical treatment.
   D) Hormone replacement therapy – Incorrect. HRT actually results in increased size of uterine fibroids. HRT is used in women suffering with postmenopausal symptoms but not for a treatment of fibroids.
   E) Danazol – Correct. Danazol is a treatment which can cause fibroid regression, likely mediated by an anti-oestrogenic effect. However, its use is limited by its androgenic sided effects.

> **❗ KEY POINT**
>
> Other medical options include iron tablets for managing anaemia, NSAIDs for pain relief and oral contraceptives to reduce menorrhagia.

5. Which of the following is/are potential interventional management options for uterine fibroids?
   The correct answers are **B) Uterine artery embolisation, C) Hysterectomy, D) Myomectomy and E) MR-guided focused ultrasound**.
   Interventional procedures are aimed at shrinking or removing fibroids. The risks of the procedures need to be weighed against the potential benefits for each patient.
   A) Radiotherapy – Incorrect. Radiotherapy is not indicated in the management of uterine fibroids.
   B) Uterine artery embolisation – Correct. Uterine artery embolisation is an interventional radiology technique. The uterine arteries are catheterised and an embolic agent is injected to cut-off the blood supply to the fibroids. It is not suitable for pedunculated fibroids as the stalk may become necrotic, causing the fibroid to separate from the uterus and incite an inflammatory response within the peritoneal cavity.
   C) Hysterectomy – Correct. Hysterectomy may be required to manage a symptomatic large fibroid uterus where other options have failed.
   D) Myomectomy – Correct. The technique essentially involves shelling out the fibroids from the myometrium. Myomectomy is intended to preserve fertility.
   E) MR-guided focused ultrasound – Correct. This is a new noninvasive, outpatient procedure. Ultrasound energy is used to heat and ablate the fibroid. It is done under MRI guidance, to allow accurate targeting of the fibroid.

> **❗ KEY POINTS**
>
> 1. There are a variety of interventional and surgical techniques to manage uterine fibroids. Not all approaches are suitable for all types of fibroid.
> 2. Post embolisation syndrome is a potential complication following fibroid embolisation. It usually presents 24 to 48 hours after the embolisation with pain, fever, malaise and raised inflammatory markers. It is a self-limiting entity and the treatment is conservative. It usually settles within 5 to 7 days.

> **IMPORTANT LEARNING POINTS**
>
> - Uterine fibroids are a common benign tumour of the uterus.
> - Most patients are asymptomatic.
> - When symptomatic, imaging involves ultrasound and MRI.
> - There are a variety of medical, interventional and surgical methods available for the treatment of uterine fibroids.
> - The classic finding of punctate 'popcorn'-like calcification in the pelvis on an abdominal X-ray is consistent with a calcified uterine fibroid, although most fibroids are not visible on X-rays.

CASE **3.14**

A 65-year-old man presents with nausea and vomiting. He has a past history of alcohol excess. An abdominal X-ray is performed to exclude bowel obstruction.

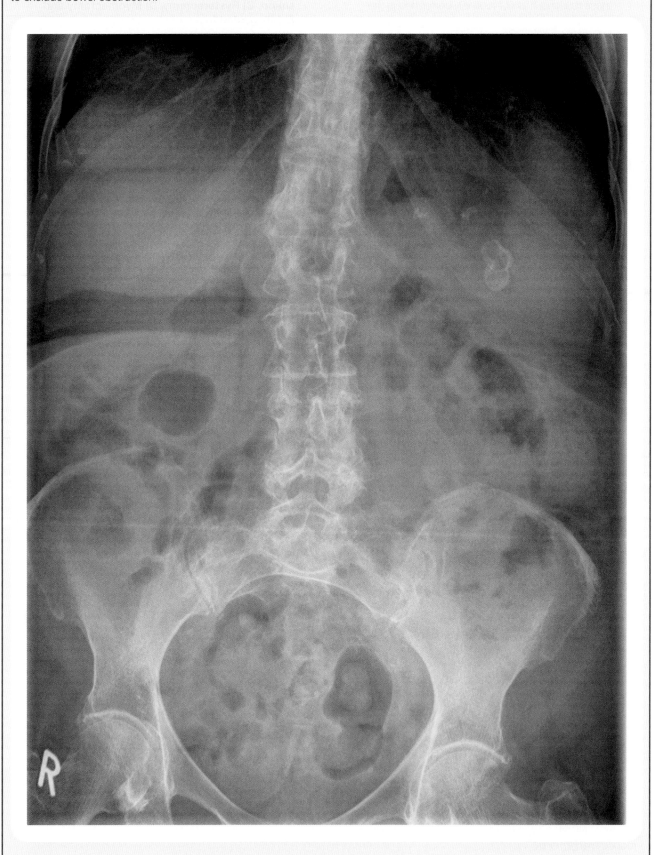

ANNOTATED X-RAY

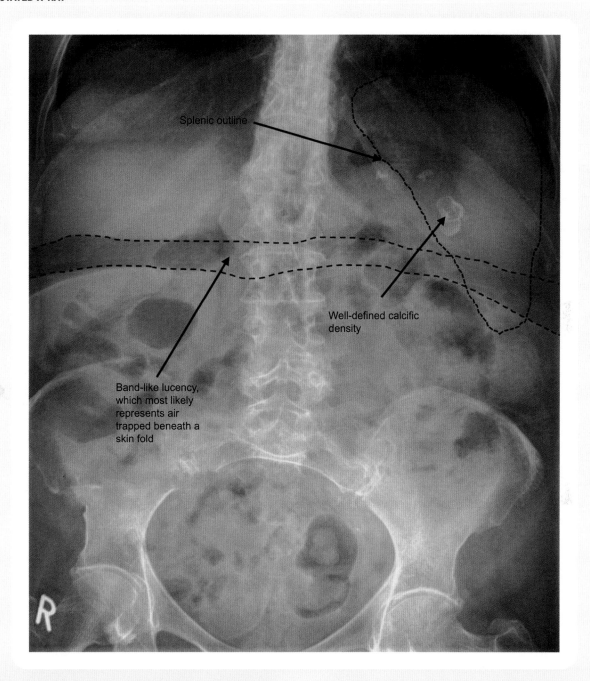

Splenic outline

Well-defined calcific density

Band-like lucency, which most likely represents air trapped beneath a skin fold

R

🔍 PRESENT YOUR FINDINGS

- This is a supine AP abdominal X-ray.
- There are no patient identifiable data on the X-ray but I would like to confirm the patient's name, date of birth and date and time that the X-ray was performed before making further assessment.
- The diaphragms have been imaged but the pubic symphysis is not visualised. Consequently, this is technically inadequate as the hernial orifices have not been complete visualised.
- The most striking abnormality is well-defined smooth calcific densities projected over the left upper quadrant.

They are overlying the region of the splenic hilum and likely represent a calcified splenic artery aneurysm. The spleen appears slightly enlarged.

- The bowel gas pattern is normal, with no plain film evidence of obstruction, perforation or mucosal oedema.
- The linear band of air density across the central abdomen may relate to air trapped beneath a fold of anterior abdominal subcutaneous tissue.
- There is no other significant abnormality of the visible abdominal organs.
- No skeletal abnormality demonstrated.

Continue

CASE **3.14** *Contd.*

IN SUMMARY – This abdominal X-ray demonstrates no evidence of bowel obstruction. There is a calcific entity in the left upper quadrant which may represent a splenic artery aneurysm. The history of alcohol excess and presence of splenomegaly raise the possibility of portal hypertension which may be implicated in the aetiology of the aneurysm. I would examine for the signs of portal hypertension. A CT scan could be performed to clarify the diagnosis and accurately determine the size.

QUESTIONS

1. Which of the following is/are causes of calcification in the left upper quadrant on abdominal X-ray?
   A) Acute pancreatitis
   B) Renal calculi
   C) Calcified lymph nodes
   D) Sickle cell anaemia
   E) Splenic artery aneurysm

2. Which of the following favours the diagnosis of splenic artery aneurysm over splenic artery pseudoaneurysm?
   A) Recent pancreatitis
   B) Recent peptic ulcer disease
   C) Recent abdominal trauma
   D) Presenting as an incidental finding with no associated symptoms
   E) Lack of peripheral calcification around the aneurysm

3. Which of the following is/are risk factors for the formation of a splenic artery aneurysm?
   A) Hypertension
   B) Portal hypertension
   C) Pregnancy
   D) Liver transplantation
   E) Male sex

4. Which of the following are true regarding portal hypertension?
   A) Splenomegaly may result
   B) Ascites may be present
   C) It can cause oesophageal varices
   D) Dilated blood vessels may be evident around the umbilicus
   E) The liver is always shrunken

5. Which of the following are true regarding treatment of splenic artery aneurysms?
   A) Symptomatic patients should be treated
   B) Asymptomatic pregnant women or women of child-bearing age should be treated
   C) Asymptomatic aneurysms <2 cm may be managed with surveillance
   D) Endovascular embolisation is not a treatment option as it causes splenic infarction
   E) Splenectomy may be required

ANSWERS TO QUESTIONS

1. Which of the following is/are causes of calcification in the left upper quadrant on abdominal X-ray?

   The correct answers are **B) Renal calculi, C) Calcified lymph nodes, D) Sickle cell anaemia and E) Splenic artery aneurysm**.

   There are a variety of causes of calcification in the left upper quadrant on abdominal X-ray. If you are stuck for this differential, first think of all the organs that are located in this area and then think of a disease process which can affect them.

   A) Acute pancreatitis – Incorrect. Calcification in the tail of the pancreas can result in calcification in the left upper quadrant on abdominal X-ray. However, this is a complication of chronic pancreatitis and is not seen in acute pancreatitis (unless there is acute-on-chronic pancreatitis).

   B) Renal calculi – Correct. Calcification in the left upper quadrant may relate to calcification in the renal pelvicalyceal system (renal stones) or within the renal parenchyma (nephrocalcinosis). However, plain X-rays of the abdomen are no longer routinely indicated in the investigation of suspected renal colic as low-dose noncontrast CT has largely replaced the historical KUB X-ray.

   C) Calcified lymph nodes – Correct. There are multiple lymph nodes in the mesentery in the abdomen. Following infection or inflammation, the nodes may calcify and be evident on the abdominal X-ray.

   D) Sickle cell anaemia – Correct. Sickle cell anaemia can result in vaso-occlusive crises in the spleen. Multiple attacks result in an atrophic spleen which may contain foci of calcification due to infarction.

   E) Splenic artery aneurysm – Correct. Splenic artery aneurysm is a rare cause of calcification in the left upper quadrant.

❶ KEY POINTS

1. There are multiple causes of calcification in the left upper quadrant on abdominal X-ray.
2. Splenic artery aneurysms are the third most common abdominal aneurysm after aortic and iliac aneurysms, and the most common type of abdominal visceral artery aneurysm. With the increasing use of CT, the detection of splenic artery aneurysms is on the increase. They are usually small (2–4 cm), solitary, fusiform and located to the middle/distal splenic artery.

2. Which of the follow favours the diagnosis of splenic artery aneurysm over splenic artery pseudoaneurysm?

   The correct answer is **D) Presenting as an incidental finding with no associated symptoms**.

   As with any true aneurysm, a splenic artery aneurysm involves all three layers of the arterial wall (intima, media and adventitia), whereas pseudoaneurysms do not have a true wall. They consist of a defect in the arterial wall confined by haematoma and the surrounding soft tissues.

   A) Recent pancreatitis – Incorrect. The release of pancreatic enzymes during an episode of acute pancreatitis can result in damage to the splenic artery wall and cause the formation of a splenic artery pseudoaneurysm.

   B) Recent peptic ulcer disease – Incorrect. Peptic ulcer disease has been described in the aetiology of splenic artery pseudoaneurysm formation, albeit rarely.

   C) Recent abdominal trauma – Incorrect. Both blunt and penetrating abdominal trauma can result in splenic artery pseudoaneursym formation. Iatrogenic postoperative causes are also recognised.

   D) Presenting as an incidental finding with no associated symptoms – Correct. If a splenic artery aneurysm ruptures, it will present with pain and possibly evidence of hypovolaemic shock. However, true aneurysms rupture less commonly than pseudoaneurysms. Furthermore, an unruptured true aneurysm usually does not invoke any symptoms, whereas unruptured pseudoaneurysms still usually result in symptoms such as abdominal pain or gastrointestinal bleeding.

   E) Lack of peripheral calcification around the aneurysm – Incorrect. True splenic artery aneurysms often have a calcific rim, as opposed to pseudoaneurysms which do not.

❶ KEY POINT

True splenic artery aneurysms are more common than pseudoaneurysms. However, pseudoaneurysms are more likely to result in symptoms and are at higher risk of rupture. Therefore, splenic artery pseudoaneurysms require urgent treatment.

3. Which of the following is/are risk factors for the formation of a splenic artery aneurysm?

   The correct answers are **A) Hypertension, B) Portal hypertension, C) Pregnancy and D) Liver transplantation**.

   Hypertension, portal hypertension, pregnancy and liver transplantation are risk factors. Splenic artery aneurysms are four times more common in women than in men.

❶ KEY POINTS

1. Other less common conditions associated with splenic artery aneurysm formation include collagen vascular disorders, arteritis and arterial fibrodysplasia.
2. Although there may be histological evidence of atherosclerosis affecting splenic artery aneurysms, this is believed to be a secondary phenomenon following primary degeneration of the media, rather than the underlying cause of the aneurysm formation. In contrast, atherosclerosis is the main risk factor for abdominal aortic aneurysm formation.

4. Which of the following are true regarding portal hypertension?

   The correct answers are **A) Splenomegaly may result, B) Ascites may be present, C) It can cause oesophageal varices and D) Dilated blood vessels may be evident around the umbilicus**.

   Portal hypertension is the elevation of blood pressure within the portal system (portal vein and its tributaries such as the splenic and superior mesenteric veins). The diagnosis of portal hypertension is usually based on characteristic clinical and ultrasound findings; however, it is possible to directly measure the blood pressure in

Continue

CASE 3.14 *Contd.*

the portal system using interventional radiology. The normal pressure of blood flow in the portal vein should be less than 10 mmHg. Portal hypertension is present when pressures are in excess of 12 mmHg.

A) Splenomegaly may result – Correct. The upper limit of the spleen in most adult patients is approximately 12 cm in maximal bipolar diameter. Portal hypertension is one cause of splenomegaly.

B) Ascites may be present – Correct. Ascites can result from elevated portal venous pressure. This may be evident on clinical examination of the patient with shifting dullness. The causes of ascites can be split into transudates (e.g. liver failure, heart failure, kidney failure, Budd–Chiari and constrictive pericarditis) and exudates (e.g. infection such as spontaneous bacterial peritonitis, malignancy, pancreatitis and serositis).

C) It can cause oesophageal varices – Correct. Portal hypertension may result in the formation of portosystemic collateral vessels. Oesophageal varices, gastric varices and haemorrhoids are examples of such collateral vessels.

D) Dilated blood vessels may be evident around the umbilicus – Correct. This sign is termed 'caput medusae' – i.e. Medusa's head. It represents tortuous dilated para-umbilical veins resulting from recanalisation of the umbilical vein due to portal hypertension.

E) The liver is always shrunken – Incorrect. Liver cirrhosis is the most common cause of portal hypertension. In established cirrhosis, the liver is shrunken and nodular. However, there are many other causes of portal hypertension. They can be divided into prehepatic, hepatic and posthepatic causes (Table C3.14.1). Portal vein thrombosis is an example of prehepatic portal hypertension where the size of the liver may not necessarily be affected. Right heart failure can cause backpressure on the hepatic veins and result in an engorged, pulsatile liver and is an example of a posthepatic cause. A rare posthepatic cause is Budd–Chiari syndrome which results from obstruction of the hepatic veins.

Table C3.14.1   Causes of Portal Hypertension

PREHEPATIC	HEPATIC	POSTHEPATIC
Portal vein thrombosis (causes include malignancy, chronic pancreatitis, hepatitis, hypercoagulable states)	Cirrhosis (causes include alcoholic, non-alcoholic fatty liver disease, hepatitis, primary biliary cirrhosis, primary sclerosing cholangitis, haemochromatosis)	Congestive heart failure
Extrinsic compression of the portal vein (e.g. from lymph nodes or pancreatic mass)	Hepatic fibrosis (congenital, myelofibrosis, Wilson disease) Infection (malaria, schistosomiasis)	Budd–Chiari syndrome

❶ KEY POINTS

1. The causes of portal hypertension can be divided into prehepatic, hepatic and posthepatic causes. Hepatic causes in the form of cirrhosis are the most common.

2. The clinical signs of portal hypertension depend on the underlying aetiology but include splenomegaly, ascites and evidence of porto-systemic collaterals, e.g. caput medusa around the umbilicus and oesophageal/splenic varices. Many of these signs can be confirmed with ultrasound. As alcoholic cirrhosis is the most common cause, clinical signs of chronic liver disease, such as flapping tremor, spider naevi and jaundice may also be evident.

---

5. Which of the following are true regarding treatment of splenic artery aneurysms?
The correct answers are **A) Symptomatic patients should be treated, B) Asymptomatic pregnant women or women of childbearing age should be treated, C) Asymptomatic aneurysms <2 cm may be managed with surveillance and E) Splenectomy may be required**.

A) Symptomatic patients should be treated – Correct. Uncomplicated splenic artery aneurysms do not usually present with symptoms. Any patient with symptoms or evidence of rupture requires treatment.

B) Asymptomatic pregnant women or women of childbearing age should be treated – Correct. Pregnancy is a risk factor for growth of splenic artery aneurysms. Ideally, they should be treated in women of childbearing age before they attempt to have a family.

C) Asymptomatic aneurysms <2 cm may be managed with surveillance – Correct. The risk of rupture of splenic artery aneurysms less than 2 cm in dimension is small. The risks of treatment need to be considered. Such aneurysms may be managed with surveillance, usually with CT.

D) Endovascular embolisation is not a treatment option as it causes splenic infarction – Incorrect. Interventional radiology has an established role in the management of splenic artery aneurysms with embolisation. Embolisation of the splenic artery does not result in splenic infarction because the spleen receives collateral arterial supply from the short gastric arteries. It is important to realise that both the arteries distal and proximal to the aneurysm need to be embolised. If the distal artery is not occluded, blood can still flow into the artery from the splenic collaterals (i.e. both the 'front and back doors' need to be closed!).

E) Splenectomy may be required – Correct. Surgical resection of the aneurysm and ligation of the splenic artery is an alternative management option. The spleen remains viable in such circumstances due to the short gastric collaterals. However, this technique may not be feasible in splenic artery aneurysms involving the distal third of the splenic artery, and splenectomy may be required.

IMPORTANT LEARNING POINTS

- Splenic artery aneurysms are the third most common abdominal aneurysm and the most common visceral artery aneurysm in the abdomen.
- True aneurysms should be distinguished from pseudoanuerysms. The latter have a high rupture rate and require urgent treatment.
- Treatment of true aneurysms can be endovascular or surgical and depends on the size of the aneurysm and patient factors.

CASE 3.15

A 67-year-old man presented to A&E with nausea and bloating. He has not opened his bowels for 5 days. He has no pain and is haemodynamically stable. You are concerned he may have developed a bowel obstruction and request an abdominal X-ray.

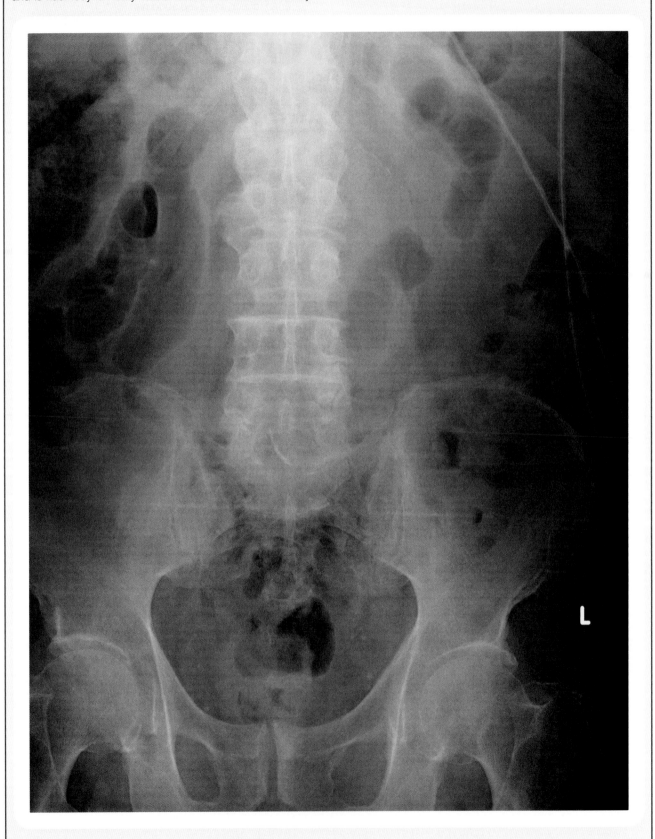

ANNOTATED X-RAY

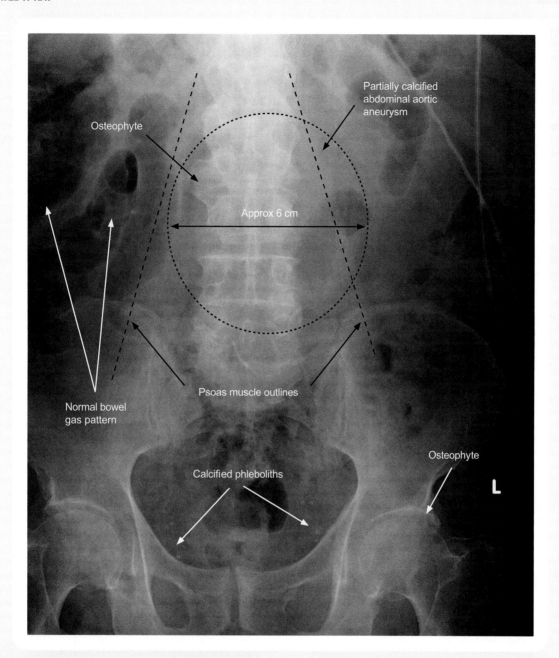

Osteophyte

Partially calcified
abdominal aortic
aneurysm

Approx 6 cm

Normal bowel
gas pattern

Psoas muscle outlines

Osteophyte

Calcified phleboliths

L

🔍 PRESENT YOUR FINDINGS

- This is a supine AP radiograph of the abdomen.
- It has been anonymised and the timing of the examination is not available. I would like to confirm this is the correct patient, as well as checking the time and date the X-ray was performed.
- The hemidiaphragms and the right flank have not been fully imaged. It is therefore a technically inadequate X-ray.
- There is a subtle rounded and partially calcified structure projected over the lumbar spine which measures approximately 6 cm in lateral diameter.
- Given its position and appearance, it is most in keeping with a partially calcified abdominal aortic aneurysm.

- The outlines of both psoas major muscles are visible, suggesting there is no large retroperitoneal collection/ haematoma.
- The bowel gas pattern is normal, with no plain film evidence of bowel obstruction, perforation or mucosal oedema.
- There are multiple rounded densities projected over the pelvis in keeping with calcified phleboliths.
- There is no obvious abnormality of the visible solid abdominal organs.
- There are degenerative changes in the lumbar spine and hip joints. However, no significant abnormality of the imaged skeleton is identified.

Continue

CASE **3.15**   *Contd.*

IN SUMMARY – This abdominal X-ray shows a partially calcified AAA. I would review the patient urgently for clinical signs of a leaking aneurysm. I would assess any previous imaging to determine whether this is a new finding, and determine whether further imaging is necessary.

QUESTIONS

1. What is the most common underlying cause of an AAA?
   A) Infection (mycotic)
   B) Trauma
   C) Atherosclerosis
   D) Connective tissue diseases
   E) Vasculitis

2. Which of the following is/are clinical findings/complications associated with an AAA?
   A) Lower limb ischaemia
   B) Hydronephrosis
   C) Transient ischaemic attack/cerebrovascular accident
   D) Syncope and shock
   E) Retroperitoneal fibrosis

3. An AAA is usually defined as the AP diameter of the abdominal aorta exceeding what?
   A) 10 mm
   B) 20 mm
   C) 25 mm
   D) 30 mm
   E) 40 mm

4. Which of the following is the most appropriate management for a patient with an asymptomatic 4-cm AAA?
   A) Ultrasound follow-up
   B) CT follow-up
   C) Angiography follow-up
   D) Urgent open repair
   E) EVAR

5. Which of the following is the most appropriate imaging in a case of possible rupture of an AAA?
   A) Abdominal X-ray
   B) Urgent MRI aortic angiogram
   C) Urgent angiography
   D) Urgent ultrasound
   E) Urgent CT

ANSWERS TO QUESTIONS

1. **What is the most common underlying cause of an AAA?**
The correct answer is **C) Atherosclerosis**.
Aneurysms can be categorised according to their aetiology, site and morphology. Around 90% of aortic aneurysms will be confined to the infrarenal segment of the abdominal aorta. Aneurysms can be fusiform or saccular in shape. True aneurysms involve all three layers of the arterial wall, whereas a false or pseudoaneurysm does not involve all the layers of the arterial wall. False aneurysms are usually the result of trauma (including iatrogenic), which allows blood to leak from the arterial lumen, through the wall, with the haematoma being contained by the adventitia or adjacent perivascular soft tissues.

   A) Infection (mycotic) – Incorrect. Infection, usually by *Staphylococcus* or *Salmonella*, is an uncommon cause of abdominal aortic aneurysm. Mycotic aneurysms are usually false aneurysms and tend to be saccular in shape. They are more common in immunosuppressed patients, intravenous drug users and patients with bacterial endocarditis.

   B) Trauma – Incorrect. Trauma is a major risk factor for developing a pseudo or false aneurysm. The common femoral artery is the most common site for pseudoaneurysms due to instrumentation (access for interventional radiology/cardiology procedures, arterial lines and accidental puncture by intravenous drug users). The abdominal aorta is much less frequently involved.

   C) Atherosclerosis – Correct. Atherosclerosis is by far the commonest cause of abdominal aortic aneurysms. Such aneurysms tend to be fusiform in shape.

   D) Connective tissue diseases – Incorrect. Connective tissue disorders, such as Marfan and Ehlers–Danlos Syndrome are rare causes of aneurysms.

   E) Vasculitis – Incorrect. Inflammatory conditions, such as Takayasu's arteritis and giant cell aortitis, are rare causes of abdominal aortic aneurysms.

❗ KEY POINT

There are a variety of causes of AAA, but atherosclerosis is by far the commonest. Consequently AAAs tend to occur more commonly with increasing age, male sex, hypertension, smoking and other risk factors for atherosclerosis.

2. **Which of the following is/are clinical findings/complications associated with an AAA?**
The correct answers are **A) Lower limb ischaemia, B) Hydronephrosis, D) Syncope and shock and E) Retroperitoneal fibrosis**.
Abdominal aortic aneurysms can produce a variety of symptoms and complications. Most patients are asymptomatic, with the AAA detected incidentally on clinical examination or imaging. AAAs are however often difficult to detect clinically and a normal clinical examination does not exclude it. An AAA can cause pain in the back, central abdomen or flanks.

   A) Lower limb ischaemia – Correct. Thrombus within the aneurysm can lead to distal embolisation and acute lower limb ischaemia. Popliteal artery aneurysms also frequently cause distal embolisation with acute ischaemia of the foot.

   B) Hydronephrosis – Correct. Inflammatory AAAs can cause retroperitoneal fibrosis, with resultant extrinsic compression of one or both ureters, resulting in hydronephrosis.

   C) Transient ischaemic attack/cerebrovascular accident – Incorrect. Whilst AAAs are associated with distal embolisation, they occur distal to the origins of the vessels supplying the brain (carotid and vertebral arteries). Therefore, they do not cause transient ischaemic attacks or strokes. However, remember that aneurysms and dissection of the ascending aorta and aortic arch may result in cerebrovascular accidents and transient ischaemic attacks.

   D) Syncope and shock – Correct. Fifty percent of patients with AAA initially present with rupture of the aneurysm. This usually results in collapse and shock. The degree of blood loss is determined in part by the location of the rupture (the retroperitoneal space can tamponade the leak, as opposed to free uncontained intraperitoneal haemmorhage). Ruptured AAAs are associated with high mortality.

   E) Retroperitoneal fibrosis – Correct. Inflammatory AAA can cause retroperitoneal fibrosis.

❗ KEY POINT

AAAs can present in a variety of ways. However, the most common presentations are as an incidental finding or rupture of the aneurysm.

3. **An AAA is usually defined as the AP diameter of the abdominal aorta exceeding what size?**
The correct answer is **D) 30 mm**.
An aneurysm is defined as an abnormal focal and permanent dilatation of an artery by at least 50% of the expected normal diameter. The upper limit of normal for the AP diameter of the abdominal aorta is 20 mm. Therefore an AAA is usually diagnosed once the AP diameter exceeds 30 mm.

4. **Which of the following is the most appropriate management for a patient with an asymptomatic 5.1-cm AAA?**
The correct answer is **A) Ultrasound follow-up**.
One of the main factors that influence the management is the risk of aneurysm rupture versus the risk of treatment. Trials have shown that in patients with asymptomatic AAA less than 5.5 cm in diameter, the risks of surgery outweigh the risks of rupture. It is important to remember, however, that all patients with symptomatic AAAs, regardless of size, should be considered for repair. This is because pain from an aneurysm often precedes a rupture and distal embolisation can result in limb loss.

   A) Ultrasound follow-up – Correct. Ultrasound provides an accurate, reproducible assessment of aneurysm size. It is noninvasive, cheap, readily available and does not involve ionising radiation. Asymptomatic patients with AAA less than 5.5 cm usually undergo

Continue

annual follow-up of their aneurysm with ultrasound. If the aneurysm enlarges to greater than 5.5 cm or they develop symptoms, the patient should be considered for repair.

B) CT follow-up – Incorrect. CT angiography provides an accurate and reliable assessment of the aneurysm size. However, it uses ionising radiation and intravenous contrast material, which make it less suitable than ultrasound for routine follow-up. CT is often used in preoperative planning and in the assessment of potentially ruptured AAAs.

C) Angiography follow-up – Incorrect. Angiography is an invasive technique that uses ionising radiation and contrast material. It is not as reliable as CT or ultrasound for assessing the size of an aneurysm. However, it permits accurate assessment of the mesenteric, renal and pelvic arteries and is occasionally used in preoperative planning.

D) Urgent open repair – Incorrect. The risk of morbidity and mortality from an open repair outweighs the risk of rupture in an asymptomatic patient with an aneurysm of this size. Therefore, emergency or elective surgery is not required in this case.

E) EVAR – Incorrect. EVAR is a less invasive technique for treating AAAs. The shape of the aneurysm and aorta and location of arterial branches (e.g. renal arteries) determine whether a patient would be suitable for EVAR. However in this case, as mentioned earlier, the risks of treatment outweigh the risks of aneurysm rupture.

❗ KEY POINT

Treatment is determined by the size of the AAA, whether the patient is symptomatic and the presence of other comorbidities (although the exact thresholds depend on local guidelines).

- Asymptomatic AAAs <5.5 cm in diameter are usually kept under ultrasound surveillance and managed conservatively (smoking cessation and modification of other risk factors such as hypertension).
- Asymptomatic AAAs which are <5.5 cm in size but have increased by >1 cm in a year, those >5.5 cm and all sympomatic AAAs (regardless of size) should be considered for repair (open or endovascular).

5. Which of the following is the most appropriate imaging in a case of possible rupture of an AAA?
The correct answer is **E) Urgent CT**.
Ruptured or leaking AAAs are a surgical emergency with high mortality. Rapid accurate assessment and early intervention help to improve the prognosis. Urgent imaging has an important role to play in confirming the diagnosis and excluding differential diagnoses.

A) Abdominal X-ray – Incorrect. Partially calcified AAAs can be visible on abdominal X-rays (as in this case). However, many AAAs (approximately 50%) are not visible on plain X-ray. Furthermore, abdominal X-rays cannot reliably demonstrate rupture or leak of an AAA (loss of the lateral psoas margin can occur with large retroperitoneal collections, such as from a ruptured AAA; however, this sign is neither sensitive nor specific for ruptured AAA).

B) Urgent MRI aortic angiogram – Incorrect. MRI can accurately assess AAAs without the need for iodinated contrast or ionising radiation. Additionally, MRI can diagnose intramural haematoma and dissection. However, compared with CT, MRI takes longer to perform, is not as reliable for identifying other causes of abdominal pain and is more sensitive to movement artefact. These factors, along with the requirement of all equipment to be MR compatible, make emergency assessment of potentially ruptured AAA impractical.

C) Urgent angiography – Incorrect. Angiography is an invasive procedure that can demonstrate the presence of an aneurysm and active extravasation. However, if there is no active haemorrhage (due to the formation of a clot or tamponade), then angiography may not allow the diagnosis of a ruptured aneurysm to be made. Additionally, angiography has limited ability in excluding other differential diagnoses.

D) Urgent ultrasound – Incorrect. Ultrasound can provide a rapid assessment of the abdominal aorta. Additionally, free fluid/haemorrhage from aneurysm rupture may be identified. However, ultrasound cannot exclude the diagnosis of a ruptured AAA, particularly if performed in suboptimal conditions (e.g. a portable ultrasound in A&E). Furthermore, body habitus and overlying bowel gas can make assessment of the entire aorta difficult or impossible.

E) Urgent CT – Correct. Urgent CT is the imaging modality of choice. It is quick, readily available and provides an accurate assessment of the aorta, allowing the diagnosis of rupture to be made. Additionally, it can identify features that are associated with an impending rupture. Initially, a noncontrast CT is performed. This may demonstrate an AAA and the presence of an intramural haematoma or surrounding haemorrhage within the retroperitoneum. Arterial phase CT can provide additional information, such as assessing for active haemorrhage, demonstrating the size of the aortic lumen and highlighting the relationship of the aneurysm to the aortic branches. Additionally, it can demonstrate the presence of an aortic dissection. A portal venous phase scan may be performed to exclude other differential diagnoses, such as diverticulitis, appendicitis or bowel obstruction.

👥 IMPORTANT LEARNING POINTS

- An AAA is defined as a focal dilatation of the abdominal aorta which measures >3 cm in AP diameter.
- The commonest cause of AAA is atherosclerosis. Consequently, AAAs occur more frequently in elderly men with other risk factors for atherosclerotic disease.
- AAAs can cause a variety of symptoms but are usually either identified incidentally or when they rupture.
- Management depends on the size of the aneurysm, the presence of symptoms and the patient's other comorbidities.
- Ruptured AAAs are associated with high mortality. CT is the imaging investigation of choice, and open surgery or endovascular repair are the treatment options.

CASE 3.16

A 73-year-old man with known metastatic prostate cancer has presented to A&E with abdominal pain, nausea and vomiting. He has not opened his bowels for 4 days. An abdominal X-ray is requested to exclude bowel obstruction.

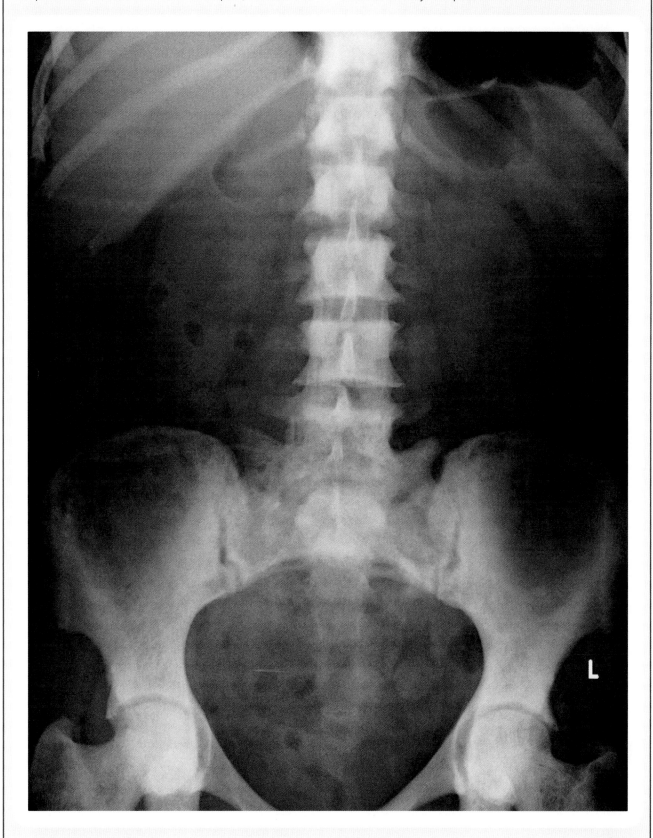

Continue

CASE 3.16 *Contd.*

ANNOTATED X-RAY

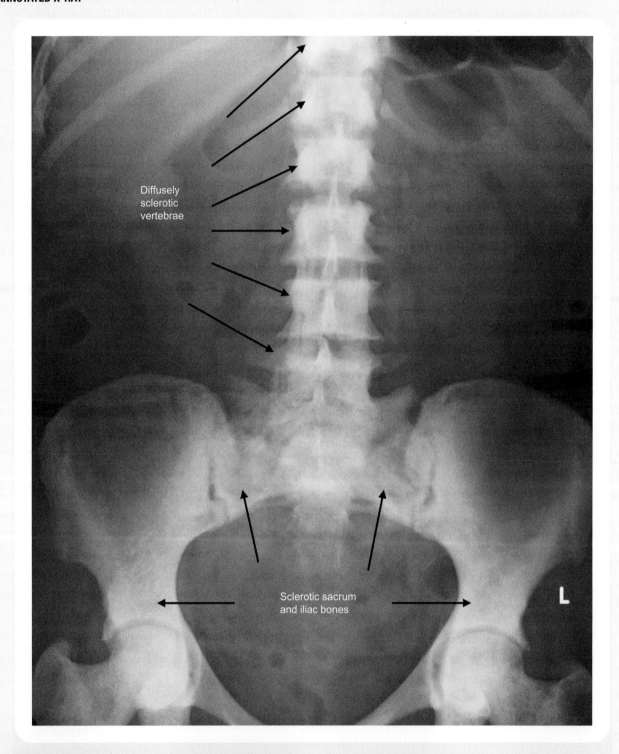

Diffusely
sclerotic
vertebrae

Sclerotic sacrum
and iliac bones

L

🔍 **PRESENT YOUR FINDINGS**

- This is a supine AP radiograph of the abdomen.
- It has been anonymised and the timing of the examination is not available. I would like to confirm this relates to the correct patient and check the time and date it was performed.
- The hemidiaphragms and hernia orifices have not been fully included in the film. Consequently, it is a technically inadequate X-ray.

- The bowel gas pattern is normal with no plain film evidence of bowel obstruction, perforation or mucosal oedema.
- There is no obvious abnormality of the visible abdominal organs.
- The imaged skeleton is diffusely sclerotic. Given the past medical history, these changes are most likely due to diffuse sclerotic bone metastases from prostate cancer.

IN SUMMARY – This abdominal X-ray shows a normal bowel gas pattern but diffuse sclerotic bone metastases are noted, in keeping with the known history of metastatic prostate cancer.

QUESTIONS

1. Which of the following clinical findings is/are associated with bone metastases?
   A) Bone pain
   B) Fractures
   C) Spinal cord compression
   D) Constipation
   E) All of the above
2. Which of the following is the commonest cause of sclerotic bone metastases?
   A) Thyroid cancer
   B) Breast cancer
   C) Lung cancer
   D) Renal cell carcinoma
   E) Transitional cell carcinoma
3. Which of the following is most commonly used to identify bony metastatic disease when staging prostate cancer?
   A) CT chest, abdomen and pelvis
   B) Skeletal survey

C) Bone scan
D) Whole body MRI
E) PET/CT

4. What is the most useful investigation for a patient with bony metastatic disease who is suspected to have developed spinal cord compression?
   A) X-rays of the spine
   B) CT whole spine
   C) MRI whole spine
   D) Bone scan
   E) No imaging is required as spinal cord compression is a clinical diagnosis
5. What is the most appropriate initial management of a patient diagnosed with spinal cord compression secondary to bony metastatic disease?
   A) Analgesia, dexamethasone and consideration of urgent radiotherapy
   B) Analgesia and outpatient radiotherapy
   C) Urgent chemotherapy
   D) Urgent surgery
   E) Analgesia and physiotherapy

Continue

CASE 3.16 *Contd.*

ANSWERS TO QUESTIONS

1. Which of the following clinical findings is/are associated with bone metastases?
   The correct answer is **E) All of the above**.
   Bone metastases can cause a variety of symptoms and clinical findings, either through direct effects on bone or via secondary metabolic effects.
   A) Bone pain – Incorrect. Bone metastases affect the local extracellular matrix of the bone and one of the consequences of this is chronic pain.
   B) Fractures – Incorrect. Bone metastases weaken the structural integrity of the bone and as a result are a frequent cause of pathological fractures.
   C) Spinal cord compression – Incorrect. Spinal cord compression can result from expansile bone metastases or pathological fractures of the vertebral column. Spinal cord compression can cause significant morbidity and urgent diagnosis and management is required.
   D) Constipation – Incorrect. Bone metastases are one of the commonest causes of hypercalcaemia, which can present in a variety of ways, including renal calculi, abdominal pain, nausea, vomiting, constipation, polyuria and depression.
   E) All of the above – Correct. Bone metastases can cause a variety of symptoms. They are also frequently asymptomatic, being diagnosed by staging investigations.

2. Which of the following is the commonest cause of sclerotic bone metastases?
   The correct answer is **B) Breast cancer**.
   Bony metastatic disease can be sclerotic, lytic or mixed.
   A) Thyroid cancer – Incorrect. Thyroid cancer typically causes lytic bone metastases. The metastases are often large and expansile.
   B) Breast cancer – Correct. The common causes of sclerotic bone metastases include prostate and breast cancer. Breast cancer can also cause lytic bone metastases. Rarer causes of sclerotic bone metastases include transitional cell carcinoma, Hodgkin lymphoma, carcinoid tumours and neuroblastoma.
   C) Lung cancer – Incorrect. Lung cancer typically causes lytic bone metastases.
   D) Renal cell carcinoma – Incorrect. Renal cell carcinoma typically causes lytic bone metastases. The metastases are often large and expansile.
   E) Transitional cell carcinoma – Incorrect. Transitional cell carcinoma can cause sclerotic bone metastases, but breast cancer is a much more common cause.

❶ KEY POINTS

1. Breast cancer is another common cause of sclerotic bone metastases, whilst carcinoid tumours and medulloblastoma are rarer causes. Other causes of diffusely dense bones include myelofibrosis, Paget disease and renal osteodystrophy.
2. It can be difficult to identify sclerotic bone metastases, particularly if they are diffuse, as in this case. Compare the appearance of the skeleton in this case with the other abdominal X-rays in the book and hopefully you'll be able to appreciate a subtle but definite difference.

3. Which of the following is most commonly used to identify bony metastatic disease when staging prostate cancer?
   The correct answer is **C) Bone Scan**.
   Like many other malignancies, prostate cancer is staged using the TNM system. T stands for tumour, N for nodes and M for metastases. Various imaging modalities are used when staging prostate cancer. For example, MRI of the pelvis is used to assess the local extent of prostate cancer and any regional nodes. Bony metastatic disease is usually assessed by bone scan.
   A) CT chest, abdomen and pelvis – Incorrect. CT is less accurate than MRI in the assessment of the prostate gland and any local malignant disease. CT is used for distant staging of prostate cancer, identifying distant lymph node involvement and metastatic disease. This includes detecting bony metastases. However, bone scans are a more sensitive imaging investigation for this.
   B) Skeletal survey – Incorrect. Skeletal surveys involve multiple X-rays of the skeleton. They are usually employed in the assessment of multiple myeloma (bone scans are poor at detecting myeloma). Plain X-rays are not a sensitive method for diagnosing bone metastases.
   C) Bone scan – Correct. Bone scanning is a type of nuclear medicine imaging commonly used in the staging of prostate cancer. It involves the intravenous injection of a radiopharmaceutical agent (Technetium 99 methylene diphosphate – a radionuclide attached to a bisphosphonate analogue). The bisphosphonate analogue component is adsorbed onto hydroxyapatite (a constituent of bone), concentrating in areas of increased osteoblastic activity. The radioactive component (technetium 99) is detected by the gamma and allows localisation. It is useful for detecting bone metastases, as well as osteomyelitis, occult fractures and other bone conditions, such as Paget disease. As this technique relies on osteoblastic activity, it is very good for detecting sclerotic bone metastases. However, bone metastases which are typically lytic, such as renal cell carcinoma, thyroid cancer and multiple myeloma, can be missed.
   D) Whole body MRI – Incorrect. MRI of the pelvis is used for assessing the local extent of prostate cancer. MRI also allows accurate assessment of the bone marrow and can identify bone metastases (the replacement of normal fatty bone marrow by tumour tissue can be detected). Although some specialist cancer centres perform whole body diffusion-weighted MRI for bone metastases, it is not currently routine clinical practice.
   E) PET/CT – Incorrect. Positron emission tomography (PET) uses a radionuclide attached to a glucose analogue to assess for areas of increased metabolism. It is used for assessing and staging certain tumours. It can help identify bony metastatic disease but may give a false positive result, requiring the need for further imaging modalities. It is not frequently used in staging prostate cancer.

4. Which is the most useful investigation for a patient with bony metastatic disease who is suspected to have developed spinal cord compression?

The correct answer is **C) MRI whole spine**.

Spinal cord compression from any cause is a medical emergency that requires accurate and timely assessment and management to reduce morbidity. Imaging plays a key role in the diagnosis.

A) X-rays of the spine – Incorrect. X-rays are an insensitive method for assessing bony metastatic disease (approximately 50% of the bone must be destroyed before a lesion will be visible on X-ray). Additionally, they only provide a limited assessment of the spinal canal and cannot exclude spinal cord compression. Therefore, X-rays are not indicated in suspected spinal cord compression.

B) CT whole spine – Incorrect. CT can identify bone metastases but is less sensitive than MRI. It permits assessment of the bony spinal canal but only limited information on the spinal cord and surrounding soft tissues can be obtained. CT myelography (CT scan is performed after the injection of contrast material into the subarachnoid space) can be used to identify spinal cord compression, but has been superseded by MRI. It is usually reserved for patients who cannot undergo MRI, such as those with certain types of pacemakers or intracranial aneurysm clips.

C) MRI whole spine – Correct. MRI is a sensitive and specific technique for assessing bone metastases. In addition, it allows the soft tissues of the spinal canal, such as the spinal cord and the surrounding cerebrospinal fluid and epidural fat, to be imaged in detail. MRI is therefore the imaging modality of choice to diagnose or exclude spinal cord compression.

D) Bone scan – Incorrect. Bone scans are often used to identify bony metastatic disease when staging malignancies. However, they provide no information on the spinal cord and therefore do not have a role in the imaging of potential spinal cord compression.

E) No imaging is required as spinal cord compression is a clinical diagnosis – Incorrect. Accurate clinical assessment is required to identify those patients who may potentially have spinal cord compression. However, imaging, in the form of MRI, is required to confirm or refute the diagnosis and guide treatment.

---

❶ KEY POINT

The spinal cord ends at roughly L1/2 in adults. Below this, it becomes the cauda equina, which is composed of nerve roots (L2–L5, S1–S5 and the coccygeal nerve). Compression of the spinal cord will cause upper motor neurone signs (increased tone, hyperreflexia and upgoing plantars (known as a positive Babinski sign), as well as weakness and sensory loss), whereas compression of the cauda equina will result in lower motor neurone signs (hypotonia, hyporeflexia and downgoing plantars, as well as weakness and sensory loss). Additionally, bowel, bladder and sexual dysfunction occur earlier in cauda equina compression compared to spinal cord compression.

5. What is the most appropriate initial management of a patient diagnosed with spinal cord compression secondary to bony metastatic disease?

The correct answer is **A) Analgesia, dexamethasone and consideration of urgent radiotherapy**.

Malignant spinal cord compression is a medical emergency that requires timely assessment and management to reduce its morbidity.

A) Analgesia, dexamethasone and consideration of urgent radiotherapy – Correct. The initial management in patients with suspected malignant spinal cord compression includes appropriate analgesia and high-dose dexamethasone (if there is no contraindication). Dexamethasone may help preserve neurological function in the acute setting. Radiotherapy can help shrink the culprit malignant lesion, helping to restore neurological function and reduce pain.

B) Analgesia and outpatient radiotherapy – Incorrect. Whilst analgesia and radiotherapy play key roles in the management, malignant spinal cord compression is a medical emergency and the management needs to be instigated urgently as an inpatient to try to preserve neurological function.

C) Urgent chemotherapy – Incorrect. Chemotherapy does not commonly play a role in the management of malignant spinal cord compression.

D) Urgent surgery – Incorrect. Urgent surgery may be required if there is spinal instability. However, it is not commonly required in the initial management of malignant spinal cord compression. It may be required in cord compression related to degenerative disc disease.

E) Analgesia and physiotherapy – Incorrect. Analgesia and physiotherapy is useful in the management of patients with noncompressive intervertebral disc herniations. However, it is not appropriate initial management in malignant spinal cord compression.

👥 IMPORTANT LEARNING POINTS

- Bony metastatic disease can be sclerotic, lytic or mixed.
- Causes of diffusely sclerotic bones include metastases (prostate and breast), Paget disease, myelofibrosis and renal osteodystrophy.
- X-rays have limited sensitivity for detecting bone metastases – MRI and nuclear medicine bone scans are much better.
- MRI has an important role in the assessment of patients with potential spinal cord or cauda equina compression because it allows accurate assessment of these and other related structures within the spinal canal.
- Spinal cord and cauda equina compression are medical emergencies and urgent treatment is required to prevent loss of function. The initial management of malignant compression includes analgesia, dexamethasone and consideration for urgent radiotherapy.

A 34-year-old man has presented with acute colicky abdominal pain, nausea and vomiting. He has not moved his bowel for 3 days. As part of his investigations he undergoes an abdominal X-ray to exclude obstruction.

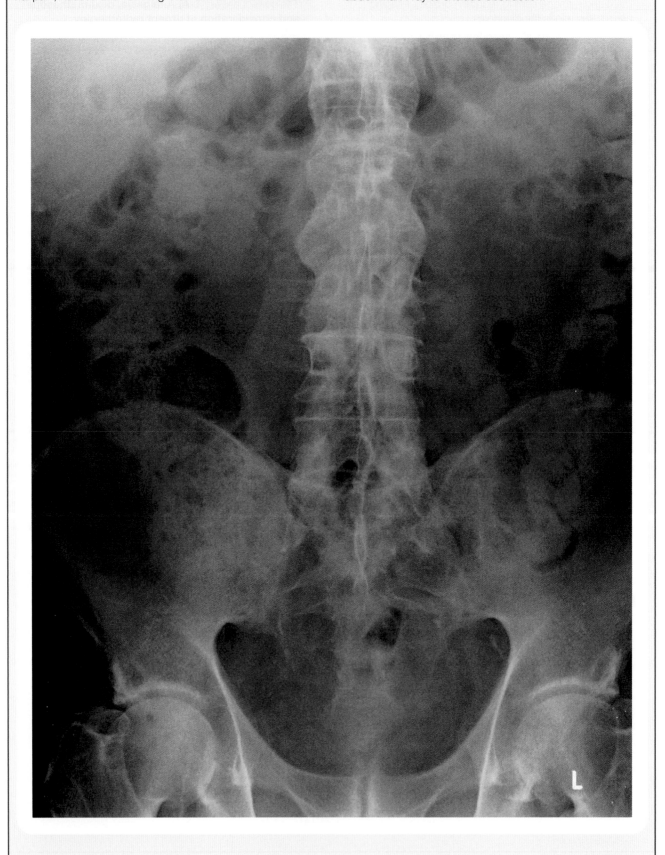

ANNOTATED X-RAY

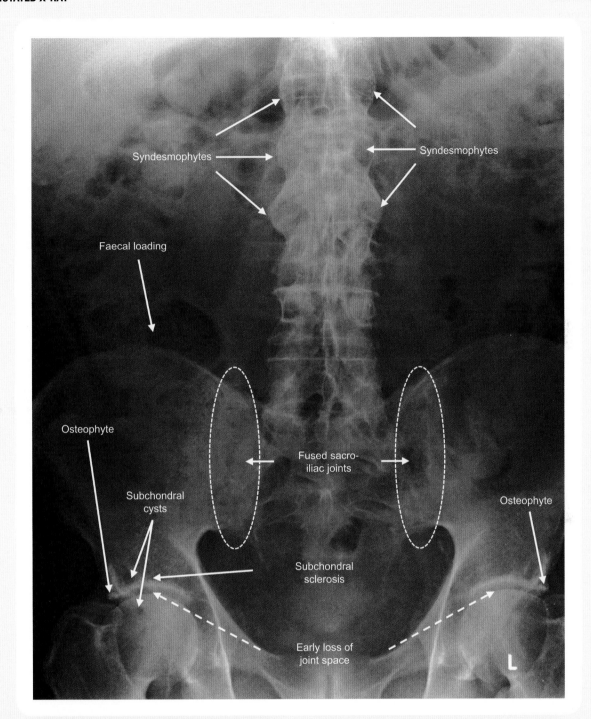

Syndesmophytes

Syndesmophytes

Faecal loading

Osteophyte

Subchondral cysts

Fused sacro-iliac joints

Osteophyte

Subchondral sclerosis

Early loss of joint space

L

🔍 PRESENT YOUR FINDINGS

- This is a supine AP X-ray of the abdomen.
- It has been anonymised and the timing of the examination is not available. I would like to ensure this is the correct patient and check the time and date the examination was performed.
- The hernial orifices, hemidiaphragms and left flank have not been included in the film. It is therefore a technically inadequate X-ray.
- Faeces are noted within the colon; the gas pattern is otherwise normal, with no plain film evidence of bowel obstruction, perforation or mucosal oedema.

- There is no obvious abnormality of the visible abdominal organs.
- Both SI joints are fused. There is fusion of the upper lumbar spine, with contiguous syndesmophytes. The hip joints show loss of joint space, subchondral sclerosis, subchondral cysts and osteophyte formation, in keeping with degenerative change.

IN SUMMARY – This abdominal X-ray shows typical features of ankylosing spondylitis. Faeces are noted within the colon but there is no evidence of obstruction, perforation or mucosal oedema.

Continue

CASE 3.17   *Contd.*

QUESTIONS

1. Which of the following is/are commonly associated with ankylosing spondylitis?
   A) Back pain
   B) Stiffness
   C) Male preponderance
   D) Typically presents in middle age (50–60s)
   E) Strongly associated with HLA-B27

2. Which of the following X-ray signs is/are associated with ankylosing spondylitis?
   A) Rugger jersey spine
   B) Ivory vertebral body
   C) Bamboo spine
   D) Squaring of the anterior vertebral margins
   E) Bone-in-bone appearance

3. Which extraspinal joint is most frequently involved in ankylosing spondylitis?
   A) Shoulders
   B) Hips
   C) Knees
   D) Elbows
   E) Ankles

4. Which of the following extraskeletal manifestations is least commonly associated with ankylosing spondylitis?
   A) Ulcerative colitis
   B) Iritis
   C) Aortitis
   D) Pulmonary fibrosis
   E) Hepatic fibrosis

5. Which of the following is/are used in the treatment of ankylosing spondylitis?
   A) Analgesia
   B) Physiotherapy
   C) Hip replacements
   D) Infliximab
   E) Radiotherapy

ANSWERS TO QUESTIONS

1. Which of the following is/are commonly associated with ankylosing spondylitis?

   The correct answers are **A) Back pain, B) Stiffness, C) Male preponderance and E) Strongly associated with HLA-B27**.

   Ankylosing spondylitis is a generalised chronic inflammatory disease (seronegative spondyloarthropathy) which predominantly affects the spine and SI joints.

   A) Back pain – Correct. The classic symptoms of ankylosing spondylitis are persistent back pain and stiffness. These are usually worse after inactivity and first thing in the morning.

   B) Stiffness – Correct. See A.

   C) Male preponderance – Correct. Males are more frequently affected (4:1 to 10:1 male:female). Ankylosing spondylitis is more common in White northern Europeans.

   D) Typically presents in middle age (50–60s) – Incorrect. Ankylosing spondylitis usually presents in young males, between the ages of 15 and 25 years. New-onset back pain in patients over the age of 50 is a red flag and should raise the suspicious of sinister underlying pathology, such as malignancy or infection.

   E) Strongly associated with HLA-B27 – Correct. Ankylosing spondylitis often runs in families and there is a very strong association with HLA-B27 (95%).

❗ KEY POINTS

1. The wall test is a useful clinical test for ankylosing spondylitis – A patient should be able to stand with their back against the wall and their heels, buttocks, scapulae and occiput should all be in contact with the wall. Failure to perform this implies loss of extension of the spine, which is often the earliest sign in ankylosing spondylitis.

2. Mechanical back pain is common. Red flags are a set of symptoms and signs which indicate there may be serious underlying pathology, and urgent investigations are needed in these patients (Table C3.17.1).

Table C3.17.1 Red Flags in Back Pain

CLINICAL FINDINGS	POSSIBLE CAUSE
Urinary or faecal incontinence, saddle anaesthesia, lower limb motor or sensory deficit	Cauda equina compression
Weight loss or previous history of cancer	Malignancy
Significant trauma or chronic steroid use	Fracture
Fever, immunosuppression, IV drug user, urinary tract infection or recent back surgery	Infection

2. Which of the following X-ray signs is/are associated with ankylosing spondylitis?

   The correct answer is **C) Bamboo spine and D) Squaring of the anterior vertebral margins**.

The inflammatory processes seen in ankylosing spondylitis progress through various stages. Initially, there is inflammation with granulation tissue formation, erosions and fibrous tissue deposition. Later, the fibrous tissue ossifies and ankylosis occurs. This progression can be seen radiologically at the sacroiliac joints – early in the disease, there may be fuzziness of the SI joints with bone erosions due to inflammation, while later there is sclerosis and eventually ankylosis and fusion.

A) Rugger jersey spine – Incorrect. A Rugger jersey spine is a classic finding in renal osteodystrophy. It is a result of secondary hyperparathyroidism in renal failure and causes dense, sclerotic vertebral body endplates in the thoracolumbar spine. This leads to a dense lucent pattern of consecutive vertebral bodies, giving the appearance of a striped rugby jersey.

B) Ivory vertebral body – Incorrect. An ivory vertebra is one which has diffuse dense and homogenous increased opacity/sclerosis, with the normal size and contours of the vertebral body being preserved. Bone metastases (prostate and breast cancer), lymphoma and Paget disease are causes, but not ankylosing spondylitis.

C) Bamboo spine – Correct. Ossification of the outer fibres of the intervertebral discs produce syndesmophytes (bony bridges). On AP views of the spine, such as an abdominal X-ray, continuous syndesmophytes give the appearance of a stick of bamboo.

D) Squaring of the anterior vertebral margins – Correct. Osteitis of the anterior corners of vertebral bodies can result in squaring of the vertebral bodies. This is one of the earlier signs of ankylosing spondylitis.

E) Bone-in-bone appearance – Incorrect. Bone-in-bone appearance (a descriptive term describing bones that on X-ray look like they have another bone within them) is classically seen with osteopetrosis, a rare inherited disorder in which the bones become denser and harder. Paradoxically, it can lead to increased fracture risk as the bones are more brittle. As the bone expands, there is contraction of the bone marrow, which can result in anaemia.

❗ KEY POINTS

1. The difference between syndesmophytes seen in ankylosing spondylitis and osteophytes associated with degenerative change is not necessarily obvious at first. Syndesmophytes are the result of calcification of the outer portion of the intervertebral discs (annulus fibrosis), whereas osteophytes are extensions of the vertebral endplates. As a result, syndesmophytes run vertically from one vertebral body to the next, whereas osteophytes have a more horizontal orientation.

2. Psoriatic arthritis and Reiter disease are other seronegative spondyloarthropathies which can affect the spine. These conditions typically produce bulky asymmetric syndesmophytes compared with the symmetrical nonbulky syndesmophytes seen in ankylosing spondylitis.

Continue

3. Which extra-spinal joint is most frequently involved in ankylosing spondylitis?
   The correct answer is **B) Hips**.
   The spine and SI joints are most commonly affected. Ankylosing spondylitis usually starts distally in the spine and SI joints, and progresses proximally through the spine. Arthritis of the proximal extra-spinal joints (hips and shoulders) occurs in approximately half of the patients.
   A) Shoulders – Incorrect. After hips, the shoulder joints are the second most frequently involved joints outside the spine and SI joint.
   B) Hips – Correct. The hip is the most commonly affected joint outside the spine and SI joints. Changes include joint space narrowing, osteophytes and erosions. Severe cases of ankylosing spondylitis may require hip replacements.
   C) Knees – Incorrect. The knees are not commonly affected.
   D) Elbows – Incorrect. The elbows are not commonly affected.
   E) Ankles – Incorrect. The ankles are not commonly affected.

❗ KEY POINT

If peripheral joints are involved, they may show a degenerative arthropathy, like osteoarthritis or an erosive arthritis, mimicking rheumatoid arthritis. The hips and shoulders are the most frequently affected peripheral joints.

4. Which of the following extraskeletal manifestations is least commonly associated with ankylosing spondylitis?
   The correct answer is **E) Hepatic fibrosis**.
   Ankylosing spondylitis is a multisystem disorder which can have extra-skeletal manifestations.
   A) Ulcerative colitis – Incorrect. The HLA-B27 haplotype, which is associated with ankylosing spondylitis, is also associated with inflammatory bowel disease, such as ulcerative colitis.
   B) Iritis – Incorrect. Iritis is found in 25% of patients with ankylosing spondylitis.
   C) Aortitis – Incorrect. Five percent of ankylosing spondylitis patients have aortitis, which can result in aortic valve insufficiency.
   D) Pulmonary fibrosis – Incorrect. Ankylosing spondylitis is a recognised cause of upper lobe pulmonary fibrosis.
   E) Hepatic fibrosis – Correct. Ankylosing spondylitis has been very rarely associated with hepatic fibrosis. The other conditions listed are far more common associations.

5. Which of the following is/are used in the treatment of ankylosing spondylitis?
   The correct answers are **A) Analgesia, B) Physiotherapy C) Hip replacements and D) Infliximab**.

There is no cure for ankylosing spondylitis; treatment is aimed at controlling symptoms and managing complications.
A) Analgesia – Correct. Back pain is one of the commonest symptoms of ankylosing spondylitis. NSAIDs, such as diclofenac, are commonly used to help reduce inflammation and ease pain. However NSAIDs have many potential side effects, including gastro-intestinal bleeding and renal impairment, which may restrict the choice and dose for a particular patient.
B) Physiotherapy – Correct. Physiotherapy is an important management option to maintain function and mobility, whilst reducing symptoms. Advice on postural control helps prevent the development of an exaggerated thoracic kyphosis.
C) Hip replacements – Correct. Patients who have involvement of the hip joints may benefit from bilateral hip replacements. Replacement of other involved joints may be indicated.
D) Infliximab – Correct. Second-line medications which can be used to treat ankylosing spondylitis include TNF-alpha antagonists, such as infliximab and adalimumab. Significant side effects of these medications include increased risk of bacterial and fungal infections and reactivation of latent tuberculosis.
E) Radiotherapy – Incorrect. Radiotherapy was widely used in the 1930s to 1950s in the treatment of ankylosing spondylitis, with very good effect on symptoms. However, radiotherapy is associated with a significant risk of cancer induction and this treatment is no longer used due to the risk of leukaemia, colorectal cancer and other malignancies.

❗ KEY POINT

Although associated with potentially significant morbidity, ankylosing spondylitis is a benign condition. Therefore, the risks of malignancy from radiotherapy outweigh the benefits of symptom improvement.

📖 IMPORTANT LEARNING POINTS

- Always assess the bony skeleton on an abdominal X-ray. Pathology may be the cause of the clinical findings, a complication of the underlying pathology or completely incidental.
- Ankylosing spondylitis typically presents in young males with back pain and stiffness.
- X-ray findings include fusion of the sacroiliac joints, spinal fusion and syndesmophytes.
- The hips and shoulder can also be affected.
- It is associated with a variety of other conditions, most notably inflammatory bowel disease.
- Treatment is symptomatic, with physiotherapy, analgesia and occasionally surgery.

CASE 3.18

A 7-year-old boy has been brought in by his parents after they saw him swallowing some small objects. An abdominal X-ray was performed.

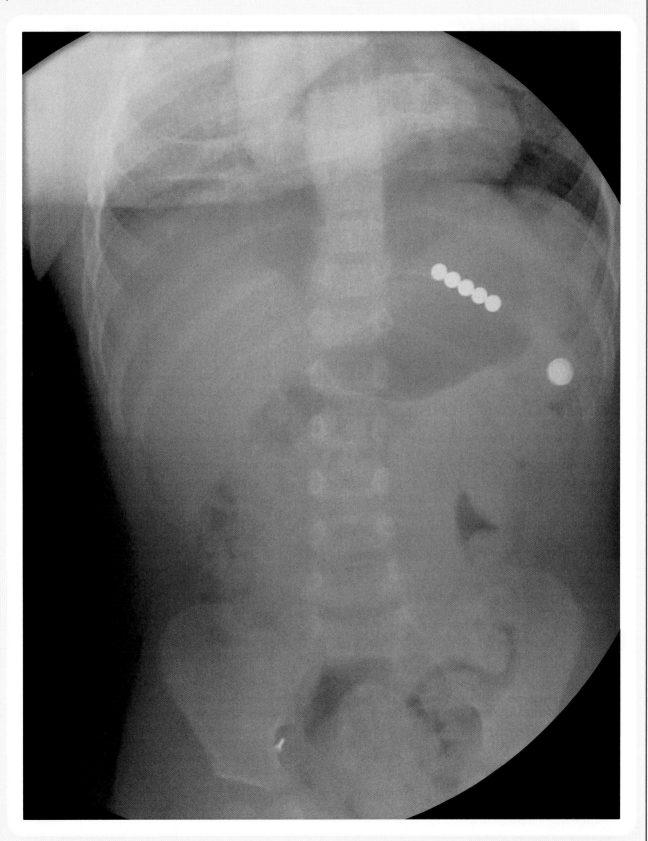

Continue

CASE **3.18**   *Contd.*

ANNOTATED X-RAY

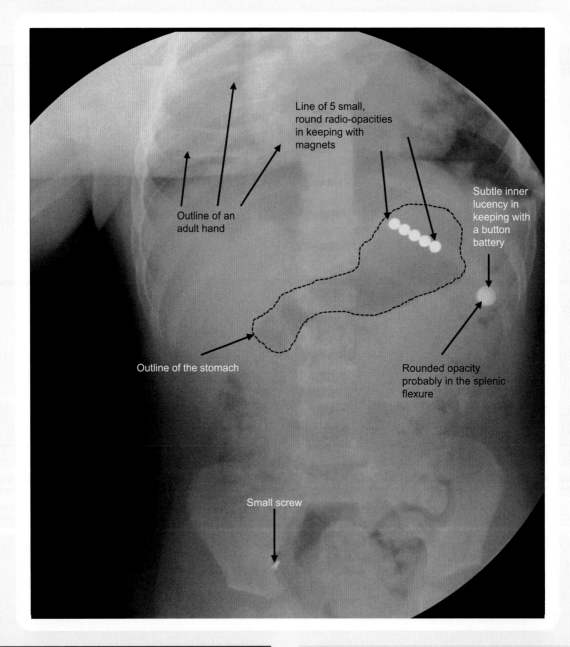

Line of 5 small, round radio-opacities in keeping with magnets

Subtle inner lucency in keeping with a button battery

Outline of an adult hand

Outline of the stomach

Rounded opacity probably in the splenic flexure

Small screw

🔍 **PRESENT YOUR FINDINGS**

- This is a supine AP abdominal X-ray of a young child.
- There are no patient identifiable data, nor a date or time marking. I would check this X-ray relates to the correct patient and the time it was performed.
- The hernial orifices have not been fully included on this image, but otherwise this is an adequate X-ray of the abdomen in this case.
- The most striking abnormalities are the radio-opaque foreign bodies projected over the abdomen. Within the left upper quadrant, there are five small circular radio-opaque foreign bodies in a line. Given their configuration they are most in keeping with magnets. It is difficult to be certain of locations on this single view but they are projected over the stomach.

- There is another larger round radio-opaque foreign body in the left upper quadrant which is out with the stomach. This is projected over the splenic flexure. Given its size and shape, this may represent a button battery or coin. Closer inspection shows it has an inner lucent rim. This is typical of a button battery.
- In the right lower quadrant, there is a further small radio-opaque foreign body which is in keeping with a small screw.
- Normal bowel gas pattern with no evidence of obstruction, perforation or mucosal oedema.
- There is no obvious abnormality of the visible solid abdominal organs.
- An adult hand can be seen projected over the thorax.
- The bones are within normal limits for age.

IN SUMMARY – This X-ray shows several radio-opaque foreign bodies in different parts of the abdomen. There appears to be a line of magnets within the stomach, a button battery probably in the splenic flexure and a small screw in the bowel in the right lower quadrant. Given the presence of both magnets and a battery I would refer this child urgently to the surgeons.

QUESTIONS

1. In which age group is ingested foreign bodies most common?
   A) 0 to 6 months
   B) 6 months to 5 years
   C) 5 to 10 years
   D) 10 to 14 years
   E) >14 years
2. What is the most common site for ingested foreign bodies to become trapped?
   A) Mouth
   B) Oropharynx (at the level of the cricopharyngeus)
   C) Lower oesophageal sphincter
   D) Gastric antrum/pylorus
   E) Ileocaecal valve
3. Which of the following is/are appropriate in the assessment of a child who has swallowed a foreign body?
   A) Assessment of vital signs
   B) Inspection of the mouth and oropharynx
   C) Chest examination
   D) Abdominal examination
   E) Rectal examination

4. Which of the following is the most appropriate management option for a button battery that is stuck in the midoesophagus?
   A) Conservative approach with serial X-rays to monitor its passage through the gastrointestinal tract
   B) Encourage the child to drink large quantities of water to flush it into the stomach
   C) Urgent endoscopy
   D) Urgent surgery
   E) Repeat X-ray in 2 to 3 days; if it has not passed through the oesophagus, then it should be removed endoscopically on the next elective list
5. Which of the following are recognised complications of ingested foreign bodies?
   A) Oesophageal perforation
   B) Tracheo-oesophageal fistula
   C) Bowel perforation
   D) Bowel obstruction
   E) Appendicitis

Continue

CASE **3.18** *Contd.*

ANSWERS TO QUESTIONS

1. In which age group is ingested foreign bodies most common?
   The correct answer is **B) 6 months to 5 years**.
   Children (and adults) of all ages can ingest foreign bodies.
   A) 0 to 6 months – Incorrect. Children of this age are not able to ingest foreign bodies themselves. However older children whilst playing may feed them small objects. Additionally, abusive parents or adults may intentionally feed young infants foreign bodies.
   B) 6 months to 5 years – Correct. Young children use their hands and mouth to explore and consequently are the most likely group to ingest foreign bodies.
   C) 5 to 10 years – Incorrect. Older children and adults can rarely ingest foreign bodies accidentally. This usually occurs with food-related foreign bodies, such as chicken or fish bones, or in the older population, parts of dentures may be ingested. Ingestion of foreign bodies can also be intentional in those with mental health issues and drug traffickers (a method of concealing illegal drugs within the gastrointestinal tract). Ingestion of hair can result in a ball of hair within the stomach, otherwise known as a trichobezoar.
   D) 10 to 14 years – Incorrect.
   E) >14 years – Incorrect.

> ❶ KEY POINT
>
> Ingested foreign bodies can occur in any age group, but is most common in children aged 6 months to 5 years of age.

2. What is the most common site for ingested foreign bodies to become trapped?
   The correct answer is **B) Oropharynx (at the level of the cricopharyngeus)**.
   Ingested foreign bodies can become stuck at various anatomical sites of narrowing in the gastrointestinal tract.
   A) Mouth – Incorrect. Foreign bodies are unlikely to be trapped in the mouth. However, toothpicks and fish bones can often be lodged in the oropharynx, between the posterior tongue to the cricopharyngeus.
   B) Oropharynx (at the level of the cricopharyngeus) – Correct. The level of the cricopharyngeus, at the thoracic inlet, is the location of the upper oesophageal sphincter, an anatomical and physiological site of narrowing, and the most common site for ingested foreign bodies to become stuck. Approximately 50% to 60% of foreign bodies become stuck at this level. The patient will often have a sensation of something stuck and may not be able to swallow. Large objects stuck at this level may compromise the airway.
   C) Lower oesophageal sphincter – Incorrect. The lower oesophageal sphincter is a physiological narrowing at the level of the gastro-oesophageal junction. Approximately 10% to 15% of ingested foreign bodies become stuck at this site. Another 15% of foreign bodies get stuck at the midoesophageal level, where there is extrinsic narrowing of the oesophagus by the aortic arch, trachea and carina.
   D) Gastric antrum/Pylorus – Incorrect. If a foreign body has passed through into the stomach it is much less likely to become stuck. The pylorus is able to distend, allowing most foreign bodies through, although a large object (>6 cm long or 2 cm wide) may become stuck at this site.
   E) Ileocaecal valve – Incorrect. Occasionally objects become stuck at the ileocaecal valve, although this is a much less frequent site than the oropharynx or oesophagus.

> ❶ KEY POINTS
>
> 1. Other sites of narrowing, such as a stricture within the oesophagus or bowel, can cause foreign bodies to be stuck.
> 2. Sharp objects, such as pins, can become lodged in the mucosa anywhere in the gastrointestinal tract, especially the oesophagus.

3. Which of the following is/are appropriate in the assessment of a child who has swallowed a foreign body?
   The correct answers are **A) Assessment of vital signs, B) Inspection of the mouth and oropharynx, C) Chest examination and D) Abdominal examination**.
   Patients may be asymptomatic after ingestion of a foreign body. Alternatively, there may be drooling due to an inability to swallow, gagging, vomiting or pain. Clinical assessment is often not useful for identifying the location of the foreign body. However, it has an important role in identifying any serious complications.
   A) Assessment of vital signs – Correct. Ingested foreign bodies can cause serious complications, such as airway obstruction or perforation of the gastrointestinal tract. In these cases, patients can be extremely unwell. Routine observations (oxygen saturations, pulse, blood pressure, respiratory rate) will help identify and monitor the condition of acutely unwell children.
   B) Inspection of the mouth and oropharynx – Correct. The oropharynx is the commonest site for foreign bodies to become lodged. Inspection of the mouth and oropharynx with a bright torch may demonstrate the culprit object, which can then be removed.
   C) Chest examination – Correct. Airway compromise can occur with an ingested foreign body. Additionally, a foreign body may be inhaled and result in lobar collapse or consolidation. Therefore, examination of the chest is important.
   D) Abdominal examination – Correct. Foreign bodies can result in obstruction or perforation of the bowel – particularly in cases of ingested button batteries and magnets. An abdominal examination is required to identify evidence of either of these two complications.
   E) Rectal examination – Incorrect. A rectal examination is unlikely to provide any useful information and is distressing for a child. It may be useful for parents to monitor the child's stools to confirm whether the swallowed foreign body has been passed. If a foreign body has been inserted into the rectum, then an examination under anaesthesia can be performed to remove the offending item.

❗ KEY POINT

The main aim of clinical assessment is to identify complications associated with ingestion of a foreign body. Imaging is used to help identify where the foreign body is within the body. Most ingested foreign bodies are radio-opaque (coins, magnets, screws, batteries). Therefore, X-rays can be used to identify its location. A single AP X-ray including the neck, chest and abdomen is often sufficient to locate the foreign body. If it has passed into the bowel, further views may be needed to determine its location. If it is not radio-opaque, CT may be able to locate the foreign body. CT is also useful for detecting complications such as perforation.

4. Which of the following is the most appropriate management option for a button battery that is stuck in the midoesophagus?
   The correct answer is **C) Urgent endoscopy**.
   The management of ingested foreign bodies depends on the type of foreign body, its location and whether any complications have occurred. Button batteries lodged in the oesophagus can cause necrosis of the oesophageal wall within as little as 2 hours, particularly if they contain lithium. This occurs as a result of a local current set up by the battery. If this process Continue, there is a risk of perforation in the acute setting or stricture formation later in life. Therefore, button batteries lodged in the oesophagus need to be removed urgently.
   A) Conservative approach with serial X-rays to monitor its passage through the gastrointestinal tract – Incorrect. A button battery impacted in the oesophagus is an emergency and must be removed urgently to prevent morbidity and potentially death. A conservative approach is therefore not appropriate.
   B) Encourage the child to drink large quantities of water to flush it into the stomach – Incorrect. The button battery will probably be adherent to the mucosal surface. It is unlikely to be flushed into the stomach by oral fluids. Additionally, if the battery is obstructing the oesophagus, there is a significant risk of aspiration if large quantities of oral fluids are consumed.
   C) Urgent endoscopy – Correct. Urgent endoscopy is the preferred option for visualising and removing the foreign body.
   D) Urgent surgery – Incorrect. Endoscopy is usually employed to retrieve foreign bodies in the oesophagus or stomach as it is associated with fewer risks. Surgery is considered if the foreign body becomes lodged more distally in the gastrointestinal tract, or if the oesophagus perforates.
   E) Repeat X-ray in 2 to 3 days; if it has not passed through the oesophagus, then it should be removed endoscopically on the next elective list – Incorrect. Any foreign body trapped in the oesophagus requires urgent removal, particularly button batteries.

❗ KEY POINT

Other types of impacted foreign bodies in the oesophagus can potentially cause significant morbidity and even mortality. Therefore, urgent removal of all foreign bodies trapped in the oesophagus should be considered.

5. Which of the following are recognised complications of ingested foreign bodies?
   The correct answers are **A) Oesophageal perforation, B) Tracheo-oesophageal fistula, C) Bowel perforation, D) Bowel obstruction and E) Appendicitis**.
   Ingested foreign bodies may be asymptomatic and pass through the gastrointestinal tract without causing any problems. However, there are several significant complications that can occur.
   A) Oesophageal perforation – Correct. Button batteries can cause perforation as a result of local current formation leading to necrosis of the oesophageal wall. Necrosis can start within 2 hours and perforation can occur as soon as 6 hours after ingestion. For this reason, they should be urgently removed by endoscopy.
   B) Tracheo-oesophageal fistula – Correct. As mentioned earlier – button batteries can erode through the oesophageal wall resulting in tracheo-oesophageal or aorto-oesophageal fistulas. The latter can result in rapid exsanguination.
   C) Bowel perforation – Correct. Sharp objects may perforate the bowel. Magnets can also lead to perforation – if magnets in different bowel loops join together or adhere to other magnetic foreign bodies, they can result in perforation and fistulation of the bowel. In these cases, an operation is required.
   D) Bowel obstruction – Correct. Acute intestinal obstruction can occur. Later, a stricture may develop at the site of mucosal inflammation caused by a foreign body, and lead to bowel obstruction.
   E) Appendicitis – Correct. There have been case reports of foreign bodies being lodged in the appendix, leading to appendicitis. Similarly, foreign bodies can become trapped in a Meckel's diverticulum.

🔖 IMPORTANT LEARNING POINTS

- Ingested foreign bodies can occur at any age but most frequently occur in children aged between 6 months and 5 years.
- The oropharynx is the most likely site an ingested foreign body will become stuck.
- Imaging, primarily with X-rays, is aimed at identifying the location of the foreign body within the gastrointestinal tract.
- Foreign bodies stuck in the oesophagus are usually removed; those that have passed through the pylorus of the stomach are usually treated conservatively – except in cases of ingested multiple magnets and batteries.
- Button batteries, sharp objects and magnets are the most frequent types of foreign bodies to result in complications.

CASE 3.19

A 1-day-old neonate presents with abdominal distension and bilious vomiting. There was an antenatal history of polyhydramnios (excess amniotic fluid in the amniotic sac). An abdominal X-ray is performed.

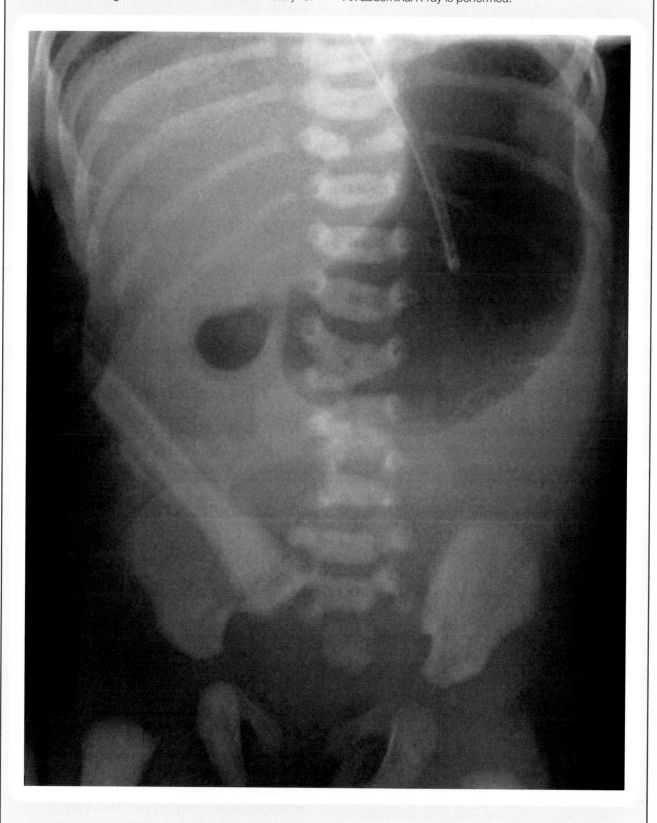

ANNOTATED X-RAY

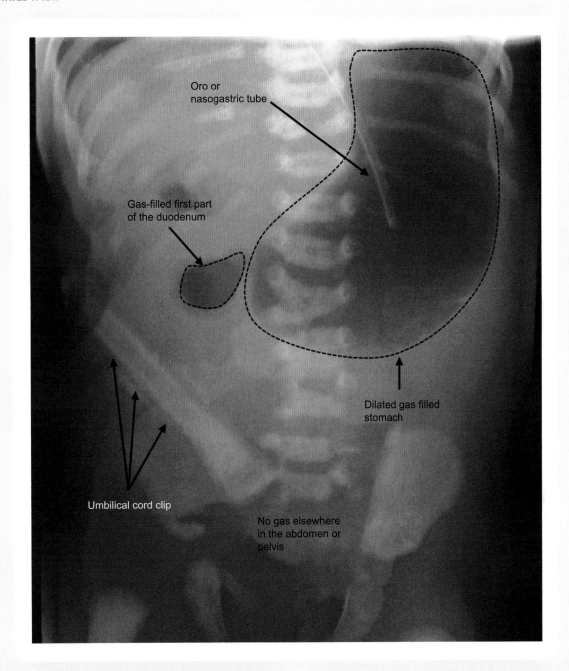

Oro or
nasogastric tube

Gas-filled first part
of the duodenum

Dilated gas filled
stomach

Umbilical cord clip

No gas elsewhere
in the abdomen or
pelvis

🔍 PRESENT YOUR FINDINGS

- This is a supine AP abdominal X-ray of a neonate.
- There are no patient identifiable data, nor a date or time marking. I would ensure this X-ray relates to the neonate in question before making any further assessment.
- The left hemidiaphragm has been partially imaged, but overall, this is an adequate X-ray of the abdomen.
- The most striking abnormality is of a dilated gas-filled viscus in the left upper quadrant extending into the central abdomen, which presumably represents a

dilated stomach. There is a further air density bubble in the right flank consistent with a dilated first part of the duodenum but no bowel gas is demonstrated distal to this point.
- A tube is projected over the gas-filled stomach. This represents an orogastric or nasogastric tube.
- The linear structure running obliquely across the patient's right iliac bone is likely an umbilical cord clip.
- There is no obvious abnormality of the visible solid abdominal organs.
- The bones are within normal limits for age.

Continue

CASE **3.19**   *Contd.*

IN SUMMARY – This abdominal X-ray of a neonate demonstrates the 'double bubble' sign suggestive of dilated stomach and first part of the duodenum. The most common cause for this appearance is duodenal atresia. I would request an urgent paediatric surgical opinion.

QUESTIONS

1. Which of the following is/are part of the differential diagnosis for the appearance of this abdominal radiograph?
   A) Duodenal atresia
   B) Duodenal stenosis
   C) Annular pancreas
   D) Preduodenal portal vein
   E) Hypertrophic pyloric stenosis
2. Which of the following is/are true regarding the signs and symptoms of duodenal atresia?
   A) Antenatal polyhydramnios is a feature
   B) Abdominal distension occurs
   C) Vomiting is always bilious
   D) Bowel motions are absent
   E) It presents in the first few days of life
3. Which of the following is/are recognised associations with duodenal atresia?
   A) Down syndrome
   B) Neonatal Bartter syndrome
   C) VACTERL (Vertebral, Anorectal, Cardiac, Tracheal, Oesophageal, Renal, Limb anomalies) association
   D) Malrotation
   E) Annular pancreas
4. Which of the following is/are correct regarding the radiological investigation of patients with duodenal atresia?
   A) The dilated stomach and duodenum may be evident on antenatal ultrasound
   B) Air injection via an orogastric tube under fluoroscopy can confirm the diagnosis
   C) An upper gastrointestinal contrast study may be performed
   D) Gas is seen distally to the level of obstruction
   E) Abdominal ultrasound is a useful test
5. Which of the following is/are part of the management of a patient with duodenal atresia?
   A) Placement of a gastric tube
   B) Making the patient nil by mouth
   C) Commence IV fluids
   D) Endoscopic duodenal stent placement
   E) Surgical duodenoduodenostomy

ANSWERS TO QUESTIONS

1. Which of the following is/are part of the differential diagnosis for the appearance of this abdominal radiograph?
The correct answers are **A) Duodenal atresia, B) Duodenal stenosis, C) Annular pancreas and D) Preduodenal portal vein**.
The double bubble sign refers to gas within the stomach and the first part of the duodenum. The pyloric sphincter results in separation of the two. The level of obstruction is therefore distal to the first part of the duodenum.
A) Duodenal atresia – Correct. Duodenal atresia is the most common cause for the double bubble sign on abdominal X-ray in a neonate.
B) Duodenal stenosis – Correct. Duodenal stenosis is less common than duodenal atresia but can present with similar radiographic findings, although there may be some gas in distal bowel.
C) Annular pancreas – Correct. An annular pancreas can cause extrinsic duodenal compression and contribute to a degree of duodenal obstruction.
D) Preduodenal portal vein – Correct. Preduodenal portal vein is a normal anatomical variant which can also exert extrinsic mass effect on the duodenum.
E) Hypertrophic pyloric stenosis – Incorrect. In hypertrophic pyloric stenosis, the level of obstruction is at the pylorus. The stomach may be distended but the duodenum will not be. In addition, the patient will present with projectile non-bilious vomiting because the obstruction is proximal to the ampulla of Vater.

> **KEY POINT**
>
> Duodenal atresia is the most common cause of the double bubble sign on abdominal X-ray in a neonate. However, there are other entities that can cause/contribute to the level of duodenal obstruction which need to be considered.

2. Which of the following is/are true regarding the signs and symptoms of duodenal atresia?
The correct answers are **A) Antenatal polyhydramnios is a feature, B) Abdominal distension occurs, D) Bowel motions are absent and E) It presents in the first few days of life**.
A) Antenatal polyhydramnios is a feature – Correct. In utero, the developing foetus cannot swallow amniotic fluid as normal due to the duodenal obstruction. This can result in polyhydramnios.
B) Abdominal distension occurs – Correct. The duodenal obstruction results in abdominal distension.
C) Vomiting is always bilious – Incorrect. Although the level of atresia is usually distal to the ampulla of Vater, in some cases the atretic segment is proximal, in which case the vomiting is nonbilious.
D) Bowel motions are absent – Correct. Nothing is able to pass distally to the atretic segment of proximal small bowel. Consequently, bowel motions are absent.

E) It presents in the first few days of life – Correct. Duodenal atresia presents early in life. In contrast, hypertrophic pyloric stenosis usually presents after 3 to 6 weeks of life.

> **KEY POINT**
>
> Nonbilious vomiting does not exclude the diagnosis of duodenal atresia as the atretic segment can occur proximally to the ampulla of Vater. However, nonbilious vomiting occurs more frequently with hypertrophic pyloric stenosis.

3. Which of the following is/are recognised associations with duodenal atresia?
The correct answers are **A) Down syndrome, C) VACTERL (Vertebral, Anorectal, Cardiac, Tracheal, Oesophageal, Renal, Limb anomalies) association, D) Malrotation and E) Annular pancreas.**
A) Down syndrome – Correct. Down syndrome is present is 30% of patients with duodenal atresia. Approximately 3% of patients with Down syndrome have duodenal atresia.
B) Neonatal Bartter syndrome – Incorrect. Neonatal Bartter syndrome is a rare inherited defect in the thick ascending limb of the loop of Henle. It results in polyhydramnios but is not associated with duodenal atresia.
C) VACTERL (Vertebral, Anorectal, Cardiac, Tracheal, Oesophageal, Renal, Limb anomalies) association – Correct. VACTERL association consists of vertebral, anal, cardiac, trachea-oesophageal fistula, renal and limb defects. It is associated with duodenal atresia.
D) Malrotation – Correct. Malrotation is present in 20% to 30% of patients.
E) Annular pancreas – Correct. An annular pancreas is associated with duodenal atresia.

> **KEY POINT**
>
> The most frequent association with duodenal atresia is Down syndrome. In addition, congenital heart disease is present in 20% to 30% patients.

4. Which of the following is/are correct regarding the radiological investigation of patients with duodenal atresia?
The correct answers are **A) The dilated stomach and duodenum may be evident on antenatal ultrasound, B) Air injection via an orogastric tube under fluoroscopy can confirm the diagnosis, C) An upper gastrointestinal contrast study may be performed and E) Abdominal ultrasound is a useful test**.
A) The dilated stomach and duodenum may be evident on antenatal ultrasound – Correct. A dilated stomach and duodenum in combination with polyhydramnios raises the possibility of the diagnosis of duodenal atresia antenatally. There may also be evidence of other associations, e.g. congenital cardiac disease.
B) Air injection via an orogastric tube under fluoroscopy can confirm the diagnosis – Correct. Occasionally the stomach and duodenum are decompressed due to

Continue

CASE **3.19** *Contd.*

vomiting or the placement of a naso- or orogastric tube. In this situation, air can be injected down the tube to demonstrate the double bubble sign with fluoroscopy.

C) An upper gastrointestinal contrast study may be performed – Correct. An upper gastrointestinal study may be performed to distinguish duodenal atresia from duodenal stenosis. In the latter, there may be a narrowing on the second part of the duodenum with a thin filling defect across the lumen which represents a duodenal web. In duodenal atresia the obstruction is complete.

D) Gas is seen distally to the level of obstruction – Incorrect. There is a complete obstruction, and therefore gas should not pass distally until surgical correction has been performed.

E) Abdominal ultrasound is a useful test – Correct. Ultrasound can confirm the abdominal radiographic findings represent dilated stomach and proximal duodenum. It can also assess for any associated pathology.

❗ KEY POINT

Fluoroscopy and ultrasound are useful investigations to confirm the diagnosis of duodenal atresia. It should be remembered that in cases of complete atresia, fluoroscopy and ultrasound cannot exclude a concomitant midgut malrotation prior to surgery.

5. Which of the following is/are part of the management of a patient with duodenal atresia?
The correct answers are **A) Placement of a gastric tube, B) Making the patient nil by mouth, C) Commence IV fluids and E) Surgical duodenoduodenostomy**.

A) Placement of a gastric tube – Correct. An orogastric or nasogastric tube should be sited to decompress the stomach.

B) Making the patient nil by mouth – Correct. No oral intake should be administered prior to the surgery or immediately postoperatively. Feeding can usually commence 2 to 3 days following treatment.

C) Commence IV fluids – Correct. It is important to rehydrate the neonate and correct any biochemical derangement prior to surgery.

D) Endoscopic duodenal stent placement – Incorrect. There is no role for endoscopic stenting of the duodenum in duodenal atresia or stenosis.

E) Surgical duodenoduodenostomy – Correct. The definitive treatment is to remove the obstruction. This can be performed via open laparotomy or by laparoscopic approach.

❗ KEY POINT

Although surgery is the definitively treatment, there is no requirement for this to happen straight away. It is better to adequately hydrate and correct any metabolic derangement prior to conducting semielective surgery within a couple of days of diagnosis, rather than emergency surgery in an unstable patient at the time of diagnosis.

👥 IMPORTANT LEARNING POINTS

- Duodenal atresia is the commonest cause of a double bubble appearance on abdominal X-ray in a neonate.
- There are many associations with duodenal atresia but Down syndrome is the most common.
- Definitive treatment requires surgical excision of the obstructing segment of duodenum.

CASE 3.20

A 7-day-old premature baby who has developed abdominal distension and bloody stools. Please comment on his abdominal X-ray.

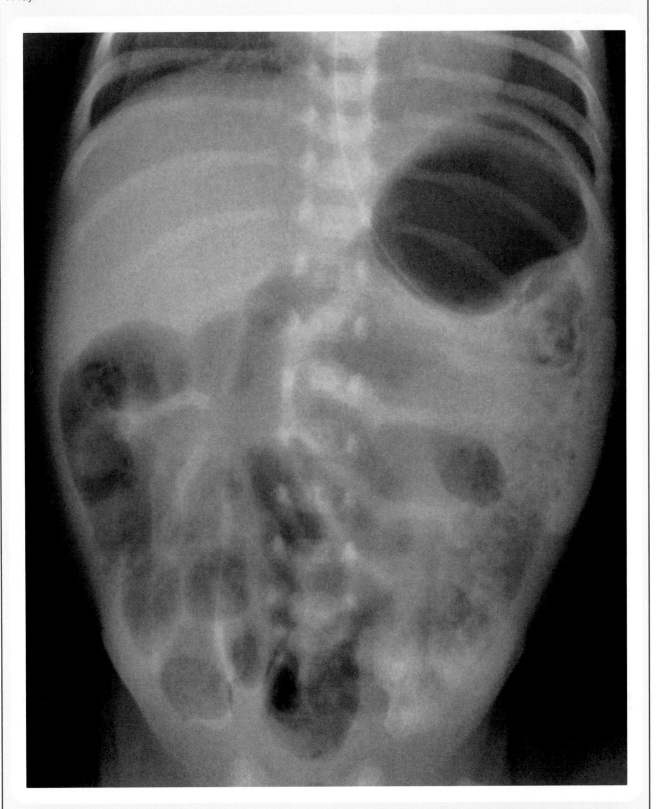

Continue

CASE **3.20**   *Contd.*

ANNOTATED X-RAY

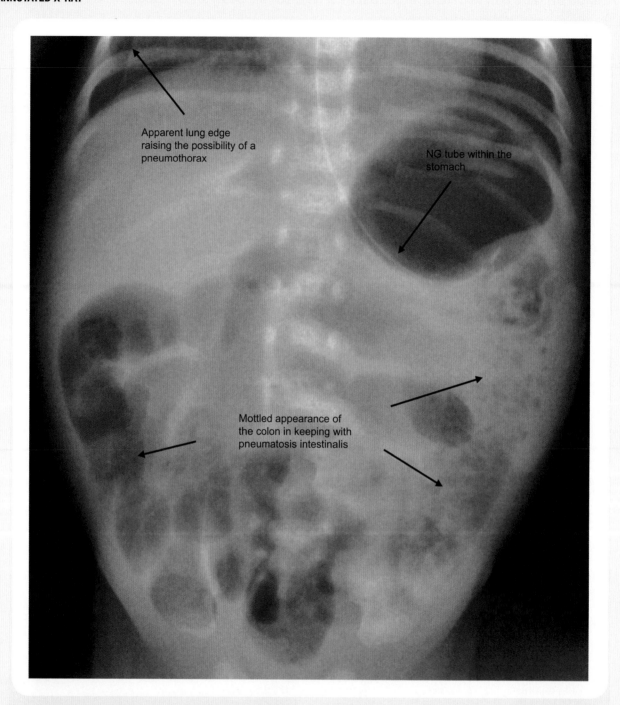

Apparent lung edge
raising the possibility of a
pneumothorax

NG tube within the
stomach

Mottled appearance of
the colon in keeping with
pneumatosis intestinalis

🔍 PRESENT YOUR FINDINGS

- This is a supine AP abdominal X-ray.
- There are no patient identifiable data on the X-ray. I would like to confirm the patient's name, date of birth and the date and time the X-ray was performed before making further assessment.
- The hernial orifices are not demonstrated. Consequently, this is technically inadequate as the entire abdomen has not been adequately visualised.
- There is a naso- or orogastric tube in situ, with its tip projected over the stomach.

- The descending and ascending colons have a mottled appearance. These findings are suspicious of pneumatosis intestinalis.
- There is no evidence of bowel dilatation or perforation. There is no visible portal venous gas.
- A line is visible at the right costophrenic angle, beyond which the lungs markings are not seen. This raises the possibility of a pneumothorax.
- There is no obvious abnormality of the visible solid abdominal organs.
- No skeletal abnormality.

IN SUMMARY – The findings are in keeping with pneumatosis intestinalis. Given the clinical scenario, these findings are suspicious for necrotising enterocolitis. Additionally, there appears to be a right-sided pneumothorax. I would like to review a chest X-ray to confirm or refute this.

QUESTIONS

1. Which of the following is/are recognised risk factors for necrotising enterocolitis?
   A) Prematurity
   B) Low birth weight
   C) Male sex
   D) Breast feeding
   E) Prolonged antibiotic exposure
2. Which of the following investigations are commonly used in the diagnosis of necrotising enterocolitis?
   A) Full blood count
   B) Blood cultures
   C) Barium enema
   D) Abdominal X-ray
   E) Abdominal CT
3. What is the commonest X-ray finding in acute necrotising enterocolitis?
   A) Dilated small bowel
   B) Dilated large bowel
   C) Pneumatosis intestinalis
   D) Pneumoperitoneum
   E) Portal vein gas
4. Which of the following form part of the management of necrotising enterocolitis?
   A) IV fluids
   B) Enteral feeding
   C) Air enema
   D) IV antibiotics
   E) Surgery
5. Which of the following is/are recognised complications of necrotising enterocolitis?
   A) Perforation
   B) Disseminated intravascular coagulation
   C) Enterocolic fistulae
   D) Short bowel syndrome
   E) Abscess formation

Continue

CASE **3.20**   *Contd.*

ANSWERS TO QUESTIONS

1. Which of the following is/are recognised risk factors for necrotising enterocolitis?

   The correct answers are **A) Prematurity, B) Low birth weight and E) Prolonged antibiotic exposure**.

   Necrotising enterocolitis is the commonest gastrointestinal emergency in neonates. It is characterised by necrosis of the mucosa or submucosa. It can affect any part of the gastrointestinal tract. The exact aetiology is not fully understood although it is likely to be multifactorial and may involve ischaemia, inflammation, antigen exposure and infection. Various risk factors for the development of necrotising enterocolitis have been identified.

   A) Prematurity – Correct. Prematurity is a well-established risk factor. The age of onset is inversely related to the gestational age at birth; i.e. full-term babies tend to present with the disease within the first few days of life, whilst premature babies have increasingly delayed presentations. Premature neonates with a patent ductus arteriosus are at even higher risk of developing necrotising enterocolitis.

   B) Low birth weight – Correct. Low birth weight is a recognised risk factor for necrotising enterocolitis.

   C) Male sex – Incorrect. No consistent association between sex and risk of developing necrotising enterocolitis has been established.

   D) Breast feeding – Incorrect. Human breast milk reduces the risk of necrotising enterocolitis by 5- to 10-fold compared to formula milk. Human milk contains secretory IgA which helps prevent the transmural migration of gut bacteria. Oligofructose, a component of human milk, aids the normal colonisation of the gut by bifidobacteria. These factors, along with other components of breast milk, are believed to help modulate the inflammatory response in the gut and protect against necrotising enterocolitis.

   E) Prolonged antibiotic exposure – Correct. Prolonged antibiotic exposure, particularly if given empirically to low birth weight babies without any indication of infection, is a risk factor for the development of necrotising enterocolitis. It is believed this is a result of altered gastrointestinal flora in the neonate.

   ❶ KEY POINT

   Prematurity and low birth weight are the most well-recognised risk factors for the development of necrotising enterocolitis.

2. Which of the following are commonly used in the diagnosis of necrotising enterocolitis?

   The correct answers are **A) Full blood count, B) Blood cultures and D) Abdominal X-ray**.

   The diagnosis of necrotising enterocolitis is made using a combination of clinical features, blood tests and imaging.

   A) Full blood count – Correct. Routine blood tests are not specific in necrotising enterocolitis but are useful in helping assess the response to treatment. Severe thrombocytopaenia, neutropaenia, coagulopathy or acidosis may indicate severe disease.

   B) Blood cultures – Correct. Sepsis often mimics necrotising enterocolitis. Therefore, it is advisable to obtain blood cultures prior to commencing antibiotics in suspected cases of necrotising enterocolitis.

   C) Barium enema – Incorrect. Generally, barium enema is contraindicated in suspected necrotising enterocolitis. Water-soluble contrast should be used if a contrast study is required (e.g. to exclude Hirschsprung disease).

   D) Abdominal X-ray – Correct. Abdominal X-ray is used to confirm the diagnosis and assess response to treatment. Typical features include ileus which does not change appearance over serial examinations, pneumatosis intestinalis, bowel wall oedema, portal venous gas and perforation. Pneumatosis intestinalis occurs in approximately 80% of cases and consists of gas within the bowel wall. This can give a mottled appearance, which may be confused with faecal material. It can also result in a tram-track-like lucency within the bowel wall.

   E) Abdominal CT – Incorrect. Whilst abdominal CT can demonstrate the features of necrotising enterocolitis more accurately than abdominal X-ray, it involves a significant radiation dose and is therefore not commonly used for diagnostic purposes.

   ❶ KEY POINTS

   1. The diagnosis of necrotising enterocolitis is based on clinical findings, blood results and imaging, such as abdominal X-rays.
   2. Ultrasound is more sensitive than abdominal X-ray for detecting portal venous gas. Ultrasound can also identify bowel wall oedema, bowel wall gas and free fluid within the abdomen.

3. What is the commonest X-ray finding in acute necrotising enterocolitis?

   The correct answer is **A) Dilated small bowel**.

   A) Dilated small bowel – Correct. A small bowel ileus, leading to bowel dilatation, is often the earliest and commonest X-ray finding in necrotising enterocolitis. It is a nonspecific finding and clinical correlation is required.

   B) Dilated large bowel – Incorrect. Stricture formation is a recognised complication of necrotising enterocolitis. Strictures tend to form at the splenic flexure and can result in large bowel obstruction. However, they occur later in life and therefore large bowel dilatation is not a common feature in the acute setting.

C) Pneumatosis intestinalis – Incorrect. Pneumatosis intestinalis is a characteristic feature of necrotising enterocolitis. It is a result of gas (produced by bacteria) within the bowel wall. It can give the bowel a bubbly appearance, or look like tram-tracks if the bowel wall is viewed side on. Pneumatosis is not specific for necrotising enterocolitis, and is also seen in cystic fibrosis, Hirschsprung disease, milk intolerance, collagen vascular disease, leukaemia and with steroid use.

D) Pneumoperitoneum – Incorrect. Necrotising enterocolitis can result in a bowel perforation. This may be visible on a supine abdominal X-ray as the football sign (elliptical central lucency as a result of gas rising up centrally within the peritoneal cavity and free fluid (ascites) lying dependently around the periphery of the abdominal cavity) if there is a large volume of free gas. Other X-ray signs of perforation include Rigler's sign (gas on both sides of the bowel outlines the bowel wall) and the falciform ligament sign (free gas outlining the falciform ligament). A lateral decubitus X-ray, with the patient rolled onto their left side, is more sensitive for detecting small quantities of free of gas.

E) Portal vein gas – Incorrect. Gas may spread from the bowel wall into the portal venous system. This portal vein gas can sometimes be seen on abdominal X-rays as branching linear lucencies projected over the liver, extending from the porta hepatis towards the periphery. However, ultrasound is more sensitive than abdominal X-rays for detecting portal venous gas.

KEY POINTS

1. Pneumatosis intestinalis and portal vein gas are characteristic X-ray findings of necrotising enterocolitis; however, small bowel dilatation is the earliest and commonest radiological sign.
2. Only 50% to 75% of neonates with perforation secondary to necrotising enterocolitis will have visible free gas on their abdominal X-ray.

4. Which of the following are parts of the management of necrotising enterocolitis?
The correct answers are **A) IV fluids, D) IV antibiotics and E) Surgery**.
The management of necrotising enterocolitis depends on the severity of the disease. The Bell classification system is one method for stratifying necrotising enterocolitis. It has three stages (Table C3.20.1). In stages 1 and 2, the management is generally nonsurgical, with surgical options considered in stage 3 disease.
A) IV fluids – Correct. IV fluids are needed to replace losses and provide ongoing maintenance fluids and electrolytes. More aggressive fluid resuscitation and inotropic support may be required for very sick neonates (stage 3).

Table C3.20.1 The Bell Classification System for Necrotising Enterocolitis

STAGE	FEATURES
1	Suspected necrotising enterocolitis. Mild, nonspecific clinical and radiological signs (bradycardia, mild abdominal distension, AXR – normal or mild bowel dilatation)
2	Definite necrotising enterocolitis with characteristic clinical and radiological signs (clinical signs as stage 1 with addition of abdominal tenderness and absent bowel sounds. AXR – small bowel dilatation and/or pneumatosis intestinalis). 2A is mild disease, 2B moderate
3	Advanced necrotising enterocolitis (as stage 2 but also hypotension, bradycardia, respiratory failure, coagulopathy). 3A = no perforation. 3B = perforation

B) Enteral feeding – Incorrect. One of the key treatments for necrotising enterocolitis is resting the gastrointestinal tract to help the inflammatory process resolve. Patients should therefore be kept nil by mouth, with enteral feeding being contraindicated. Instead, nutrition is provided via a central line (total parenteral nutrition). A large-bore NG tube is needed to decompress the stomach and bowel.

C) Air enema – Incorrect. Air enema is a nonsurgical method of treating intussusception. It is not used in the management of necrotising enterocolitis.

D) IV antibiotics – Correct. Broad-spectrum antibiotics are initiated after culture samples have been obtained. The choice of antibiotics is determined by the most common nosocomial organism in that particular hospital/area. Doses are adjusted depending on weight and age of the neonate.

E) Surgery – Correct. Most neonates respond to medical management. Surgery is considered for patients who deteriorate despite optimal medical therapy and for patients with necrotic bowel or perforation. A paediatric surgeon should be involved in the care of neonates with necrotising enterocolitis at an early stage. Surgery usually involves the resection of necrotic bowel and the formation of a stoma. Primary anastomosis (the anastomosis is formed during the initial operation) is usually avoided due to the high risk of anastomotic breakdown. Instead, the end of the proximal part of bowel is initially brought out as a stoma, with a delayed anastomosis performed at a later date once the patient has recovered.

Continue

CASE 3.20   *Contd.*

KEY POINT

The management of NEC involves:
- Gut rest: Making the patient nil by mouth and providing nutrition through total parenteral nutrition.
- Intravenous antibiotics: Broad-spectrum antibiotics to cover possible infection.
- Cardiac and ventilatory support: Neonates may become haemodynamically unstable, requiring fluid boluses, and possibly inotropes, especially in severe cases. Intubation may be required for ventilatory support.
- Surgery: For patients who deteriorate despite optimal medical management and for those with perforation or necrotic bowel.

5. Which of the following are recognised complications of necrotising enterocolitis?
   The correct answers are **A) Perforation, B) Disseminated intravascular coagulation, C) Enterocolic fistulae, D) Short bowel syndrome and E) Abscess formation**.
   The complications of necrotising enterocolitis can be acute or chronic and be due to the underlying inflammatory process or iatrogenic in nature.
   A) Perforation – Correct. Perforation is a well-recognised complication of necrotising enterocolitis. Many patients with necrotising enterocolitis can be managed conservatively with medical therapy but those who perforate will usually require surgery. Surgery is also indicated for patients who are not improving despite optimal medical therapy. Such patients often have necrotic bowel which requires resection.
   B) Disseminated intravascular coagulation – Correct. Disseminated intravascular coagulation is the pathological activation of the coagulation systems. It typically occurs in severely unwell and shocked patients, such as those with stage 3 necrotising enterocolitis. There is widespread intravascular clot formation, which can obstruct small blood vessels, leading to organ impairment. As this pathological process progresses, there is consumption of clotting factors which in turns impairs normal coagulation. The result is haemorrhage from various areas

of the body, such as the gastrointestinal tract and surgical wounds. Management is aimed at treating the underlying cause.
   C) Enterocolic fistulae – Correct. Necrotising enterocolitis, like Crohn's disease, can result in transmural inflammation of the bowel. There is therefore a risk of fistula formation, particularly between loops of small and large bowel (enterocolic).
   D) Short bowel syndrome – Correct. Short bowel syndrome is caused by malabsorption usually secondary to surgical small bowel resection. Patients with necrotising enterocolitis who develop necrotic bowel will require the necrotic area to be resected. If a significant length of small bowel is removed, small bowel syndrome may occur. Clinical features include weight loss, malnutrition and diarrhoea.
   E) Abscess formation – Correct. Bowel perforation can result in abscess formation. Treatment includes antibiotics, percutaneous drainage and/or surgery.

KEY POINTS

1. Acute complications of necrotising enterocolitis include perforation, abscess formation, disseminated intravascular coagulation and multiorgan failure.
2. Longer-term complications include stricture formation, fistula formation and short bowel syndrome.

IMPORTANT LEARNING POINTS

- Necrotising enterocolitis is the commonest gastrointestinal emergency in neonates.
- Prematurity and low birth weight are the main risk factors.
- The clinical and biochemical findings are nonspecific.
- Abdominal X-rays allow confirmation of the diagnosis and help assess the response to treatment.
- Necrotising enterocolitis is graded according to the Bell classification system.
- Treatment is often supportive, with gut rest, IV fluids, total parenteral nutrition and IV antibiotics. Surgery is reserved for severe cases.

4

Orthopaedic X-rays

Christopher Gee

Chapter Outline

INTRODUCTION

This introduction to this chapter is aimed at providing a systematic framework for approaching orthopaedic X-rays. Further details and examples of the specific X-ray findings discussed next are covered more extensively in the example cases later in the chapter and the bonus X-ray chapter.

> **! KEY POINT**
>
> Systematic approach to orthopaedic X-rays
> 1. Projection
> 2. Patient details
> 3. Technical adequacy
> 4. Obvious abnormalities
> 5. Systematic review of the X-ray
> 6. Summary

PROJECTION

- Assessment of any bone or joint in general requires at least two views – *'one view is one too few!'* These normally consist of AP and lateral X-rays (Fig. 4.1).
- For some sites, such as the scaphoid, where fractures are difficult to detect, it is routine to obtain more than two views.

- For some patients in whom the clinical suspicion of a fracture is high but is not evident on the usual two views, additional views may be requested, such as internal rotation views of the hip.
- If the shaft of a long bone is fractured it is imperative to X-ray the joint above and below because of the potential for additional injuries (fracture or dislocation) at these sites.
- Comment on whether the patient is skeletally mature (fused epiphyses/growth plates). This is useful because the types of injury and pathology vary between skeletally immature and mature patients.

> **! KEY POINT**
>
> Remember: children develop and mature at different rates and therefore the age of a patient does not tell you whether they are skeletally mature or not.

PATIENT DETAILS

- It is important to check you are looking at the correct X-ray of the correct patient.
- The patient details should be listed on the X-ray.

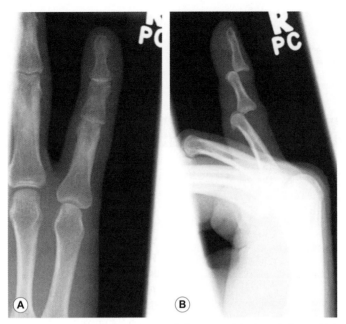

Fig. 4.1 **(A)** AP view of this finger shows apparently normal alignment of the interphalangeal joints. **(B)** The lateral view shows posterior dislocations at both of these joints! These X-rays dramatically show why one view is one too few!

- State the name, age (or date of birth) and the date on which the X-ray was taken.

TECHNICAL ADEQUACY

- The entire area of concern should be included in the X-ray. This is particularly important with X-rays of the cervical spine.
- Are the X-rays adequately exposed so that bone and soft tissues can be seen and differentiated?
- Is the patient rotated? Sometimes a small amount of rotation, which results in a nonstandard view, can make accurate assessment difficult. If the patient is significantly rotated, then the X-rays may need to be repeated.

OBVIOUS ABNORMALITIES

- If there is an obvious abnormality, such as fractures, subluxations/dislocations or bone lesions, comment on this before conducting your systemic review of the X-ray.

SYSTEMATIC REVIEW OF THE X-RAY (FIGS 4.2–4.5)

- Look around the edges of all the bones for fractures. The cortex should be a smooth, continuous line. Any disruption to, or, irregularity of this may represent a fracture.
- Also look at the medulla for evidence of fractures – look for disruption to the trabeculations and for lucent and sclerotic lines.

- Displaced fractures appear as black lines, whereas impacted or overlapping fractures usually result in areas which appear sclerotic.
- Assess for soft tissue swelling and joint effusion (knee and elbow joints), if appropriate. Such findings may represent soft tissue injury or can be indirect evidence of a fracture.
- Look at the joint surfaces for any evidence of subluxation or dislocation.
- Assess joints for degenerative (loss of joint space, subchondral sclerosis, subchondral cysts and osteophytes) and inflammatory changes (periarticular osteoporosis, soft tissue swelling and bony erosions).
- Review the bone density and texture looking for any abnormal lucent or sclerotic areas.

SUMMARY

- State your key findings (either as a description or a diagnosis), put forward a differential diagnosis, suggest any further relevant imaging and suggest an appropriate initial management plan.

DESCRIBING FRACTURES

- Being able to accurately describe a fracture is vital for conveying the correct information to other members of the team (e.g. an on-call consultant who is at home during the night). See Fig. 4.6 for an example. When describing a fracture, you need to comment on:
- Which bone is involved
- Which part of the bone is fractured
  - Proximal third.
  - Middle third.

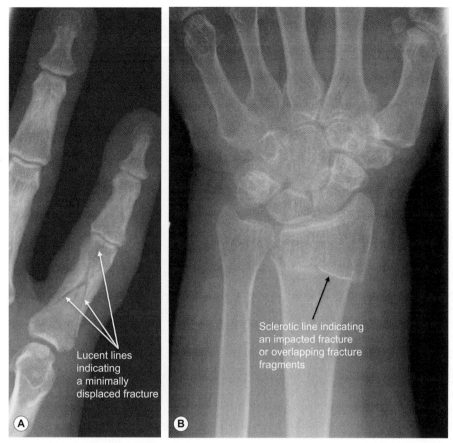

Fig. 4.2 The appearances of fractures. **(A)** A minimally displaced fracture of the proximal phalanx which extends to the proximal interphalangeal joint. This fracture is indicated by the lucent lines. **(B)** A distal radius fracture with either impaction or overlapping fragments, resulting in a sclerotic line.

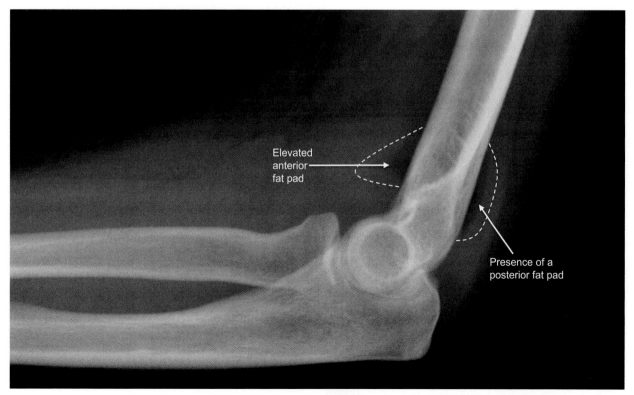

Fig. 4.3 A lateral elbow X-ray showing a joint effusion (elevated anterior fat pad and the presence of a posterior fat pad). There are a variety of causes of any joint effusion, but an elbow effusion in the context of trauma suggests an underlying fracture, which may or may not be visible. A fracture is difficult to see on this X-ray.

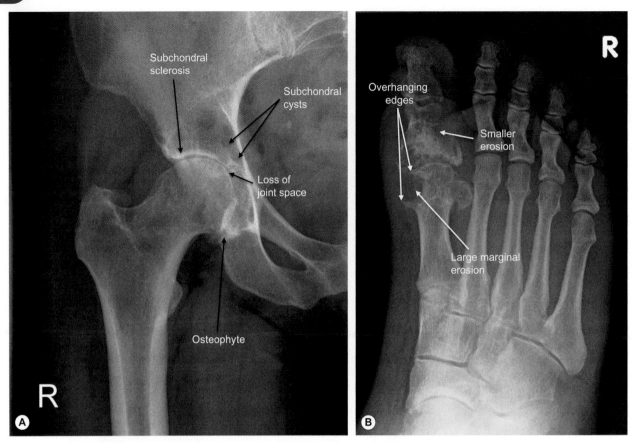

Fig. 4.4 **(A)** AP X-ray of the right hip showing the classic findings of osteoarthritis. **(B)** Oblique X-ray of the right foot showing an erosive/inflammatory arthropathy involving the 1st metatarsal phalangeal joint. The marginal erosions with overhanging edges are typical of gout.

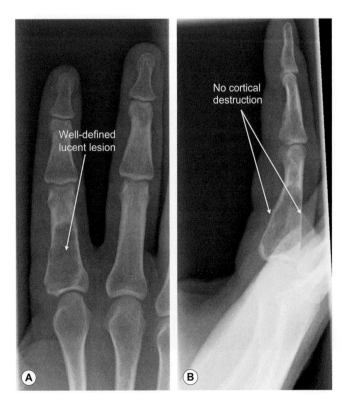

Fig. 4.5 AP **(A)** and lateral **(B)** X-rays of an index finger showing a well-defined, slightly expansile lucent lesion. It appears uniformly lucent with no cortical destruction. These features are consistent with a benign bone lesion. In combination with its position, this is in keeping with an enchondroma (a benign cartilaginous tumour). Whilst benign, there is a risk of a pathological fracture.

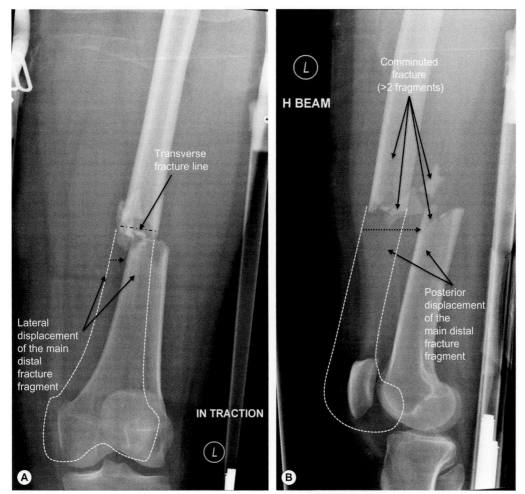

Fig. 4.6 A comminuted transverse fracture involving the middle third (diaphysis) of the left femur. **(A)** AP and **(B)** lateral. There is marked posterior displacement with minor lateral displacement. No significant angulation, rotation or shortening is present. The background bone texture and the knee joint look normal.

- Distal third.
- Intraarticular.

(The bone can also be subdivided into the epiphysis, metaphysis and diaphysis.)

- Fracture pattern
  - Simple (skin is intact) or open (skin not intact).
  - Comminuted (more than two fragments of bone).
  - Impacted (when bone fragments are driven into each other).
- Type of fracture
  - Transverse (i.e. perpendicular to the long axis of the bone).
  - Oblique (i.e. angled less than 90 degrees to the long axis of the bone).
  - Spiral (i.e. curving around the bone).
  - Greenstick (occurs in children, break in one cortex with the other cortex remaining intact, often associated with angulation).
  - Vertical (i.e. parallel to the long axis of the bone).
- Translational displacement
  - Relationship of distal fragment to proximal fragment.
  - Nondisplaced or anterior, posterior, medial, lateral displacement.
  - It is essential to use both X-rays to assess this.
- Angulation
  - The angulation of the distal fragment relative to the proximal bone in degrees.
  - Again, it is essential to use both X-rays to fully assess this.
- Rotation
  - Measured along the long axis of the bone.
  - Generally more easily assessed on clinical examination but may be diagnosed on X-rays.
  - Requires knowledge of normal anatomical alignment.
  - Either internal or external rotation.
  - Important to assess all long bone fractures for rotation.
- Shortening
- Joint space
  - May be smaller than it should be, asymmetrical or bone fragments/foreign bodies may be present.

- Joint cartilage
  - Look for symmetry of the outline of the cartilage and any fractures on the surface of the bones.
- Bone texture
  - If most of the bone is radiolucent (dark) and the cortices appear thinned, then consider whether the patient has osteopaenia.
  - Radiolucency just around the joint suggests inflammatory/infected joint.
  - Focal lucent areas may indicate an underlying bone lesion (primary or secondary bone tumour, infection). Sclerotic (radioopaque) areas are rarer (Paget's disease, osteochondritis, sclerotic bone metastases). Fractures related to bone lesions should be considered to be pathological fractures.

> ❗ KEY POINT
>
> Some fractures have eponymous names, such as Colles', Smith's, Monteggia, etc. They are useful as they convey a lot of information – the appearance of the fracture, likely mechanism of injury, treatment options and prognosis. However, they refer to a specific fracture pattern and are commonly misused. Therefore, if you are not certain whether a fracture fits a specific eponymous term, then it is best to just describe the fracture as outlined earlier.

SUBLUXATION VERSUS DISLOCATION

The difference between these two terms may not appear obvious in the first instance (Fig. 4.7).

- Subluxation
  - The normal anatomy of the joint is disrupted but there remains some contact between the articular surfaces of the joint.
- Dislocation
  - Complete disruption of the joint with no contact between the joint surfaces.

CERVICAL SPINE

First, check the X-rays adequately cover the cervical spine. The importance of adequate views is demonstrated in Fig. 4.8.

- For trauma, at least three views are required:
  - Lateral, which must show all seven cervical vertebrae and the top of the 1st thoracic vertebra (Figs 4.9A, 4.10 and 4.11A).
  - AP (Figs 4.9B and 4.11B).
  - Open mouth AP/Peg view (named peg since you can visualise the odontoid peg), to view C1 and C2 (Fig. 4.9C).
- If any of these are inadequate, then repeat views or alternative views (such as a Swimmer's view

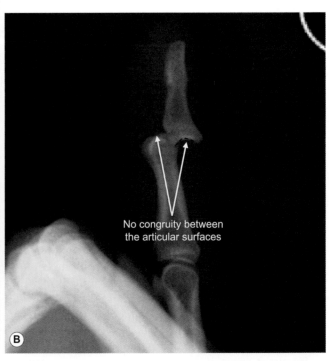

Some congruity between the articular surfaces remains

No congruity between the articular surfaces

Fig. 4.7 X-rays illustrating the difference between subluxation **(A)**, where some contact between the articular surfaces remains, and dislocation **(B)**, where there is no congruity between articular surfaces.

to try to better image the C7/T1 junction) should be considered. In this image, the patient is placed in a swimmer's position with one arm back and one arm forward to try and take the shoulders out of view. Even with additional views, a CT scan may be required to adequately assess the cervical spine.

> **❶ KEY POINT**
>
> The lateral X-ray is the most useful for detecting cervical spine injuries. Most of the injuries occur at C1/2 or C5-T1 region. This is why the lateral X-ray must include the C7/T1 junction (see Fig. 4.8).

LATERAL X-RAY

- Vertebral alignment
  - Anterior vertebral line
  - Posterior vertebral line
  - Spinolaminar line
  - Spinous processes

These curves should be smooth and unbroken.
- Vertebral bodies
  - From the third cervical vertebrae downwards, the vertebral bodies should have a regular rectangular shape.
  - There should be no wedging (i.e. the height of the anterior and posterior aspects of the vertebral bodies should be roughly equal).
  - The intervertebral discs should be approximately the same size.
- C1/2 articulation
  - The distance between the posterior aspect of the anterior arch of C1 and the anterior aspect of the peg should be <3mm in adults (5mm in children) – if this distance is increased, you should consider displacement/subluxation of the C1/2 articulation, which may be due to a fracture and/or ligament damage.
- Posterior elements
  - The facet joints should overlap each other like slates on a roof – if this is not the case, you must consider a facet joint subluxation/dislocation.

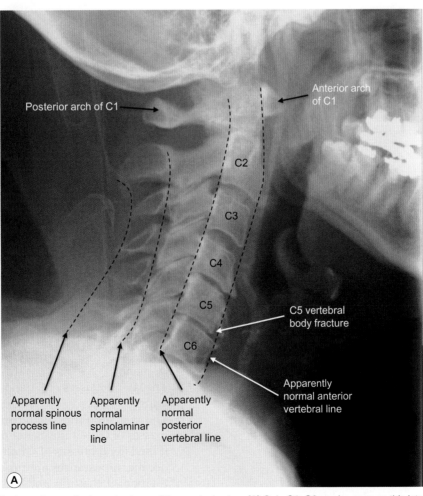

Fig. 4.8 The importance of adequate views of the cervical spine. **(A)** Only *C1–C6* can be seen on this lateral view on the left. There is a fracture through the *C5* vertebral body but the vertebral alignment appears normal.

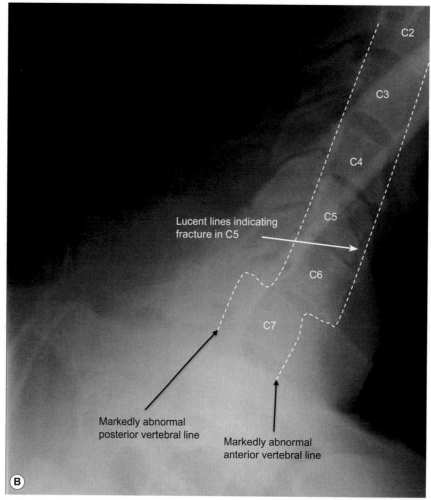

Fig. 4.8, Cont'd **(B)** The Swimmer's view X-ray shows (in addition to the *C5* fracture) markedly abnormal vertebral alignment with anterior subluxation of *C6* on *C7*, demonstrated by the abnormal anterior and posterior vertebral lines (the *spinolaminar* and *spinous process* lines are not clearly visible).

- The gap between adjacent spinous processes should be roughly equal – if this is not the case, you should consider a dislocation or ligamentous injury.
- Prevertebral soft tissues
  - The distance between the anterior vertebral line and the edge of the prevertebral soft tissues should be <7 mm between C1-C4 (or less than one-third of the adjacent vertebral body) and <22 mm between C5-C7 (or less than the width of the adjacent vertebral body).
  - Increase in these distances suggests the presence of a haematoma and thus an important underlying injury. Remember: not all fractures will result in significant soft tissue swelling; therefore, its absence does not exclude significant underlying injury.

AP VIEW

- Alignment
  - The spinous processes should follow a straight line – if this is not the case, you should consider a

rotational abnormality, such as a unilateral facet joint dislocation – go back and check the alignment of the facet joints on the lateral view.
- Spacing
  - The spinous processes should be roughly equidistant – if this is not the case, you should consider an anterior cervical dislocation or ligamentous injury.
  - The intervertebral disc spaces should be a uniform height.

PEG VIEW

- Alignment
  - The lateral masses of C1 and C2 should line up.
- Spacing
  - The peg should be equidistant from the lateral masses of C1 – if this is not the case, check to see if the lateral masses of C1 and C2 line up. If they do, the appearances are probably due to patient rotation; if they do not line up, you must consider a fracture or ligament damage involving C1 and C2.

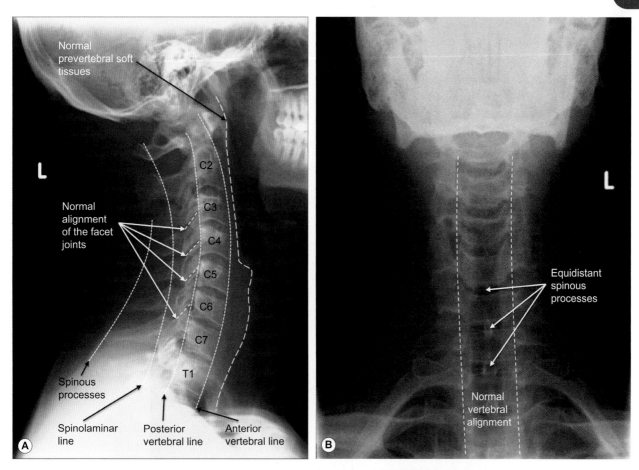

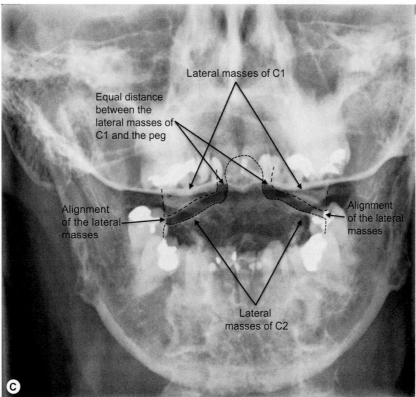

Fig. 4.9 Normal cervical spine X-rays: Lateral **(A)**, AP **(B)** and Peg **(C)** views.

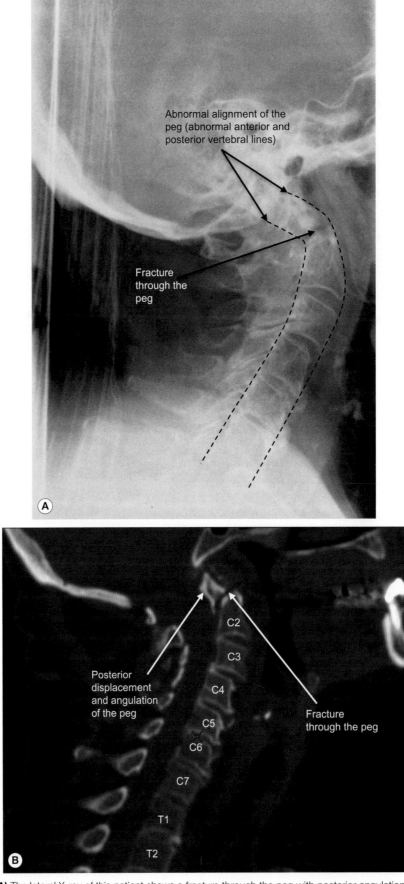

Fig. 4.10 (A) The lateral X-ray of this patient shows a fracture through the peg with posterior angulation of the proximal fracture. **(B)** CT in the same patient confirms the X-ray findings.

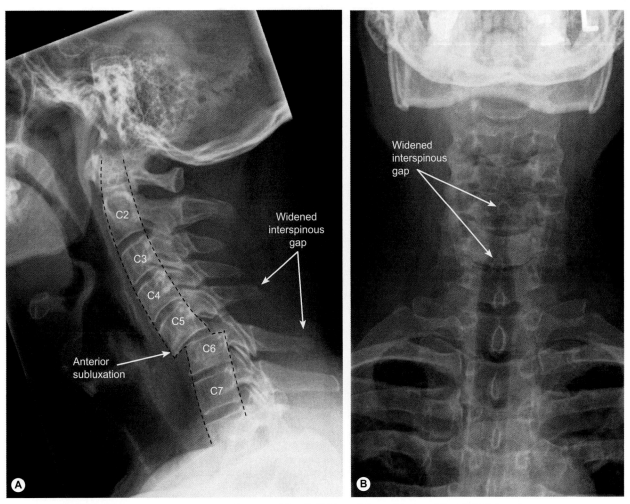

Fig. 4.11 (A) Lateral X-ray showing subluxation of the *C5/C6* facet joints, widening of the *C5/C6* interspinous gap and anterior subluxation of *C5* on *C6*. **(B)** AP X-ray confirming a widened interspinous gap.

❗ KEY POINTS

1. Roughly 10% of patients with a C-spine fracture have a second noncontiguous vertebral column fracture. Therefore, if you see one abnormality, make sure you look carefully for a second.
2. Assessing cervical spine X-rays can be difficult, so make sure you ask an experienced doctor to review the X-rays as well.
3. There is usually a low threshold to perform a CT in cases of suspected or confirmed cervical spine injuries.

THORACOLUMBAR SPINE

The three vertebral columns concept is an important concept regarding the spine (Fig. 4.12). This approach is helpful for determining whether a spinal injury is stable or unstable. The three columns consist of:

- Anterior
  - Anterior longitudinal ligament, the anterior half of the vertebral body and the anterior part of the annulus fibrosus.
- Middle

- Posterior half of the vertebral body, the posterior part of the annulus fibrosus and the posterior longitudinal ligament.
- Posterior
  - Posterior ligaments and bone arch.

Each column should be assessed. Instability is present if two of the three columns are disrupted (fractures, steps or kinks).

First assess the lateral X-ray:

- Alignment
  - Smooth, unbroken contour on both the AP and lateral X-rays.
  - The thoracic spine normally has a kyphosis, whereas the lumbar spine normally has a lordosis.
  - Straightening of the lumbar lordosis is often related to pain and muscle spasm.
  - Displacement of one vertebra in relation to the vertebra below is known as spondylolisthesis. If the superior vertebra has moved anteriorly, this is an anterolisthesis. This can be related to defects in the pars interarticularis (this is referred to as a spondylolysis), to facet joint degeneration or to trauma.

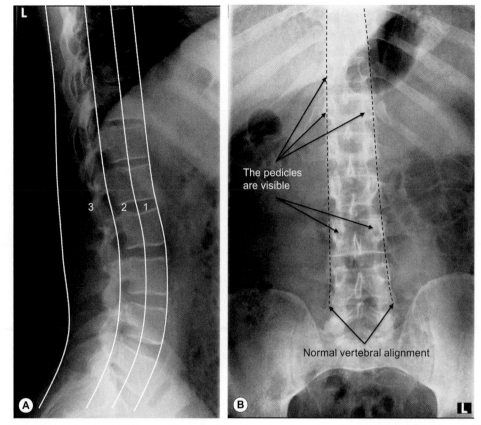

Fig. 4.12 Normal lateral and AP X-rays of the lower thoracic and lumbar spine. **(A)** On the left, the positions of the three vertebral columns is illustrated (*1* = anterior, *2* = middle, *3* = posterior). Note the normal lumbar lordosis, and the normal appearance of the vertebral bodies (square shape) and intervertebral disc spaces. **(B)** The AP X-ray on the right shows the normal appearance of the vertebral bodies including the pedicles.

- Posterior displacement of one vertebra in relation to the vertebra below is known as retrolisthesis.
- No breaks, steps or kinks should be present in any of the three vertebral columns.
- Vertebral bodies
  - Anterior and posterior margins should be equal in height. Anterior wedge fractures (Figs 4.13 and 4.14) are a common type of fracture, particularly in those with osteoporosis.
  - The superior and inferior endplates are often slightly concave but should have smooth surfaces.
  - The posterior margin is normally slightly concave – loss of this may be due to retropulsion of fracture fragments or tumour infiltration into the vertebral body.
  - Thinning of the vertebral body cortices and increased lucency in the medulla are in keeping with osteopaenia.

Then, look at the AP view:
- Alignment:
  - The vertebral bodies and spinous processes should follow a straight line.
  - A scoliosis results in an abnormal lateral curvature of the spine on the AP view. This can be due to congenital bony abnormalities, idiopathic (commonest cause in adolescents) or due to

degenerative changes (commonest cause in middle and old age).
- Pedicle:
  - The pedicles should be visible – if a pedicle is not visible, you must consider whether it eroded due to a pathological process (e.g. by a bone metastasis).

Specific features to look for include:
- Fractures: look at the height of the vertebral bodies, comparing each side and comparing above and below, as crush/osteoporotic wedge fractures are common.
  - Most fractures will be evident on the lateral X-ray.
- Stability: if a fracture is present, comment on whether the abnormality is stable or unstable (by assessing the columns of the spine as mentioned earlier).
- Disc space narrowing is common and a sign of degenerative disease.
- Comment on:
  - Lordosis (anterior convexity; i.e. inward curvature of the spine. Normally there is a cervical and lumbar lordosis).
  - Kyphosis (anterior concavity; i.e. outward curvature of the spine. Normally there is a thoracic and sacral kyphosis).

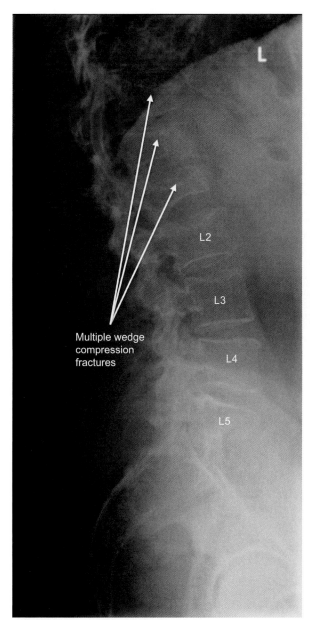

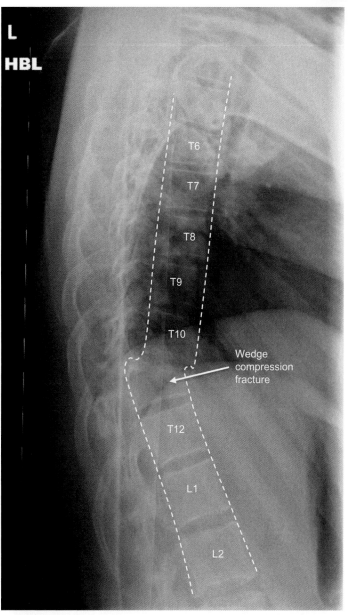

Fig. 4.13 Lateral X-ray of the lumbar spine showing multiple wedge compression fractures. The cortices of the vertebral bodies are thinned and the medulla appears relatively lucent, in keeping with osteopaenia.

Fig. 4.14 Lateral X-ray of the mid and lower thoracic/upper lumbar spine. There is a serious injury with anterior displacement of *T10* on *T11*. There is a wedge compression fracture of *T11*. With this displacement the wedge fracture is part of a more significant injury that needs further assessment. This should also raise concerns about neurological compromise.

- Scoliosis (side-to-side (lateral) curvature of the spine).
- Osteoporosis is also common in the spine.

SHOULDER

X-rays of the shoulder will include an AP X-ray. Additional views vary, but may include axial, Y or apical oblique views and all essentially attempt to get a tangential view of the shoulder. There are pros and cons to each of these views and the choice of view used varies from hospital to hospital. You should familiarise

yourself with the type of second view used in the hospital in which you train/work.

First, look at the AP view (Fig. 4.15A):
- Trace around the cortices for disruption and look for lucent or sclerotic lines within the medulla, signifying a fracture. Fractures through the surgical neck (proximal humeral shaft) and humeral head are more common with increasing age.
- Assess the alignment of the glenohumeral (shoulder) joint.
  - The articular surfaces of the humeral head and glenoid should be parallel.

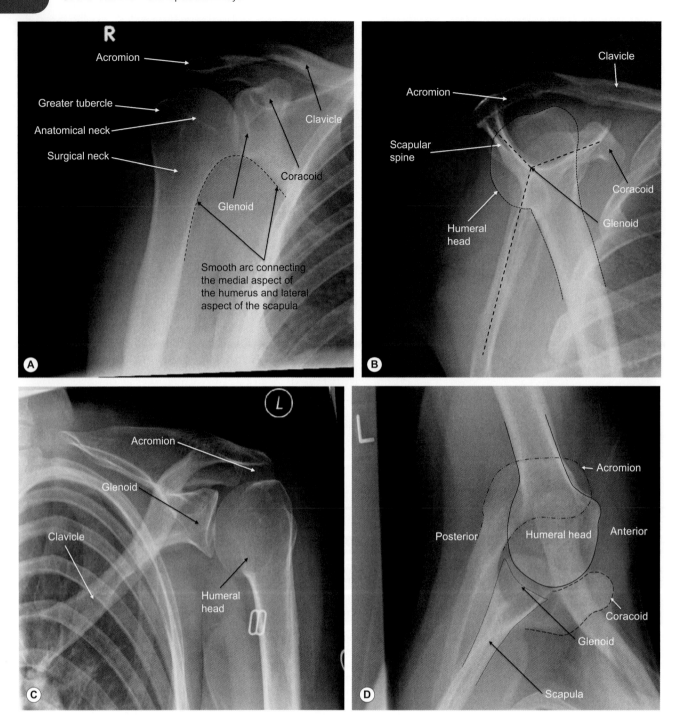

Fig. 4.15 (A) Normal AP shoulder X-ray showing the normal articulation between the humeral head and glenoid. **(B)** Normal Y view. The scapular spine, coracoid and scapula blade forming the Y are shown. The glenoid lies at the centre of the Y and the humeral head is projected over this position. **(C)** A normal apical oblique X-ray showing the normal articulation between the humeral head and glenoid. **(D)** Normal axial X-ray showing the humeral head sitting on top of the glenoid like a golf ball on a tee. The acromion and coracoid point anteriorly.

- There should be a smooth arch running from the medial aspect of the proximal humerus to the lateral aspect of the scapula.
- Anterior dislocations are the commonest type of dislocation (Fig. 4.16A). The humeral head will adopt a typical subcoracoid location. Look for associated fractures (bony Bankart – fracture of the inferior glenoid, and Hill–Sachs

deformity – compression fracture of the postero-lateral humeral head).
- Posterior dislocations are rare and easily over-looked on the AP view (Fig. 4.16B). The humeral head will have an abnormal symmetrical appear-ance (like a light bulb). This is because the patient will be unable to externally rotate their shoulder to adopt the usual position for a shoulder X-ray.

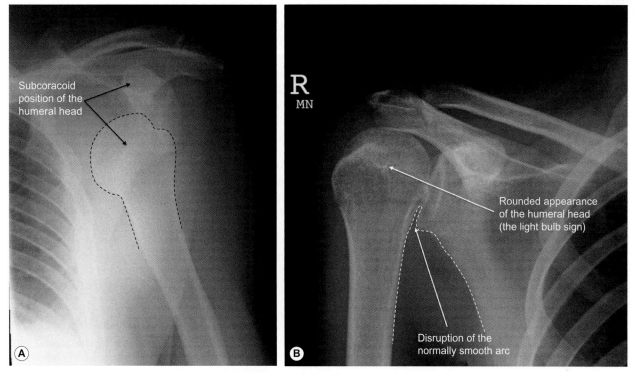

Fig. 4.16 (A) AP X-ray of the left shoulder showing the typical subcoracoid location of the anteriorly dislocated humeral head. **(B)** AP X-ray of the right shoulder showing a posterior dislocation – rounded appearance of the humeral head and disruption to the normally smooth arch connecting the medial humerus to the lateral scapula. These appearances are subtle and easily overlooked.

The smooth arch connecting the medial humeral shaft and lateral scapula will be disrupted.
- Assess the alignment of the acromioclavicular joint.
  - The inferior surfaces of the distal clavicle and acromion should align. Remember: thorough assessment of the acromioclavicular joint requires a specific acromioclavicular joint X-ray.
- Look for fractures of the clavicles, scapula or ribs.
- Assess the visible lung for pathology, such as a pneumothorax or lung nodule.

Then, look at the second view:

If the AP shows a typical anterior dislocation, then there is often no need for a second view to be performed.

The second view is helpful for confirming the normal or abnormal articulation of the glenohumeral joint. In particular, posterior dislocations are easier to identify on the second view. The second view is also helpful for detecting fractures.
- Axial view (Fig. 4.15D)
  - The patient needs to abduct their arm. The X-ray plate is placed below their armpit and an X-ray is taken from above the shoulder down towards the armpit.
  - The humeral head should sit on the glenoid (like a golf ball sitting on a golf tee).
  - The coracoid and acromion point anteriorly.

- An anterior dislocation is present if the humeral head lies anterior to the glenoid. Conversely, with a posterior dislocation, the humeral head will be positioned posterior to the glenoid.
- Y view (Fig. 4.15B)
  - The patient extends their upper arm and the X-ray is taken from the medial aspect of the scapula, obliquely, towards the humeral head.
  - The coracoid, scapular spine/acromion and scapular blade form a Y shape and the humeral head should sit directly over the centre of the Y.
  - If the humeral head lies anterior (towards the ribs and coracoid), then there is an anterior dislocation. If it lies posteriorly (towards the acromion), there is a posterior dislocation.
- Apical oblique (Fig. 4.15C)
  - The same patient positioning as for an AP X-ray. The difference is the X-ray tube is elevated approximately 45 degrees to the horizontal.
  - With anterior dislocations, the humeral head will lie anteroinferior to the glenoid, whereas it will lie posteriorly in posterior dislocations.

❶ KEY POINT

A shoulder joint effusion can result in the inferior displacement of the humeral head, which may give the impression of a dislocation.

ELBOW

X-rays of the elbow consist of an AP and lateral view.
Look at the AP view (Fig. 4.17A):
- Trace around the cortices for disruption and look for lucent or sclerotic lines within the medulla, signifying a fracture.
- Assess the radiocapitellar line (a line drawn along the neck of the radius should intersect the midpoint of the capitellum). Disruption of this line indicates a dislocated radial head.
  Assess the lateral view (Fig. 4.17B):
- Trace around the cortices for disruption and look for lucent or sclerotic lines within the medulla, signifying a fracture. The 'champagne flute' within the distal humerus should be intact (Fig. 4.18) – a break in the stem of the 'champagne flute' indicates a supracondylar fracture.
- Assess the radiocapitellar line, as mentioned earlier. Again, disruption to this indicates a radial head dislocation.
- Assess the anterior humeral line (a line drawn down the anterior aspect of the distal humerus intersecting the capitellum, with at least one-third of the capitellum anterior to it). You must consider a supracondylar fracture if less than one-third of the capitellum is anterior to the anterior humeral line (Fig. 4.19).
- Look for evidence of an effusion by assessing the fat pads. Normally, a thin anterior fat pad (lucent area anterior to the distal humerus) is visible. If this is elevated, resulting in a triangular appearance (the sail sign), or a posterior fat pad is visible, then an elbow effusion is present (see Fig. 4.18).

> **❗ KEY POINT**
>
> In the context of trauma, an elbow effusion suggests there is likely to be an underlying fracture (usually radial head in adults and supracondylar fracture of the humerus in children). The joint effusion may be reactive as a result of a soft tissue injury around the elbow, but if there are concerns of a fracture then either further imaging is needed, such as a CT, or the patient should be treated as having a presumed fracture.

> **❗ KEY POINT**
>
> Fractures of the forearm bones can be associated with a second injury at the elbow or wrist. Ulnar shaft fractures with associated radial head dislocation are known as a Monteggia fracture, whereas a radial fracture with disruption of the DRUJ is known as a Galeazzi fracture.

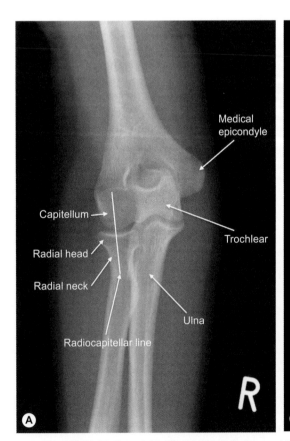
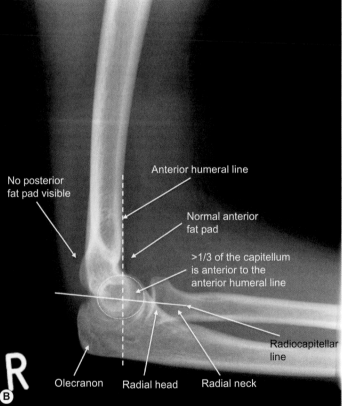

Fig. 4.17 Normal AP **(A)** and lateral **(B)** X-rays of the elbow, demonstrating the normal appearance of the radiocapitellar lines, the anterior humeral line and the anterior fat pad.

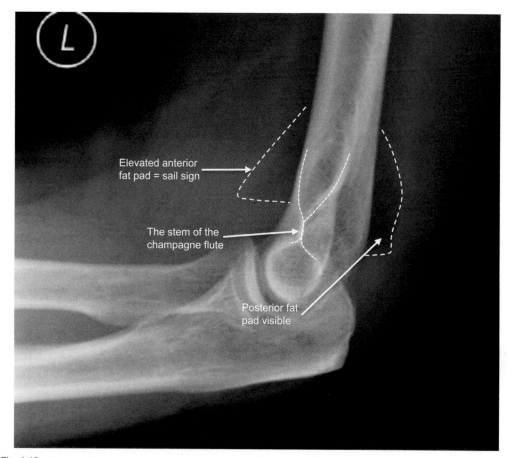

Fig. 4.18 A lateral elbow X-ray demonstrating elevation of the anterior fat pad (forming the sail sign) and the presence of a posterior fat pad, indicating an elbow joint effusion. In the context of trauma, an underlying occult fracture should be suspected. The stem of the 'champagne flute' is intact.

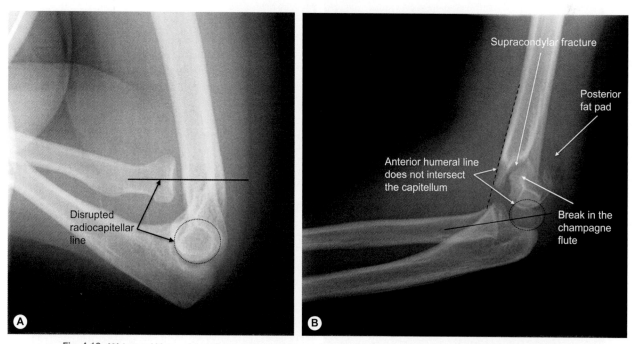

Fig. 4.19 **(A)** Lateral X-ray of the elbow demonstrating a disrupted radiocapitellar line, indicating dislocation of the radial head. **(B)** Lateral X-ray of the elbow showing an abnormal anterior humeral line as a result of a supracondylar fracture. The posterior fat pad is visible, indicating a joint effusion.

Ossification centres:

Ossification centres are present in children, and simply put, they are sites of bone formation (Fig. 4.20). There are six ossification centres around the elbow, which can make interpreting a child's X-ray a little more difficult. The order in which these ossification centres appear is fairly constant and can be remembered by the acronym CRITOE (Capitellum (aged 1), Radial head (aged 3), Internal/medial epicondyle (aged 5), Trochlear (aged 7), Olecranon (age 9), External epicondyle (age 11)).

Knowing the order of ossification is helpful. The most important reason for this is that the site of an ossification centre may be mistaken for a fracture. It is also important in the diagnosis of an avulsion injury to the internal/medial epicondyle (the ossification centre which appears at approximately age 5). This is the site of the origin of the elbow flexors. Avulsion injuries can occur here, particularly in children.

If completely avulsed, the medial epicondyle may lie in the joint and might be easily overlooked as you may think that the medial epicondyle is not present on the X-ray because it has not yet ossified. Consider both the age of the patient, and the presence of other ossification centres. If the trochlear ossification centre (or the olecranon/external epicondyle) is visible but the medial epicondyle centre is not present, then it is possible that the medial epicondyle is in an abnormal position. You must therefore suspect an avulsion of the medial epicondyle.

The Gartland classification system is useful for categorising the severity of supracondylar fractures, and the X-ray features are summarised in Table 4.1. It relates to 'extension type' supracondylar injury, where the distal fragment is displaced posteriorly. Flexion type injuries comprise 5% of supracondylar fractures, and are classified separately.

WRIST

The standard X-rays are a PA and lateral view.

Look at the PA X-ray (Fig. 4.21A):

- Trace around the cortices of the bones, looking for evidence of irregularity/disruption and look for lucent or sclerotic lines within the medulla, signifying a fracture. An ulnar styloid fracture is commonly seen with a distal radius fracture.
- There should be a uniform gap between the carpal bones. If this is not the case, you should suspect a fracture/ligament injury (Fig. 4.22). The commonest injury is to the scapholunate ligaments and results in a widening of the scapholunate joint.
- The proximal and distal rows of carpal bones should form smooth arcs.

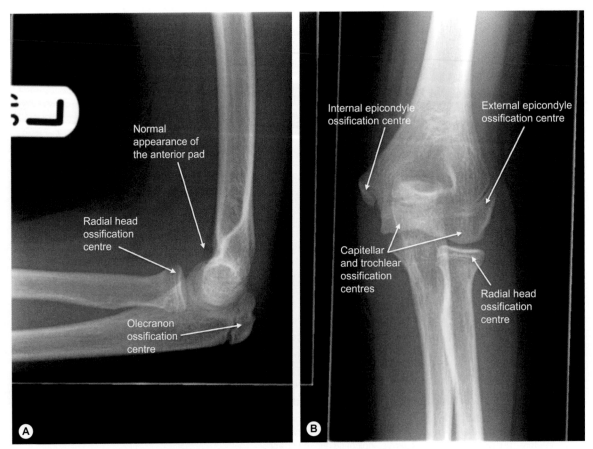

Fig. 4.20 Lateral **(A)** and AP **(B)** elbow X-rays demonstrating the various ossification centres (CRITOE). *CRITOE,* Capitellum, Radial head, Medial/Internal epicondyle, Trochlear, Olecranon, External/Lateral epicondyle.

Table 4.1   The Gartland Classification for Supracondylar Fractures

GARTLAND 1	GARTLAND 2	GARTLAND 3
Anterior humeral line. Humerus Capitellum Radius Ulna	Posterior cortex intact Anterior humeral line doesn't transect capitellum	Complete displacement
An **undisplaced** supracondylar fracture. A line drawn along the anterior edge of the humerus (anterior humeral line) transects the capitellum.	This is a displaced supracondylar fracture but the **posterior cortex of the distal humerus is intact.** However, the anterior humeral line now does not transect the capitellum.	This is a **completely displaced** supracondylar fracture, and the posterior cortex of the distal humerus is not intact. These are the injuries most often associated with neurovascular compromise and compartment syndrome.

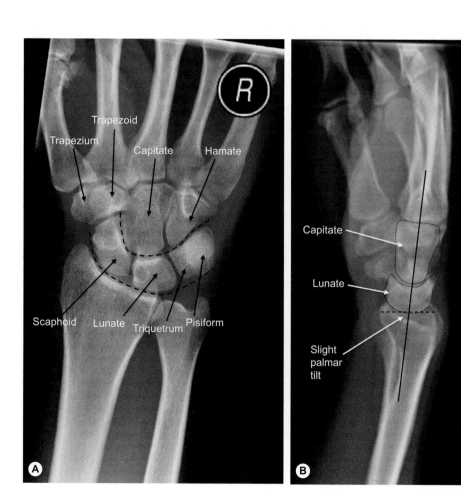

Fig. 4.21 Normal X-rays of the wrist. **(A)** The PA X-ray shows the normal alignment of the proximal and distal rows of the carpal bones. **(B)** The lateral X-ray shows the normal alignment of the distal radius, lunate and capitates. The normal slight volar/palmar angulation of distal radius is also demonstrated.

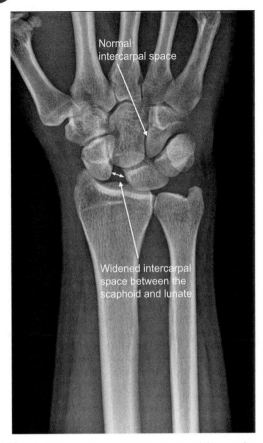

Fig. 4.22 This PA X-ray may initially appear normal, but on closer inspection, the intercarpal space between the scaphoid and lunate is widened (compare this to the space between the other carpal bones). This indicates damage to the scapholunate ligaments and is a serious injury requiring orthopaedic assessment.

- Remember to look at the imaged metacarpals for evidence of fractures.
  On the lateral view (Fig. 4.21B):
- Trace around the cortices for disruption and look for lucent or sclerotic lines within the medulla, signifying a fracture. In particular, the dorsal surface of the distal radius should be smooth – an irregularity here may be the only evidence of an undisplaced fracture (Fig. 4.23).
- The articular surface of the distal radius should have a slight volar angulation. If this is not the case, you should again suspect a distal radial fracture (distal radial fractures typically result in dorsal angulation).
- The distal radius, lunate and capitate should line up in a straight line. A lunate dislocation results in the anterior (palmar) dislocation of the lunate, whereas a perilunate dislocation results in the dorsal dislocation of the capitate, with the lunate remaining in its anatomical position.
- There should be no bone fragments over the dorsal surface of the carpal bones. If you see any bone fragments in this position, you should suspect a triquetral fracture (Fig. 4.24).

ULNAR VARIANCE, RADIAL INCLINATION AND VOLAR ANGULATION

These measurements are helpful for assessing if there is pathology (Fig. 4.25). They are also used by orthopaedic surgeons when assessing the severity of a fracture and adequacy of the subsequent reduction. They are not core knowledge for medical students but useful principles to understand (Table 4.2).

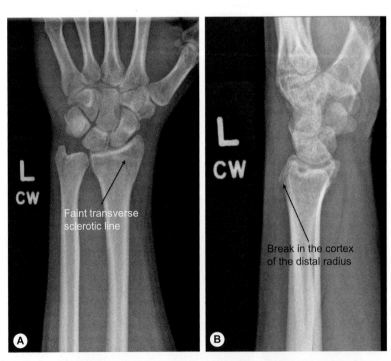

Fig. 4.23 Most distal radius fractures are obvious; however, these X-rays show how subtle they can be. **(A)** The PA X-ray is normal, apart from the faint sclerotic line in the distal radius. **(B)** The lateral view reveals a break in the dorsal cortex of the distal radius, confirming a minimally displaced fracture.

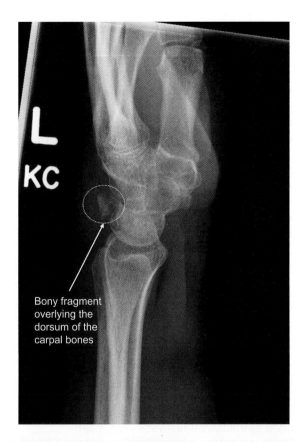

Fig. 4.24 This lateral wrist X-ray shows a bone fragment over the dorsum of the carpal bones. A fracture fragment in this location is pathognomonic of a triquetral fracture.

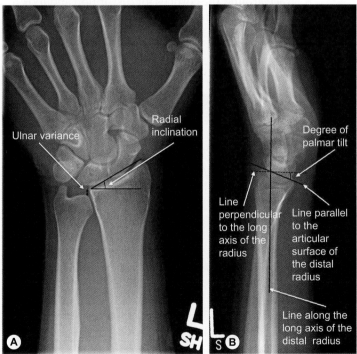

Fig. 4.25 PA and lateral views of a normal left wrist. **(A)** shows how to assess the ulnar variance and radial inclination. **(B)** demonstrates how to calculate the palmar (or dorsal) tilt.

Table **4.2**	Radiological Parameters of the Distal Radius	
TERM	**DEFINITION**	**NORMAL**
Ulna Variance	Difference in height between ulna and radius visible on AP X-ray	Normally the ulna is between 2 mm longer and 2 mm shorter than the radius
Radial Inclination	Angle between tip of radial styloid and distal radioulnar joint visible on AP X-ray	Normal is approximately 22 degrees
Volar Angulation	Describes the tilt/angulation of the distal radius visible on lateral X-ray	Normal is approximately 12 degrees volar (palmar) angulation

In a Colles' fracture, the radius will shorten, increasing the ulna variance (making the ulna relatively long); the radial styloid will lose its shape and reduce the radial inclination; and the radius will have a dorsal tilt rather than the normal palmar tilt.

PELVIS AND HIP

The standard view of the pelvis is the AP X-ray. If there is concern regarding a femoral neck fracture, a lateral view of that hip should also be performed.

On the AP pelvis view (Fig. 4.26A):

- Trace around the cortices for disruption and look for lucent or sclerotic lines within the medulla, signifying a fracture.
- The three bony rings (main pelvic ring and two smaller obturator rings formed by the pubic rami) in the pelvis should be intact.
- The ilioischial and iliopubic lines should be continuous and smooth with no breaks (Fig. 4.27).
- The sacroiliac joints should be of equal width. The arcuate lines of the sacrum (curved horizontal lines on the left and right sides of the sacrum which represent the superior aspect of the sacral nerve exit foramina) should be intact – these can be difficult to assess on X-ray and are better demonstrated on CT.
- The pubic symphysis should be less than 5 mm wide.

- Most neck of femur fractures are displaced and easy to detect.
- Characterise the site of fracture as this affects management and prognosis (Figs 4.28–4.29):
  - Draw a line between the greater and lesser trochanters.
  - A fracture proximal to this line is intracapsular.
  - A fracture distal is extracapsular (roughly speaking).
- If you cannot identify a fracture, look closely for:
  - Disruption to the cortex – look for a step, buckle or gap.
  - Interrupted trabecular pattern.
  - A transverse region of sclerosis (caused by impacted fracture).
  - Shenton's line (normally a smooth curve composed of the inferior edge of the superior pubic ramus and the medial side of the femur); if Shenton's line shows a sudden sharp angle, the fracture is nearby.
  - Changes on the lateral view (more easily missed than on the AP view).
- Look for acetabular and pubic rami fractures which can present with similar symptoms to neck of femur fractures.

Look at the lateral hip view (Fig. 4.26B):

- Trace around the cortices for disruption and look for lucent or sclerotic lines within the medulla, signifying a fracture.

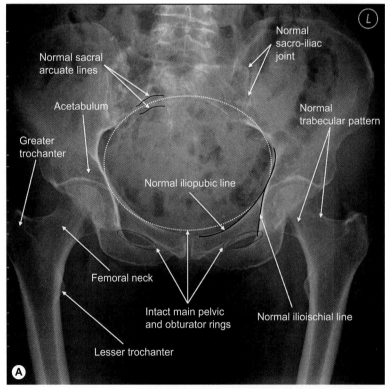
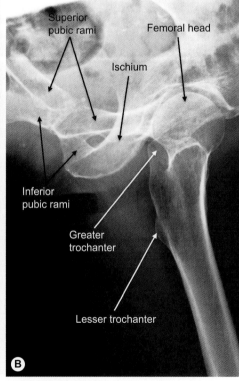

Fig. 4.26 **(A)** Normal AP X-ray of the pelvis. **(B)** Normal lateral X-ray of the hip.

Classification systems are useful for grading the severity, and choosing appropriate management for intracapsular and extracapsular fractures. The X-ray features in the Garden classification for intracapsular neck of femur fractures is summarised in Table 4.3. The X-ray features in the 2 to 4 parts classification of extracapsular neck of femur fractures (this is specific for intertrochanteric fractures) are summarised in Table 4.4.

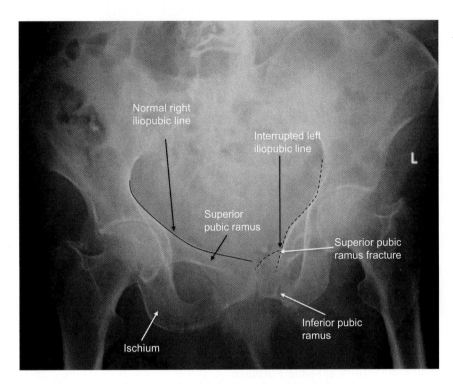

Fig. 4.27 AP pelvis X-ray showing interruption of the left iliopubic line due to a superior pubic ramus fracture.

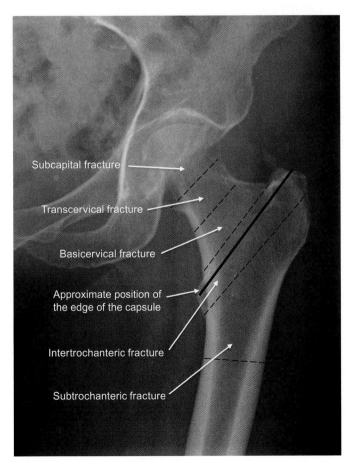

Fig. 4.28 The AP view of the left hip demonstrates the locations of different types of femoral neck fractures. The important distinction is between an intracapsular and extracapsular fracture. Subcapital and transcervical are intracapsular fractures. Intertrochanteric and subtrochanteric are extracapsular. Basicervical fractures can be intra- or extracapsular depending on their exact position.

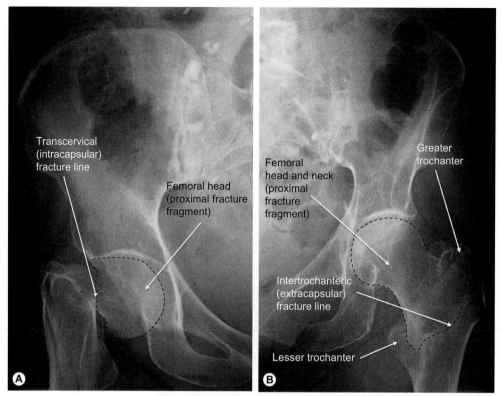

Fig. 4.29 (A) AP X-ray showing a displaced right intracapsular (transcervical) fracture. **(B)** AP X-ray showing a minimally displaced extracapsular (intertrochanteric) fracture.

Table **4.3**	The Garden Classification for Intracapsular Neck of Femur Fractures

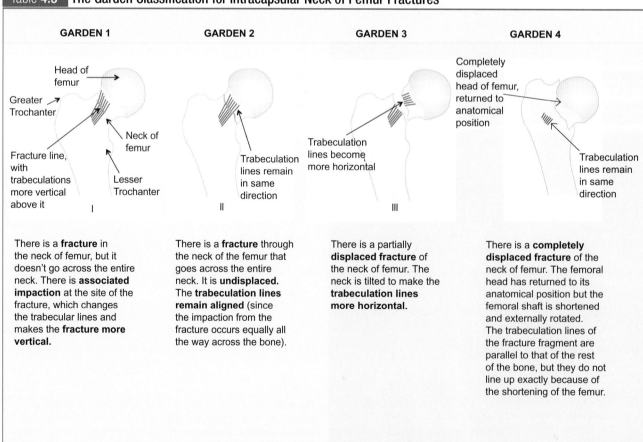

GARDEN 1	GARDEN 2	GARDEN 3	GARDEN 4
There is a **fracture** in the neck of femur, but it doesn't go across the entire neck. There is **associated impaction** at the site of the fracture, which changes the trabecular lines and makes the **fracture more vertical.**	There is a **fracture** through the neck of the femur that goes across the entire neck. It is **undisplaced.** The **trabeculation lines remain aligned** (since the impaction from the fracture occurs equally all the way across the bone).	There is a partially **displaced fracture** of the neck of femur. The neck is tilted to make the **trabeculation lines more horizontal.**	There is a **completely displaced fracture** of the neck of femur. The femoral head has returned to its anatomical position but the femoral shaft is shortened and externally rotated. The trabeculation lines of the fracture fragment are parallel to that of the rest of the bone, but they do not line up exactly because of the shortening of the femur.

Table 4.4 The 2 to 4 Parts Classification of Intertrochanteric (Extracapsular) Neck of Femur Fractures

2 PARTS	3 PARTS	4 PARTS

Neck of Femur · Greater Trochanter · Head of Femur · Lesser Trochanter · Two parts · Three parts · Four parts

There are **two parts** to the fracture.

There is the fragment which includes the **femoral head and neck** and the part which includes the **shaft of the femur**.

There are **three parts** to the fracture.

There is now a fracture of the **lesser trochanter.**

This can be a single fragment - as shown here, or may be comminuted (so although it is '3 parts' there may be more pieces).

There are **four parts** to the fracture.

There is now also a fracture of the **greater trochanter.**

This can be a single fragment or may be comminuted.

KNEE

The standard X-rays are AP and lateral views (Figs 4.30–4.31).
Assess the AP view:
- Trace around the cortices for disruption and look for lucent or sclerotic lines within the medulla, signifying a fracture.
- Look specifically for tibial plateau fractures – these are often depressed and difficult to identify. A vertical line drawn along the lateral margin of the lateral femoral condyle should have no more than 5 mm of the lateral tibial plateau outside it. If this rule is broken, you should suspect a tibial plateau fracture.
- Ensure that you look at the fibular neck for evidence of a fracture.

Look at the lateral view:
- Trace around the cortices for disruption and look for lucent or sclerotic lines within the medulla, signifying a fracture.
- Look for evidence of an effusion. The suprapatellar pouch should contain only fat density. An almond-shaped soft tissue shadow projected over this site is in keeping with an effusion.
- A fat–fluid level in the suprapatellar pouch indicates a lipohaemarthrosis, which implies there is an intraarticular fracture.
- Patellar fractures are often most easily seen on the lateral view.
- Ensure that you look at the fibular neck for evidence of a fracture.

> **KEY POINT**
>
> A normal knee X-ray does not exclude significant ligamentous or cartilage injury.

ANKLE

The standard views are an AP mortice view (an AP X-ray with approximately 15 degrees internal rotation) and a lateral view (Figs 4.32–4.33).
Look at the AP mortice view:
- Trace around the cortices for disruption and look for lucent or sclerotic lines within the medulla, signifying a fracture.
- The ankle joint space should be equal all around the talus. The medial clear space is the distance

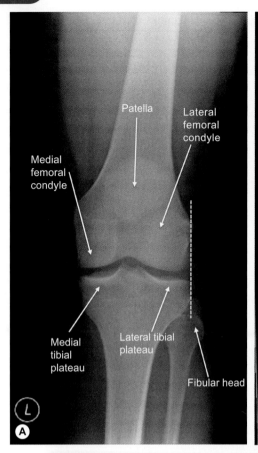

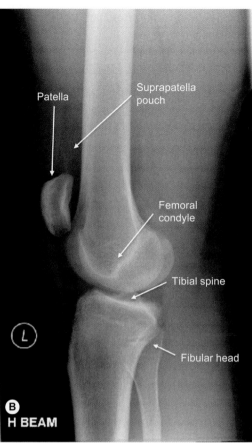

Fig. 4.30 (A) Normal AP X-ray of the left knee. A vertical line (*dotted line*) drawn along the lateral aspect of the lateral femoral condyle should have no more than 5 mm of the lateral tibial plateau outside it. (B) Normal lateral X-ray. Note the suprapatellar pouch has a homogenous lucency. Any ovoid soft tissue density in this area is suggestive of an effusion.

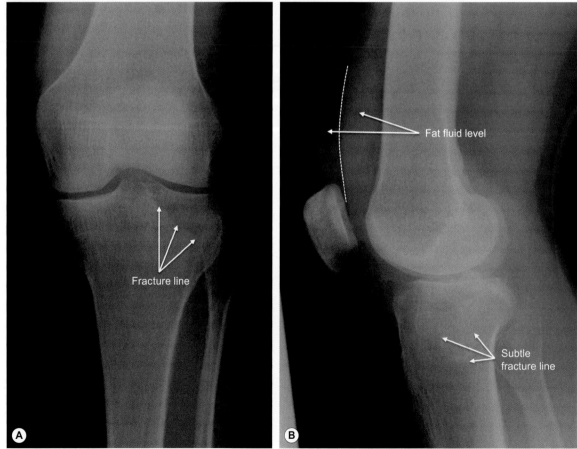

Fig. 4.31 (A) AP knee X-ray showing a subtle fracture line in the lateral tibial plateau. (B) Lateral knee X-ray showing a joint effusion with a fat–fluid level, indicating a lipohaemarthrosis. A subtle area of sclerosis is visible in the proximal tibia, in keeping with a fracture.

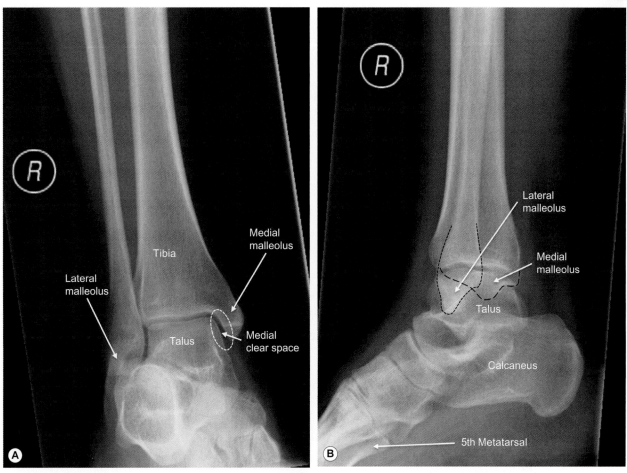

Fig. 4.32 Normal AP **(A)** and lateral **(B)** ankle X-rays. The medial clear space is shown on the AP X-ray.

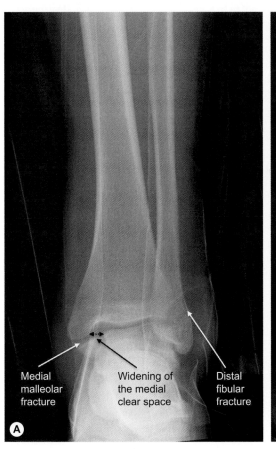

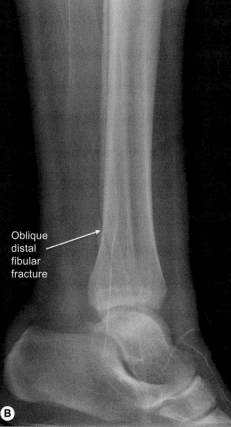

Fig. 4.33 **(A)** AP view of the left ankle showing a fracture through the medial malleolus with medial displacement of the distal fragment. A fracture through the distal fibula, at the level of the syndesmosis, is also visible (Weber B). There is some rotation of the patient's ankle making assessment difficult but the medial clear space appears widened, in keeping with talar shift. **(B)** Lateral view showing the minimally displaced oblique distal fibular fracture more clearly.

between the talus and medial malleolus. If the space is greater than 4 mm, this suggests there is talar shift.

- The top of the talus bone (talar dome) should have a smooth surface.

Assess the lateral view:

- Trace around the cortices for disruption and look for lucent or sclerotic lines within the medulla, signifying a fracture.
- Look particularly at the posterior tibial surface (the 'posterior malleolus') and the base of the 5th metatarsal.
- Fractures of the calcaneus may be visible.

The Weber classification is useful for categorising lateral malleolar fractures, and the X-ray features are summarised in Table 4.5.

GROWTH PLATE FRACTURES

These are specific to fractures in children, and can potentially occur in any bone where the growth plates are not fused. Growth plates are areas of cartilage tissue near the end of long bonus, such as the ulna. Damage to the growth plate can potentially impair long-term bone development, and therefore appropriate recognition and management of growth plate fractures is important. Table 4.6 summarises the X-ray features of growth plate fractures based on the Salter–Harris classification.

Tables 4.7 and 4.8 summarise the important eponymous fractures and eponymous X-ray terminology. You can use the checklist in Table 4.9 to assess the musculoskeletal X-rays shown in this chapter.

Case examples follow (Case 4.1–Case 4.20).

Table **4.5** | Weber Classification of Ankle Fractures

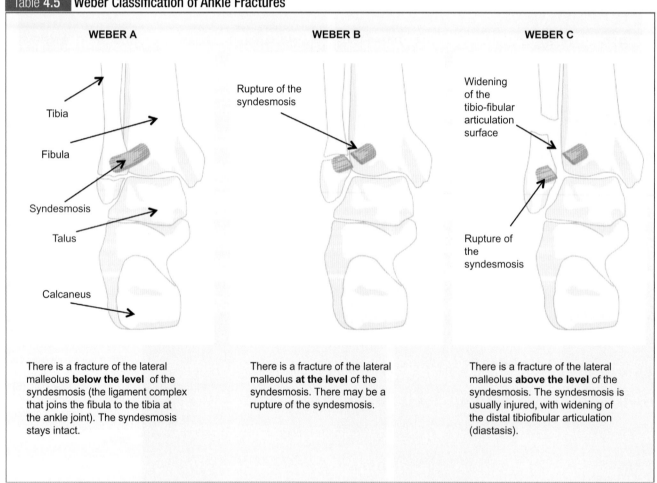

WEBER A	WEBER B	WEBER C

Tibia

Fibula

Syndesmosis

Talus

Calcaneus

Rupture of the syndesmosis

Widening of the tibio-fibular articulation surface

Rupture of the syndesmosis

There is a fracture of the lateral malleolus **below the level** of the syndesmosis (the ligament complex that joins the fibula to the tibia at the ankle joint). The syndesmosis stays intact.

There is a fracture of the lateral malleolus **at the level** of the syndesmosis. There may be a rupture of the syndesmosis.

There is a fracture of the lateral malleolus **above the level** of the syndesmosis. The syndesmosis is usually injured, with widening of the distal tibiofibular articulation (diastasis).

Table **4.6**   Salter–Harris Classification of Growth Plate Fractures

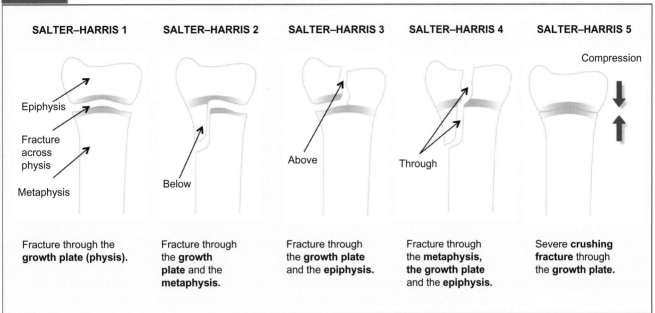

SALTER–HARRIS 1	SALTER–HARRIS 2	SALTER–HARRIS 3	SALTER–HARRIS 4	SALTER–HARRIS 5
Fracture through the **growth plate (physis)**.	Fracture through the **growth plate** and the **metaphysis**.	Fracture through the **growth plate** and the **epiphysis**.	Fracture through the **metaphysis, the growth plate** and the **epiphysis**.	Severe **crushing fracture** through the **growth plate**.

Table **4.7**   Eponymous Fractures

NAME	X-RAY APPEARANCE	DESCRIPTION OF INJURY
Bennett's fracture	There is an intraarticular fracture through the base of the thumb.	Intraarticular fracture at the base of thumb. There is often associated subluxation of the thumb metacarpophalangeal joint, which needs reduction and fixation.
Burst fracture	There is loss of the vertebral height of both the anterior and middle columns of the vertebral body best seen on the lateral X-ray.	An unstable fracture of the vertebral column following compression/axial loading type injury, such as a fall from height. It is similar to a Jefferson fracture but can occur anywhere in the spine.
Chance fracture	There is a transverse fracture line running through a vertebral body and there is loss of the normal alignment of the vertebral column.	An unstable fracture of the spinal column. It follows a flexion type injury and is often associated with lap belt injuries. There is a compression fracture of the vertebral body with a transverse fracture through the posterior vertebral elements.
Colles' fracture	There is dorsal angulation and shortening of the distal radius.	A fracture of the distal radius which is extraarticular and typically occurs in osteoporotic bone following a low-energy fall onto an outstretched hand.
Galeazzi fracture	The ulna dislocates at the distal radio-ulnar joint and there is an associated fracture of the radial shaft.	Pain and soft tissue swelling in the distal third of the radius, and around the wrist. May be associated with an anterior interosseous nerve palsy.
Hangman's fracture	There is a subluxation of C2 on C3 with disruption of the anterior vertebral line.	An unstable fracture of C2 resulting from hyperextension and traction-type injury, such as hanging. There are bilateral fractures of both of the C2 pars interarticularis or pedicles with anterior subluxation/dislocation of the C2 vertebral body.
Hill–Sachs lesion	There is an impacted fracture of the humeral head.	A lesion seen on the humeral head following an anterior shoulder dislocation. This is an impacted fracture which looks like a divot on X-ray and occurs as the humeral head impacts on the glenoid during the dislocation.
Holstein–Lewis fracture	There is a fracture through the junction between the middle/distal third of the humerus which is most commonly spiral in nature.	Fracture of the middle/distal third junction of the humeral shaft. There is an association with a radial nerve palsy as the radial nerve is very close to the bone at this point.

Continue

Table **4.7**   **Eponymous Fractures –** *Contd.*

NAME	X-RAY APPEARANCE	DESCRIPTION OF INJURY
Jefferson fracture	The odontoid peg view shows a lateral displacement of the lateral masses of C1.	An unstable fracture of C1 following compression/axial loading type injury. There are fractures of both the anterior and posterior arches of C1. It can be unilateral or bilateral, so check carefully for a bilateral injury if a unilateral injury is seen.
Jones fracture	There is a fracture through the base of the fifth metatarsal.	This is an avulsion fracture through the base of the fifth metatarsal and is associated with an increased incidence of nonunion. However, surgical fixation is generally unnecessary.
Lisfranc injury	There is disruption of the normal alignment between the 1st and 2nd metatarsals and the medial and intermediate cuneiforms, respectively.	This is a complex injury where there is disruption of the Lisfranc ligament which attaches from the second metatarsal base to the medial cuneiform. The structure stabilises the joint between the metatarsal bones and the tarsal bones (cuneiforms, cuboid). The injury can be very subtle on X-ray but CT usually shows multiple small fractures to the metatarsal bases as well as the tarsal bones.
Maisonneuve injury	There is disruption of the ankle mortice (the bony arch formed by the tibia and the two malleoli) with no fracture on ankle X-rays. X-rays of the knee reveal a proximal fibula fracture.	This is an injury which is sometimes missed and very important. The ankle mortice may look abnormal without any fracture on the ankle X-rays. There is, however, a fracture of the proximal fibula. The ankle joint is unstable and requires fixation.
Monteggia fracture	The radial head is dislocated and the ulna is fractured proximally.	A fracture of the proximal ulna with dislocation of the radial head.
Rolando's fracture	There is a comminuted intraarticular fracture through the base of the thumb.	This is a more serious injury than a Bennett's fracture. The fracture often occurs following higher-energy injury and generally requires surgical fixation.
Smith's fracture	There is volar angulation and shortening of the distal radius.	A fracture of the distal radius which is extraarticular. This is the opposite of a Colles' fracture and there is volar displacement of the distal fragment. This is a result of a fall onto the back of the hand.
Thurstan Holland fragment	There is a fracture of a growth plate (for example the distal radius). There is an associated metaphyseal fragment which is the Thurstan Holland fragment.	This is a fracture fragment associated with Salter–Harris type 2 fractures. The fracture line goes through the growth plate (physis) and then through the metaphysis. The metaphyseal fragment is the Thurstan Holland fragment.
Segond fracture	There is a small avulsion fracture fragment seen on the lateral aspect of the knee on the AP X-ray.	An avulsion fracture of the lateral tibial plateau which when seen following a knee injury is suggestive of an injury to the anterior cruciate ligament.
Volar Barton's fracture	There is a volarly displaced partially intraarticular fracture with radial shortening.	This fracture occurs at the distal radius. The fracture is partially intraarticular and the fracture fragment displaces volarly.

Table **4.8**   **Eponymous X-ray Terminology**

NAME	DESCRIPTION
Klein's line	This is a line drawn along the superior border of the femoral neck and is used to assess whether there may be a slipped upper femoral epiphysis (SUFE).
Shenton's line	A line drawn along the inferior border of the superior pubic ramus and the medial aspect of the femoral neck. If this line is disrupted, it suggests a fracture of the neck of femur.
Trethowan's sign	If Klein's line does not transect the femoral head, this is Trethowan's sign, and it is indicative of SUFE.
Wackenheim's line	This is a line used on the lateral X-ray of the cervical spine to assess the atlantooccipital joint. The line is drawn along the clivus and should transect the odontoid peg. If it does not, this suggests a possible atlantooccipital subluxation/dislocation.

Table **4.9**   Checklist for Assessing an X-ray

Technical Aspects	
Checks patient details (name, date of birth, hospital number)	✓
Checks the date of the X-rays	✓
Identifies the projections of the X-rays	✓
Assesses technical quality of X-ray (entire bone/joint included, adequate views)	✓
Obvious Abnormalities	
Describes any obvious abnormality	✓
Systematic Review of the Film	
Assesses the bones for fractures (cortical step, buckle, gap, disruption of the trabeculae)	✓
Comments on the joints (dislocation/subluxation)	✓
Assesses for joint effusions if appropriate (e.g. knee or elbow)	✓
Comments on degenerative joint changes	✓
Comment on abnormal bone texture (e.g. radiolucency consistent with osteopaenia)	✓
Describing fractures (if relevant)	✓
Which bone	✓
Which part of the bone (proximal, middle, distal third, intraarticular)	✓
Fracture pattern (simple/open, comminuted, impacted)	✓
Fracture type (transverse, oblique, spiral, greenstick)	✓
Displacement	✓
Angulation	✓
Rotation	✓
Shortening	✓
Summary	
Presents findings	✓
Reviews relevant previous imaging if appropriate	✓
Provides a differential diagnosis where appropriate	✓
Suggests appropriate further imaging/investigations if relevant	✓

CASE EXAMPLES

CASE **4.1**

A 49-year-old female presents to A&E with a 3-day history of progressive weakness of her right leg. This is associated with severe back pain and a feeling of difficulty passing urine. X-rays have been performed in A&E.

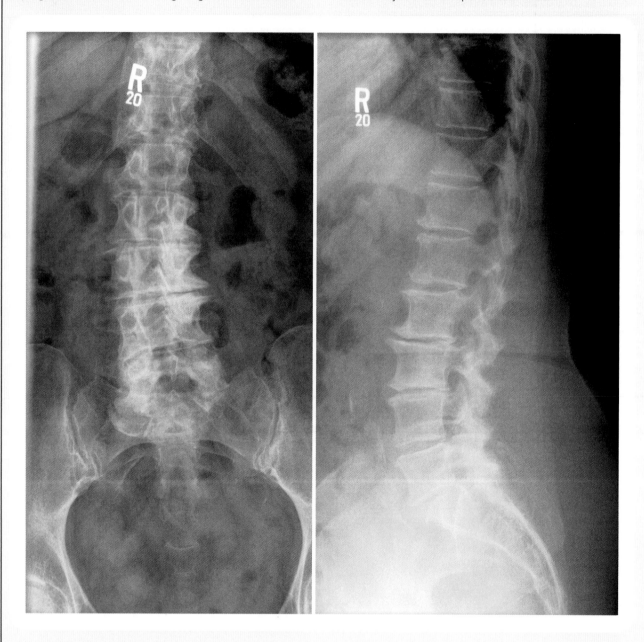

ANNOTATED X-RAY

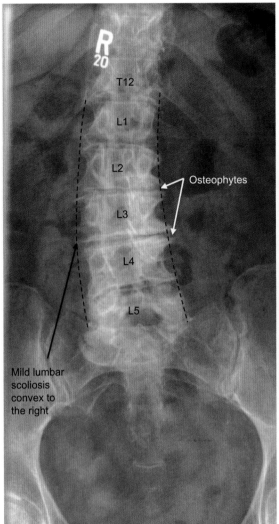

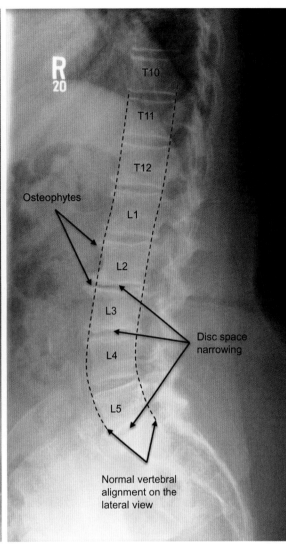

PRESENT YOUR FINDINGS

- These are AP and lateral X-rays of the lumbar spine in a skeletally mature patient.
- They have been anonymised and the timing of the examination is not available. I would like to confirm the patient's details and timing of the examination before I make any further assessment.
- The X-rays are adequately exposed, with no important areas cut off.
- There is a mild lumbar scoliosis convex to the right evident on the AP X-ray, which is probably degenerative in aetiology.
- The alignment of the imaged spine is otherwise normal.
- No evidence of a fracture.

- There are degenerative changes in the lumbar spine with loss of the normal disc height L2/3, L3/4 and L5/S1 and osteophyte formation most marked at L2/3.
- The sacroiliac joints appear normal.
- The bone texture is normal, with no lucent or sclerotic areas.

IN SUMMARY – These X-rays of the lumbar spine show lumbar degenerative changes, with a mild degenerative scoliosis. However, to exclude the diagnosis of cauda equina syndrome, further imaging in the form of an MRI will be required.

Continue

CASE **4.1**   *Contd.*

QUESTIONS

1. Which one of these features in a history of back pain is most suggestive of a cauda equina syndrome?
   A) Unilateral sciatica
   B) New urinary incontinence
   C) Altered sensation in the right leg
   D) Severe back pain
   E) Ineffective analgesia

2. Which of these examination findings is most suggestive of cauda equina syndrome?
   A) Altered sensation of the right leg in the L4 distribution
   B) Normal lower limb neurology
   C) Positive right leg sciatic stretch test
   D) Saddle anaesthesia
   E) Normal tone on digital rectal examination

3. What is the investigation of choice for diagnosing cauda equina syndrome?
   A) Lumbar spine X-rays
   B) Full blood count and CRP
   C) MRI lumbar spine
   D) CT myelogram
   E) Bladder scan

4. Which of these is a clear indication for emergency surgical decompression for cauda equina syndrome secondary to an acutely herniated disc?
   A) 12-hour history of severe back pain with bilateral sciatica, saddle anaesthesia and loss of anal tone, with a central disc compressing the cauda equina on MRI
   B) A 5-week history of dribbling urinary incontinence with bilateral sciatica and neurological findings
   C) Right-sided sciatica with progressive weakness of the right leg over 3 days with normal bowel and bladder function
   D) Persistent, unremitting back pain
   E) 5 weeks of unilateral sciatica with an L5 nerve root compression on MRI and normal bowel and bladder function

5. How is chronic simple back pain best managed?
   A) Elective spinal surgery
   B) Analgesia alone
   C) Physiotherapy alone
   D) Urgent spinal decompression
   E) A multidisciplinary approach including physiotherapists and specialists based in the community

ANSWERS TO QUESTIONS

1. Which one of these features in a history of back pain is most suggestive of cauda equina syndrome?
The correct answer is **B) New urinary incontinence**.
The vast majority of people will experience back pain at some point in their life. A group of these patients will go on to develop sciatica, which can be troubling. These patients complain of a shooting pain down their leg all the way to the foot like an electric shock. Back pain and sciatica can be managed without significant urgency. However, cauda equina syndrome is an emergency and if missed can lead to permanent loss of neurological function, including bowel and bladder function.

A) Unilateral sciatica – Incorrect. Sciatica is defined as a shooting pain which travels down the leg and below the knee. It is caused by irritation/compression of one of the spinal nerve roots which forms the sciatic nerve (L4 to S3) or the sciatic nerve itself. Unilateral sciatica suggests the nerve root rather than the cauda equina is being compressed. These cases are usually managed conservatively and most resolve spontaneously. Bilateral sciatic is more worrying. This suggests a central pathology (such as an intervertebral disc herniation) is compressing both nerve roots and therefore possibly the cauda equina as well.

B) New urinary incontinence – Correct. The cauda equina is the collection of nerve roots within the spinal canal below the termination of the spinal cord (conus medullaris). Cauda equina syndrome is caused by the compression of the cauda equina. This can be a result of intervertebral disc herniation, tumours, trauma, inflammatory conditions and spinal stenosis. It is characterised by bilateral sciatica and neurological symptoms such as altered sensation, urinary dysfunction and bowel incontinence. Not all of the symptoms may be present, and given the potential severity of the syndrome, it is important to have a high index of suspicion in all patients presenting with back pain and sciatica.

C) Altered sensation in the right leg – Incorrect. Altered sensation in the right leg suggests a nerve root irritation or possibly a central nervous system abnormality, such as a stroke. On its own, it is not suggestive of cauda equina compression.

D) Severe back pain – Incorrect. A portion of people who develop back pain find the pain uncontrollable and severe. This can have a huge impact on their life, and persistent severe pain warrants further investigation. However, severe back pain itself is not the most suggestive symptom of cauda equina syndrome. Such patients need to be managed with pain relief, not an emergency admission to hospital.

E) Ineffective analgesia – Incorrect. Back pain can be very troublesome and sometimes patients find they get very little relief from analgesia. However, this in itself is not especially suggestive of cauda equina compression.

> **KEY POINT**
>
> Back pain is common and most cases have a benign aetiology (although they can still be very debilitating). The history and examination are essential for identifying those patients with potentially sinister underlying causes. The red flags in the history for cauda equina syndrome are:
> - Bilateral sciatica
> - Saddle anaesthesia
> - Reduced anal tone
> - Urinary retention or incontinence
> - Faecal incontinence

2. Which of these examination findings is most suggestive of cauda equina syndrome?
The correct answer is **D) Saddle anaesthesia**.
There are several examination findings which suggest a possible cauda equina syndrome. These are saddle anaesthesia, loss of anal tone, bilateral abnormal neurological findings in the lower limbs and contralateral sciatica on straight leg raise. A careful examination with clear documentation is important for all patients with a possible cauda equina syndrome.

A) Altered sensation in the right leg in the L4 distribution – Incorrect. This is suggestive of an L4 nerve root compression rather than cauda equina syndrome.

B) Normal lower limb neurology – Incorrect. This finding suggests no nerve root involvement. However, make sure you examine for evidence of bowel or bladder dysfunction.

C) Positive right leg sciatic stretch test – Incorrect. This suggests nerve root compression rather than a cauda equina syndrome.

D) Saddle anaesthesia – Correct. Anaesthesia of the saddle area (perineum) is a worrying finding. Together with urinary incontinence or retention and reduced anal tone, this finding is suggestive of possible cauda equina syndrome. Some patients, however, will develop urinary symptoms secondary to severe pain without cauda equina compression. Regardless, if the symptoms are present, then cauda equina syndrome must be definitively excluded.

E) Normal tone on digital rectal examination – Incorrect. Digital rectal examination is an important part of examining the patient referred with possible cauda equina syndrome. Reduced anal tone is a worrying sign.

Continue

CASE **4.1**   *Contd.*

❶ KEY POINT

The cauda equina is composed of nerves and therefore lower motor neurones. Therefore the expected findings on examination in cauda equina syndrome include:

- Reduced tone
- Reduced power and altered sensation
- Reduced or absent reflexes
- Down-going plantar reflexes
- Bowel, bladder and sexual dysfunction occurring early in the course of the pathology

In contrast, the spinal cord is part of the central nervous system and composed of upper motor neurones. Therefore, spinal cord compression will lead to upper motor signs such as:

- Increased tone
- Reduced power and altered sensation
- Increased reflexes
- Up-going plantar reflexes
- Bowel, bladder and sexual dysfunction occurring relatively late in the course of the pathology

3. What is the investigation of choice for diagnosing cauda equina syndrome?

   The correct answer is **C) MRI lumbar spine**.

   Cauda equina syndrome is associated with significant morbidity. It is essential that it is diagnosed quickly and managed appropriately. Clinical assessment is important for identifying patients with possible compression of the cauda equina; however, imaging is needed to confirm the diagnosis and identify the underlying aetiology.

   A) Lumbar spine X-rays – Incorrect. Lumbar spine X-rays have specific uses, such as identifying fractures in patients following trauma. They can also show loss of the normal lumbar lordosis in patients with back pain. However, they provide little, if any, information about the spinal canal and they do not allow any assessment of the cauda equina. Therefore, they cannot diagnose or exclude cauda equina syndrome and are not indicated in such cases. In fact, the X-rays in this case should not have been performed as they are added radiation without providing any diagnostic information.

   B) Full blood count and CRP – Incorrect. Blood tests cannot diagnose cauda equina syndrome. However, if the concern is one of infection, such as osteomyelitis or discitis, then these tests have a role.

   C) MRI lumbar spine – Correct. MRI provides detailed images of the soft tissues of the spinal canal, including the thecal sac (dura surrounding the spinal cord/cauda equina), spinal cord, cauda equina, exiting nerve roots and the intervertebral discs. A noncontrast MRI can accurately demonstrate compression of the cauda equina and identify the underlying aetiology. It can also show compression of the nerve roots, which may result in sciatica. Examples of MRI scans of the spine are given (Chapter 6).

   D) CT myelogram – Incorrect. CT myelography (a CT scan performed after the injection of contrast material into the subarachnoid space) can be used to identify cauda equina compression in these patients; however, it involves ionising radiation and has been superseded by MRI. In patients with MRI-incompatible metalwork, such as certain metallic heart valves, CT myelography can be used.

   E) Bladder scan – Incorrect. A bladder scan is a useful, noninvasive bedside test for assessing the volume of the bladder. It is possible to look for incomplete emptying of the bladder or urinary retention, both of which may result from cauda equina syndrome. However, there are several other causes for these findings, plus bladder function may be normal. Therefore, it is not specific or sensitive for the diagnosis of cauda equina syndrome.

❶ KEY POINT

X-rays of the lumbar spine have no role in the diagnosis of patients with cauda equina compression. If you suspect cauda equina syndrome, you should request an urgent MRI of the lumbar spine (or whole spine, if the patient has known metastatic disease).

4. Which of these is a clear indication for emergency surgical decompression for cauda equina syndrome secondary to an acutely herniated disc?

   The correct answer is **A) 12-hour history of severe back pain with bilateral sciatica, saddle anaesthesia and loss of anal tone, with a central disc compressing the cauda equina on MRI**.

   Cauda equina syndrome needs urgent referral to a neurosurgeon for consideration of surgical decompression to prevent permanent loss of neurological function. Without this, the likelihood of bowel and bladder function returning to normal will reduce dramatically.

   A) 12-hour history of severe back pain with bilateral sciatica, saddle anaesthesia and loss of anal tone, with a central disc compressing the cauda equina on MRI – Correct. This is the clinical picture of a cauda equina syndrome. Their symptoms are very acute and with an emergency decompression, there is a good chance of return of normal/near normal neurological function. However, after 24 hours the likelihood of normal neurological returning reduces significantly.

   B) A 5-week history of dribbling urinary incontinence with bilateral sciatica and neurological findings – Incorrect. Acute cauda equina syndrome is thankfully rare. However, a lot of people with chronic back pain may develop urinary symptoms or may present having had these symptoms for some time. This is not an emergency, although it requires urgent investigation. The 24-hour window has passed and therefore the patient can have an MRI scan within 48 hours. It is, however, worth discussing the case with a neurosurgeon.

   C) Right-sided sciatica with progressive weakness of the right leg over 3 days with normal bowel and bladder function – Incorrect. This is not in keeping with a cauda equina syndrome. However, progressive weakness of a limb with sciatica and suspected nerve root compression is a relative emergency and some neurosurgeons will consider early intervention. Therefore, patients with motor loss on examination should be considered for an urgent MRI.

D) Persistent, unremitting back pain – Incorrect. Surgery in the presence of back pain alone can make things much worse. It should not be performed as an emergency, but instead only be considered in specialised cases after careful assessment of and discussion with the patient.

E) Five weeks of unilateral sciatica with an L5 nerve root compression on MRI and normal bowel and bladder function – Incorrect. This is not an emergency but may be a suitable case for decompression of the nerve root. Decompression involves removing a small piece of bone around the nerve root (laminectomy) and removing the offending piece of disc which is causing the compression (discectomy). However, there is no need to rush as timing of surgery in this situation does not significantly affect the success rate of the surgery.

🛈 KEY POINT

Cauda equina is a syndrome characterised by bowel and bladder disturbance and sciatica, not by back pain. In fact, the patient with a true cauda equina syndrome may not have back pain. Cauda equina syndrome from a herniated disc also tends to present in younger patients who have developed all the red flags rapidly over 12 or 24 hours.

5. How is chronic simple back pain best managed?
The correct answer is **E) A multidisciplinary approach including physiotherapists and specialists based in the community**.

Simple back pain is a huge burden on those who suffer it. A further burden is placed on healthcare systems, and society in general. By managing these patients appropriately in the community, you can improve their symptoms, help them return to work and reduce ED and hospital admissions.

A) Elective spinal surgery – Incorrect. Surgery may make the back pain worse and is reserved for particular causes of back pain, such as cauda equina compression, some symptomatic disc herniations and some patients with spinal canal stenosis.

B) Analgesia alone – Incorrect. Adequate analgesia is important to allow the patient to remain mobile and prevent the patient from becoming bed bound. Analgesia alone is often not sufficient for those patients with ongoing problematic back pain.

C) Physiotherapy alone – Incorrect. Physiotherapy is an important part of treating back pain. Physiotherapists can help keep patients mobile, help reduce the pain and perform daily activities. However, in isolation, it is not the best management for back pain.

D) Urgent spinal decompression – Incorrect. This is only indicated for cauda equina syndrome and not simple back pain.

E) A multidisciplinary approach including physiotherapists and specialists based in the community – Correct. This is the approach of choice for back pain. Most hospitals and the surrounding community have a team which manages these patients to limit the burden on the acute hospital and allow patients to remain at work. Often the cause of chronic back pain is uncertain. The team will involve specialist doctors, physiotherapists, occupational therapists, pain specialists and surgeons.

👥 IMPORTANT LEARNING POINTS

- Back pain is common and is a large burden on the patient and health service.
- Most causes of back pain are benign; however, those with a sinister aetiology need to be recognised and treated appropriately.
- Cauda equina syndrome is a serious condition caused by compression of the cauda equina, usually by a herniated intervertebral disc.
- It is characterised not by back pain but by lower motor neurone signs in the perineum and lower limbs, including saddle anaesthesia and bladder and bowel disturbance.
- If suspected, an urgent MRI should be performed; X-rays have no role in the diagnosis of cauda equina syndrome.
- Cauda equina syndrome is an emergency. When secondary to a herniated disc, it warrants urgent referral to a neurosurgeon for consideration of surgical decompression. Malignant deposits causing cauda equina syndrome are often managed with corticosteroids and radiotherapy.

CASE **4.2**

A 35-year-old woman has been thrown from her horse at high speed. She landed on her back and was trampled by the horse. She has been brought to A&E, where she is complaining of severe pain in her lumbar spine.

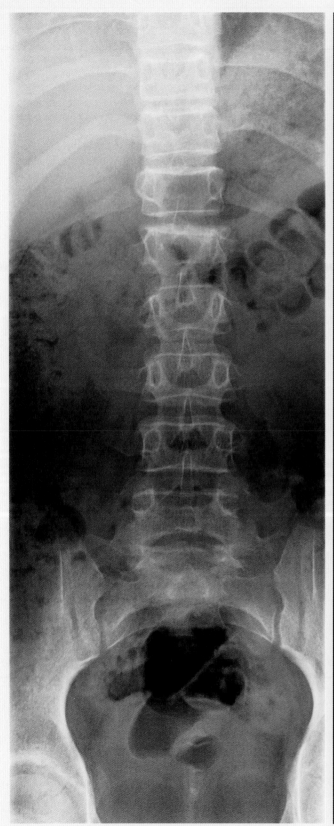
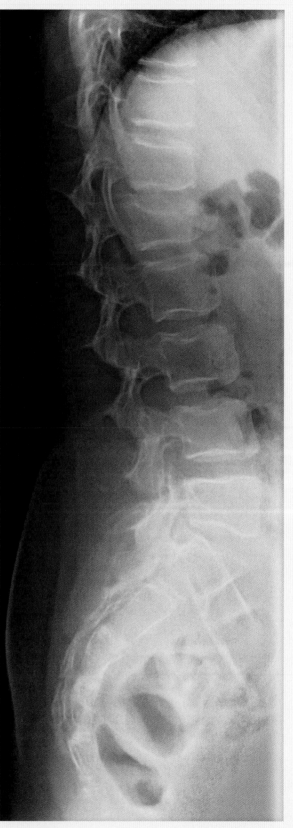

ANNOTATED X-RAY

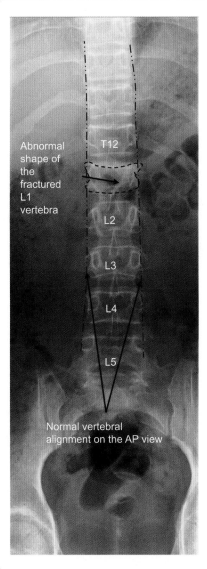

Abnormal shape of the fractured L1 vertebra

T12

Possible minor retropulsion of the posterior cortex

L2

L3

L4

L5

Normal vertebral alignment on the AP view

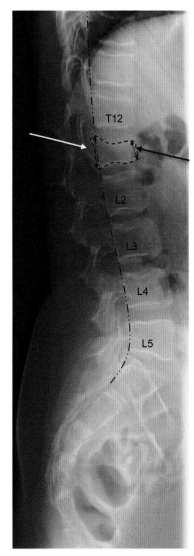

T12

Anterior wedge compression fracture with ~50% loss of height

L2

L3

L4

L5

PRESENT YOUR FINDINGS

- These are AP and lateral X-rays of the lumbar spine in a skeletally mature patient.
- They have been anonymised and the timing of the examination is not available. I would like to confirm the patient's details and timing of the examination before I make any further assessment.
- The X-rays are adequately exposed, with no important areas cut off.
- There is a fracture of L1. There is a reduction in height of the anterior cortex (of approximately 50%), in keeping with a wedge fracture. There is a suspicion of minor retropulsion of the posterior cortex of L1 into the spinal canal.
- The alignment of the spine is otherwise normal.
- No other fractures are visible.
- The bone texture appears normal, with no areas of lucency or sclerosis.
- The sacroiliac joints appear normal.
- There are no soft tissue abnormalities.

IN SUMMARY – These X-rays show an anterior wedge compression fracture of L1 with collapse of approximately 50%. I am also concerned there may be some retropulsion of the posterior cortex. Therefore, the fracture should be considered unstable and a CT is required for further assessment. Prior to CT, I would like to fully assess the patient using the ABCDE ATLS approach to ensure she is stable and identify any other areas which may require further imaging.

Continue

CASE **4.2**   *Contd.*

QUESTIONS

1. Which of these is a stable fracture of the spine?
   A) Anterior wedge fracture with 10% wedging
   B) Burst fracture
   C) Chance fracture
   D) Fracture dislocation of L2
   E) Jefferson fracture
2. Which type of injury is most commonly associated with Chance fractures?
   A) Pneumothorax
   B) Aortic transection
   C) Major head injury
   D) Abdominal and retroperitoneal injuries
   E) Bilateral calcaneal fractures
3. A patient suffers a spinal fracture and has no sensation from the umbilicus down, no lower limb reflexes or lower limb motor activity bilaterally. Upper limb motor, sensory and reflexes are intact. What is the likely level of injury?
   A) L4
   B) T5
   C) L5
   D) S1
   E) T10
4. What is the definition of spinal shock?
   A) Hypotension with a spinal injury
   B) Loss of sensation, motor function and reflexes following spinal injury
   C) No tachycardia in association with hypovolaemia
   D) Bradycardia with a spinal injury
   E) Hypoventilation
5. What is the central cord syndrome?
   A) Ipsilateral loss of power and proprioception with contralateral loss of pain and temperature sensation
   B) Motor loss with altered sensation but preserved proprioception
   C) Greater loss of motor strength in the upper limbs than the lower limbs with variable sensory loss
   D) Pure loss of proprioception
   E) Pure motor loss

ANSWERS TO QUESTIONS
1. Which of these is a stable fracture of the spine?
The correct answer is **A) Anterior wedge fracture with 10% wedging**.

Fractures of the spine vary in severity from major fracture dislocations, which are often associated with dramatic neurological deficit, to slight anterior wedging or a small avulsion fracture of the vertebral body. One important aspect when assessing a spinal fracture is determining whether it is a stable or unstable fracture. Stable fractures can usually be treated conservatively, whereas unstable fractures usually require consideration of surgical fixation.

X-ray, CT or MRI can be used to infer the stability of a spinal fracture by determining how many columns of the spine are involved. The vertebral column is divided into three columns. The anterior column is the anterior longitudinal ligament and the anterior 50% of the vertebral body; the middle column is the posterior 50% of the vertebral body and the posterior longitudinal ligament; and the posterior column includes all the posterior structures (pedicles, facet joints, laminae and spinous process) and the interspinous ligaments. If two or more columns are affected, then the fracture is considered to be unstable.

A) Anterior wedge fracture with 10% wedging – Correct. An anterior wedge fracture with <50% wedging is a stable injury. With this injury, only the anterior column is affected and so the injury is stable.

B) Burst fracture – Incorrect. A burst fracture is a more serious injury caused by axial compression of the spine. The vertebral body is compressed by the force and 'bursts' apart, with both the anterior and middle columns being involved. Consequently, this is an unstable fracture. Importantly bone fragments from the comminuted vertebral body may be located in the spinal canal, resulting in potential spinal cord injury.

C) Chance fracture – Incorrect. A Chance fracture is typically seen in patients following a road traffic accident. It is caused by a hyperflexion injury which occurs most commonly from a restraining lap belt (they are otherwise known as lap belt fractures) and usually involves the L2 and L3 levels. They are transverse fractures through the vertebral body (anterior and middle columns) and involve the posterior elements as well (posterior column). This makes the injury unstable. The fracture line may run through the intervertebral disc space rather than the vertebral body. These fractures are often associated with other injuries, especially small bowel and colonic injuries.

D) Fracture dislocation of L2 – Incorrect. Fracture dislocation injuries are a very serious type of injury. They usually involve relatively minor fractures, such as transverse or spinous process fractures. However, spinal cord injury is common due to the dislocation with potential for transection of the spinal cord at the level of the injury. In the thoracic and upper lumbar spine, the spinal canal is relatively small, with the spinal cord filling most of the canal. Therefore, there is only a small amount of free space and a fracture dislocation at this site is likely to lead to a significant cord injury. In the upper cervical spine, the spinal canal is relatively larger, so injuries to the cord are not as common at this site.

E) Jefferson fracture – Incorrect. This is a fracture of C1 where there are fractures of the anterior and posterior arches of C1, with displacement of the lateral masses on the odontoid peg view. This is an unstable injury which requires stabilisation.

KEY POINTS

1. The patterns of injury described here are common and relate to severity of injury and likelihood of spinal cord injury.
2. Spinal fractures and cord injuries are associated with significant morbidity. All patients suffering significant trauma should be assumed to have a spinal injury until proven otherwise. Patients should be treated lying supine with C-spine immobilisation and log rolling to prevent spinal cord injury until a spinal injury can be excluded.
3. Patients who have suffered significant trauma usually now have a CT scan, rather than X-rays, to assess their injuries. This allows accurate assessment of the organs as well as the bones, including the spine. MRI is used to assess the spinal cord and surrounding soft tissue structures if there is clinical or radiological suspicion of a spinal cord injury.

2. Which type of injury is most commonly associated with Chance fractures?
The Correct answer is **D) Abdominal and retroperitoneal injuries**.

Chance fractures are also known as lap belt injuries. Intraabdominal pressure is raised significantly with these hyperflexion injuries and there is a high risk of associated intraabdominal or retroperitoneal injuries.

A) Pneumothorax – Incorrect. A pneumothorax may occur in any patient involved in a road traffic accident and so all patients should have a chest examination and X-ray following major trauma. However, a pneumothorax is not specifically associated with Chance fractures.

B) Aortic transection – Incorrect. Aortic transection is caused by rapid deceleration. The aorta is torn usually just distal to the origin of the left subclavian artery, at the site of the ligamentum arteriosum, as this point is relatively fixed. Although seen in trauma patients, it is not specifically associated with Chance fractures.

C) Major head injury – Incorrect. Although there is an association between head injury and spinal injuries, there is not a specific relationship between a Chance fracture and head injuries.

Continue

CASE **4.2**   *Contd.*

D) Abdominal and retroperitoneal injuries – Correct. All patients with a Chance fracture need to have a careful assessment of their abdomen to ensure there is no intra- or retroperitoneal injuries. The patient may initially be stable but if there is doubt, then a CT scan of the patient is indicated (remember: the patient will need a CT for further assessment of the Chance fracture in any case; however, a larger area will be imaged and IV contrast given if intraabdominal injuries are to be excluded).

E) Bilateral calcaneal fractures – Incorrect. Bilateral calcaneal injuries suggest a fall from height. There is therefore a risk of associated injuries to the long bones, pelvis and spine and these need to be examined. However, these patients are more likely to have sustained a burst fracture as a result of axial compression rather than a Chance fracture.

❶ KEY POINT

Remember that spinal injuries usually occur after significant trauma. Remember to examine the rest of the patient, using the ATLS algorithm (ABCDE) to assess for other injuries. In addition to the chest X-ray (which is part of the ATLS algorithm), such patients may require CT scanning (noncontrast CT of the head and cervical spine followed by a contrast enhanced CT of the chest, abdomen and pelvis) to accurately and fully assess their injuries.

3. A patient suffers a spinal fracture and has no sensation from the umbilicus down, no lower limb reflexes or lower limb motor activity bilaterally. Upper limb motor, sensory and reflexes are intact. What is the likely level of injury?
The correct answer is **E) T10**.

It is important in all patients with spinal injuries to perform a complete neurological examination once the patient is stabilised (Table C4.2.1). Spinal injuries can be complete or incomplete. Complete injuries are where there is total loss of sensation and power below a level. It is therefore important to document whether there is motor or sensory loss or both.

A) L4 – Incorrect. A complete injury at the L4 level will result in loss of knee (L4) and ankle (S1) reflexes. Sensation will be affected from the L4 dermatome distally. The L4 dermatome is the medial part of the calf. There would be hip flexion and perhaps knee extension but no other lower limb motor function below the knee.

B) T5 – Incorrect. A T5 level injury would result in lower limb paralysis and loss of sensation from the nipples down.

C) L5 – Incorrect. An injury to the L5 level would result in loss of the ankle reflex and loss of plantar and dorsiflexion. The knee reflex (L4) should be preserved. The L5 dermatome gives sensation to the lateral aspect of the calf and most of the dorsum of the foot.

D) S1 – Incorrect. An S1 level would result in loss of the ankle reflexes, but the knee reflexes would be intact.

E) T10 – Correct. The clue to the level in this pattern of injury is the level of sensation. This patient has lost sensation at T10 and has a complete spinal injury from T10 down.

❶ KEY POINT

Knowledge of the dermatomes and myotomes is essential when assessing spinal injuries.

Table C4.2.1   Dermatomes, Myotomes and Reflexes for Different Spinal Nerve Levels

SPINAL NERVE	DERMATOME	MYOTOME	REFLEX
T5	Nipple level	–	–
T10	Umbilicus level	–	–
L1	Anterior medial thigh (proximal third)[a]	Hip flexion	Cremasteric reflex
L2	Anterior medial thigh (middle third)[a]	Hip flexion	–
L3	Medial femoral condyle	Knee extension	Patella reflex
L4	Medial malleolus	Knee extension and ankle dorsiflexion	Patella reflex
L5	Dorsum of foot (3rd MTPJ[b])	Hip extension, knee flexion, great toe extension	–
S1	Lateral aspect of calcaneus	Hip extension, knee flexion, ankle plantarflexion	Ankle jerk
S2	Popliteal fossa	Ankle plantarflexion	–
S3	Ischial tuberosity	–	–
S4 and 5	Perianal region	–	–

[a]The sites of these dermatomes are variable and there is no reliable anatomical landmark.
[b]Metatarsophalangeal joint.

4. What is the definition of spinal shock?

The correct answer is **B) Loss of sensation, motor function and reflexes following spinal injury**.

Understanding the difference between spinal and neurogenic shock is important. Neurogenic shock refers to patients with a spinal injury who are hypotensive, may be bradycardic and are unable to mount a tachycardic response to hypovolaemia; this condition is potentially life-threatening. It most commonly occurs with spinal cord injuries above the level of T5 and is a result of disruption to the autonomic nervous system. Spinal shock is the loss of sensation, motor function and reflexes that initially occurs following a spinal injury.

A) Hypotension with a spinal injury – Incorrect. This is part of neurogenic shock. Hypovolaemia from haemorrhage must be excluded as a cause of hypotension in trauma patients before presuming a neurogenic cause.

B) Loss of sensation, motor function and reflexes following spinal injury – Correct. This is the definition of spinal shock following spinal injury. Remember that upper motor neurone lesions (such as spinal cord injuries) are expected to result in loss of power and sensation but increased reflexes. However, in spinal shock, there is an initial loss of reflexes, along with power and sensation. After 1 to 3 days, the reflexes usually return to normal, before becoming permanently increased after a week or so.

C) No tachycardia in association with hypovolaemia – Incorrect. A patient with neurogenic shock (not spinal shock) has disruption to the autonomic nervous system. Therefore, they cannot mount the usual sympathetic response to hypovolaemia and will not become tachycardic.

D) Bradycardia with a spinal injury – Incorrect. Bradycardia is sometimes part of neurogenic shock.

E) Hypoventilation – Incorrect. Hypoventilation is not a feature of either neurogenic or spinal shock. However, patients with an upper thoracic or cervical spine injury may struggle with breathing as a result of paralysis of the diaphragm or accessory respiratory muscles.

❶ KEY POINT

Neurogenic shock may cause hypotension in the trauma patient but it is important to exclude hypovolaemia first, as missing this can be rapidly fatal. It is also important to appreciate that neurogenic shock may mask the expected tachycardic response to hypovolaemia.

5. What is central cord syndrome?

The correct answer is **C) Greater loss of motor strength in the upper limbs than the lower limbs with variable sensory loss**.

There are several spinal cord syndromes which are complex but it is useful to know about them. They can occur with or without spinal column injury and are forms of incomplete spinal cord injuries.

Central cord syndrome is caused by an acute cervical spinal cord injury (typically high force trauma in young patients or hyperextension injuries in elderly patients with preexisting cervical spondylosis). There will be greater motor loss in the upper limbs than in the lower limbs and sensory loss is variable.

A) Ipsilateral loss of power and proprioception with contralateral loss of pain and temperature sensation – Incorrect. This is the description of the rare Brown–Sequard syndrome. There is hemisection of the spinal cord with ipsilateral motor and proprioceptive loss, but contralateral pain and temperature sensory loss. This pattern of neurological findings is due to the levels at which the neurones in the different spinal tracts decussate. It is usually the result of a penetrating spinal injury.

B) Motor loss with altered sensation but preserved proprioception – Incorrect. This is the anterior cord syndrome. This syndrome is characterised by infarction of the cord in the region of the anterior spinal artery. This has the lowest rate of recovery in comparison to the other syndromes.

C) Greater loss of motor strength in the upper limbs than the lower limbs with variable sensory loss – Correct. This accurately describes the central cord syndrome and is most often seen in hyperextension injuries of the cervical spine with some degree of preexisting spinal canal stenosis. The central part of the spinal cord is injured. As the motor supply to the upper limb is more central than the motor supply to the lower limbs the patient loses more power from the upper limbs.

D) Pure loss of proprioception – Incorrect. Pure loss of proprioception does not fit any of the spinal cord syndromes.

E) Pure motor loss – Incorrect. Pure motor loss does not fit any of the spinal cord syndromes.

👥 IMPORTANT LEARNING POINTS

- All patients suspected of having a spinal injury should be immobilised until this is confirmed or excluded.
- Spinal fractures are often the result of significant trauma – associated injuries must be excluded using the ABCDE ATLS approach.
- Unstable spinal fractures are fractures which involve at least two of the three vertebral columns and include Chance fractures, burst fractures and fracture dislocations.
- Spinal cord injury is more likely with unstable spinal fractures.
- Neurogenic shock refers to patients with a spinal injury who are hypotensive, bradycardic and are unable to mount a tachycardic response to hypovolaemia. Spinal shock is the loss of sensation, motor function and reflexes that initially occurs following a spinal injury.
- There are several spinal cord incomplete injury syndromes with specific neurological findings which you need to know about.

A 73-year-old woman presents to the hospital with fatigue, weight loss and neck pain. There is no history of trauma. X-rays of the cervical spine have been performed.

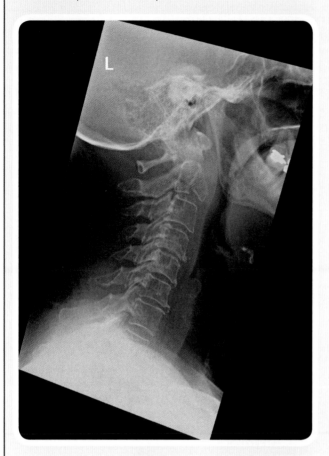

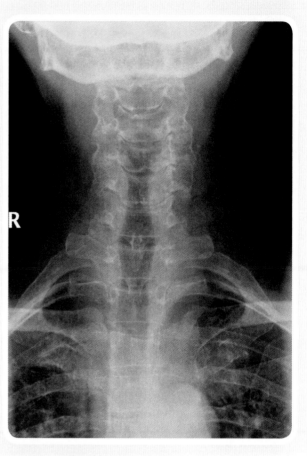

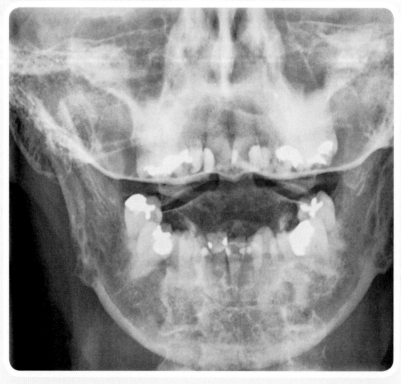

ANNOTATED X-RAY

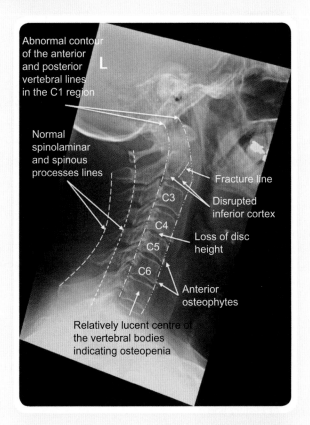

Abnormal contour of the anterior and posterior vertebral lines in the C1 region

L

Normal spinolaminar and spinous processes lines

C3

C4

C5

C6

Fracture line

Disrupted inferior cortex

Loss of disc height

Anterior osteophytes

Relatively lucent centre of the vertebral bodies indicating osteopenia

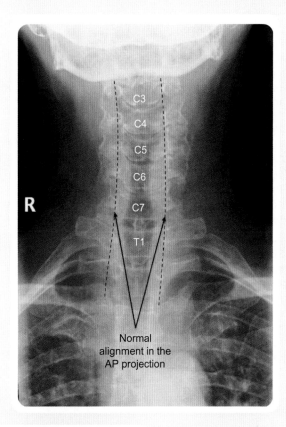

R

C3
C4
C5
C6
C7
T1

Normal alignment in the AP projection

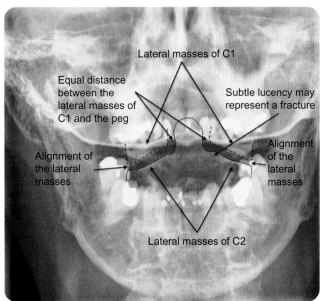

Lateral masses of C1

Equal distance between the lateral masses of C1 and the peg

Subtle lucency may represent a fracture

Alignment of the lateral masses

Alignment of the lateral masses

Lateral masses of C2

PRESENT YOUR FINDINGS

- These are AP, lateral and peg X-rays of the cervical spine in a skeletally mature patient.
- They have been anonymised and the timing of the examination is not available. I would like to confirm the patient's details and timing of the examination before I make any further assessment.

- It is difficult to clearly see the margins of the left lateral mass on the peg view. The X-rays are otherwise adequate, with the lateral view covering C1 to the C7/T1 intervertebral disc space.
- There is a fracture through the base of the odontoid peg (C2), visible on the lateral X-ray. It is difficult to assess the bone texture of the odontoid peg on these

Continue

CASE 4.3 *Contd.*

views, but given the history, I am concerned this is a pathological fracture.

- The anterior and posterior vertebral lines are abnormal in the region of C1/2, with the peg, C1 vertebral body and skull being angulated posteriorly in relation to the lower cervical vertebral bodies. The spinolaminar line and the line of the spinous processes are normal.
- There is no soft tissue swelling.
- Elsewhere, there are degenerative changes with anterior osteophytes and disc space narrowing at the C4/C7 levels. The alignment and appearance of the remaining cervical spine is unremarkable.
- There is generalised osteopaenia of the vertebral bodies.

IN SUMMARY – These X-rays of the cervical spine show a fracture through the base of the odontoid peg, with posterior angulation of the C1 vertebral body and skull. There are degenerative changes at the C4/C7 levels, and generalised osteopaenia of the vertebral bodies. Given the history, I am concerned this may be a pathological fracture. A full history and examination in addition to further imaging will be required.

QUESTIONS

1. What is the most important initial aspect of the management of this patient?
   A) Pain relief
   B) Stabilisation of the cervical spine with in-line immobilisation
   C) Full history and examination to identify any underlying malignancy
   D) Trauma assessment
   E) Referral to neurosurgeons

2. What lines is/are useful for assessing the cervical spine on the lateral X-ray?
   A) Anterior vertebral line
   B) Posterior vertebral line
   C) Klein's line
   D) Line of the spinous processes
   E) Spinolaminar line

3. Which of these may indicate an unstable Jefferson fracture on odontoid peg view?
   A) Normal Wackenheim's line
   B) 1-mm gap between the peg and the lateral masses
   C) >7-mm displacement of lateral masses
   D) A type 2 fracture of the odontoid peg
   E) C1/C2 subluxation

4. Which of these is/are likely to be initially required when investigating a suspected pathological fracture of the cervical spine?
   A) History and examination
   B) CT scan
   C) MRI scan
   D) PET/CT scan
   E) Ultrasound of the neck

5. Where would you assess sensation for the C7 dermatome?
   A) Radial border of the forearm
   B) Thumb
   C) Ulnar border of the little finger
   D) Middle finger
   E) Area over the deltoid

ANSWERS TO QUESTIONS

1. What is the most important initial aspect of the management of this patient?

   The correct answer is **B) Stabilisation of the cervical spine with in-line immobilisation**.

   This patient has presented with a cervical spine fracture without trauma. This is uncommon (most fractures of the cervical spine occur following trauma). In patients with a pathological fracture, it is important to consider the cause of the fracture. However, regardless of whether the fracture occurred following trauma or not, it first requires stabilisation to prevent any (further) damage to the spinal cord.

   A) Pain relief – Incorrect. Although this is always important for patients with pain, it is more important to focus on stabilising a potentially unstable cervical spine injury.

   B) Stabilisation of the cervical spine with in-line immobilisation – Correct. Any patient with a cervical spine injury should be immobilised with a hard collar and blocks to prevent flexion, extension or rotation of the cervical spine and potential damage to the spinal cord. In trauma patients, the patient may arrive in the A&E department immobilised. If not, it may be appropriate to immobilise the cervical spine before further assessment, such as X-rays.

   C) Full history and examination to identify any underlying malignancy – Incorrect. This patient has presented with an atraumatic cervical spine fracture. The likelihood is that this is a pathological fracture. A full history and examination is therefore especially important. In this age group, the two most likely diagnoses are either secondary metastases or multiple myeloma. By fully assessing the patient, you may identify the primary tumour – lung, breast and prostatic cancer are the most common primaries, so request a chest X-ray, and examine the breasts in females and the prostate in males. Serum electrophoresis and urine Bence Jones proteins should be performed to assess for myeloma.

   D) Trauma assessment – Incorrect. This is not a trauma patient and therefore this is not necessary. However, if a patient presents following trauma, it is important to follow the ATLS protocol. This is ABCDE followed by a secondary survey. Cervical spine injuries are serious enough that ATLS suggest that as part of the airway assessment, there is control of the cervical spine with in-line immobilisation.

   E) Referral to neurosurgeons – Incorrect. This patient should be discussed with the neurosurgeons but stabilisation of the cervical spine and further investigations are required first. An MRI will demonstrate whether this is a pathological fracture and will also guide potential surgical management. Treatment options include surgical stabilisation or radiotherapy.

KEY POINTS

1. All patients presenting with significant trauma should be treated as if they have a cervical spine injury until it can be safely excluded.

2. The five tumours which commonly metastasise to bone are: breast, lung, prostate, thyroid and renal. Primary bone tumours are much less common than bone metastases, and the commonest primary bone tumour in adults is myeloma.

---

2. What lines is/are useful for assessing the cervical spine on the lateral X-ray?

   The correct answers are **A) Anterior vertebral line, B) Posterior vertebral line, D) Line of the spinous processes and E) Spinolaminar**.

   Cervical spine X-rays can be difficult to interpret. When assessing the X-rays you should follow a standard pattern (see the introduction of this chapter for further details). First, assess whether the X-rays are adequate. In particular, the C7/T1 junction is often poorly visualised in adults and additional X-rays may be required. Assess the overall alignment of the bones, the bones individually, looking for fractures and abnormal bone texture, and the soft tissue structures that surround the bones. There are some measurements which can be helpful. Here, we discuss the four lines which are useful for assessing the overall alignment of the cervical spine.

   A) Anterior vertebral line – Correct. This line is drawn down the anterior aspect of the vertebral bodies of C2 to T1. The line should be a smooth curve with no steps in it. If steps are evident, this suggests that there is displacement of the vertebral body and therefore an underlying cervical spine injury.

   B) Posterior vertebral line – Correct. This line is drawn down the posterior aspect of the vertebral bodies. If there is a step in this line, there may be a fracture which is being pushed posteriorly into the spinal canal, potentially compressing the spinal cord. We call this retropulsion and it is often seen with burst fractures.

   C) Klein's line – Incorrect. Klein's line is used to assess the alignment of the upper femoral epiphysis in cases of suspected SUFE.

   D) Line of the spinous processes – Correct. This is not a straight line, as C6 and C7 have prominent spinous processes. However, you may identify any displacement by assessing this line and you can also assess for widening of the interspinous gap (the gap between two adjacent spinous processes).

   E) Spinolaminar line – Correct. This line follows the anterior part of the spinous processes. Assessing this line may demonstrate a fracture of the posterior elements of the cervical spine. It is also important to look for widening of the gap between the spinous processes, which occurs with injuries to the interspinous ligaments.

Continue

CASE **4.3** *Contd.*

Cervical spine X-rays can be difficult to assess. Using the lines described earlier allows for the safe assessment of the lateral X-ray of the cervical spine.

3. Which of these may indicate an unstable Jefferson fracture on odontoid peg view?
   The correct answer is **C) >7-mm displacement of lateral masses**.
   Jefferson fractures are burst fractures (fractures where there is significant compression of a vertebra, which then 'bursts') of C1 (atlas). They occur following axial loading; for example, if someone falls from a height and lands on their head. Fortunately, at C1, the spinal canal is relatively wide and there is therefore a low incidence of associated neurological injury. However, a Jefferson fracture is an unstable fracture and will need urgent referral to the neurosurgeons for further management. Additionally, there are often injuries to other parts of the cervical spine and elsewhere in the patient which will need managing.
   A) Normal Wackenheim's line – Incorrect. Wackenheim's line is assessed on the lateral X-ray of the cervical spine. It is used to assess the atlantooccipital joint. A line drawn down the posterior part of the clivus (in the middle of the skull) should not intersect the peg. If it does, then this suggests atlantooccipital instability.
   B) 1-mm gap between the peg and the lateral masses – Incorrect. If there is lateral displacement of the lateral masses (see later), then this is suggestive of a potential Jefferson fracture. However, a 1-mm gap between the lateral masses and the peg is within normal limits (>2mm is considered abnormal).
   C) More than 7-mm displacement of lateral masses – Correct. This is the definition of an unstable Jefferson fracture. With this degree of displacement, the transverse ligament is likely ruptured and the cervical spine is unstable. This patient will then require further immobilisation, potentially through the use of a Halo. This is a form of external fixation for the cervical spine.
   D) A type 2 fracture of the odontoid peg – Incorrect. The Jefferson fracture is a fracture of C1, whereas the odontoid peg is a process of C2. Fractures of the odontoid peg are potentially visible on the odontoid peg view or on the lateral X-ray. Odontoid peg fractures are classified into 1, 2 and 3. Type 1 fractures occur at the very tip of the peg and are very rare. Type 2 fractures are the most common and occur through the base of the peg. Type 3 fractures extend through the vertebral body of C2.
   E) C1/C2 subluxation – Incorrect. This is a ligamentous injury, and not a fracture, which more frequently occurs in children. This is best assessed on the lateral X-ray. If the gap between the odontoid peg (C2) and the anterior arch of the atlas (C1) is greater than 3mm in adults or 5mm in children, then this suggests a possible C1/C2 subluxation.

A Jefferson fracture is most easily diagnosed on the peg view. Look for widening of the gap between the peg and the lateral masses (>2mm) and overhanging of the lateral margins of C1 in relation to C2.

4. Which of these is/are likely to be initially required when investigating a suspected pathological fracture of the cervical spine?
   The correct answers are **A) History and examination, B) CT scan and C) MRI scan**.
   Fractures which occur with no or minimal trauma raise the suspicion of an underlying abnormality of the bone. This may represent a sinister cause, such as a malignancy, or a benign cause such as osteoporosis. It is important to thoroughly assess such patients as it may affect the treatment of the fracture and the patient may require additional treatment of the underlying condition.
   A) History and examination – Correct. A full history should include asking about systemic features of malignancy, such as loss of appetite and weight loss. Ask about smoking, environmental exposures (such as asbestos) and a family history of cancer. They may also have impending pathological fractures at other locations, so ask about any pain they may be experiencing. A thorough examination, including the breasts, is required to assess the overall condition of the patient and the potential primary source of the pathological fracture. The urine should be tested as part of a myeloma screen and bloods tests should include an FBC, U&Es, LFTs, calcium/bone profile and serum electrophoresis. Tumour markers may be required following a discussion with a senior doctor.
   B) CT scan – Correct. A CT scan is a useful modality for accurately assessing the pathological fracture. Additionally, many patients will also have a CT scan of the chest, abdomen and pelvis to identify the primary tumour and assess for other metastatic disease (stage the tumour).
   C) MRI scan – Correct. MRI is better than CT for assessing the spine for metastatic deposits. It also allows an accurate assessment of the spinal canal and cord which may be affected by bony metastatic disease. Additionally, some tumours, such as rectal tumours and tumours of the prostate, are better assessed with MRI than CT.
   D) PET/CT scan – Incorrect. A PET/CT scan uses a radionuclide to assess for areas of increased metabolic activity (tumours often have increased metabolic activity). It is a specialised investigation with only very specific indications. It may be used in the investigation of a patient with a pathological fracture but this depends on the underlying tumour. Therefore, it is not likely to be an initial investigation.
   E) Ultrasound of the neck – Incorrect. Ultrasound of the neck provides an assessment of the soft tissue structures, such as the thyroid, salivary glands and lymph nodes. It is not useful for assessing the cervical spine.

5. Where would you assess sensation for the C7 dermatome?

   The correct answer is **D) Middle finger**.

   It is important that you have a full understanding of the dermatomes of the body when assessing anyone with a potential neurological injury, such as a spinal fracture (Table C4.3.1). The dermatomes are areas of skin consistently supplied by specific nerve roots, which help to assess the level of cord injury. It is always important to document your findings accurately. If you find that the patient's neurological assessment does not fit a recognisable pattern, then document this as well. Remember: patients can find it difficult to be sure of what does or does not feel normal in the presence of trauma and pain.

   A) Radial border of the forearm – Incorrect. This is part of the C6 dermatome. It is also part of the sensory distribution of the lateral cutaneous nerve of the forearm, which is the end branch of the musculocutaneous nerve. Remember that as well as the dermatomes there are individual nerves which correspond to the dermatomes.

   B) Thumb – Incorrect. This is part of the C6 dermatome, and is a more commonly used site to assess C6 nerve sensation than the radial border of the forearm. In addition, while examining sensation to the first webspace dorsally you can assess the sensory branch of the radial nerve.

   C) Ulnar border of the little finger – Incorrect. This is the area where you should examine for the sensory branch of the ulnar nerve and also for the C8 dermatome.

   D) Middle finger – Correct. The C7 dermatome is relatively small and essentially the middle finger is the only definitive place to examine for this dermatome. To examine for median nerve sensation, you should examine the radial border of the index finger.

   E) Area over the deltoid – Incorrect. This is the area of the C5 dermatome which corresponds to the C5 myotome which supplies the deltoid. The deltoid is supplied by the axillary nerve and sensation over this area (the regimental badge patch) may be lost in injuries to this nerve.

KEY POINTS

1. Dermatomes are areas of skin consistently supplied by specific nerve roots, whereas myotomes are muscles supplied by specific nerve roots.
2. Dermatomes are related to the central nervous system, whereas areas of skin supplied by named nerves are used to assess the peripheral nervous system.

Table C4.3.1 Upper Limb Dermatomes, Myotomes and Reflexes

SPINAL NERVE	DERMATOME	MYOTOME	REFLEX
C2	Occiput	Neck flexion/ extension	–
C3	Supraclavicular fossa	Lateral neck flexion	–
C4	Over the acromioclavicular joint	Shoulder elevation	–
C5	Lateral aspect of the antecubital fossa	Shoulder abduction, elbow flexion	Biceps, brachioradialis
C6	Thumb	Elbow flexion	Biceps, brachioradialis, triceps
C7	Middle finger	Elbow extension, wrist flexion, wrist extension, finger extension	Brachioradialis, triceps
C8	Little finger	Thumb extension, wrist flexion	Triceps
T1	Medial aspect of the antecubital fossa	Finger abduction	–
T2	Apex of the axilla	–	–

IMPORTANT LEARNING POINTS

- Always immobilise a suspected cervical spine injury.
- The standard three-view assessment of the cervical spine consists of lateral and AP X-rays, including C1 and the C7/T1 junction, and an open mouth peg view.
- Interpreting cervical spine X-rays can be daunting. Assess:
  - Alignment of the bones.
  - The individual bones looking for fractures and abnormal bone texture.
  - The soft tissues that surround the bones.
- Pathological fractures can occur in the cervical spine and are commonly the result of bony metastatic disease or multiple myeloma.
- A thorough knowledge of the dermatomes and myotomes is needed for assessing potential spinal cord injuries.

CASE 4.4

A 20-year-old woman has fallen off her bike. She developed immediate severe pain in the left shoulder and a deformity. She has been brought to the A&E department by ambulance and has required morphine to make her comfortable. X-rays have been taken and the patient is referred to you.

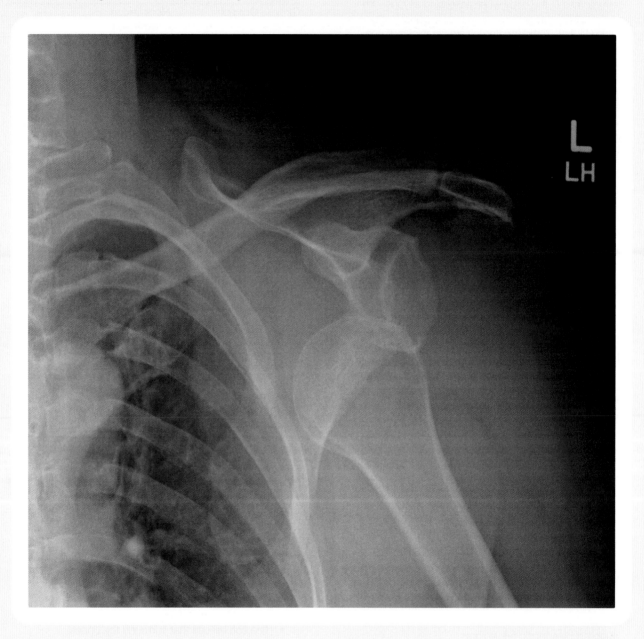

ANNOTATED X-RAY

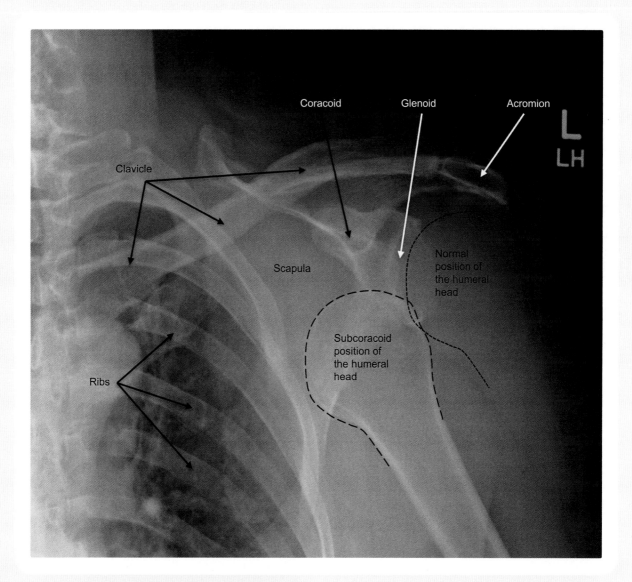

Coracoid   Glenoid   Acromion

Clavicle

Scapula

Normal position of the humeral head

Subcoracoid position of the humeral head

Ribs

L
LH

PRESENT YOUR FINDINGS

- This is an AP X-ray of the left shoulder of a skeletally mature patient.
- It has been anonymised and the timing of the examination is not available. I would like to confirm the patient's details and timing of the examination before I make any further assessment.
- The X-ray is adequately exposed, with no important areas cut off.
- The most striking abnormality is the abnormal location of the humeral head, lying in a subcoracoid position. This finding is in keeping with an anterior glenohumeral joint (shoulder) dislocation.

- There is no associated fracture visible.
- The bones have a normal appearance, with no areas of lucency or sclerosis.
- No rib fractures are visible and the partially imaged left lung is unremarkable.
- There are no soft tissue abnormalities.
- I would want to see a second view, such as scapula Y view, to complete my radiological assessment.

IN SUMMARY – This single AP view of the left shoulder shows an anterior dislocation of the glenohumeral joint. There is no associated fracture.

Continue

CASE **4.4**　*Contd.*

QUESTIONS

1. Excluding anterior dislocations, what are the two other types of shoulder dislocation?
   A) Superior and inferior
   B) Inferior and posterior
   C) Posterior and superior
   D) Lateral and medial
   E) Posterior and medial

2. Which of these is/are methods for reducing shoulder dislocations?
   A) Kocher's
   B) Hippocratic
   C) Ledbetter's manoeuvre
   D) Sudden forced traction
   E) General anaesthesia

3. What nerve is most commonly injured following shoulder dislocation or reduction?
   A) Radial nerve
   B) Axillary nerve
   C) Long thoracic nerve
   D) Phrenic nerve
   E) Musculocutaneous nerve

4. Which bony abnormalities is/are commonly seen with anterior dislocations?
   A) Reverse Hill–Sachs
   B) Hill–Sachs
   C) Bony Bankart
   D) Bankart
   E) Monteggia fracture

5. Which of the following complications most commonly occurs following anterior shoulder dislocations in young patients?
   A) Pain
   B) Arthritis
   C) Instability
   D) Rotator cuff tear
   E) Stiffness

ANSWERS TO QUESTIONS

1. Excluding anterior dislocations, what are the two other types of shoulder dislocation?

   The correct answer is **B) Inferior and posterior**.

   The anterior shoulder dislocation is the most common, accounting for 90% to 95% of shoulder dislocations. It is seen frequently in A&E, in fracture clinics and in examination questions! In the anterior dislocation, the humeral head is displaced anteriorly into the axilla. The normal contour of the shoulder is lost and the most lateral bony structure palpable is the acromion. If in doubt, compare the injured side to the normal.

   Anterior shoulder dislocations are comparatively easy to identify on X-ray; on the AP view, the humeral head will be in a subcoracoid position, no longer articulating with the glenoid. A second view can confirm anterior dislocation.

   A) Superior and inferior – Incorrect. A superior shoulder dislocation does not exist. There is a type of shoulder dislocation in which the humeral head dislocates inferiorly, called Luxatio Erecta. This is very rare and unmistakable. The patient presents in severe pain, with their arm held above their head. These are the most difficult types of dislocation to reduce and have the highest incidence of nerve or vessel injury. Urgent referral to orthopaedics is advised.

   B) Inferior and posterior – Correct. As well as the inferior dislocation, a posterior dislocation is also possible. It is rare, accounting for about 5% of shoulder dislocations, and classically occurs in patients who have had a seizure or been electrocuted. It can occur with trauma. The patient holds the arm in internal rotation and it is locked in this position. On the AP X-ray, the shoulder may appear to be in joint. However, the humeral head appears abnormal (it looks like a light bulb rather than its normal appearance). The second view helps confirm the diagnosis and will demonstrate the posteriorly displaced humeral head.

   C) Posterior and superior – Incorrect. This is the incorrect combination. Posterior dislocations can occur; however, a superior shoulder dislocation does not exist.

   D) Lateral and medial – Incorrect. These are not types of shoulder dislocation.

   E) Posterior and medial – Incorrect. Only the posterior dislocation is a type of shoulder dislocation; a medial dislocation does not exist.

❗ KEY POINT

Have a high index of suspicion for a posterior dislocation in patients who present with shoulder pain following a seizure. Make sure you have adequate X-rays (it can be subtle on the AP X-ray, but usually obvious on the second view), and if in doubt, ask for help. Missing this injury leads to significant morbidity, including the need for an open reduction and stabilisation, stiffness and recurrent dislocations.

2. Which of these is/are methods for reducing shoulder dislocations?

   The correct answers are **A) Kocher's and B) Hippocratic**.

   There are multiple described methods for reducing an anteriorly dislocated shoulder. The aim of the reduction is to restore anatomical congruity of the joint without causing further injury. The inappropriate use of force or performing these methods incorrectly can actually lead to a fracture and nerve injury. Medications such a midazolam or propofol are required for the procedure, to ensure the patient is appropriately relaxed. It is useful to have an assistant.

   A) Kocher's – Correct. This is the most well-known method for reducing a dislocated shoulder. The patient is relaxed and with the elbow flexed to 90 degrees the shoulder is slowly externally rotated. If resistance is felt, wait for this to subside before continuing with further external rotation. This may often be enough and the shoulder joint may reduce. However, if this is not successful, you need to then adduct whilst internally rotating the shoulder. This can be done as one quick smooth movement and this should reduce the joint. Whilst this is the most well-known method for shoulder reduction, it is falling out of favour due to the small associated risk of nerve/brachial plexus injury.

   B) Hippocratic – Correct. Hippocratic is the other commonly used method which you may have seen. The person reducing the dislocation holds the arm slightly abducted with the elbow fully extended. Traction is then applied, with counter traction applied by a second person holding a sheet around the axilla. This method works for both anterior and posterior dislocations and is associated with a lower incidence of nerve injury than the Kocher's method.

   C) Ledbetter's manoeuvre – Incorrect. Ledbetter's manoeuvre is used for reducing displaced intracapsular neck of femur fractures. There are many slight variations to the technique but the hip is flexed to 90 degrees and is slightly adducted. The hip is then put into internal rotation. Finally, the hip is further flexed before being brought down into slight abduction and extension. The internal rotation must be held to keep the reduction.

   D) Sudden forced traction – Incorrect. A sudden forced traction to the limb, rather than a more measured approach, may lead to a nerve injury or a fracture. Care must be taken when reducing these dislocations.

   E) General anaesthesia – Incorrect. Although conscious sedation is required, general anaesthesia is only rarely needed. A technique for reducing the shoulder will also be needed.

❗ KEY POINT

Appropriate conscious sedation and correct technique are both important for successfully reducing dislocated joints. It is difficult to understand the manoeuvres mentioned earlier from the text descriptions alone; try to observe these techniques in practice in A&E.

Continue

3. What nerve is most commonly injured following shoulder dislocation or reduction?

The correct answer is **B) Axillary nerve**.

The axillary nerve is the most commonly injured nerve following a shoulder dislocation. It is therefore important to assess the neurovascular status of the limb as part of your standard work up. This must be done both before and after attempted reduction and clearly documented.

A) Radial nerve – Incorrect. The radial nerve is not commonly injured in dislocations of the shoulder. In the rare Luxatio Erecta dislocation, the brachial plexus may be injured. Therefore, it is important to assess all the nerves of the arm in cases of shoulder dislocation, not just the axillary nerve.

B) Axillary nerve – Correct. The axillary nerve wraps very closely around the surgical neck of the humerus. The axillary nerve supplies the deltoid muscle and the sensation to the regimental badge patch on the outer aspect of the upper arm. The nerve can be injured either during the initial dislocation or during reduction. Fortunately, the majority of these nerve injuries are minor with good recovery.

C) Long thoracic nerve – Incorrect. The long thoracic nerve is a very important nerve which supplies the serratus anterior muscle. This muscle pulls the scapula to the thorax when contracted. A long thoracic nerve injury can occur in various sports, following a blow to the axilla, for example, or in axillary surgery, such as breast cancer surgery or lymph node dissection. Such injury will lead to winging of the scapula. It is not usually injured in shoulder dislocations.

D) Phrenic nerve – Incorrect. The phrenic nerve is a very important nerve which supplies the diaphragm. Its nerve roots are C3, 4 and 5. Hence, the phrase '3, 4 and 5 keeps the diaphragm alive'. It can be injured at any point on its course; for example, from a spinal cord injury above the levels C3-5 or from a mass compressing it as it passes anteriorly over the mediastinum. However, the phrenic nerve is away from the shoulder joint and is not injured with shoulder dislocations. Injury results in paralysis of the hemidiaphragm. Injury to both phrenic nerves can result in paralysis of the entire diaphragm, which can lead to asphyxia and respiratory arrest.

E) Musculocutaneous nerve – Incorrect. The musculocutaenous nerve supplies the muscles of the anterior compartment of the arm. It can be injured in the surgical approach for neck of humerus fractures but not commonly following a dislocation of the shoulder.

❗ KEY POINT

The anatomy and sensory area of the axillary nerve is a very common exam question. Make sure you have this question clear in your revision notes before continuing.

4. Which bony abnormalities is/are commonly seen with anterior dislocations?

The correct answer is **B) Hill–Sachs and C) Bony Bankart**.

Anterior dislocations of the shoulder in the young are often associated with a couple of common findings on X-ray. The Hill–Sachs lesion is a depressed fracture created in the cortex of the posterolateral aspect of the humeral head. It occurs as the dislocated humeral head impacts against the inferior edge of the glenoid. As the head of the humerus dislocates, it often injures the labrum (the fibrocartilaginous rim attached around the margin of the glenoid cavity). If the labrum comes away from the glenoid with a small fragment of bone, this may be visible on X-ray and represents a bony Bankart lesion. It is therefore vital to assess for these associated injuries.

A) Reverse Hill–Sachs – Incorrect. The Reverse Hill–Sachs lesion is a defect caused by an anterior compression fracture of the humeral head in posterior shoulder dislocation. It may be predictive of ongoing instability.

B) Hill–Sachs – Correct. The Hill–Sachs lesion is described earlier. If large, it can cause ongoing instability. These patients may therefore require surgery to minimise the risk of recurrent dislocation. As discussed earlier, a bony Bankart lesion is also a commonly associated finding.

C) Bony Bankart – Correct. The bony Bankart lesion is described earlier. If large, it may be necessary to repair this arthroscopically to reduce the risk of recurrent dislocations and ongoing instability. As discussed earlier, a Hill–Sachs lesion is also a commonly associated finding.

D) Bankart – Incorrect. The Bankart lesion represents a tear in the labrum without bony injury. It is therefore not visible on X-ray. This can be identified by MRI.

E) Monteggia fracture – Incorrect. This is a type of forearm injury which involves a fracture of the ulna and dislocation of the radial head.

5. Which of the following complications most commonly occurs following anterior shoulder dislocations in young patients?

The correct answer is **C) Instability**.

All these options can potentially occur. The patient may have some pain in the shoulder for some time after the injury and may require physiotherapy to help improve the pain and function of the shoulder. Similarly, the shoulder may be stiff initially following the injury. However, the main concern following this injury in a young person is instability. It is likely some of the stabilising structures of the shoulder have been injured and a percentage of these patients will develop symptomatic instability and recurrent dislocations.

A) Pain – Incorrect. Pain often takes weeks to months to settle down. Although pain may be a feature of instability, most patients find the pain settles down with time.

B) Arthritis – Incorrect. Arthritis is not a common problem following this injury. If the rotator cuff has also been injured, as can occur in the elderly, there may be a resultant rotator cuff arthropathy (arthritis secondary to a rotator cuff tear).

C) Instability – Correct. Instability can be an ongoing problem following this injury. The shallow glenoid of the shoulder allows the wide range of movement, but makes the shoulder an unstable joint. If the stabilising structures are injured, the shoulder may give ongoing symptoms of instability with clicking and clunking and the feeling that the shoulder will dislocate in various positions. There will have been an injury to the capsule, and the labrum may have been injured. If the labrum has come off with a piece of bone, this represents the bony Bankart lesion. Some patients will require an arthroscopy if instability is a problem.

D) Rotator cuff tear – Incorrect. The rotator cuff is a stabilising structure of the shoulder. It is not commonly injured in young patients. The rotator cuff is more prone to injury in shoulder dislocations occurring in elderly patients. This is because age-related degeneration in the rotator cuff predisposes it to injury. A rotator cuff tear should be assessed clinically and further investigations, such as ultrasound, may be required. Patients with a postdislocation rotator cuff tear should be considered for arthroscopic repair of the rotator cuff.

E) Stiffness – Incorrect. Stiffness is less of a problem than instability. However, if the patient does not undergo physiotherapy, then an adhesive capsulitis (frozen shoulder) may occur. This can be very painful and stiff, but with time, up to 18 months, it does fortunately settle in the majority of patients.

 IMPORTANT LEARNING POINTS

- Anterior shoulder dislocations are the most common type of shoulder dislocation – the humeral head usually adopts a subcoracoid position on the AP view.
- Associated injuries, such as a Hill–Sachs or a bony Bankart lesion should be assessed for on the X-rays.
- Reduction techniques include Kocher's and the Hippocratic method. These techniques can result in nerve damage, particularly the axillary nerve. Distal neurovascular assessment is therefore needed before and after attempted relocation/reduction.
- Posterior dislocations are rare, more difficult to diagnose and can be easily missed – look for the light bulb sign on the AP X-ray and use a second view to confirm the posterior position of the humeral head.
- Instability can occur following shoulder dislocation and this needs to be assessed by a shoulder surgeon.

An 8-year-old boy has fallen off a trampoline. He is brought into hospital. He is in severe discomfort with a deformed right arm. His hand is white and there is no pulse. His X-rays are shown here.

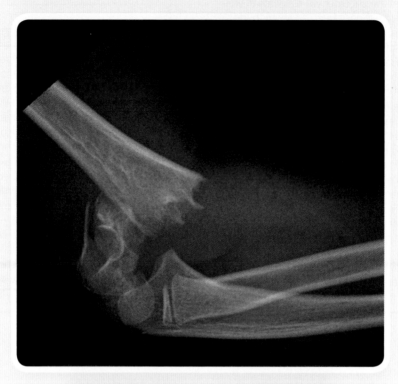

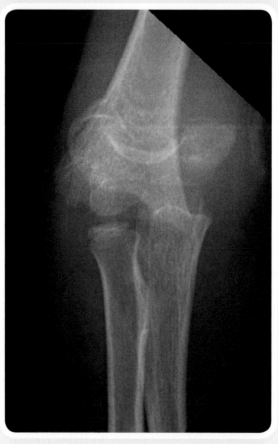

ANNOTATED X-RAY

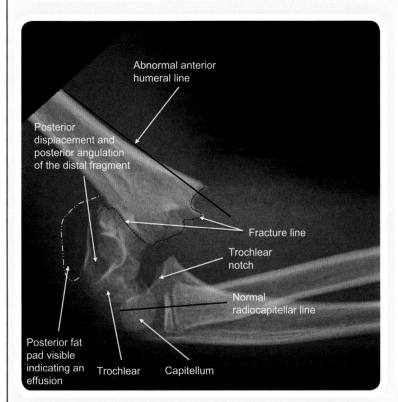

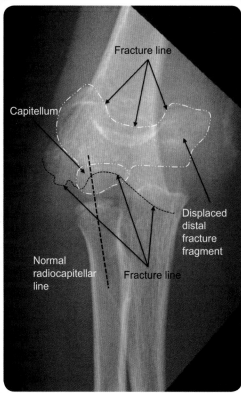

PRESENT YOUR FINDINGS

- These are AP and lateral X-rays of the elbow of a skel-etally immature patient.
- They have been anonymised and the timing of the examination is not available. I would like to confirm the patient's details and timing of the examination before I make any further assessment.
- The X-rays are technically adequate with no important areas cut off.
- The most obvious abnormality is a markedly displaced supracondylar fracture of the distal humerus.
- The distal fragment is displaced and angulated posteriorly, with subluxation of the trochlear and trochlear notch.
- Normal articulation of the radiocapitellar joint is preserved.

- There is associated soft tissue swelling and evidence of an elbow joint effusion.
- The bones are skeletally immature, but have a normal density with no lucent or sclerotic changes to suggest a pathological fracture.
- There is no evidence on X-ray that this is an open fracture.

IN SUMMARY – These X-rays show a markedly displaced and angulated supracondylar fracture with subluxation of the trochlear. These appearances, in addition to the clinical findings of a white, pulseless hand, mean this patient needs urgent referral to orthopaedics and a vascular surgeon.

Continue

CASE **4.5**   *Contd.*

QUESTIONS

1. Which of these is/are important for assessing a patient with this fracture?
   A) Check neurovascular status
   B) Assess whether there is an open fracture
   C) Check for signs of compartment syndrome
   D) Examine for other injuries
   E) Take a history

2. What is the classification system for this fracture and what would this be classified as?
   A) Garden 3 fracture
   B) Gartland 3 fracture
   C) Garden 4 fracture
   D) Gartland 2 fracture
   E) Milch 1 fracture

3. Which nerve is most commonly injured in supracondylar fractures?
   A) PIN
   B) Radial nerve
   C) Median nerve
   D) AIN
   E) Lateral cutaneous nerve of the forearm

4. Which of these is the correct order of the three main structures of the cubital fossa from lateral to medial?
   A) Biceps tendon, brachial artery, median nerve
   B) Brachial artery, median nerve, radial nerve
   C) Radial nerve, lateral cutaneous nerve of the forearm, median nerve
   D) Biceps tendon, ulnar nerve, AIN
   E) Brachial artery, biceps tendon, median nerve

5. What is the common potential deformity of the arm which results if a supracondylar fracture is not accurately reduced?
   A) Gunstock deformity
   B) Cubitus valgus
   C) Cubitus varus
   D) Hyperextension of the elbow
   E) Stiffness of the elbow

ANSWERS TO QUESTIONS

1. Which of these is/are important for assessing a patient with this fracture?

   The correct answers are **A) Check neurovascular status, B) Assess whether there is an open fracture, C) Check for signs of compartment syndrome, D) Examine for other injuries and E) Take a history**.

   This is potentially a very serious injury. It is difficult to manage and can develop significant complications. Supracondylar fractures need early recognition and early thorough assessment. The ABCDE method from the ATLS algorithm is a useful approach for assessing any trauma patient, including children, and has been covered elsewhere in this chapter. Further specific features important to assess are discussed next.

   A) Check neurovascular status – Correct. A displaced supracondylar fracture like this example can easily cause neurovascular compromise. All relevant nerves must be assessed individually for motor and sensory function. The pulse must be assessed together with the capillary refill. There is a difference between a pulseless pink hand and a pulseless white hand. In the former, the pulse generally returns with reduction and fixation of the fracture, although the patient should be taken straight to theatre. The latter, however, is an emergency which needs immediate theatre and input from vascular surgeons.

   B) Assess whether there is an open fracture – Correct. Fractures that are significantly displaced can be open. Open fractures need immediate recognition, removal of gross contamination, intravenous antibiotics according to local policy, photos to prevent repeated exposure of the wound and wound coverage with saline soaked gauze. Also remember that tetanus prophylaxis may be required.

   C) Check for signs of compartment syndrome – Correct. These fractures can swell rapidly and lead to compartment syndrome. If identified in time, patients will have a compartment decompression; however, they will be left with large scars. If missed, the patient may develop a Volkmann's ischaemic contracture which causes variable contracture of the flexor muscles of the forearm depending on the severity of ischaemia to the muscles. This can lead to long-term deformity and loss of function of the limb. Multiple further operations may be required in an attempt to reverse the contractures or preserve function. Therefore, assessing for compartment syndrome is important.

   D) Examine for other injuries – Correct. It is very important to assess for other injuries. Life-threatening injuries should be identified and managed on the primary survey, whereas any other injury should be picked up on the secondary survey.

   E) Take a history – Correct. The anaesthetists will want to know when the child last ate and drank, what allergies they have and if they have any past medical history. The child may have had a reaction to a previous anaesthetic and it could be disastrous to miss

this in the rush of getting the patient with a pulseless white hand to theatre.

> ## ❶ KEY POINT
>
> It is important to check for the presence of distal pulses, not just capillary refill, even if the A&E doctors have already put a plaster on. Expose the wrist and feel for the pulse. If the pulse is not palpable, you can use a handheld Doppler probe to listen for the pulse. An oxygen saturation probe on one of the fingers distal to the fracture can be used to assess for degree of vascular compromise. If you are concerned, do not hesitate to call your senior.

2. What is the classification system for this fracture and what would this be classified as?

   The correct answer is **B) Gartland 3 fracture**.

   The correct classification for this fracture is the Gartland classification. It is very useful if describing the fracture over the phone. The classification is only used for supracondylar fractures where the distal fragment is displaced posteriorly (also known as extension type supracondylar fractures), as in this case. The Gartland classification goes from 1 to 3, increasing in severity. Five percent of supracondylar fractures are flexion type, where the distal fragment is displaced anteriorly. Such fractures are not part of the Gartland classification.

   A) Garden 3 fracture – Incorrect. This is the classification used for intracapsular neck of femur fractures.

   B) Gartland 3 fracture – Correct. Gartland 3 fractures are the most serious. The posterior cortex is completely displaced and the fracture is 'off-ended'. This phrase means there is no contact at all between the two fracture fragments. These are the fractures that can often cause neurovascular compromise and compartment syndrome.

   C) Garden 4 fracture – Incorrect. This is the classification used for intracapsular neck of femur fractures.

   D) Gartland 2 fracture – Incorrect. This is the correct classification system but the wrong grade. A Gartland 2 fracture is only partially displaced, with the posterior cortex of the humerus, visible on the lateral X-ray, still intact. Although neurovascular injury is less common, it can still occur. Gartland 1 fractures are undisplaced and are often difficult to detect. In these cases, you may have clinical suspicion of a fracture but no clear fracture is seen. Assessing for the presence of an elbow effusion is very helpful. When there is a fracture, the bleeding causes an effusion which elevates the anterior and posterior fat pads. A dark area is just visible around the distal end of the humerus on the lateral X-ray.

   E) Milch 1 fracture – Incorrect. The Milch classification refers to fractures of the lateral condyle of the humerus. If this fracture is missed or not properly reduced, it can lead to a cubitus valgus deformity where the arm below the elbow deviates away from the body, which can affect function and lead to an ulna nerve palsy.

Continue

! KEY POINTS

It is useful to assess the following three features in all elbow X-rays (paediatric and adult):

1. The anterior humeral line is a useful method for detecting supracondylar fractures. It is assessed on the lateral X-ray. In normal patients, approximately one-third of the capitellum should be anterior to a line drawn down the anterior cortex of the humerus. If less than one-third lies anterior to this line, then, in the context of trauma, you must suspect a supracondylar fracture.

2. The radiocapitellar line is assessed on both the AP and lateral X-rays. A line drawn along the shaft of the radial neck should intersect the capitellum on both the AP and lateral views. If this is not the case, then you must suspect dislocation or subluxation of the radio-capitellar joint.

3. Look for the presence of an elbow joint effusion by assessing the anterior and posterior fat pads on the lateral view. The anterior fat pad is often visible in a normal person as a thin area of lucency anterior to the distal humerus. The posterior fat pad should not be visible in normality. An effusion is present if there is elevation of the anterior fat pad or if the posterior fat pad is visible. You must suspect a fracture if there is an elbow effusion in the context of trauma (typically supracondylar in children and radial head in adults).

3. Which nerve is most commonly injured in supracondylar fractures?

The correct answer is **D) AIN**.

Nerve injury is very rare with undisplaced fractures (Gartland 1). If there is some displacement (Gartland 2), then there is a small risk of nerve injury. However, the most concerning fracture is the completely 'off-ended' Gartland 3 fracture in the child with a white hand, as described earlier. Not only may they have a vascular injury that needs immediate exploration, but they may have significant nerve damage. Knowing which nerves run around the elbow, their anatomical course and how to test for them is therefore crucial for the assessment of this child.

A) PIN – Incorrect. The PIN is a branch of the radial nerve and begins distal to the elbow. It wraps around the neck of the radius and can be injured in fractures or surgery to this area. It supplies the forearm extensors and injury to this nerve will lead to a wrist drop.

B) Radial nerve – Incorrect. The radial nerve can be injured with fractures around the elbow. Just proximal to the elbow, the nerve goes from the PA compartment of the arm. It runs deep in the tissues at the elbow and is therefore at risk of injury during this fracture; however, it is not the most commonly injured nerve.

C) Median nerve – Incorrect. The median nerve passes anteriorly through the elbow and can be injured in supracondylar fracture. It supplies sensation to the thumb, index and middle fingers as well as the radial border of the ring finger. The nerve also supplies most

of the flexors of the forearm except the ulnar one-third of FDP, and flexor carpi ulnaris, which are supplied by the ulnar nerve.

D) AIN – Correct. The AIN is the nerve most likely to be injured in supracondylar fractures. It is a branch of the median nerve and is the motor branch of the median nerve to the flexors of the forearm. This nerve can be tested by assessing FPL and FDP to the index finger. This is achieved by asking the patient to make the 'OK sign' (partially flexing the index finger and thumb so that the tips of both come together).

E) Lateral cutaneous nerve of the forearm – Incorrect. The lateral cutaneous nerve of the forearm is a superficial nerve which supplies sensation to the lateral border of the forearm. It is the end branch of the musculocutaneous nerve which supplies the muscles of the anterior compartment of the forearm. It is not commonly injured in these fractures.

! KEY POINT

Although the AIN is the nerve most likely to be injured, remember to check all the nerves individually to ensure there is no neurological deficit. Other structures can be injured as well!

4. Which of these is the correct order of the three main structures of the cubital fossa from lateral to medial?

The correct answer is **A) Biceps tendon, brachial artery, median nerve**.

The structures of the cubital fossa are very important both clinically and for exams. TAN or tendon, artery, nerve is a useful mnemonic for remembering this. As described in the following list, the cubital fossa, however, contains additional important structures.

A) Biceps tendon, brachial artery, median nerve – Correct. Using this order allows you to palpate the brachial artery easily and also allows you to consider what may have been injured if there is an injury to this area.

B) Brachial artery, median nerve, radial nerve – Incorrect. Although not mentioned as one of the three key structures of the cubital fossa, the radial nerve is also present and is found deep and lateral to the biceps tendon.

C) Radial nerve, lateral cutaneous nerve of the forearm, median nerve – Incorrect. The lateral cutaneous nerve of the forearm is a superficial structure of the cubital fossa.

D) Biceps tendon, ulnar nerve, AIN – Incorrect. The ulnar nerve is found away from the cubital fossa running in the cubital tunnel, posterior to the medial epicondyle of the humerus. The AIN is a structure which begins distal to the cubital fossa and is the motor branch of the median nerve.

E) Brachial artery, biceps tendon, median nerve – Incorrect. These are three main structures but in the incorrect order. As detailed earlier, the cubital fossa also contains the radial nerve and the lateral cutaneous nerve of the forearm, as well as lymph nodes.

KEY POINT

Knowledge of the anatomy of the cubital fossa is important for clinical assessment and surgery.

5. What is the common potential deformity of the arm which results if a supracondylar fracture is not accurately reduced?
The correct answers are **A) Gunstock deformity and C) Cubitus varus**.
Cubitus varus is the deformity of the elbow acquired through malunion of a supracondylar fracture. Fortunately, the deformity is more cosmetic than functionally limiting. However, the deformity can cause compression of the ulna nerve which will lead to a tardy ulnar nerve palsy. There are two correct answers because the same deformity has two names!
A) Gunstock deformity – Correct. This is the common name given to the cubitus varus deformity but it is better to describe the deformity accurately as this allows you to understand exactly what the deformity is.
B) Cubitus valgus – Incorrect. This is the deformity associated with malunion following a lateral epicondyle fracture of the humerus (which is difficult to see on X-ray and is therefore often missed). The forearm is deviated laterally when the elbow is extended.
C) Cubitus varus – Correct. Varus means deviation towards the midline. Therefore a cubitus varus deformity is deviation of the forearm towards the midline when the elbow is extended and occurs most commonly from supracondylar fractures. It is crucial that the fracture is accurately reduced to stop this deformity from occurring. Two and sometimes three pins are used to hold the fracture in the right position while it heals. These wires can then be removed either in fracture clinic or under an anaesthetic. Care must be taken

by the surgeon when placing the wire on the medial side as the ulnar nerve is very near the entry point.
D) Hyperextension of the elbow – Incorrect. This is a normal variant and some people have lax joints normally. This injury will not lead to increased joint laxity.
E) Stiffness of the elbow – Incorrect. Although not a deformity, if this injury is complicated by malunion, nerve injury, Volkmann's contracture or tardy (late onset) ulnar nerve palsy, then there may be loss of function in the arm and stiffness. Fortunately, however, children are quite resilient to developing stiffness following an injury and most recover good function.

KEY POINT

Supracondylar fractures need accurate reduction. As these fractures often result in a lot of swelling, the sooner the patient is taken to theatre, the easier it will be to reduce the fracture before swelling causes a problem. Therefore, do not leave a supracondylar fracture until the next morning without discussing with a senior.

IMPORTANT LEARNING POINTS

- Displaced fractures can lead to neurovascular compromise.
- The most common nerve to be injured is the AIN.
- Remember the mnemonic TAN (biceps Tendon, brachial Artery, median Nerve) for the main structures of the cubital fossa.
- These fractures need accurate reduction to prevent deformity.
- This type of supracondylar fracture is classified by the Gartland classification.

An 8-year-old boy has been brought into hospital having fallen off the monkey bars onto his right wrist. It is painful and there is a deformity. X-rays have been taken and are displayed here.

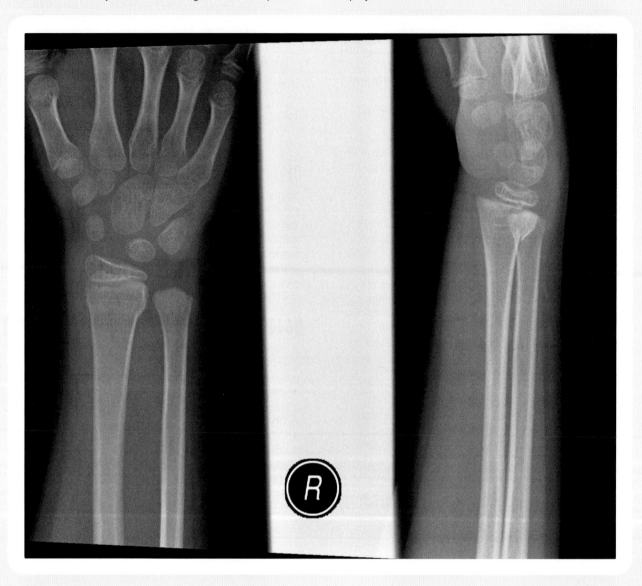

ANNOTATED X-RAY

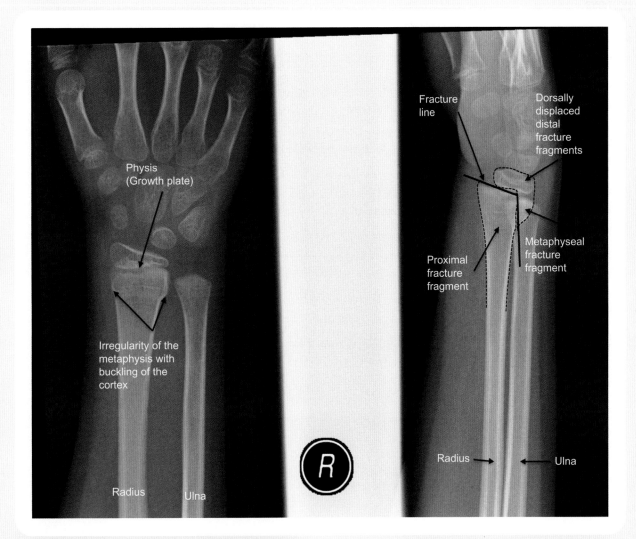

Physis
(Growth plate)

Irregularity of the
metaphysis with
buckling of the
cortex

Radius   Ulna

Fracture
line

Dorsally
displaced
distal
fracture
fragments

Proximal
fracture
fragment

Metaphyseal
fracture
fragment

Radius   Ulna

R

PRESENT YOUR FINDINGS

- These are AP and lateral X-rays of the right wrist of a skeletally immature patient.
- They have been anonymised and the timing of the examination is not available. I would like to confirm the patient's details and timing of the examination before I make any further assessment.
- The X-rays are adequately exposed displaying the abnormality. No important areas are cut off.
- There is a fracture through the distal radial metaphysis and physis, with dorsal displacement of the distal fragments (metaphyseal fragment and epiphysis). The fracture pattern is consistent with a Salter–Harris type 2 fracture of the distal radius.

- The lateral X-ray is rotated, making it difficult to comment on the degree of angulation of this fracture.
- There is mild associated soft tissue swelling.
- No other fractures are identified.
- There are no areas of lucency or sclerosis within the bones.

IN SUMMARY – These X-rays show a Salter–Harris type 2 fracture of the distal radius, with dorsal displacement of the metaphyseal fragment and epiphysis.

Continue

CASE 4.6 *Contd.*

QUESTIONS

1. What is the medical term for the growth plate?
   A) Epiphysis
   B) Physis
   C) Metaphysis
   D) Diaphysis
   E) Megaphysis

2. What type of Salter–Harris fracture is shown in the previously mentioned example?
   A) 1
   B) 3
   C) 2
   D) 4
   E) 5

3. Which Salter–Harris fractures are most associated with a growth disturbance?
   A) 1
   B) 2
   C) 3
   D) 4
   E) 5

4. What is the definitive management of this injury?
   A) Plaster alone
   B) Intramedullary nail
   C) Plate fixation
   D) Manipulation and percutaneous wires
   E) Manipulation and plaster

5. Where would you find the triplane fracture?
   A) Wrist
   B) Shoulder
   C) Toe
   D) Ankle
   E) Knee

ANSWERS TO QUESTIONS

1. What is the medical term for the growth plate?
   The correct answer is **B) Physis**.
   When assessing the fractures around the growth plate in children, it is very important to be able to describe clearly the different parts of the bone as the location of the fracture determines the best treatment option.
   A) Epiphysis – Incorrect. The epiphysis is the name given to the part of the bone next to the joint. At the joint end, the epiphysis is covered by cartilage. Depending on which bone you are describing, the epiphysis may be proximal or distal to the growth plate, so you can see it is very important to describe these areas correctly.
   B) Physis – Correct. The physis is the correct name. The surrounding structures have names that relate to the physis. The physis consists of hyaline cartilage and is the area of long bones where growth occurs. Some long bones, such as the radius and femur, have a physis at each end, whereas others only have one physis, such as the phalanges. The physis fuses once growth has been completed.
   C) Metaphysis – Incorrect. The metaphysis is the area of bone where the shaft of the bone meets the growth plate (physis).
   D) Diaphysis – Incorrect. The diaphysis is the shaft of the bone.
   E) Megaphysis – Incorrect. This is a made-up term.

❗ KEY POINT

Make sure you understand fully the correct names of the bone in relation to the growth plate. These terms are needed for describing fractures in children. They can also be used to describe fractures in adults, remembering that the physis will no longer be present. However, it is often easier to refer to adult fractures as being intra- or extraarticular and occurring in the proximal, middle or distal third of a bone.

2. What type of Salter–Harris fracture is shown in the example?
   The correct answer is **C) 2**.
   The Salter–Harris classification describes fractures around the growth plate and is very important. Using the classification not only immediately tells the senior what the fracture is but also gives an idea on potential management. The correct management of these fractures is particularly important as these injuries have the potential to close the physis and arrest growth prematurely. The types of Salter–Harris fractures are numbered in worsening prognosis (i.e. type 1 has the best prognosis and type 5 the worst).
   A) 1 – Incorrect. The Salter–Harris type 1 fracture is a transverse fracture through the growth plate. This is not very common (only 6% of Salter–Harris fractures are type 1) and is often difficult to see on the X-ray if there is no displacement. If displaced, this fracture will usually need to be reduced to ensure that there is no persistent deformity.
   B) 3 – Incorrect. The Salter–Harris type 3 fracture is a fracture through the growth plate and through the epiphysis into the joint. Eight percent of Salter–Harris

fractures are type 3. As this is an intraarticular fracture there is the risk of affecting joint function in the future. These fractures need to be accurately reduced and may well require surgical fixation.
   C) 2 – Correct. The Salter–Harris type 2 fracture is a fracture through the growth plate with a small metaphyseal fragment called the Thurstan Holland fragment. This is a common injury, accounting for 75% of Salter–Harris type fractures. It has a good prognosis but if displaced, it will require reduction.
   D) 4 – Incorrect. This is an uncommon injury (10% of Salter–Harris type fractures) with a fracture straight through the growth plate with a fracture of the metaphysis and the epiphysis. This is an intraarticular fracture which requires careful reduction to preserve joint function.
   E) 5 – Incorrect. Type 5 fractures are compression fractures of the physis. They are rare, accounting for 1% of Salter–Harris fractures, and have a poor prognosis. They can be very difficult to identify as there is no epiphyseal or metaphyseal component; the only abnormality is a reduced distance between the metaphysis and epiphysis.

❗ KEY POINT

1. A useful mnemonic for Salter–Harris fractures is SALTR.
   • Type 1: S = Slipped or Straight across the physis
   • Type 2: A = Above the physis in the metaphysis or Away from the joint
   • Type 3: L = Lower – fracture below the physis
   • Type 4: T = Through the metaphysis, physis and epiphysis
   • Type 5: R = Rammed or Ruined physis (compression of the physis)

3. Which Salter–Harris fractures are most associated with a growth disturbance?
   The correct answer is **C) 3, D) 4 and E) 5**.
   Fractures through the growth plate can cause a growth disturbance which is worrying for the child, the parents and doctors. By understanding the different zones of the growth plate and how these are affected in the different Salter–Harris injuries, it is possible to know which fractures are likely to cause a problem. The four main zones of the growth plate are the resting zone, proliferative zone, calcifying zone and ossification zone. These zones are in order from closest to the epiphysis to nearest the metaphysis. If the resting zone is affected (i.e. the zone closest to the epiphysis), this can result in growth arrest.
   A) 1 – Incorrect. This fracture is often very difficult to diagnose and is not associated with growth disturbance. This is because the resting zone is not damaged.
   B) 2 – Incorrect. This is the most common type of fracture around the growth plate. The fracture line goes through the proliferative zone (and down through the metaphysis), leaving the resting zone untouched and

Continue

CASE **4.6**   *Contd.*

therefore undamaged. No growth disturbance should occur.

C) 3 – Correct. This is a fracture through the growth plate and through the epiphysis. The resting zone is affected, and growth may be affected. In addition, this is an intraarticular fracture; therefore, if it is not accurately reduced, then the joint may become abnormal, leading to complications such as posttraumatic arthritis in later life.

D) 4 – Correct. This is a fracture through both the metaphysis and the epiphysis. The fracture line goes through the resting zone and growth can potentially be affected.

E) 5 – Correct. This is the severest type of growth plate injury/fracture and is a crush injury of the growth plate. The resting zone is severely damaged and so growth is often affected.

❗ KEY POINT

The Salter–Harris classification is arranged in increasing severity/worsening prognosis. Types 3, 4 and 5 are most commonly associated with growth disturbance, with type 5 having the worst prognosis.

4. What is the definitive management of this injury?
The correct answer is **E) Manipulation and plaster**.
Displaced Salter–Harris type 2 fractures of the distal radius are best managed with gentle manipulation under anaesthesia followed by application of a plaster cast. They reduce easily if identified acutely and do not need overzealous manipulation, which may cause an iatrogenic growth plate injury. The given answers cover a wide range of options which can be used for any fracture. Any fracture can be treated conservatively or with an operation. Conservative measures, broadly speaking, may include traction, plaster, analgesia, physiotherapy and injections. Operative options include manipulation, percutaneous wires, plates and intramedullary nails. If you get asked a difficult question, then use this sieve and you can answer any question on how to manage an orthopaedic problem.

A) Plaster alone – Incorrect. Failing to manipulate the fracture will leave it displaced, leading to a deformity. It is therefore appropriate to attempt to reduce the fracture first through gentle manipulation.

B) Intramedullary nail – Incorrect. The use of intramedullary nails in growing bones is generally contraindicated. Placing a large nail down the centre of the bone through the growth plates will lead to growth disturbance. There are, however, some small flexible nails which can be inserted into the metaphysis along the diaphysis without damaging the growth plate and these are often used in forearm and femoral fractures in children.

C) Plate fixation – Incorrect. Using a plate around the growth plate will affect growth and is not recommended. However, plates are often used in displaced

fractures of the forearm in children. These are sometimes removed once the fracture has healed, to reduce the risk of a later fracture around the plate.

D) Manipulation and percutaneous wires – Incorrect. Although not recommended, if the surgeon wants to stabilise the growth plate, then a percutaneous wire with manipulation is the least invasive surgical option after manipulation.

E) Manipulation and plaster – Correct. This patient should be taken to theatre at the next available opportunity when safe to do so and have a gentle manipulation under general anaesthesia, followed by a below-elbow plaster which is moulded and well fitted. It is also possible for this to be done in EDs with modern analgesia/techniques.

❗ KEY POINT

Premature growth arrest can cause significant morbidity and can be related to the fracture directly, or result from inappropriate management. Therefore, the treatment of fractures in patients who are skeletally immature often differs from that used in adults. This needs to be taken into account when considering operative intervention.

5. Where would you find the triplane fracture?
The correct answer is **D) Ankle**.
This is a very complex fracture to understand and if suspected, the child will often require a CT scan to further delineate the injury, so do not worry if you find this difficult. This fracture is actually made of three fractures; hence, the name triplane. First, there is a fracture through the growth plate in the axial plane. Second, there is a metaphyseal fracture in the coronal plane. Finally, there is an epiphyseal fracture in the sagittal plane. These are severe ankle injuries that need early recognition and reduction. They occur in children aged 12 to 15 as the growth plate fuses, so fortunately are not associated with too much growth disturbance. However, the intraarticular component needs careful reduction and fixation, usually with a few percutaneous screws.

A) Wrist – Incorrect. Although growth plate injuries/fractures may occur in the wrist, this combination is not an injury of the wrist.

B) Shoulder – Incorrect. This fracture pattern does not occur at the shoulder. Fractures of the proximal humerus are almost always treated without an operation in children. They remodel significantly and any residual deformity is not associated with a loss of function.

C) Toe – Incorrect. This fracture pattern does not occur in toes. Toe fractures are common but generally do not require surgical intervention. Weight bearing can begin as normal and the fracture treated with buddy strapping. Occasionally, toe fractures in children will have displacement but these can be reduced and held with strapping with little further complication.

D) Ankle – Correct. We have discussed at length this difficult fracture. When assessing the X-rays of a child's ankle, be sure to look carefully for this injury. It needs further assessment and likely surgical intervention.

E) Knee – Incorrect. This injury does not occur at the knee. However, children can get fractures of the tibial tuberosity or the tibial spine. Look for these injuries if a child presents with knee pain following trauma.

IMPORTANT LEARNING POINTS

- There are four main zones in the physis and the position of these explains how the fracture pattern may injure the growing potential of a bone.
- The Salter–Harris classification is used for fractures around the physis. The mnemonic SALTR can be used to help remember the different types of Salter–Harris fractures.
- The higher the number, the higher the risk of injury to the growth plate and the worse the prognosis.
- Salter–Harris type 2 fractures are by far the commonest type. They have a good prognosis but need gentle manipulation to reduce the fracture and not damage the physis if they are displaced.

CASE 4.7

An 18-year-old man has fallen off his mountain bike. He presents to A&E with a painful right wrist. This is his X-ray.

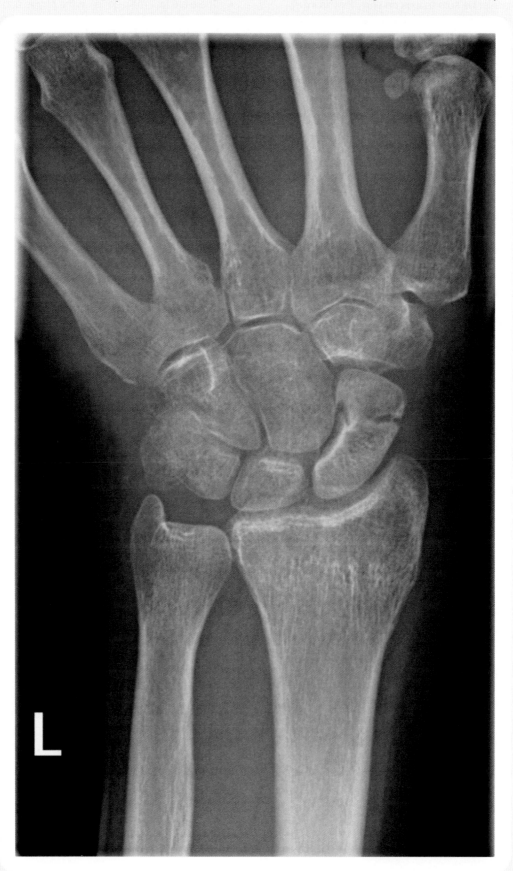

ANNOTATED X-RAY

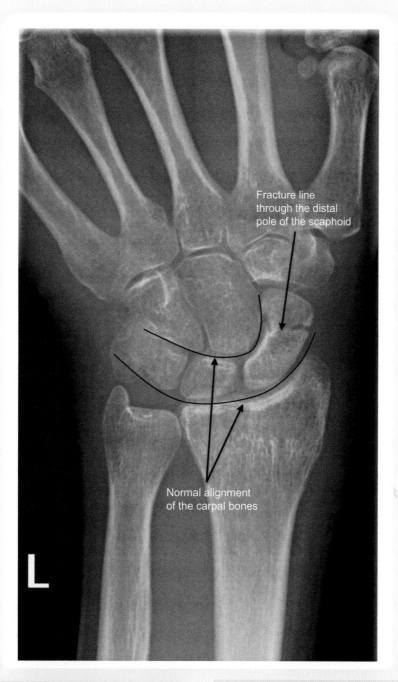

Fracture line
through the distal
pole of the scaphoid

Normal alignment
of the carpal bones

L

🔍 PRESENT YOUR FINDINGS

- This is a single AP view of the left wrist of a skeletally mature patient.
- It has been anonymised and the timing of the examination is not available. I would like to confirm the patient's details and timing of the examination before I make any further assessment.
- The X-ray is adequately exposed, with no important areas cut off.
- There is a transverse fracture through the distal pole of the scaphoid.
- On this X-ray, the fracture appears to be minimally displaced.

- No other fractures are visible, although I would like to view the other X-rays of the wrist/scaphoid.
- Normal alignment of carpal and metacarpal bones is evident on this single view.
- The bone shows normal density, with no areas of lucency or sclerosis.

IN SUMMARY – This single AP view of the wrist shows a minimally displaced transverse fracture through the distal pole of the scaphoid. I would like to review other views of the scaphoid (lateral and obliques) to complete my radiological assessment.

Continue

CASE 4.7 *Contd.*

QUESTIONS

1. Where is the typical location for pain following a scaphoid fracture?
   A) Over the ulna
   B) Over the radius
   C) In the anatomical snuff box
   D) Over the hamate
   E) At the 1st (thumb) carpometacarpal joint
2. Which of these carpal bones is most frequently associated with AVN?
   A) Lunate
   B) Scaphoid
   C) Hamate
   D) Pisiform
   E) Trapezium
3. Which imaging modality is least useful for diagnosing a fracture of the scaphoid?
   A) CT
   B) PET scan
   C) Bone scan
   D) Scaphoid series of X-rays
   E) MRI
4. Which of these is the best management for this fracture?
   A) 2 weeks in a wrist splint
   B) Surgical fixation
   C) 6 weeks in plaster and then mobilisation
   D) 6 weeks in a scaphoid cast with repeat X-rays at 6 weeks out of plaster
   E) 12 weeks in plaster
5. Which of the following structures does not run through the carpal tunnel?
   A) FDP tendons
   B) FDS tendons
   C) Median nerve
   D) FPL tendon
   E) Flexor carpi radialis tendon

ANSWERS TO QUESTIONS

1. Where is the typical location for pain following a scaphoid fracture?

   The correct answer is **C) In the anatomical snuff box**.

   Scaphoid fractures typically occur when a patient FOOSH, with their weight being transmitted through the palm and carpal bones to the distal radius. They can occur in all age groups but are most common in young adults.

   A) Over the ulna – Incorrect. Ulna fractures or injuries to the soft tissues overlying the ulna will produce pain here. Injuries to the DRUJ may also cause pain at this site.

   B) Over the radius – Incorrect. Pain over the distal radius is associated with fractures here; however, sometimes the patient may find it difficult to accurately localise the pain. Therefore, a scaphoid fracture should be considered in these patients.

   C) In the anatomical snuff box – Correct. The anatomical snuff box is formed by the boundaries of extensor pollicis longus, extensor pollicis brevis and abductor pollicis longus. If you extend your thumb, you will see a divot created dorsally at the base of the thumb (the anatomical snuff box). This is a common site for pain in scaphoid fractures.

   D) Over the hamate – Incorrect. This is associated with fractures of the hamate. These fractures can cause subluxation between the hamate and the 5th metacarpal base, so it is important to examine this joint.

   E) At the 1st (thumb) carpometacarpal joint – Incorrect. It is very difficult to distinguish whether someone has pain from their carpometacarpal joint or from their scaphoid, as they are very close on examination. X-rays, however, will hopefully help differentiate between a scaphoid fracture or arthritis/pathology of the first carpometacarpal joint.

❶ KEY POINTS

1. There are a few classic examination findings for a scaphoid fracture. These are pain in the anatomical snuff box, pain over the scaphoid tubercle and pain on telescoping the thumb. The scaphoid tubercle is palpable at the proximal part of the thenar eminence on the volar aspect of the wrist. If you flex your fingers, they will all point to the scaphoid tubercle.

   To telescope the thumb, take the thumb in your hand and provide axial pressure onto the base of thumb (i.e. try to push the thumb onto the trapezium). This pressure is transmitted onto the fractured scaphoid and produces pain.

2. Patients may present with distal radius pain following a fall on an outstretched hand. Make sure you examine for a scaphoid fracture, as this is the same mechanism of injury. If you have clinical concern, request scaphoid views as well as X-rays of the distal radius.

3. There are many mnemonics to help remember the order of the carpal bones. One of the less rude versions is 'Students Like Taking People To The Carlton Hotel'. To remember where the trapezium and trapezoid are found, think 'trapezium under the thumb'.

2. Which of these carpal bones is most frequently associated with AVN?

   The correct answer is **B) Scaphoid**.

   AVN is the death of bone (necrosis) secondary to a disrupted blood supply (avascular). This can occur with or without trauma. There are several bones in the body which are prone to this, including the scaphoid, lunate, femoral neck and talus. In the hand, the scaphoid is most commonly affected.

   A) Lunate – Incorrect. AVN of the lunate is a rare finding. It occurs in Kienböck disease. The cause is uncertain but may be related to previous trauma/fracture of the lunate disrupting the blood supply. This leads to pain and arthritis in the wrist.

   B) Scaphoid – Correct. The scaphoid has an end arterial blood supply from the dorsal branch of the radial artery, which enters the scaphoid via its distal pole. A fracture of the scaphoid can disrupt this tenuous blood supply, leading to AVN. Scaphoid fractures are usually classified by their location – through the distal pole, waist and proximal pole. The risk of AVN is highest in proximal fractures, due to its limited blood supply, and lowest in distal pole fractures, due to the relatively good blood supply.

   C) Hamate – Incorrect. Although it is possible to fracture the hamate, it is not a bone associated with AVN.

   D) Pisiform – Incorrect. The pisiform can rarely be fractured and AVN is not a consequence. Occasionally, a patient can develop arthritis at the joint between the pisiform and the triquetrum, but this is rare.

   E) Trapezium – Incorrect. The trapezium is often affected by arthritis not AVN, causing pain at the base of the thumb. The surgical treatment for this is excision of the trapezium.

❶ KEY POINTS

1. Scaphoid fractures need to be accurately diagnosed and appropriately managed to reduce the risk of AVN developing.

2. Consequences of AVN at any site include loss of normal bone architecture, pain and arthritis.

3. Which imaging modality is least useful for diagnosing a fracture of the scaphoid?

   The correct answer is **B) PET scan**.

   Diagnosing a fracture of the scaphoid can be difficult. Given the high risk of AVN, missed scaphoid fracture can result in significant pain and morbidity. Fortunately, if you follow the advice given here, you are much less likely to miss this fracture.

   A scaphoid series of X-rays (four views usually – AP, lateral and two obliques) will identify the majority of scaphoid fractures. However, if there is clinical concern of a scaphoid fracture (pain and an appropriate mechanism of injury) and no fracture visible on the initial scaphoid series, the patient should either undergo additional imaging or be treated empirically for a scaphoid fracture with interval imaging in 2 weeks' time. Repeat

Continue

X-rays after 2 weeks are more likely to demonstrate a fracture line.

A) CT – Incorrect. CT of the wrist is useful for identifying fractures of the scaphoid not seen on the original X-rays; however, it has a relatively high radiation dose. Bone contusions (bruising) cannot be identified on CT, but complete fractures are reliably diagnosed.

B) PET scan – Correct. PET scanning has no place in the imaging of a potential scaphoid fracture and is an imaging modality reserved for the diagnosis and management of cancer patients.

C) Bone scan – Incorrect. Bone scanning identifies areas of increased osteoblastic activity. It is usually performed 3 to 7 days after the injury and a focal hotspot over the scaphoid is considered evidence of a fracture, although some patients may have incomplete cortical fractures or bone bruising.

D) Scaphoid series of X-rays – Incorrect. These X-rays should always be performed for a suspected scaphoid fracture. Four views, instead of the usual two, are performed as the scaphoid has an unusual shape. The patient can be placed in a scaphoid plaster with the thumb immobilised and the patient referred to a fracture clinic. At clinic, the patient can be reassessed. If still tender, the X-rays can be repeated and the fracture line may have become visible. If the X-rays are normal and there is still concern, then the patient can have a CT, bone scan or MRI to identify a subtle fracture. This approach leads to overtreating many patients who do not have a scaphoid fracture. An alternative approach is to perform an MRI of the wrist at presentation if the initial X-rays are unclear. As discussed later, MRI allows identification of bone bruising and fractures, as well as other soft tissue injuries, helping to prevent overtreatment.

E) MRI – Incorrect. A focused MRI of the scaphoid can be a quick, sensitive and cost-effective imaging method for patients in whom the X-rays are inconclusive. Limited sequences are sufficient – T1 can show a fracture line, which appears as a low signal line. T2-weighted and STIR imaging are useful for identifying oedema, such as bone bruising. The limitations of MRI include its restricted availability (however, some units have dedicated miniature MRI scanners for imaging potential scaphoid fractures). The other problem is that MRI may lead to overtreatment – those patients who have bone bruising but not a cortical fracture may end up being treated for a scaphoid fracture even though they probably do not require it.

① KEY POINT

Scaphoid series of X-rays are the first-line imaging modality for potential scaphoid fractures. However, they cannot exclude a fracture and if there is clinical suspicion, then further imaging options, such as MRI, bone scanning or CT, may be required. Alternatively, the patient can be treated as a scaphoid fracture and undergo follow-up X-rays 14 days after the injury to try to confirm a fracture.

4. Which of these is the best management for this fracture?

The correct answer is **D) 6 weeks in a scaphoid cast with repeat X-rays at 6 weeks**.

A confirmed fracture of the scaphoid will require approximately 6 weeks in plaster. With the tenuous blood supply and risks of AVN or nonunion, further immobilisation may be required. To assess whether the fracture is healing, X-rays should be repeated at 6 weeks and if there is still a concern that the fracture has not healed, then a further 6 weeks in plaster may be required. A percentage of these fractures will not heal and will require surgery.

A) Two weeks in a wrist splint – Incorrect. This is the appropriate management for a patient with clinical signs of a fracture but nothing visible on X-ray. The patient can be immobilised in either a splint or plaster and reassessed at 2 weeks. X-rays should be repeated and if a fracture is suspected, the patients should be immobilised in a scaphoid cast. If repeat X-rays are normal but the patient has ongoing clinical signs of a fracture, then further imaging is required. There is also an increasing number of centres offering further imaging from the outset to avoid over- or undertreatment and delays in reaching a definitive diagnosis.

B) Surgical fixation – Incorrect. Surgical fixation is occasionally required for fractures of the scaphoid. All fractures of the proximal pole of the scaphoid should be considered for fixation as there is a high risk of nonunion and AVN. Displaced fractures of the waist (middle) of the scaphoid should be considered for surgical fixation. Undisplaced fractures of the waist of the scaphoid which are not healing should be considered for surgical fixation. Very few fractures of the distal pole of the scaphoid require fixation.

C) Six weeks in plaster and then mobilisation – Incorrect. Although it is right to treat the fracture with 6 weeks of plaster immobilisation, it is important to ensure the patient is in the correct plaster cast and the patient requires X-rays after 6 weeks to assess whether the fracture has healed.

D) Six weeks in a scaphoid cast with repeat X-rays at 6 weeks out of plaster – Correct. A confirmed fracture of the scaphoid is treated with plaster immobilisation for at least 6 weeks, with repeated X-rays at 6 weeks to check for X-ray signs of union. The scaphoid plaster is a plaster extending from the forearm past the thumb up to the level of the MCPJs and incorporating the thumb up to the level of the thumb interphalangeal joint.

E) Twelve weeks in plaster – Incorrect. Some scaphoid fractures take a prolonged time to heal and some patients will require a longer period of immobilisation than 6 weeks. However as this patient has a relatively distal fracture, it is likely this will go on to heal and require 6 weeks immobilisation.

5. Which of the following structures does not run through the carpal tunnel?

The correct answer is **E) Flexor carpi radialis tendon**. The carpal tunnel contains nine tendons and one nerve. There are the four tendons of FDP (causing flexion at the DIPJ), four tendons of FDS (causing flexion at the proximal interphalangeal joint) and the one tendon of FPL (causes thumb flexion). Compression of the medial nerve in the tunnel causes carpal tunnel syndrome. This is characterised by altered sensation in the median nerve distribution (thumb, index, middle and radial half of the ring finger), together with pain at night and weakness, often reported by the patient as dropping objects.

The flexor carpi radialis tendon inserts into the base of the 2nd metacarpal. It does not travel in the carpal tunnel. The flexor carpi radialis causes wrist flexion and abduction.

 IMPORTANT LEARNING POINTS

- Scaphoid fractures typically occur following a fall onto an outstretched hand, and lead to pain in the anatomical snuff box.
- They can be difficult to identify on X-ray and specific scaphoid views should be performed.
- Consider an MRI of the wrist or interval imaging with X-rays if there is clinical concern of a scaphoid fracture but no fracture visible on the initial X-rays.
- These fractures are associated with a high risk of AVN due to the end arterial supply.
- Proximal pole fractures are most likely to lead to AVN.
- Appropriate treatment reduces the risk of AVN.

CASE **4.8**

A 65-year-old woman presents to A&E, having fallen over on a slippery pavement, landing onto her outstretched right hand. She has a painful right wrist with obvious deformity. You request X-rays of the wrist.

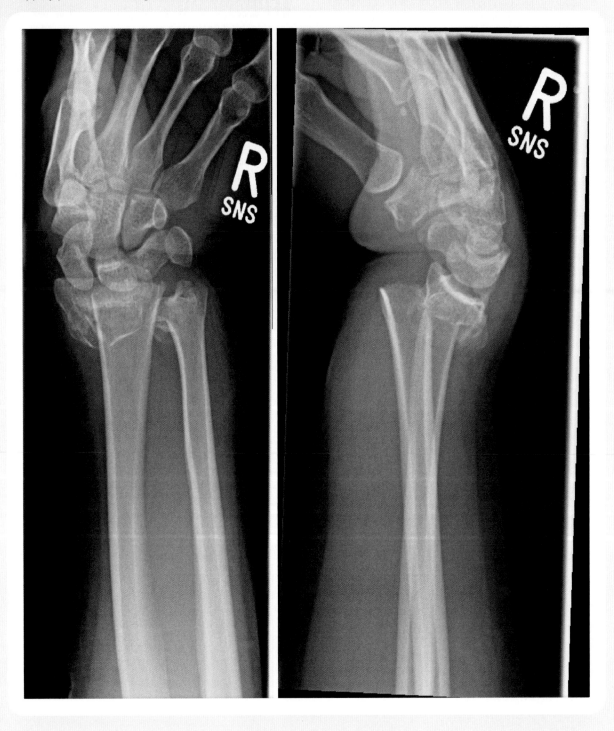

ANNOTATED X-RAY

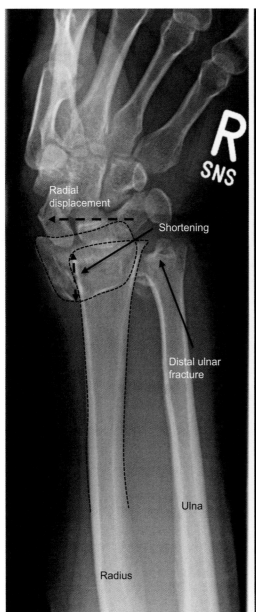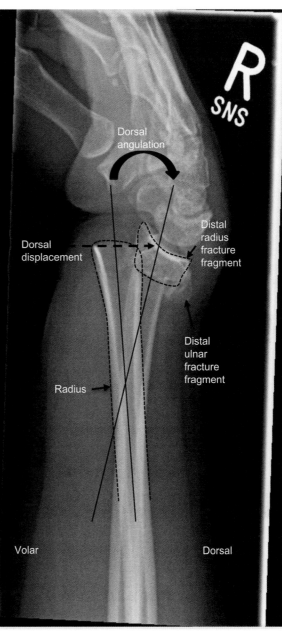

Labels on images: Radial displacement, Shortening, Distal ulnar fracture, Ulna, Radius, Dorsal angulation, Dorsal displacement, Distal radius fracture fragment, Radius, Distal ulnar fracture fragment, Volar, Dorsal, R SNS

🔍 PRESENT YOUR FINDINGS

- These are AP and lateral X-rays of the right wrist of a skeletally mature patient.
- They have been anonymised and the timing of the examination is not available. I would like to confirm the patient's details and timing of the examination before I make any further assessment.
- The X-rays are adequately exposed, with no important areas cut off.
- There is an obvious transverse fracture of the distal radius with an associated fracture of the distal ulna.
- There is dorsal angulation and displacement of the distal radial fragment, radial displacement and shortening.

- The distal ulna fracture is more difficult to assess but also appears displaced.
- No other fractures are visible.
- Bone density is normal, with no areas of lucency or sclerosis.
- There is soft tissue swelling related to the fracture but no other soft tissue abnormality.

IN SUMMARY – These X-rays show a dorsally angulated and displaced distal radius fracture, in keeping with a Colles' fracture. There is an associated fracture of the distal ulna.

Continue

CASE **4.8** *Contd.*

QUESTIONS

1. When assessing this patient, it is important to:
   - A) Take a history
   - B) Examine the joint above and below
   - C) Ensure this is not an open fracture
   - D) Check neurovascular status
   - E) Assess for other injuries

2. The nerve most likely to be affected by this fracture is:
   - A) Radial nerve
   - B) Superficial branch of the ulnar nerve
   - C) PIN
   - D) Median nerve
   - E) AIN

3. Which of the following is the most appropriate acute management of this fracture?
   - A) Take straight to theatre as this is an emergency
   - B) Put the arm in plaster and discharge the patient to fracture clinic
   - C) Immediately manipulate the fracture
   - D) Discharge the patient, with fracture clinic follow-up
   - E) Give adequate analgesia, manipulate the fracture with sedation and repeat the X-rays to confirm realignment

4. Which of these is/are eponymous fracture(s) of the distal radius?
   - A) Skier's thumb
   - B) Thurstan Holland fragment
   - C) Smith's fracture
   - D) Jones fracture
   - E) Holstein–Lewis fracture

5. The normal radiological measurements of a distal radius are:
   - A) 7 degrees of dorsal angulation, 4 mm +ve ulnar variance, radial inclination of 3 degrees
   - B) 12 degrees of volar angulation, between +2 mm and −2 mm ulnar variance, 22 degrees of radial inclination
   - C) 18 degrees volar angulation, −2 mm ulnar variance, 30 degrees of radial inclination
   - D) Neutral angulation, 0 ulna variance, 15 degrees of radial inclination
   - E) 10 degrees dorsal angulation, 0 ulnar variance, 7 degrees of radial inclination

ANSWERS TO QUESTIONS

1. When assessing this patient, it is important to:
   The correct answers are **A) Take a history, B) Examine the joint above and below, C) Ensure this is not an open fracture, D) Check neurovascular status and E) Assess for other injuries**.

   Whenever you have to assess a patient with an injury, it is important to take a history and to examine them. In the case of traumatic injury, you need to focus on the mechanism of the injury, whether the injury is open or closed and the distal neurovascular status. Remember: in high-energy injuries, there may be other more immediately life-threatening problems than a fractured wrist. Such patients should be assessed using the ATLS algorithm of ABCDE.

   A) Take a history – Correct. It is important to take a history from all patients but this is not all that is needed. The patient will hopefully be able to tell you about the mechanism of injury, such as a simple trip, as well as any other injuries. Further investigations will usually be required if the patient had a blackout/loss of consciousness leading to the injury. It is useful to know:
   - If the patient is right or left hand dominant
   - Whether they are working and if so what kind of work they do
   - The patient's functional status

   These factors may be used when determining what degree of fracture reduction /alignment would be satisfactory.

   B) Examine the joint above and below – Correct. Together with your history and examination, it is imperative to examine the joint above and below to ensure there is no missed injury. Associated injuries are common in the forearm and ankle. In trauma patients, you may need to examine the whole patient using a secondary survey. Fractures of the distal radius can occur following major trauma.

   C) Ensure this is not an open fracture – Correct. In patients where the bone is superficial (limited subcutaneous fat, thin skin) or those who have sustained a higher-energy injury, there may be an open fracture. Open fractures need to be identified and managed early to minimise the risk of infection. This should involve cleaning the wound, taking a photo of the wound, covering the wound and giving antibiotics. Taking a photo ensures the wound remains covered as much as possible as fellow doctors can look at the photo, rather than undressing the wound.

   D) Check neurovascular status – Correct. Displaced distal radius fractures can compress nerves around the wrist and significant injuries with swelling can cause a neurological deficit. It is important to examine the patient for this.

   E) Assess for other injuries – Correct. It is important to assess for other injuries. The patient may have hit their head during the fall, for example, and may require further assessment of this. Alternatively, if the fracture was caused by a high-energy injury, there may well be other fractures or internal injuries.

❶ KEY POINT

Distal radius fractures occur in two age groups. In the younger adult (20–30 years old), this is a high-energy injury and other injuries need to be excluded. In the older patient (>60 years old), this fracture is most likely a low-energy injury in an osteoporotic bone. This type of patient may need to be referred for a bone density scan (DEXA scan) to diagnose osteoporosis.

2. The nerve most likely to be affected by this fracture is:
   The correct answer is **D) Median nerve**.

   It is important for all fractures that the neurovascular status is examined thoroughly and specific nerves are examined individually (Table C4.8.1). Patients may have a neurological deficit because of a direct injury to the nerve or secondary to swelling. They may even be developing compartment syndrome.

   A) Radial nerve – Incorrect. The radial nerve divides at the elbow into the PIN and the superficial radial nerve. The radial nerve can be injured in fractures of the humerus but not the distal radius.

   B) Superficial branch of the ulnar nerve – Incorrect. It is uncommon for the superficial branch of the ulnar nerve to be injured following a distal radius fracture. It does, however, need to be identified and protected for the surgical approach to the distal ulna.

   C) PIN – Incorrect. The PIN supplies the majority of the extensors of the forearm and wrist. It has little function beyond the wrist and is not commonly injured in this fracture. This nerve can be injured in surgery to the radial head, as it wraps around the neck of the radius.

   D) Median nerve – Correct. The median nerve runs in the flexor compartment of the forearm before passing through the carpal tunnel at the wrist. When there is significant deformity or swelling, the median nerve can be compressed, giving symptoms similar to carpal tunnel syndrome.

   E) AIN – Incorrect. The AIN supplies the majority of flexors of the forearm and wrist. It has little function beyond the wrist and is not commonly injured in this type of fracture. It is, however, often injured in supracondylar fractures of the humerus in children and must be examined for in these patients.

❶ KEY POINT

To examine peripheral nerves you need to test as shown in Table C4.8.1.

Table C4.8.1   Upper Limb Motor and Sensory Functions

NERVE	MOTOR INNERVATION	SENSATION INNERVATION
Radial nerve	Wrist and finger extension	First dorsal web space
Superficial branch of ulnar nerve	–	Ulnar border of little finger

Continue

CASE 4.8 *Contd.*

Table C4.8.1   Upper Limb Motor and Sensory Functions—Cont'd

NERVE	MOTOR INNERVATION	SENSATION INNERVATION
PIN	Finger and wrist extension	–
Median nerve	Abduction of the thumb	Radial border of index finger
AIN	Difficulty making 'OK' sign. Flexion of IP joint of thumb (FPL), and DIP joints of index and middle fingers (FDP)	–

DIPJ, Distal interphalangeal joint; *FDP*, flexor digitorum profundus; *FPL*, flexor pollicis longus; *IP*, interphalangeal.

3. Which of the following is the most appropriate acute management of this fracture?

   The correct answer is **E) Give adequate analgesia, manipulate the fracture with sedation and repeat the X-rays to confirm realignment**.

   Following the initial assessment of a patient with a fracture, it is important to instigate initial management including analgesia. Displaced fractures may require manipulation with appropriate sedation. Following manipulation, repeat X-rays are necessary. A repeat assessment of the neurovascular status is important and should be clearly documented.

   A) Take straight to theatre as this is an emergency – Incorrect. It is very rare for this injury to be an emergency. This would only be the case if there was associated ischaemia or compartment syndrome. Open fractures are urgent but do not usually require immediate transfer to theatre.

   B) Put the arm in plaster and discharge the patient to fracture clinic – Incorrect. For undisplaced distal radius fractures, the only treatment required may be a plaster for splinting; however, with a displaced fracture like this, reduction is required. Not reducing the fracture can lead to further soft tissue damage, swelling and neurological compromise.

   C) Immediately manipulate the fracture – Incorrect. This fracture does need manipulation but there are other aspects to the care of this patient as well. In undisplaced fractures, a plaster and fracture clinic appointment is likely all that is required.

   D) Discharge the patient with fracture clinic follow-up – Incorrect. A displaced fracture like this cannot just be discharged to a fracture clinic. An undisplaced fracture of the distal radius can be treated nonoperatively.

   E) Give adequate analgesia, manipulate the fracture with sedation and repeat the X-rays to confirm realignment – Correct. By doing this, you may be able to provide all the treatment this patient will need and potentially avoid any operation at all.

4. Which of these is/are eponymous fracture(s) of the distal radius?

   The correct answer is **C) Smith's fracture**.

   Although it is important to describe the fracture as it appears on the X-ray, there are occasions where an eponymous name of a fracture is very useful. For example, when you describe the fracture to a senior colleague, they will immediately know what you are describing if you use the correct eponym or classification. Eponymous fractures usually have typical mechanisms of injury, management and prognosis. For the wrist, the most common fracture is a Colles' fracture.

   A) Skier's thumb – Incorrect. Skier's thumb is an injury of the ulnar collateral ligament of the thumb MCPJ. This is not necessarily a fracture but is a rupture of the ligament. There can be a small bony fragment that comes away with the ligament, a Stener lesion. This injury can cause instability of the thumb and may require repair. This injury is also known as a Gamekeeper's thumb.

   B) Thurstan Holland fragment – Incorrect. The Thurstan Holland fragment refers to a bony fragment seen in Salter–Harris 2 fractures. The Salter–Harris fracture classification is used to define fractures around the growth plate in children.

   C) Smith's fracture – Correct. A Smith's fracture is an extraarticular fracture of the distal radius with volar angulation and displacement. This is an unstable injury not to be confused with the more common dorsally angulated distal radius fracture (Colles' fracture). The patient is more likely to have fallen onto the back of their hand rather than onto an outstretched hand as is seen in Colles' fractures. This needs referral to an orthopaedic surgeon.

   D) Jones fracture – Incorrect. A Jones fracture is a fracture of the base of the 5th metatarsal. This fracture can potentially not heal (nonunion) or be slow to heal (delayed union). It can, however, be treated nonoperatively in a weight-bearing rigid soled shoe.

   E) Holstein–Lewis fracture – Incorrect. A Holstein–Lewis fracture is a fracture at the junction of the middle and distal third of the humerus. This is a very important fracture as it is where the radial nerve is most vulnerable and therefore associated with the highest incidence of a radial nerve palsy. It is important to examine patients with this fracture pre and post manipulation. If a new nerve palsy develops following manipulation, this is an indication for surgical exploration.

❗ KEY POINT

The correct use of eponymous terms can be used to convey a lot of information about a particular fracture (likely mechanism of injury, appearance and expected management and prognosis); however, they refer to particular fracture patterns. If you are unsure, it is best to describe the fracture.

5. The normal radiological measurements of a distal radius are:

The correct answer is **B) 12 degrees of volar angulation, between +2 mm and −2 mm ulnar variance, 22 degrees of radial inclination**.

The radiological measurements of the distal radius are used by orthopaedic surgeons to guide surgical management, particularly in active, fit patients. They are useful in understanding the degree of the deformity/displacement and deciding whether this is acceptable. However, these measurements do not take into account whether the fracture is intraarticular or extraarticular. Intraarticular fractures need accurate reduction to minimise the risks of posttraumatic arthritis of the wrist joint.

 IMPORTANT LEARNING POINTS

- For all fractures, you need to clinically assess whether the fracture is neurovascularly intact, open or associated with any other injuries.
- Distal radius fractures are common, and require accurate reduction to improve outcome.
- In the younger adult (20–30 years old), this is a high-energy injury and other injuries need to be excluded.
- In the older patient (>60 years old), this fracture is most likely a low-energy injury in an osteoporotic bone.
- Management depends on the degree of displacement and whether it is an open fracture.
- Intraarticular fractures need accurate reduction.

A 74-year-old lady is referred to the elective orthopaedic clinic with a 7-month history of hip pain. She says the pain is worse on the right side. An X-ray of the hips has been performed.

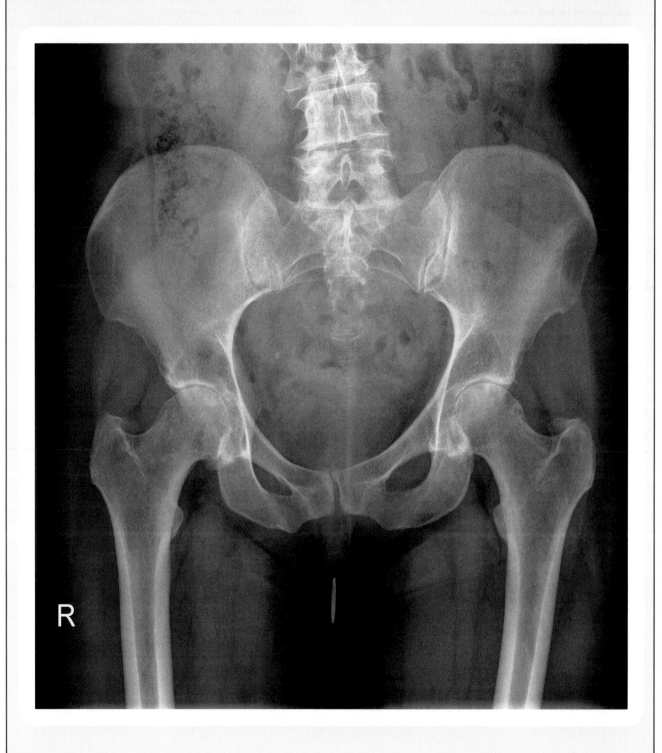

ANNOTATED X-RAY

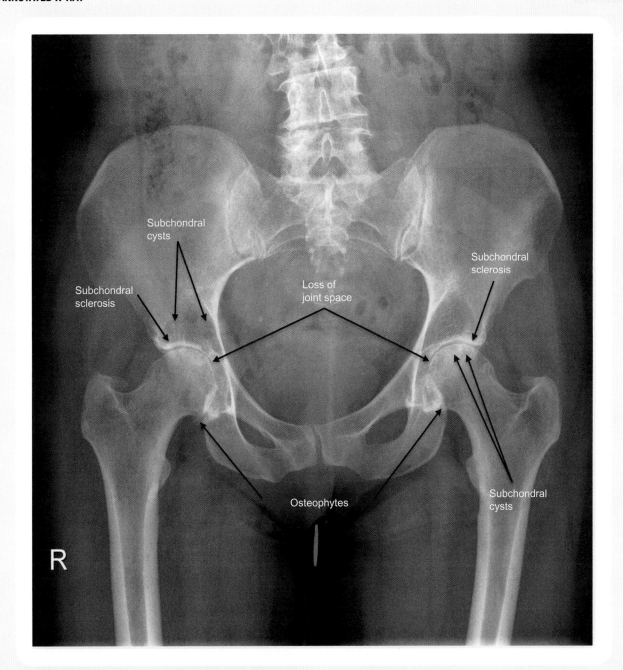

Subchondral
cysts

Subchondral
sclerosis

Subchondral
sclerosis

Loss of
joint space

Osteophytes

Subchondral
cysts

R

🔍 PRESENT YOUR FINDINGS

- This is an AP X-ray of the pelvis of a skeletally mature patient.
- It has been anonymised and the timing of the examination is not available. I would like to confirm the patient's details and timing of the examination before I make any further assessment.
- The X-ray is adequately penetrated and well centred, with no important areas cut off.
- Both hip joints are abnormal with bilateral loss of joint space, osteophytes, subchondral sclerosis and subchondral cysts. These findings are consistent with osteoarthritis of both hips.

- There is no fracture.
- The sacrum and sacroiliac joints have a normal appearance.
- Apart from the changes around the hip joints, the bone texture is normal, with no focal areas of lucency or sclerosis.
- No other abnormalities are present and the soft tissues appear normal.

IN SUMMARY – This X-ray shows bilateral hip joint osteoarthritis. I would like to review previous X-rays to assess whether these changes were previously present and whether they have progressed.

Continue

CASE **4.9** *Contd.*

QUESTIONS

1. Which of the following are X-ray features of osteoarthritis?
   A) Osteophytes
   B) Periarticular erosions
   C) Periarticular osteoporosis
   D) Loss of joint space
   E) Subchondral sclerosis

2. How do you test for a Trendelenburg sign?
   A) With the patient lying flat, place one hand under the back and ask them to flex their hips up together. Then ask then to straighten the hips in turn
   B) Ask the patient to lift the leg straight off the bed
   C) With the patient prone, lift the leg straight up
   D) Ask the patient to walk up and down
   E) Ask the patient to stand. Ask them to put their hands on your hands. Then ask them to stand on their good leg and watch for any pelvic tilt. Then do the same on the affected side

3. Which of these is/are useful for assessing the severity of osteoarthritis?
   A) Degree of pain
   B) Night pain
   C) Pain on standing from sitting
   D) X-ray changes
   E) Rheumatoid factor levels

4. What is the best management option for a fit and active 75-year old with severe debilitating osteoarthritis of the hip?
   A) Hip resurfacing
   B) Physiotherapy, weight loss and analgesia
   C) THR
   D) Hemiarthroplasty
   E) Girdlestone

5. Which of these are common approaches to the hip for joint replacement?
   A) Anterior approach
   B) Anterolateral approach
   C) Lateral approach
   D) Posterior approach
   E) Inferior approach

ANSWERS TO QUESTIONS

1. **Which of these are X-ray features of osteoarthritis?**
The correct answers are **A) Osteophytes, D) Loss of joint space and E) Subchondral sclerosis**.
Osteoarthritis is common and usually easily recognised on an X-ray. The classic findings are:
- Loss of the normal joint space
- Osteophytes, which are small bony protuberances around the edge of the joint
- Subchondral sclerosis, which is where the joint surface looks sclerotic and more white
- Subchondral cysts, which form with the sclerosis
    A) Osteophytes – Correct. Osteophytes (bony projections that occur along joint margins) are a feature of osteoarthritis. They are a useful finding as they help distinguish osteoarthritis from rheumatoid arthritis.
    B) Periarticular erosions – Incorrect. Periarticular erosions are a feature of inflammatory arthritides such as rheumatoid and psoriatic arthritis. The inflammatory process within the joint capsule (synovitis) in these conditions causes erosion of the bone. The articular surfaces are usually protected by their cartilage lining; hence, the erosions usually occur in a periarticular distribution.
    C) Periarticular osteoporosis – Incorrect. Periarticular osteoporosis is an early feature of rheumatoid arthritis. It can be difficult to spot but the bone around the affected joints will appear less dense. It is not found in psoriatic arthritis or osteoarthritis.
    D) Loss of joint space – Correct. Loss of joint space is one of earliest signs of osteoarthritis; however, it is nonspecific as it can be present in most forms of arthritis, such as rheumatoid and psoriatic arthritis.
    E) Subchondral sclerosis – Correct. Subchondral sclerosis is a common finding in osteoarthritis.

❶ KEY POINT

The X-ray findings of osteoarthritis are an extremely common question in exams. They are repeated in this chapter to ensure they are not forgotten!

2. **How do you test for a Trendelenburg sign?**
The correct answer is **E) Ask the patient to stand. Ask them to put their hands on your hands. Then ask them to stand on their good leg and watch for any pelvic tilt. Then do the same on the affected side**.
It is important to know how to examine the hip properly. There are many clinical tests of the hips to help assess for different pathologies. The Trendelenburg test is one most medical students have trouble with.
    A) With the patient lying flat, place one hand under the back and ask them to flex their hips up together. Then ask then to straighten the hips in turn – Incorrect. This is Thomas' test which is performed to assess for any fixed flexion deformity. This is an important part of hip

examination. There may be a fixed flexion deformity of the hip in osteoarthritis.
    B) Ask the patient to lift the leg straight off the bed – Incorrect. This is a straight leg raise. Straight leg raise tests quadriceps function or can be used in the examination of patients with a neck of femur fracture where there is doubt about the diagnosis of a fracture. If combined with ankle dorsiflexion followed by knee flexion, then this is a sciatic stretch test which tests for nerve root irritation.
    C) With the patient prone lift the leg straight up – Incorrect. This is the femoral stretch test, which is a sign of femoral nerve root irritation.
    D) Ask the patient to walk up and down – Incorrect. By examining a patient's gait, you may identify the cause of their pain. The Trendelenburg gait is different from the Trendelenburg sign. The Trendelenburg gait is characterised by a downward tilt of the opposite pelvis to the affected side. This is due to weakness of the hip abductors.
    E) Ask the patient to stand. Ask them to put their hands on your hands. Then ask them to stand on their good leg and watch for any pelvic tilt. Then do the same on the affected side – Correct. This accurately describes the Trendelenburg test. This tests the function of the abductor muscles (gluteus medius and minimus). These muscles normally pull the opposite side of the pelvis up, stopping it from dipping down (i.e. if the patient is standing on their right leg, their right hip abductors should contract to prevent the pelvis tilting to the left and vice versa).
In a positive test, the patient will not be able to stand on one leg. Instead, they will either lean over to the affected side or will apply pressure on your hands to steady their balance. This test can be positive for several reasons, but in a patient with osteoarthritis of the hip, it is most likely to be positive because of pain inhibiting the abductor muscles from functioning normally.

❶ KEY POINT

Orthopaedic examinations are generally simple and follow the process of look, feel, move and special tests.

3. **Which of these is/are useful for assessing the severity of osteoarthritis?**
The correct answers are **A) Degree of pain, B) Night pain, C) Pain on standing from sitting and D) X-ray changes**.
Do not rely solely on the X-ray findings when assessing a patient with osteoarthritis of the hips, as the patient's symptoms and the X-ray findings do not always correlate. Additionally, it is important to assess how the symptoms are affecting the patient's life. Some patients who are less active are more willing to accept some restriction in their activities of daily living, whereas others will be very troubled if they are unable to run a marathon.

Continue

CASE **4.9**   *Contd.*

A) Degree of pain – Correct. It is important to ask the patient how severe the pain is. They may have mild symptoms and have come to the orthopaedic clinic because they want reassurance not an operation! Asking a patient to quantify their pain (using a scale of 1–10) is useful, especially to compare pain scores pre- and postoperatively.

B) Night pain – Correct. Pain at night is a common complaint in severe osteoarthritis and is often a good marker of when to offer a hip replacement. Patients often are kept up all night by their pain and this has a major effect on their quality of life. Be sure to exclude more sinister causes of night pain, such as malignancy and infection.

C) Pain on standing from sitting – Correct. This is a common symptom of osteoarthritis and helps diagnose osteoarthritis as the cause of pain.

D) X-ray changes – Correct. The severity of X-ray changes is most important when considered with the degree of symptoms and the clinical findings. X-ray changes of osteoarthritis can be graded subjectively as mild, with little loss of joint space and only a few osteophytes, to severe where there is complete loss of joint space.

E) Rheumatoid factor levels – Incorrect. Rheumatoid factor is associated with rheumatoid not osteoarthritis. It is not used to assess the severity of osteoarthritis.

---

❶ KEY POINT

When assessing for osteoarthritis, consider the patient's wishes and expectations, the history and examination, not just the X-ray!

---

4. What is the best management option for a fit and active 75-year old with severe debilitating osteoarthritis of the hip?
The correct answer is **C) THR**.
The vast majority of patients with severe osteoarthritis who are fit and well are best treated with a THR. The head and neck of the femur are excised and replaced with a new ball and socket joint. Both the acetabular and the femoral parts of the joint are replaced. However, it is important to consider the different options available which may occasionally have use.

A) Hip resurfacing – Incorrect. Hip resurfacing is a surgical option for hip arthritis. The acetabulum is replaced and the head of the femur is not excised but resurfaced. This option is not favoured at present because of poorer long-term outcomes.

B) Physiotherapy, weight loss and analgesia – Incorrect. Hip replacement surgery is a big operation with associated risks. It is only after careful counselling that an operation should be considered. Although not appropriate for this patient, there are nonoperative measures which may delay the need for a hip replacement. Some patients will benefit from weight loss, physiotherapy and analgesia.

C) THR – Correct. THR is the best option for this patient. They are usually discharged from hospital 2 to 3 days after the operation and will be expected to have a good functional return. Most patients find their pain improves rapidly and are delighted with their results. About 5% of patients, however, develop complications such as infection, dislocation, loosening or wear. Currently, it is expected that most hip replacements will last at least 15 to 20 years.

D) Hemiarthroplasty – Incorrect. A hemiarthroplasty is only a surgical option for fractures of the neck of femur. A hemiarthroplasty is essentially a half hip replacement. The acetabulum is not replaced and instead just the femoral head and neck is replaced. This reduces the risk of dislocation, is a quicker operation and is better suited to frail patients with a fracture of the neck of the femur.

E) Girdlestone – Incorrect. This is a salvage procedure in unwell patients or those who have had complications from their THR. The hip joint is excised, leaving the leg shortened. The neck of the femur then forms a pseudoarticulation with the superior lip of the acetabulum. The functional outcome from this is surprisingly good, with some patients able to walk afterwards (all be it with a shoe raise).

5. Which of these are common approaches to the hip for joint replacement?
The correct answers are **A) Anterior approach B) Anterolateral approach, C) Lateral approach and D) Posterior approach**.
There are several surgical approaches to the hip joint. Some of these are used for joint replacement surgery while others are used in different operations. It is useful to know that these approaches exist and the anatomy of these approaches.

A) Anterior approach – Correct. The anterior approach is being used increasingly for arthroplasty around the world. This approach is between tensor fascia lata and sartorius and care needs to be taken to protect the femoral nerve, artery and vein and the lateral cutaneous nerve of the thigh. The approach has also more traditionally been used in paediatric orthopaedics for septic arthritis or development dysplasia.

B) Anterolateral approach – Correct. The anterolateral approach is commonly used for hip replacements. The fascia lata is opened and the anterior third of the abductors is taken off the greater trochanter. If the abductors (gluteus medius and gluteus minimus) are not carefully repaired at the end of the operation, the patient will develop a Trendelenburg gait.

C) Lateral approach – Correct. The lateral approach is a more traditional approach in which the abductors are taken off the greater trochanter with or without a greater trochanter osteotomy (where the bone is purposely broken). This approach is not as commonly used now and has been modified into the anterolateral approach.

D) Posterior approach – Correct. The posterior approach is one of the standard approaches for accessing the hip joint. The abductors are not disturbed; therefore, the patient does not develop a postoperative Trendelenburg gait. However, this approach takes the surgeon very close to the sciatic nerve which must be protected. Additionally, there is a slightly increased risk of posterior dislocation postoperatively with this approach.

E) Inferior approach – Incorrect. This approach does not exist.

IMPORTANT LEARNING POINTS

- Osteoarthritis of the hip is a common finding in the ageing population. It is important to know for examinations and for clinical practice.
- A thorough history and examination are as important, if not more so, than an X-ray for assessing the most appropriate treatment.
- When examining the hip look, feel and move the hip and include the special tests discussed, such as Trendelenburg test.
- The four X-ray features of osteoarthritis (of any joint) are loss of joint space, osteophytes, subchondral sclerosis and subchondral cyst formation.
- Osteoarthritis of the hip can be managed conservatively, with weight loss, physiotherapy and analgesia or operatively, usually with a THR.

CASE **4.10**

A 6-year-old boy presents to your clinic with an 8-week history of a limp. His X-ray is shown here.

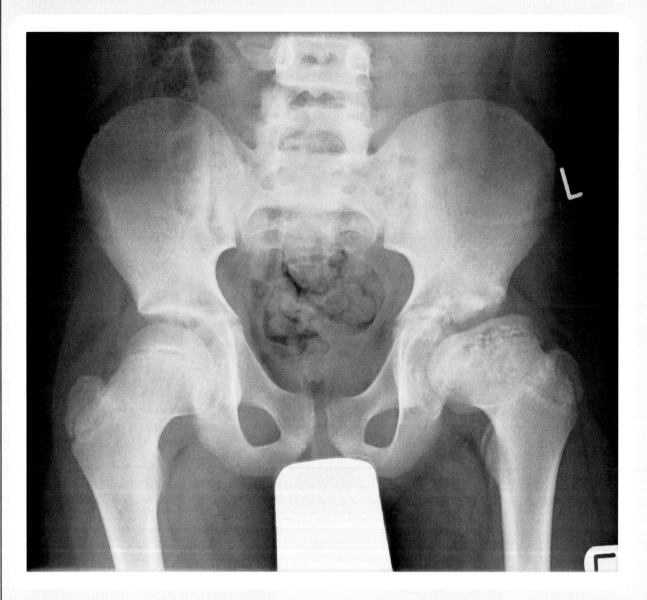

ANNOTATED X-RAY

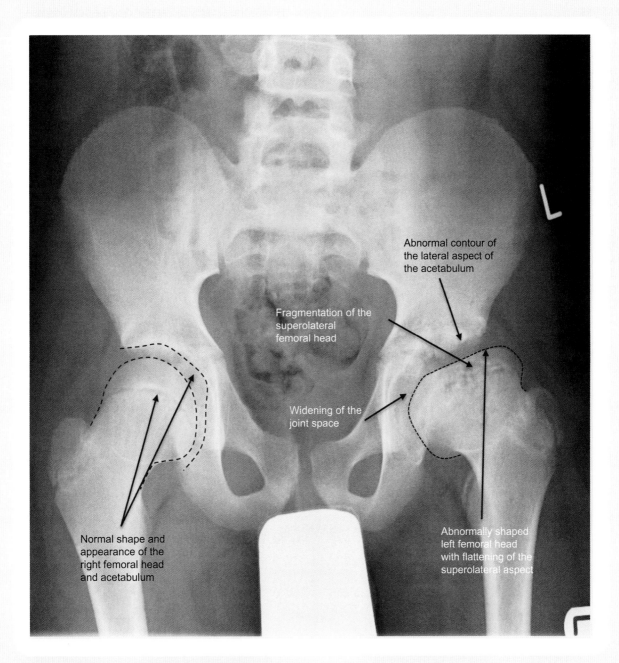

Abnormal contour of
the lateral aspect of
the acetabulum

Fragmentation of the
superolateral
femoral head

Widening of the
joint space

Normal shape and
appearance of the
right femoral head
and acetabulum

Abnormally shaped
left femoral head
with flattening of the
superolateral aspect

🔍 PRESENT YOUR FINDINGS

- This is an AP X-ray of the pelvis of a skeletally immature patient.
- It has been anonymised and the timing of the examination is not available. I would like to confirm the patient's
  details and timing of the examination before I make any
  further assessment.
- The X-ray is adequately exposed to display the pathology, with no important areas cut off the X-ray.
- The left hip joint is abnormal. There is flattening and
  fragmentation of the left femoral head and widening of
  the joint space.

- The left acetabulum is also abnormal with an irregular
  appearance to its lateral aspect.
- The right hip joint has a normal appearance.
- There are no lytic lesions or fractures.
- There is no associated soft tissue abnormality.

IN SUMMARY – The findings on the X-ray are in keeping
with AVN of the left hip. The right hip is normal. The findings
are consistent with Perthes disease.

CASE **4.10**   *Contd.*

QUESTIONS

1. What imaging modality is most commonly used for assessing a child with suspected Perthes disease?
   A) X-ray
   B) MRI
   C) Ultrasound
   D) Bone scan
   E) CT

2. The features of Perthes disease on X-ray include which of the following?
   A) Widening of the joint space
   B) Increased density of the ossification centre of the femoral head
   C) Flattening of the femoral head
   D) Fragmentation
   E) Narrowing of the joint space

3. The differential diagnosis for Perthes disease includes which of the following?
   A) Septic arthritis of the hip
   B) Osteomyelitis of the femur
   C) NAI
   D) DDH
   E) All of the above

4. How is the severity of Perthes disease best assessed?
   A) Using clinical examination
   B) The use of close clinical monitoring
   C) Age of presentation
   D) Changes on X-ray
   E) Family history

5. Which of the following is/are treatment options for Perthes disease?
   A) Reassurance and analgesia
   B) Early operative intervention
   C) Abduction brace
   D) THR
   E) Adduction brace

ANSWERS TO QUESTIONS

1. What imaging modality is most commonly used for assessing a child with suspected Perthes disease?
   The correct answer is **A) X-ray**.
   Although there are several imaging modalities available for assessing Perthes disease, the most commonly used is X-ray. X-rays will usually demonstrate the disease but will also allow specialists to decide on the management and severity of the condition.
   A) X-ray – Correct. X-rays of the hip in paediatrics requires two views. These include the AP pelvis view above and also a lateral. For children, the lateral is best obtained with a frog view lateral, where the child sits like a frog, with their hips and knees flexed and the soles of their feet touching. This allows for a lateral of both hips to be obtained simultaneously.
   B) MRI – Incorrect. MRI is actually more sensitive for detecting Perthes disease, as it can show changes long before there is any evidence of a problem on an X-ray. It also allows an assessment of the cartilaginous portion of the joint, which cannot be seen on X-ray. However, MRI is comparatively expensive and not always readily available. Furthermore, X-rays are usually sufficient for making the diagnosis and can be used for determining prognosis. MRI is reserved for patients in whom the X-rays are inconclusive or if other conditions are being considered. MRI in children can be difficult as it is noisy, in a tight space and the child has to stay completely still for a prolonged period of scanning.
   C) Ultrasound – Incorrect. Ultrasound of the hip is used to identify or exclude an effusion in a limping child or DDH. However, it is not routinely used to diagnose Perthes disease.
   D) Bone scan – Incorrect. A bone scan can identify areas of ischaemia before changes are visible on X-rays. Such areas will appear as a photopenic area on the bone scan (i.e. areas of reduced or absent osteoblastic activity). However, bone scans are not commonly used for diagnosing Perthes disease.
   E) CT – Incorrect. CT provides more information about bones and fractures than plain X-rays. However, it uses significantly higher doses of radiation and is not required for making the diagnosis.

❶ KEY POINT

X-rays are the mainstay for diagnosing and following up Perthes disease. However, MRI is a more sensitive imaging modality and allows the diagnosis to be made at an earlier stage.

2. The features of Perthes disease on X-ray include which of the following?
   The correct answers are **A) Widening of the joint space, B) Increased density of the ossification centre of the femoral head, C) Flattening of the femoral head, D) Fragmentation and E) Narrowing of the joint space**.

Perthes disease is a form of AVN where the femoral head loses its blood supply. It usually presents in children between the ages of 4 and 8 years. There is pain and a limp. The loss of blood supply to the femoral head is not permanent and there can be varying degrees of severity of the condition. There are various features on X-ray to look out for, depending on the stage and severity of the condition.
A) Widening of the joint space – Correct. Widening of the joint space may be the earliest sign of the disease. Typically, the medial joint space is widened. However, there are other X-ray features to look for.
B) Increased density of the ossification centre of the femoral head – Correct. Increased density of the bony epiphysis is the other earliest sign of Perthes disease. The ossification centre is where the necrosis occurs and this is visible on the X-ray. Remember: the cartilagenous part of the femoral head is not visible on the X-ray but it usually keeps its shape initially despite the bone necrosis. There may also be asymmetry of the epiphyses (the affected side is smaller). However, there are other X-ray features to look for.
C) Flattening of the femoral head – Correct. Flattening of the femoral head is a late sign. The necrosis of the bone has led to the femoral head losing its structural integrity and over time it loses its normal shape due to the stresses of weight bearing.
D) Fragmentation – Correct. Fragmentation is seen as the bone undergoes necrosis. Some bone will reform and some will be replaced by fibrous tissue, which gives the appearance of fragments of increased density interspersed with areas of lucency. Other associated findings include lateral displacement of the epiphysis and broadening of the metaphysis.
E) Narrowing of the joint space – Correct. Osteoarthritis is a complication of Perthes disease, and one of the radiological hallmarks of osteoarthritis is joint space narrowing.

❶ KEY POINTS

1. There are several different X-ray findings associated with Perthes disease which vary with the degree of ischaemia, the patient's age and the stage of the disease.
2. The X-ray features of Perthes disease are applicable to other causes of AVN.
3. The common causes of AVN (in adults or children) in any bone are:
   - Idiopathic
   - Alcoholism
   - Sickle cell anaemia
   - Exogenous steroids or radiotherapy
   - Pancreatitis
   - Trauma
   - Infection
   - Caisson disease (decompression sickness)
   - Perthes disease
   - SUFE

Continue

CASE 4.10 *Contd.*

3. The differential diagnosis for Perthes disease includes which of the following?

The correct answer is **E) All of the above**.

There is a wide range of differential diagnoses for a limping child. Understanding how the different conditions present will allow you to tailor your history, examination and investigations. In Perthes disease the child presents with a history over weeks of pain in the hip with a limp. Symptoms may be intermittent and on examination you will normally find a reduced range of movement in the hip joint.

A) Septic arthritis of the hip – Incorrect. Septic arthritis presents acutely with fever, inability to weight bear and raised inflammatory markers. X-rays may show an effusion of the hip. If left with pus in the joint, there will be bone destruction and early osteoarthritis.

B) Osteomyelitis of the femur – Incorrect. Osteomyelitis presents with fever and pain at the affected site. The disease is progressive rather than intermittent.

C) NAI – Incorrect. NAI must be considered when assessing all children who present to a doctor. Features include fractures at different stages of healing, bruises at different stages of healing, delayed presentation with a fracture or inconsistencies in the history. NAI is difficult to determine and has wide-reaching consequences. It is therefore essential to discuss the case with your seniors as soon as possible.

D) DDH – Incorrect. DDH is present from birth and more common in babies who are born breech. It is caused by deformity of the hip joint such that the femoral head is not held within the acetabulum – instead it subluxes or dislocates. Babies are screened for DDH and so the patient will often have a known history of DDH and may have been treated surgically already or with the use of a harness to keep the hip from dislocating. However, occasionally the diagnosis may have been missed in infancy and the child may present later with a limp and pain.

E) All of the above – Correct. These are not the only conditions to consider and others include irritable hip and SUFE.

> **❶ KEY POINT**

The differential diagnosis of a limping child is useful to know for clinical practice but also commonly assessed in exams! In addition to the history and examination, the age of the child helps to identify the most likely underlying cause:

- 0 to 4 years: DDH, transient synovitis (irritable hip)
- 4 to 10 years: Perthes disease, transient synovitis (irritable hip), juvenile rheumatoid arthritis
- 14 to 16 years: SUFE
- Fractures, infection and tumours can occur in any age group, although the types of fracture and tumours vary depending on the age of the child (e.g. toddler's fractures occur in infants, whereas stress fractures occur in adolescents)

4. How is the severity of Perthes disease best assessed?

The correct answers are **C) Age of presentation and D) Changes on X-ray**.

Perthes disease is a condition which generally resolves over approximately a 4-year period, with limited long-term functional problems. Following the onset of AVN there is new bone formation. As long as the overall shape of the cartilaginous femoral head has not been affected then the new bone will form in the femoral head without losing the normal shape and function of the hip joint. However, a proportion of patients may require further intervention and it is important to be able to recognise which patients are likely to have a worse prognosis.

A) Using clinical examination – Incorrect. Although it is important to examine the patient, clinical assessment gives few clues about the degree of the disease and prognosis, and will not guide possible intervention.

B) The use of close clinical monitoring – Incorrect. Although it is important to monitor these patients to ensure the disease is progressing appropriately, clinical monitoring alone does not suggest severity.

C) Age of presentation – Correct. It is generally accepted that Perthes disease presenting at a later age has a worse prognosis. In patients under the age of 6 the outcome is usually good regardless of treatment. Those over 6 are more likely to develop complications, especially patients older than 8 years of age.

D) Changes on X-ray – Correct. The Herring classification system looks at the degree of disintegration of the femoral epiphysis on the X-ray. It ranges from group A to C, with group C having the worst prognosis.

E) Family history – Incorrect. Family history is important to enquire about in the history but it does not affect prognosis.

5. Which of the following is/are treatment options for Perthes disease?

The correct answers are **A) Reassurance and analgesia, B) Early operative intervention, C) Abduction brace and D) THR**.

Treatment of Perthes disease can be split into medical (nonoperative) and operative options. Each case needs to be considered individually and managed appropriately. The choice of the exact treatment option is usually decided upon by the orthopaedic surgeon and beyond the knowledge expected for a medical student or junior doctor.

A) Reassurance and analgesia – Correct. For young patients with mild Perthes disease the outcome is likely to be good. Analgesia and reassurance may be all that is required although monitoring of the condition is advised.

B) Early operative intervention – Correct. Operative intervention for Perthes disease is complex and needs to involve a paediatric orthopaedic surgeon. It is however important to recognise which patients may benefit from intervention and refer on as appropriate. These include those presenting at an older age or those with more severe Perthes disease as defined by Herring's classification. There are multiple surgical options. This includes an osteotomy to ensure that the femoral head remains in the acetabulum and therefore better retains its shape. The decision on when to operate is, however, variable between surgeons.

C) Abduction brace – Correct. An abduction brace is useful for Perthes disease when the femoral head is displaced laterally. This forces the femoral head medially and holds it in the joint, reducing the loss of contour of the femoral head (in the growing hip, correct alignment of the femoral head with the acetabulum is needed for the normal development of the hip joint). Abduction is often the movement that is lost as a result of the flattened femoral head. The use of these braces again needs to be decided by a specialist.

D) THR – Correct. THR is an absolute last resort and will usually only be considered in adults or teenagers who have reached skeletal maturity. The necrosis causes flattening of the femoral head which can lead to early osteoarthritis of the hip which is then treated with a joint replacement later in life.

E) Adduction brace – Incorrect. Abduction not adduction bracing is a possible treatment option.

 IMPORTANT LEARNING POINTS

- Perthes disease is a form of AVN of the femoral head.
- It typically presents in children aged 4 to 8 years with intermittent pain and limping.
- The differential diagnosis of a limping child is partly determined by the age of the child, but fractures, infection and neoplasia can occur in any age group.
- X-rays are usually sufficient for diagnosis of Perthes disease, and the X-ray features are the same as any form of AVN.
- MRI is more sensitive for detecting early changes, but is reserved for difficult cases.
- Prognosis is determined by the age of presentation (younger age = better prognosis) and the X-ray findings including the Herring classification. Females also have a poorer outcome.
- Management depends on the likely prognosis and includes analgesia, bracing and rarely surgery.

CASE **4.11**

A 25-year-old motorcyclist has been brought to A&E after coming off her bike at 50 mph. She was wearing a helmet but no protective clothing. She is hypotensive and tachycardic, and complaining of pain all over. The A&E team are stabilising the patient. As the orthopaedic junior doctor, you have been called to review her pelvis X-ray.

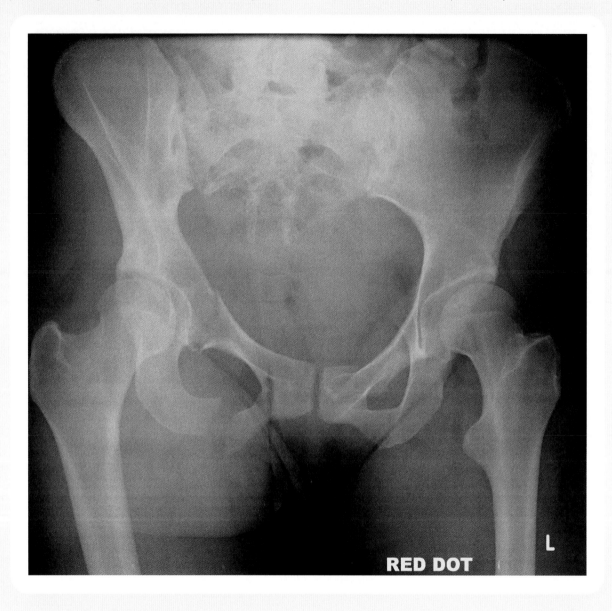

ANNOTATED X-RAY

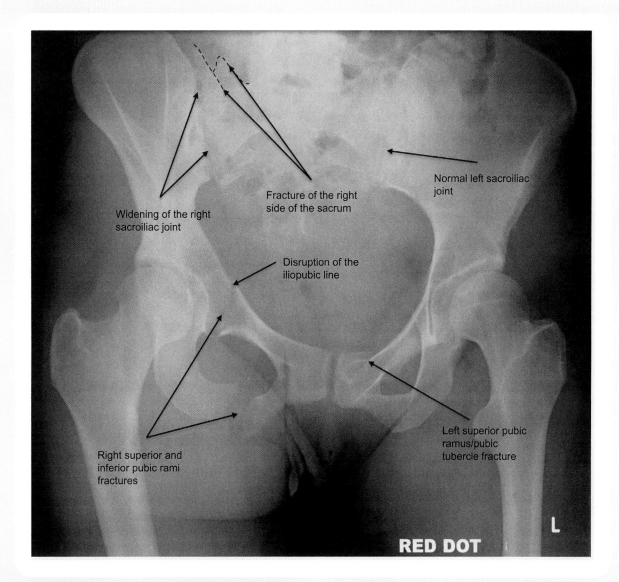

Widening of the right sacroiliac joint

Fracture of the right side of the sacrum

Normal left sacroiliac joint

Disruption of the iliopubic line

Right superior and inferior pubic rami fractures

Left superior pubic ramus/pubic tubercle fracture

L

RED DOT

🔍 PRESENT YOUR FINDINGS

- This is an AP X-ray of a pelvis in a skeletally mature individual.
- It has been anonymised and the timing of the examination is not available. I would like to confirm the patient's details and timing of the examination before I make any further assessment.
- The X-ray is adequately exposed, with no important areas cut off.
- There are multiple pelvic fractures. There are displaced fractures through the superior and inferior right pubic rami, with disruption of the right iliopubic line. There is a fracture of the left superior pubic ramus.

- There is a fracture and dislocation of the right sacroiliac joint.
- There is no soft tissue abnormality.

IN SUMMARY – This pelvic X-ray shows multiple fractures of the pelvis. There is a high risk of associated internal pelvic injuries as well as other injuries from the accident. This patient requires urgent assessment using the ATLS ABCDE approach, with early cross sectional imaging to guide definitive management.

Continue

CASE **4.11** *Contd.*

QUESTIONS

1. How is this patient best managed initially?
   A) Using an ABCDE assessment
   B) With a trauma team
   C) Take straight to theatre as she will almost certainly have life-threatening injuries
   D) Early cross sectional imaging
   E) Taking a thorough history and performing a complete examination before commencing any treatment

2. What X-rays is/are part of the initial 'trauma series'?
   A) Portable AP chest and pelvis X-rays
   B) Portable AP chest and pelvis X-rays and cervical spine X-rays
   C) Departmental PA chest X-ray and AP pelvis X-ray
   D) AP pelvis X-ray
   E) FAST scan and diagnostic peritoneal lavage

3. Which of these are types of major pelvic fracture?
   A) Lateral compression
   B) Vertical shear
   C) Closed book
   D) Avulsion fracture of the superior acetabulum
   E) Isolated pubic ramus fracture

4. Which of these injuries is/are most commonly associated with pelvic fractures?
   A) Vaginal perforation
   B) Hip dislocation
   C) Bladder and urethral injuries
   D) Rectal perforation
   E) Death

5. Which of these is/are definitive management options for this fracture?
   A) A pelvic binder
   B) Internal fixation
   C) Angiography
   D) Traction and internal rotation
   E) External fixation

ANSWERS TO QUESTIONS

1. How is this patient best managed initially?

   The correct answers are **A) Using an ABCDE assessment, B) With a trauma team and D) Early cross sectional imaging**.

   Trauma patients are often unstable and can have multiple injuries. The initial management is aimed at identifying and treating the immediate life-threatening injuries before fully assessing the patient for evidence of other injuries. Initial trauma management is guided by the ATLS guidelines. Many hospitals will have a trauma team which will assemble in the A&E resuscitation department to rapidly assess and manage a trauma patient.

   A) Using an ABCDE assessment – Correct. The ABCDE assessment is a very useful framework for assessing trauma patients.

   - **A** is for **airway with cervical spine control and external haemorrhage control**. An obstructed airway can be rapidly fatal; therefore, this must be identified and managed appropriately. Treat all trauma patients as if they have a cervical spine injury until proven otherwise. Apply pressure to sites of active haemorrhage.

   - **B** is for **breathing and ventilation**. A tension pneumothorax is a life-threatening injury and should be identified clinically. Immediate needle decompression can be lifesaving. Other treatment includes high flow oxygen and chest drain insertion (for pneumo or haemothoraces).

   - **C** is for **circulation with haemorrhage control**. This may include bleeding from intraabdominal or thoracic causes. There is a useful way of remembering where life-threatening bleeding may occur – on the floor and four more. The four more are the chest, abdomen, pelvis and thigh. Trauma patients will need large-bore IV access and fluid resuscitation, including blood products if appropriate. Urgent bloods, including a full blood count and cross match are taken at this stage.

   - **D** stands for **disability**. Assess D by using the AVPU scale. GCS can be assessed formally later. It is important to document a blood sugar and patient's body temperature (this is especially important in near-drowning accidents).

   - **E** is for **exposure**, which is crucial in trauma. A full secondary survey should be performed to identify any other injuries. You may have treated the tension pneumothorax and controlled the bleeding pelvic fracture so now you have to deal with any other injuries, such as the bilateral open femoral fractures! A brief history using the AMPLE framework (Allergies, Medications, Past illness/Pregnancy history, Last meal – in case the patient needs to be intubated, and Events around injury) may be possible.

   In practice, many of the different facets of the ABCDE assessment are performed simultaneously by different members of the trauma team. For example, whilst one member is assessing the airway and securing the cervical spine, another can gain IV access and take bloods and a third can be assessing breathing and circulation. This is important as every minute counts in trauma. If there are enough people, a designated person should take a step back and lead the resuscitation to maintain overall control of the situation.

   B) With a trauma team – Correct. The trauma team will include a trauma consultant, an anaesthetist, a general surgeon, an orthopaedic surgeon and junior doctors. In tertiary centres, there may also be early assessment from plastic surgeons, neurosurgeons, urologists, etc. depending on the injuries sustained. Such a multidisciplinary approach helps ensure a rapid and effective assessment of the trauma patient and early instigation of appropriate management.

   C) Take straight to theatre as she will almost certainly have life-threatening injuries – Incorrect. Whilst the patient is likely to need surgery for the pelvic fracture, it is important to assess for and manage other life-threatening injuries prior to theatre. For example, a pneumothorax must be identified and managed before the patient is anaesthetised as mechanical ventilation would turn it into a tension pneumothorax. The principles of ATLS are to rapidly identify and manage life-threatening injuries. This can usually be performed in the A&E department. Cross sectional imaging, in the form of CT, is increasingly performed early during the patient's assessment to clarify the extent of injuries and help plan appropriate management.

   D) Early cross sectional imaging – Correct. Early CT scanning is increasingly used in trauma situations. CT is a rapid investigation which can accurately diagnose most types of injury (it is not able to assess the spinal cord in detail). It allows the trauma team to assess all of the injuries and prioritise them, helping plan management. The source of any internal bleeding can often be identified, and thus accurately guide the interventional radiologists or trauma surgeons should an intervention be required.

   A noncontrast scan of the head and cervical spine, followed by contrast enhanced scans of the chest, abdomen, pelvis (and thighs, if required), is typically performed. Additional CT imaging, such as delayed phases and cystograms, may be required if there is suspicion of ureteric or bladder injuries.

   E) Taking a thorough history and performing a complete examination before commencing any treatment – Incorrect. The ATLS algorithm emphasises assessing and treating the patient simultaneously as the patient may have life-threatening injuries which need urgent management. Whilst this is occurring, another member of the team can be taking a history from the patient, any witnesses and the ambulance crew.

Continue

CASE **4.11** *Contd.*

1. Using ATLS will help save lives. Treat all major trauma patients the same with an ABCDE assessment and presume they have a serious injury until it has been excluded.
2. The mnemonic 'AMPLE' is helpful for remembering important points in the history (Allergies, Medications, Past illnesses/Pregnancy, Last meal (in case the patient needs surgery), Events around the injury).
3. Fractures of the pelvis such as this usually result from significant trauma and are potentially life-threatening. The patient may have other serious injuries. Appropriate timely management of all these injuries is therefore crucial and a multidisciplinary team approach is required.
4. The pelvis is a bony ring which often breaks in at least two places. So if you see one fracture involving the pelvis, look for further injuries of the pelvis. These may be fractures or dislocations of the sacroiliac joints or pubic symphysis.

---

2. What X-rays is/are part of the initial 'trauma series'?
The correct answer is **A) Portable AP chest and pelvis X-rays**.
Trauma patients need rapid assessment and resuscitation. They should be managed using the ATLS algorithm. An initial trauma series of chest and pelvic X-rays is important; however, this must not delay patient resuscitation. The patient will be too unstable for formal departmental X-rays; therefore portable X-rays will be required. The chest X-ray might reveal an immediately life-threatening diagnosis such as a tension pneumothorax, whilst a pelvic fracture usually indicates the need for early blood transfusion. The quality of the image is not crucial, so often rotated or poorly penetrated films are accepted initially if they give a clear diagnosis, as it is not safe to transfer an unwell patient to the radiology department for higher quality X-rays.
A) Portable AP chest and pelvis X-rays – Correct. As well as a pneumothorax the chest X-ray may reveal rib fractures, including a flail chest (multiple adjacent rib fractures, which results in paradoxical movement of that segment of chest wall and compromised ventilation), or an effusion which may suggest a haemothorax. The AP pelvic X-ray will demonstrate major pelvic fractures as well as hip fractures and dislocations. Pelvic fractures can cause significant haemorrhage and their presence indicates the need for early blood transfusion.
B) Portable AP chest and pelvis X-rays and cervical spine X-rays – Incorrect. Although appropriate to include chest and pelvic X-rays as part of your initial assessment, it is important not to over investigate without focussing on stabilising the patient first. Whilst cervical spine injuries are very important, they are unlikely to be immediately life-threatening. Therefore, only the chest and pelvis X-rays are performed initially during the

primary survey. Imaging of the cervical spine and other body parts is deferred until the secondary survey. In addition, it is very difficult to get adequate X-rays of the cervical spine in a trauma patient. Therefore, most of these patients usually now have an early CT which includes the cervical spine rather than X-rays.
C) Departmental PA chest X-ray and AP pelvis X-ray – Incorrect. Imaging must not delay the resuscitation process. By taking the unstable trauma patient to the radiology department for X-rays, you are risking their life. Furthermore, a trauma patient is unlikely to be able to stand/sit up for a formal PA chest X-ray!
D) AP pelvis X-ray – Incorrect. This is half of the initial trauma series of X-rays which is commonly requested.
E) FAST scan and diagnostic peritoneal lavage – Incorrect. There are many imaging modalities and investigations available to identify major injuries. FAST scanning and diagnostic peritoneal lavage are techniques for identifying occult intraabdominal haemorrhage.
FAST is a quick, portable ultrasound scan used to identify the presence of free fluid in the abdomen or pelvis, which in the context of trauma usually represents haemorrhage. It is less sensitive and specific than CT scanning, is operator dependent and usually performed under sub-optimal conditions in a bright, noisy resuscitation room. Additionally, a negative scan does not exclude serious intraabdominal injury and a positive scan often cannot identify the site of injury. Therefore, CT scanning is also often required anyway in the stable patient. If there is free fluid on FAST scan, and the patient is unstable, they may proceed straight to a laparotomy. FAST scanning is also useful in the triage of multiple trauma patients, helping to prioritise patients for further imaging and surgery.
Diagnostic peritoneal lavage is a surgical procedure performed using local anaesthetic in the resuscitation room. It involves puncturing the peritoneal cavity, instilling saline and sending a sample of the fluid for erythrocyte counts. It will not identify retroperitoneal haemorrhages and has largely been replaced by CT scanning.

1. When considering imaging for any patient, it is important you assess whether departmental or portable studies are more suitable. Departmental X-rays are better quality compared with portable examinations. However, if the patient is too unstable to be transported to the department, a portable X-ray would be more appropriate, accepting that the image quality will be reduced.
2. The initial trauma series is used to identify life-threatening injuries in patients who are usually unstable. Portable X-rays are likely to provide all the information initially required, with the added bonus of not needing to move the patient from the resuscitation room.

3. Which of these are types of major pelvic fracture?
The correct answers are **A) Lateral compression and B) Vertical shear**.

Pelvic injuries can be classified depending on the type of force leading to the injury. Open book fractures are caused by an AP compression force. There is disruption of the pubic symphysis and injury to the posterior ligaments of the pelvis. This is the injury most commonly associated with major haemorrhage. The two other types of major pelvic fracture are lateral compression fractures and vertical shear fractures. In very high-energy trauma, there may be a combination of these.

A) Lateral compression – Correct. This is a result of compression on the lateral aspect of the pelvis. This leads to a reduction in the pelvic volume and therefore haemorrhage is less common.

B) Vertical shear – Correct. These fractures are a result of falls from height or any other shearing force through the hemipelvis. These are comparatively rare.

C) Closed book – Incorrect. This type of fracture does not exist. Open book fractures are described in the introduction to this answer.

D) Avulsion fracture of the superior acetabulum – Incorrect. The rectus femoris muscle attaches in part to the superior acetabulum and can often be avulsed with a small fragment of bone causing an avulsion fracture. It is not considered a major pelvic fracture. It is more common in children/adolescents.

E) Isolated pubic ramus fracture – Incorrect. These fractures, when isolated, are generally seen in low-energy falls in the elderly. They can be managed conservatively with mobilisation.

❶ KEY POINT

Pelvic fractures can also be classified as stable or unstable.

Stable fractures involve a single break in the pelvic ring and include pubic rami fractures, avulsion fractures and isolated sacral or iliac fractures.

Unstable fractures follow the described patterns of open book, vertical shear and lateral compression fractures. These fractures need referral to specialist orthopaedic surgeons with experience in pelvic fractures for further management.

4. Which of these is/are most commonly associated with pelvic fractures?
The correct answer is **C) Bladder and urethral injuries and E) Death**.

As we have already discussed, pelvic fractures are major injuries and potentially life-threatening. They may be associated with other injuries to the pelvic organs. It is important as part of your initial assessment of a major trauma patient to meticulously assess the patient and inspect the rectum, perineum and all orifices for bleeding or bruising. Also look for evidence of an open pelvic fracture.

A) Vaginal perforation – Incorrect. This is not commonly associated with pelvic injuries but all pelvic organs can be injured in association with a pelvic fracture.

Examine for vaginal bleeding as part of your assessment of a major trauma patient.

B) Hip dislocation – Incorrect. Dislocation of a THR is common following low-energy trauma. However, it takes a huge force to dislocate a native hip. This may occur with a fracture of the pelvis but it is not the most commonly cited injury to occur with pelvic fractures.

C) Bladder and urethral injuries – Correct. These are the most common injuries to occur with pelvic fractures. Bladder injuries occur in 10% of patients with pelvic fractures. Typically, pelvic fractures injure the base of the bladder and result in an extraperitoneal bladder rupture. Such injuries are usually treated conservatively with a urinary catheter. Urethral injuries are much more common in males. Clinically, the prostate will be high riding (sitting high in the rectum and difficult to feel on PR); there may be blood at the urethral meatus or a scrotal haematoma. If you suspect a urethral rupture, do not attempt to catheterise the patient! Contact the urologists immediately.

D) Rectal perforation – Incorrect. The rectum can be perforated by bone fragments from the pelvic fracture; however, it is not the most frequently associated injury. As the bone has come into contact with faeces and a passage to the open air, pelvic fractures with rectal perforation are considered open fractures. Rectal perforation should be assessed for as part of the digital rectal examination. Blood may be visible at the anus if there has been an injury and there may be an associated perineal wound. A defunctioning colostomy may be needed to allow the rectal injury to heal.

E) Death – Correct. The mortality rate for an open pelvic fracture is 50%. Overall, however, the mortality rate for all pelvic fractures is between 5% and 30%.

❶ KEY POINT

• Make sure you examine the perineum, urethra, vagina and the rectum in all major trauma patients. Occult injuries are too frequently missed.

• CT can accurately detect and characterise bladder injuries. A retrograde urethrogram is usually required to assess for urethral injuries.

5. What of these is/are definitive management options for this fracture?
The correct answers are **B) Internal fixation and E) External fixation**.

The management of pelvic fractures can be subdivided into early and definitive. For the pelvic fracture shown, the patient is most likely going to require operative intervention either with internal fixation or external fixation.

A) A pelvic binder – Incorrect. The pelvic binder is a very useful tool in the acute setting. The binder wraps around the pelvis at the level of the greater trochanters and closes open book fractures. It helps reduce the fracture and limit haemorrhage. However, it is very tight and can cause pressure ulcers. Therefore, it can only be used temporarily and is not a definitive management option.

Continue

CASE **4.11** *Contd.*

B) Internal fixation – Correct. This is the definitive treatment method for a major pelvic fracture. It is not the only option, however, and some fractures may not require operative fixation. Furthermore, some patients may have multiple injuries and are not well enough to tolerate a complex surgery to fix a pelvic fracture.

C) Angiography – Incorrect. This is a useful tool when the patient is bleeding despite pelvic stabilisation. It is a minimally invasive technique performed through a small arterial puncture (usually at the groin in the common femoral artery). The radiologist uses catheters and wires to access different pelvic arteries and intraarterial contrast can be administered to identify bleeding vessels. These vessels can be embolised using particles or metallic coils. Whilst it can be very useful for stopping the haemorrhage, it does not treat the fracture.

D) Traction and internal rotation – Incorrect. Traction on the legs, together with internal rotation, will help reduce the fracture and potentially stop bleeding. However, it is not a suitable treatment option outside of the initial resuscitation period.

E) External fixation – Correct. This is a more definitive option for the management of the fracture. Pins and rods are used to rigidly fix the pelvis externally in a more anatomical position. Some pelvic fractures can successfully be treated this way. Others, however, will require further definitive treatment through operative fixation. Patients who are too unwell to have internal fixation of the pelvic fracture may better tolerate external fixation, which is less invasive and takes less time.

IMPORTANT LEARNING POINTS

- Pelvic fractures often occur in high-energy trauma and are commonly associated with multiple injuries.
- Rapid, systematic assessment and treatment of these patients using the ATLS algorithm will improve outcome.
- The initial trauma series consists of portable chest and pelvic X-rays; however, there is a move towards immediate CT scanning for patients involved in significant trauma.
- Bladder and urethral injuries are common complications of pelvic fractures.
- Pelvic binders can be used to rapidly stabilise an unstable pelvic fracture. Definitive treatment options include external or internal fixation. Angiography may be required to control haemorrhage if other options have failed.

CASE **4.12**

A 13-year-old girl has presented to accident and emergency with a 2-week history of left knee pain and an occasional left hip pain. A frog leg lateral X-ray has been performed.

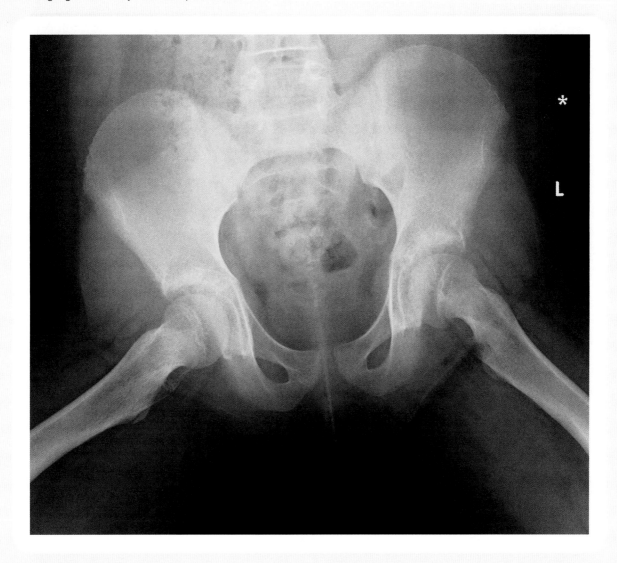

Continue

CASE 4.12 *Contd.*

ANNOTATED X-RAY

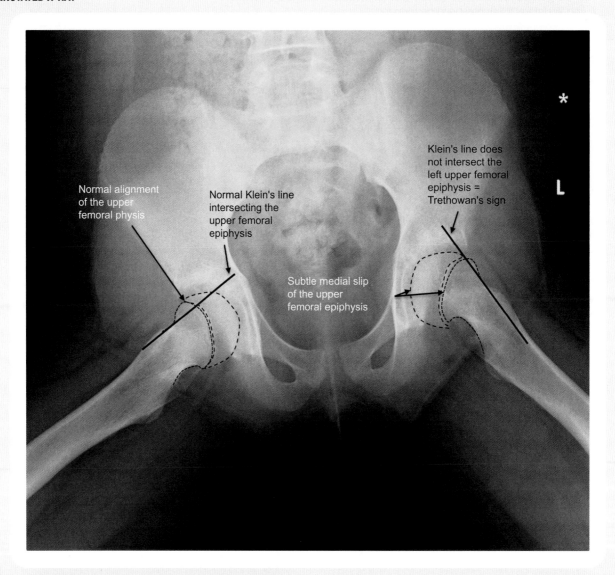

Normal alignment of the upper femoral physis

Normal Klein's line intersecting the upper femoral epiphysis

Subtle medial slip of the upper femoral epiphysis

Klein's line does not intersect the left upper femoral epiphysis = Trethowan's sign

*

L

PRESENT YOUR FINDINGS

- This is a frog leg lateral view of the pelvis of a skeletally immature patient.
- It has been anonymised and the timing of the examination is not available. I would like to confirm the patient's details and timing of the examination before I make any further assessment.
- The X-ray is adequately exposed displaying the pathology. No important areas are cut off the X-ray.
- The left hip joint is abnormal. There is a subtle slip of the left upper femoral epiphysis medially in relation to the physis and femoral neck, with a positive Trethowan's sign.

- The right hip is normal.
- Bone density is normal, with no areas of lucency or sclerosis.
- There is no soft tissue swelling.

IN SUMMARY – This frog leg lateral view of the pelvis demonstrates a subtle left SUFE.

QUESTIONS

1. Which of these may be present on examination of a patient with a SUFE?
   A) Knee pain
   B) External rotation
   C) Inability to weight bear
   D) Shortening of the femur
   E) All of the above

2. Which of these accurately describes the pathology of SUFE?
   A) Slip through the hypertrophic zone of the proximal femoral physis
   B) Slip through the resting zone of the proximal femoral physis
   C) Fracture of the femoral epiphysis
   D) Salter–Harris 2 fracture of the proximal femoral physis
   E) Salter–Harris 3 fracture of the proximal femoral physis

3. Which of these signs is/are a radiological feature of SUFE?
   A) Trethowan's sign
   B) Klein's line
   C) Wackenheim's line
   D) Shenton's line
   E) Segond fracture

4. What is the incidence of slippage of the contralateral hip in a patient presenting with SUFE?
   A) 1%
   B) 5%
   C) 20%
   D) 50%
   E) 90%

5. What is the most appropriate management of this patient?
   A) RICE
   B) DHS
   C) Open reduction and cannulated screw fixation
   D) Cannulated screw fixation in situ
   E) THR

Continue

CASE **4.12**   *Contd.*

ANSWERS TO QUESTIONS

1. Which of these may be present on examination of a patient with a SUFE?

   The correct answer is **E) All of the above**.

   A full history and examination is important for these patients. The focus of the history should be on the onset of symptoms as there may have been a minor trauma and the presence of knee pain. It is also important to ask about a family history and whether there is any history of hormonal disorders. Children who develop a SUFE tend to be overweight and tall. Underlying endocrine disorders, such as hypothyroidism, are known risk factors in the development of the SUFE.

   A) Knee pain – Incorrect. Knee pain is a common presenting feature of SUFE. Always be suspicious of a hip problem in a child presenting with knee pain as the femoral nerve supplies both joints so referred pain is common.

   B) External rotation – Incorrect. With the epiphyseal slip, the femur moves into a position of external rotation. This may be clinically obvious and should increase suspicion of a SUFE if present.

   C) Inability to weight bear – Incorrect. It is always important to ask about whether the patient can bear weight through an injured lower limb. In SUFE, the child may have a limp or may be unable to bear any weight through the hip.

   D) Shortening of the femur – Incorrect. If there is significant displacement, then the femur moves superiorly in relation to the femoral head, causing shortening of the leg.

   E) All of the above – Correct. Only once a full history and examination is performed can X-rays be properly interpreted. Never assess an X-ray in isolation.

2. Which of these accurately describes the pathology of SUFE?

   The correct answer is **A) Slip through the hypertrophic zone of the proximal femoral physis**.

   SUFE occurs in children aged between 8 and 17. Like Perthes disease, boys are more commonly affected than girls. The slip occurs during a phase of accelerated growth and therefore SUFE tends to occur earlier in girls (8–15 years versus 10–17 years in boys), as they usually go through puberty at a younger age. Endocrine disorders, obesity and Afro-Caribbean origin are recognised risk factors. SUFE can occur acutely following trauma or subacutely following a short period of pain. Classically, the child presents with referred pain in the knee, which is why you must always examine the joint above and below.

   A) Slip through the hypertrophic zone of the proximal femoral physis – Correct. During the growth spurt, the physis widens and becomes more oblique, making it more prone to shearing forces. SUFE is caused by increased forces across the hypertrophic zone of the proximal femoral physis. This is also the zone which if damaged, does not tend to lead to growth disturbance.

   B) Slip through the resting zone of the proximal femoral physis – Incorrect. The resting zone can lead to growth disturbance if injured, but is not the site of pathology in SUFE.

   C) Fracture of the femoral epiphysis – Incorrect. Fracture of the femoral epiphysis is a rare injury that occurs in high-energy trauma, often with dislocation of the hip. SUFE on the other hand is a Salter–Harris type 1 fracture through the proximal femoral physis.

   D) Salter–Harris 2 fracture of the proximal femoral physis – Incorrect. SUFE is technically a Salter–Harris 1 fracture of the physis where the femoral neck has displaced with external rotation and anterior displacement leaving the head in a more posterior position.

   E) Salter–Harris 3 fracture of the proximal femoral physis – Incorrect. SUFE is technically a Salter–Harris 1 fracture.

3. Which of these signs is/are a radiological feature of SUFE?

   The correct answer is **A) Trethowan's sign, D) Shenton's line**

   The slip in SUFE occurs posteriorly, and to a lesser extent medially. Therefore, the frog leg lateral views are the best for diagnosing SUFE. Obvious slips may be visible on the AP view but subtle slips are often only visible on the frog leg lateral view.

   The earliest finding of SUFE are widening of the physis, with irregularity of the physeal margins and osteopaenia of the metaphysis, which occur before any slipping of the epiphysis. Trethowan's sign is the sign which is most commonly used for the diagnosis of SUFE once a slip has occurred. It is assessed on the frog leg lateral view or the AP. In a chronic SUFE, the physis is widened and sclerotic.

   A) Trethowan's sign – Correct. This sign is when a line drawn along the lateral cortex of the femoral neck (Klein's line) does not intersect the epiphysis. The annotated X-ray demonstrates this sign.

   B) Klein's line – Incorrect. The line drawn along the lateral cortex of the femoral neck is Klein's line. It does not indicate a SUFE but is the line that is used to demonstrate Trethowan's sign.

   C) Wackenheim's line – Incorrect. Wackenheim's line is a radiological line used to assess whether there is subluxation of the joint between the occiput and C1.

   D) **Shenton's line – Correct. Shenton's line is a line drawn along the medial cortex of the neck of the femur. The line then continues along the inferior border of the superior pubic ramus and should be a smooth semicircle. If this line is disrupted, then this suggests a fracture of the neck of femur. Technically a SUFE is a Salter–Harris 1 fracture through the neck of femur.**

   E) Segond Fracture – Incorrect. A Segond fracture is an avulsion fracture of the lateral tibial condyle associated with rupture of the anterior cruciate ligament. There is often associated injury to the menisci. It occurs with a varus internal rotation injury.

❶ KEY POINT

A frog leg lateral view is the most commonly performed imaging test to diagnose SUFE. It is more sensitive than an AP view of the hips due to the posteromedial direction of slippage. MRI is superior to X-rays for diagnosing SUFE and can show changes suggestive of early SUFE, such as marrow oedema; however, such findings are nonspecific. Ultrasound is nonspecific in SUFE and may show a joint effusion.

4. What is the incidence of slippage of the contralateral hip in a patient presenting with SUFE?
The correct answer is **C) 20%**.
Once the SUFE has been diagnosed, it is important to ask about symptoms in the other hip and monitor the other hip on X-ray. Slippage of the contralateral hip occurs in 20%. This can actually be precipitated by treatment of the unstable side. Therefore, some surgeons will fix both sides at the same time under one anaesthetic.

5. What is the most appropriate management of this patient?
The correct answer is **D) Cannulated screw fixation in situ**.
The management of a SUFE includes analgesia and surgical management. There are several options available, but in our patient with a subtle slip, the most appropriate treatment would be cannulated screw fixation without trying to reduce the slip.
A) RICE – Incorrect. The orthopaedic mantra of RICE does not work here although there is some evidence that if the injury is not treated, patients may not be left with too much functional deficit. However, surgical management is usually recommended to prevent further displacement.
B) DHS – Incorrect. The DHS involves a large screw placed into the femoral head with a plate on the lateral border of the femur. This is used for extracapsular fractures of the femoral neck. The screw is large and would disrupt the physis unnecessarily.
C) Open reduction and cannulated screw fixation – Incorrect. If the SUFE is displaced significantly, the

only option is to reduce the SUFE and use a cannulated screw to maintain the reduction. Opening up the hip joint to reduce the slip increases the risk of AVN to the femoral head and is therefore not indicated in this case.
D) Cannulated screw fixation in situ – Correct. This is the treatment of choice for most SUFEs. This does not disturb the blood supply to the femoral head and stops the SUFE from slipping further.
E) THR – Incorrect. Unfortunately, a severe SUFE may progress to AVN if the blood supply to the femoral head has been disturbed. In time, this will lead to osteoarthritis and will require a THR. However, THR is not necessary in mild SUFE when recognised early and treated appropriately.

❶ KEY POINT

SUFE is managed surgically with cannulated screw fixation. Due to the relatively high risk of SUFE in the contralateral hip, some surgeons will fix both hips.

IMPORTANT LEARNING POINTS

- SUFE is a Salter–Harris type 1 fracture of the proximal femoral physis which typically presents in adolescents during a period of rapid growth.
- It is more common in boys, obese patients and Afro-Caribbeans.
- Presentation can be with hip or knee pain and/or a limp.
- A frog leg lateral view is the most useful investigation for diagnosing SUFE (Trethowan's sign).
- Management is surgical, with cannulated screw fixation.
- Slippage of the contralateral hip occurs in 20% – some surgeons advocate prophylactic treatment of the normal side to prevent this.
- Complications of untreated SUFE include AVN, osteoarthritis, chronic pain and gait abnormalities.

CASE 4.13

A 75-year-old man has fallen over at home. He was unable to get up and has been brought to A&E by ambulance where it was noted his left leg was shortened and externally rotated. This is his X-ray.

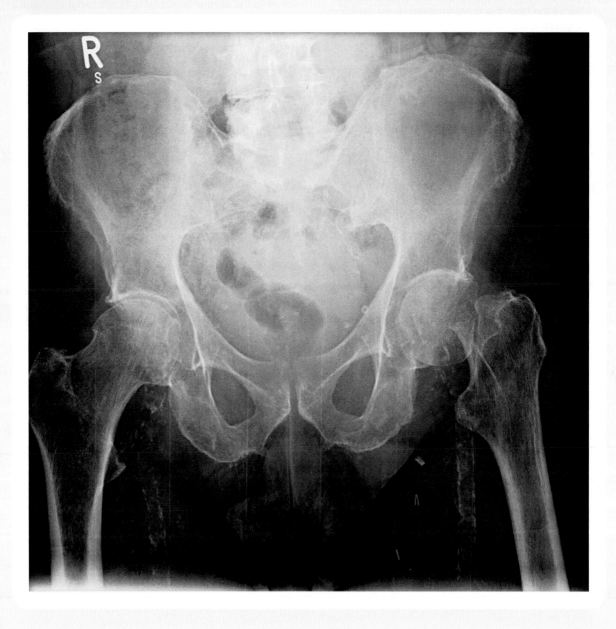

ANNOTATED X-RAY

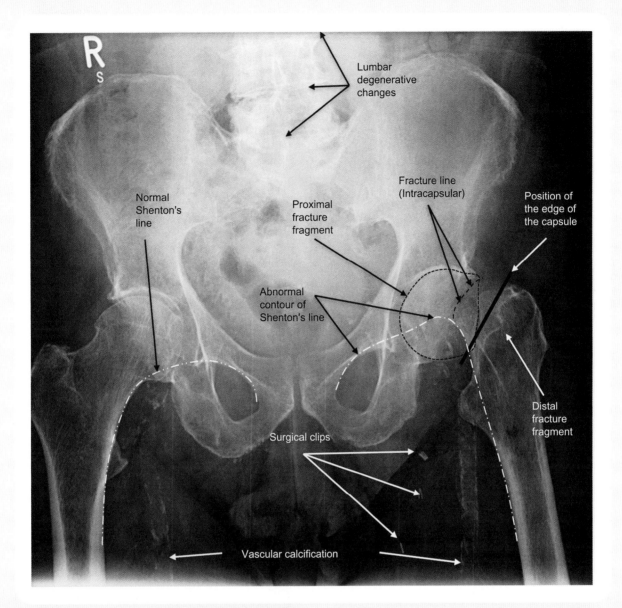

R
S

Lumbar degenerative changes

Normal Shenton's line

Proximal fracture fragment

Fracture line (Intracapsular)

Position of the edge of the capsule

Abnormal contour of Shenton's line

Distal fracture fragment

Surgical clips

Vascular calcification

🔍 PRESENT YOUR FINDINGS

- This is an AP X-ray of the pelvis of a skeletally mature patient.
- It has been anonymised and the timing of the examination is not available. I would like to confirm the patient's details and timing of the examination before I make any further assessment.
- The X-ray is adequately penetrated, with no important areas cut off.
- There is a displaced fracture of the left hip. It is an intracapsular subcapital fracture of the femoral neck.
- There is shortening and external rotation of the femur.
- No other fracture is visible.
- There are no areas of lucency or cystic changes to suggest a pathological fracture.
- There is a loss of joint space in both hips with osteophytes, subchondral sclerosis and subchondral cysts consistent with osteoarthritis.

- Degenerative changes are also visible in the lumbar spine and the lumbosacral junction.
- There is calcification of the femoral vessels bilaterally, in keeping with diabetes or renal failure.
- There are a few surgical clips projected over the left thigh suggesting previous surgery.

IN SUMMARY – This X-ray shows a displaced left intracapsular fracture of the neck of femur. I would want to see a lateral X-ray of the hip to complete my radiological assessment of the fracture. Degenerative changes of the hips and spine are evident and there is marked vascular calcification.

Continue

CASE 4.13 *Contd.*

QUESTIONS

1. The initial management of this fracture involves which of the following?
   A) Stabilise the patient
   B) Identify any medical issues
   C) Take a full history including a history of the mechanism of injury
   D) Take a full social history
   E) Request a CT of the hip to allow accurate preoperative planning

2. What grade is this fracture using the Garden classification?
   A) 1
   B) 2
   C) 3
   D) 4
   E) A

3. What is the best surgical management for this 75-year-old patient if they are independent and medically fit prior to the injury?
   A) Hemiarthroplasty
   B) THR
   C) Surgical fixation
   D) Traction and bed rest
   E) Early mobilisation

4. If this fracture occurred in a fit and well 20-year old, which would be the best surgical option?
   A) Hemiarthroplasty
   B) THR
   C) Surgical fixation
   D) Traction and bed rest
   E) Early mobilisation

5. Which of these is absolutely necessary prior to the patient having surgery?
   A) Consent from the patient
   B) Nil by mouth for 6 hours
   C) Blood cross-matched
   D) Results of a full set of bloods including urea and electrolytes
   E) None of the above

ANSWERS TO QUESTIONS

1. The initial management of this fracture involves which of the following?

The correct answers are **A) Stabilise the patient, B) Identify any medical issues, C) Take a full history including a history of the mechanism of injury and D) Take a full social history**.

A) Stabilise the patient – Correct. Stabilising all trauma patients is important; however, there are other important points to consider. Patients should be assessed using the ATLS ABCDE algorithm if there is any concern about major trauma. Stabilisation includes fluid resuscitation and early pain relief. Analgesia should be prescribed using the WHO pain ladder as a guide, starting at the most appropriate step. A nerve block is a very effective method of pain relief but should only be performed by a trained member of staff.

B) Identify any medical issues – Correct. Patients with femoral neck fractures are typically elderly and often have other medical comorbidities which must be considered. These include chronic comorbid conditions such as renal failure, COPD, ischaemic heart disease and dementia as well as acute problems which may have contributed to the fall (e.g. infection) or resulted from the fall (e.g. intracranial haemorrhage). These must be identified and treated early to optimise the patient for surgery. Patients may also be on warfarin. This will need to be reversed prior to surgery. However, the indication for warfarin must be considered before reversing it, as the risks of stopping it may be high. In these cases, or if you are in doubt, you should discuss the case with a haematologist for advice.

C) Take a full history including a history of the mechanism of injury – Correct. A full history of the mechanism of injury is very important. Did they trip or did they collapse?

D) Take a full social history – Correct. It is important to take a full social history from all patients who sustained fractures to the femoral neck. This includes where the patient lives, the requirement of assistance with their activities of daily living, the use of walking aids both in the house and outside and an AMT. The degree of independence will impact on surgical decision-making.

E) Request a CT of the hip to allow accurate preoperative planning – Incorrect. This is not required. The main questions which needs to be answered for preoperative planning are whether the fracture is intra- or extracapsular and the degree of displacement. AP and lateral X-rays can almost always answer these questions. CT of the hip can be used if there is high clinical suspicion of a hip fracture but no evidence on the X-rays. MRI is an alternate imaging strategy in such cases.

⚠ KEY POINT

Blood tests should also be performed to assess for:
A) Preoperative anaemia – patients may need a preoperative transfusion
B) Preoperative renal failure or electrolyte derangement which may affect anaesthesia and fluid management
C) Blood group and save – surgery can be associated with significant blood loss and should be prepared for
D) Inflammatory markers – patients may have sepsis
E) Clotting – drugs or liver dysfunction may affect clotting and may need to be corrected preoperatively

2. What grade is this fracture using the Garden classification? The correct answer is **C) 3**.

Intracapsular fractures often need surgery to have the femoral head replaced, but in certain cases this is not necessary, and in some cases conservative management might be considered. The Garden classification is used to categorise the degree of displacement of an intracapsular femoral neck fracture, and as such, also defines how likely it is that the blood supply to the femoral head has been disrupted.

The classification system goes from 1 to 4, where 1 and 2 are undisplaced and 3 and 4 are displaced. The subtle differences between 1/2 (undisplaced) and 3/4 (displaced) are best appreciated by looking at the trabeculation (lines seen within bone) in the different fractures. In Garden 1 fractures, the trabeculation lines in the head point vertically in comparison to the normal. In Garden 2 fractures, they are all in line. In Garden 3 fractures, the trabeculation lines in the head are more horizontal than normal. In Garden 4 fractures, the head has displaced but returned to its normal alignment and so the trabeculations are all in line.

A) 1 – Incorrect. In Garden 1 fractures, there is an incomplete fracture with impaction at the fracture site with the femoral head tilted into a valgus (more upright) position. Therefore, it is more likely that the capsule will remain intact and the risk of AVN is reduced. Surgical fixation using screws or a two-hole DHS prevents displacement of the fracture and is an option for these patients (although some form of joint replacement is normally the surgical option of choice). The advantages of surgical fixation include the patient keeping their own femoral head which reduces the risk of dislocation or need for revision arthroplasty surgery. If the patient has little pain, this fracture could potentially be treated without surgery and with full weight bearing but follow-up X-rays are needed to ensure the fracture does not displace.

B) 2 – Incorrect. In Garden 2 fractures, the fracture is complete and undisplaced and again surgical fixation is possible as the risk of AVN is low. This fracture is often grouped with Garden 1 fractures as undisplaced

Continue

and treatment is essentially the same although as the fracture is complete there is a higher risk of displacement if the fracture is treated nonoperatively.

C) 3 – Correct. This is a Garden 3 fracture. In Garden 3 fractures, there is displacement and there is a high chance of AVN. In the vast majority of patients, a hemiarthroplasty or THR is necessary.

D) 4 – Incorrect. In Garden 4, the fracture is fully displaced. For the vast majority of patients, THR or hemiarthroplasty is required.

E) A – Incorrect. The classification is from 1 to 4 not A to D.

❗ KEY POINT

Undisplaced fractures have a lower risk of AVN in comparison to displaced fractures. Use the Garden classification to consider the degree of displacement and then this will help guide your surgical decision-making.

3. What is the best surgical management for this 75-year-old patient if they are independent and medically fit prior to the injury?
The correct answer is **B) THR**.
The aim of surgery in fractures of the neck of femur should be to allow early mobilisation with limited chance of further surgery. In the elderly, most surgeons will opt for either a THR or a hemiarthroplasty for intracapsular fractures regardless of how much displacement there is present.

A) Hemiarthroplasty – Incorrect. A hemiarthroplasty is a half hip replacement. The ball of the ball and socket joint is replaced but the socket is left alone. This option has some advantages such as a low risk of dislocation. However, the implant differs from normal anatomy and patients will often not be able to return to full function. It is therefore usually reserved for patients with limited premorbid mobility. In addition, if a patient had arthritis in the joint prior to the fracture, then there is the chance of ongoing pain because the arthritis is still present in the acetabulum.

B) THR – Correct. In a THR, the ball and socket are replaced, allowing for a better correction of the prior anatomy and a better return to function. NICE guidelines state that THR should be considered for independent patients with a displaced intracapsular fracture of the neck of the femur who need no more than one stick to mobilise. This operation takes slightly longer and is therefore associated with slightly more blood loss compared with a hemiarthroplasty. There is also a higher chance of dislocation. However, by replacing both the ball and socket, it is possible to get a more anatomical implant which allows better return to function. In addition, there are further benefits for patients with a fracture and preexisting hip joint arthritis, as replacing both the femoral head and lining the acetabulum will help alleviate the symptoms of arthritis.

C) Surgical fixation – Incorrect. In this age group, it is not advisable to attempt fixation for a displaced intracapsular fracture as the risks of further surgery are too high if AVN develops. However, if the fracture is undisplaced or minimally displaced, then this may be a good option. The risk of AVN in displaced fractures is above 30%, but may be much lower in undisplaced fractures.

D) Traction and bed rest – Incorrect. Intracapsular fractures do not respond well to traction and bed rest. Although some extracapsular fractures will heal with time, as this fracture is displaced and intracapsular, the likelihood is the fracture will not heal (nonunion) and the patient will be left immobile with all the associated/related complications. This treatment option may be considered in very frail patients who are expected to die from an underlying or acute medical problem (in these patients, surgery is not appropriate).

E) Early mobilisation – Incorrect. Very occasionally, patients will present with an undisplaced intracapsular fracture where the fracture is old and healed or the patient is able to mobilise. In such circumstances, it is possible to avoid an operation. However, should further pain develop, X-rays are repeated to ensure there has been no displacement that would warrant surgical intervention.

4. If this fracture occurred in a fit and well 20-year old, which would be the best surgical option?
The correct answer is **C) Surgical fixation**.
There is a significant difference between femoral neck fractures in the elderly (>65 years) and the young. Young patients are usually fit and the fracture is often associated with high-energy trauma. They are expected to live longer and be more active. Therefore, preservation of the native femoral hip is crucial in young patients with an intracapsular fracture.

A) Hemiarthroplasty – Incorrect. This surgical option would provide a poor outcome for a 20-year old, resulting in limited mobility and future problems secondary to marked wear and tear from the metal femoral head against the patient's own acetabulum.

B) THR – Incorrect. If the femoral head does not survive or surgical fixation is not possible, then this is the best surgical option. However, a THR does not last forever and it is likely a 20-year old with a THR will need further surgery in the future. Therefore, it is usually best to attempt surgical fixation (see C) in young patients with femoral neck fractures regardless of degree of initial displacement.

C) Surgical fixation – Correct. Ideally, the patient needs to go to theatre on the next available list. The fracture can be accurately reduced and fixed with either three screws or a short DHS and a second screw. There is still a significant risk of AVN of the femoral head, which would require a further operation. However, as this patient is young and fit, the risks of further surgery are relatively low. It is therefore desirable to keep the patient's femoral head and accept the possibility of further surgery, rather than replacing it in the first instance.

D) Traction and bed rest – Incorrect. This is not appropriate for patients in this age group with this fracture.

E) Early mobilisation – Incorrect. Young patients with an intracapsular fracture are best treated by surgical fixation even if the fracture is undisplaced. It is also very unlikely for a young person to present with a healing intracapsular fracture, as this is a high-energy injury which will be picked up on initial presentation.

> **❶ KEY POINT**
>
> Patients under 50 should be considered for surgical fixation of their intracapsular neck of femur fracture within 24 hours of injury. Doing so may reduce the risk of AVN and preserve the femoral head, improving the long-term functional outcome.

5. Which of these is absolutely necessary prior to the patient having surgery?
   The correct answer is **E) None of the above**.
   None of these are absolutely necessary for a patient to have an operation. In an emergency situation, you may not be able to wait for the patient to be adequately fasted or to consent the patient if they are unconscious. Similarly, blood results may not be available in time. Although these are not absolutely necessary in such patients, they are desirable and should be considered in a 'standard' patient with a femoral neck fracture.

   A) Consent from the patient – Incorrect. Informed consent should be obtained from the patient or guardian. Ideally, the person consenting should either be the operating surgeon or someone who can perform the operation. If not, then the person consenting should have a full understanding of all the risks and benefits of a surgery together with the technical steps of the operation. The patient should be allowed sufficient time to come to a decision. In some circumstances, such as an unconscious patient requiring emergency surgery, it is not possible to obtain consent, in which case it is acceptable to perform the surgery if it is judged to be in the patient's best interests.

   B) Nil by mouth for 6 hours – Incorrect. It is generally important to make sure the patient is fasted for 6 hours prior to the operation. This reduces the risk of aspiration of gastric contents on the anaesthetic induction. Although this applies for all surgical patients, this is especially relevant in trauma, which itself delays gastric emptying. Again, in some circumstances, this may not be possible,

and emergency surgery should not be delayed if the patient is not fasted. Instead, the anaesthetic team can perform a rapid sequence induction, which minimises the risk of aspiration.

C) Blood cross-matched – Incorrect. Patients undergoing surgery for femoral neck fractures are at risk of significant intraoperative blood loss and should have a valid G&S. If there is concern that the patient is at high risk of bleeding, then they should have blood cross-matched prior to surgery. In an emergency, waiting for cross-matched blood is not necessary as O negative or type specific blood is readily available.

D) Results of a full set of bloods including urea and electrolytes – Incorrect. Elderly patients with neck of femur fractures often have multiple medical conditions and most take several medications. These can adversely affect their renal function and electrolyte balance, which needs to be recognised and addressed prior to surgery. It is therefore important to discuss such patients with the anaesthetist. If you are unsure about the patient's other co-morbid conditions or past medical history, you should seek advice from the medical registrar. In emergency situations, the full blood result may not be available at the time of surgery. In such cases, the anaesthetic team may have to correct any electrolyte abnormality during the operation.

E) None of the above – Correct. Although not absolutely necessary, these should all be done for the standard patient with a neck of femur fracture.

> **👥 IMPORTANT LEARNING POINTS**
>
> - The Garden classification helps classify intracapsular fractures based on the degree of displacement.
> - Undisplaced fractures (Garden 1 and 2) are at lower risk of AVN, as the capsular blood vessels are less likely to be damaged. These patients can be considered for surgical fixation using, for example, cannulated screws, thus preserving the patient's native femoral head.
> - Displaced fractures (Garden 3 and 4) are at significant risk of AVN and require some form of arthroplasty. Hemiarthroplasty is a good option for minimally mobile elderly patients who are frail. A THR is good for more active older patients but carries a higher risk of dislocation.
> - In younger patients, fixing the fracture improves functional outcome if the femoral head can be preserved. If the younger patient then develops AVN, they are young and fit enough to survive a second operation. A simplified algorithm is shown in Figure C4.13.1.

Continue

CASE **4.13**   *Contd.*

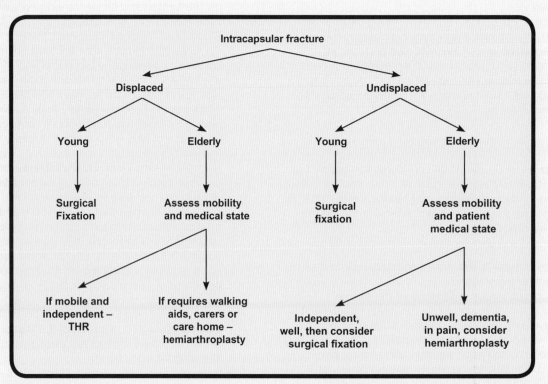

Figure C4.13.1 Simplified decision making algorithm for intracapsular hip fractures. In reality, decision-making is more complex, and each patient and their fracture need to be considered and options discussed both in the trauma meeting and with the patient.

A 99-year-old woman with dementia is brought to A&E following an unwitnessed fall in her nursing home. She is in pain and her left leg is shortened and externally rotated.

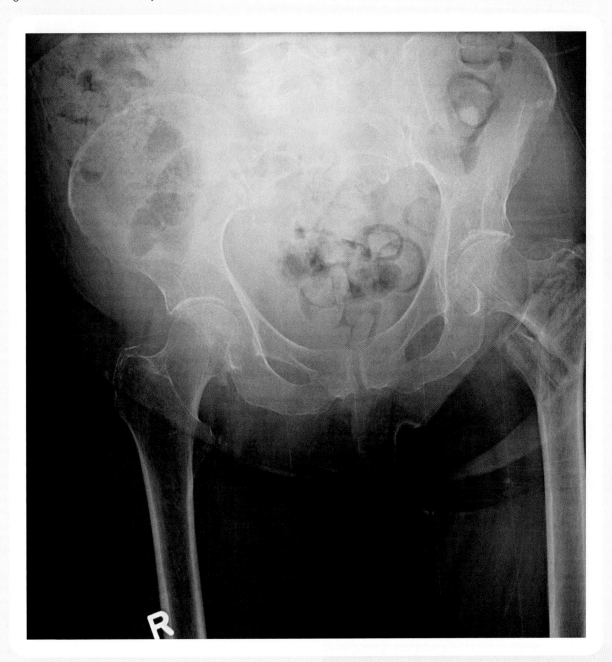

Continue

CASE **4.14** *Contd.*

ANNOTATED X-RAY

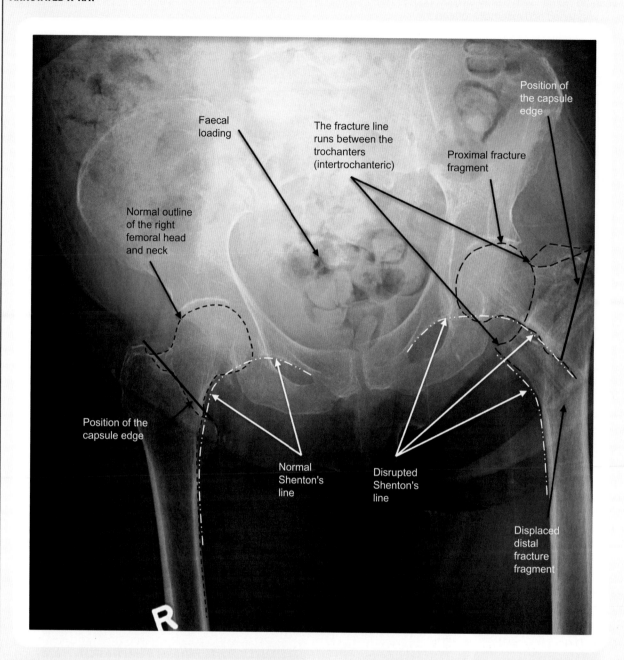

Faecal loading

The fracture line runs between the trochanters (intertrochanteric)

Position of the capsule edge

Proximal fracture fragment

Normal outline of the right femoral head and neck

Position of the capsule edge

Normal Shenton's line

Disrupted Shenton's line

Displaced distal fracture fragment

R

PRESENT YOUR FINDINGS

- This is an AP X-ray of the pelvis of a skeletally mature patient.
- It has been anonymised and the timing of the examination is not available. I would like to confirm the patient's details and timing of the examination before I make any further assessment.
- The X-ray is adequately penetrated but the patient is rotated and the tip of the left greater trochanter is not included.
- There is a fracture of the left neck of femur, which has not been fully included in the X-ray. The fracture line runs in the intertrochanteric region, making this an extracapsular fracture. It is completely displaced and two fracture fragments appear to be present.
- The femur is shortened.
- No other fracture is identified.
- The bone texture is normal with no areas of lucency or cystic changes to suggest a pathological fracture.
- There is some faecal loading in the rectum.

IN SUMMARY – This single AP X-ray of the pelvis shows a displaced extracapsular fracture of the left femoral neck. I would want to see a lateral X-ray of the left hip to complete the radiographic assessment of this injury.

QUESTIONS

1. Why is it important to know the mechanism of injury in patients with neck of femur fractures?
   A) To help exclude any other injury
   B) To ensure the mechanism fits the injury
   C) To ensure this was a mechanical fall and no underlying medical problems led to the fall
   D) To make sure the patient is not a vulnerable adult
   E) To help prevent further falls

2. In relation to hip fractures, what does the term extracapsular mean?
   A) The fracture is outside of the capsule of the joint
   B) The capsule of the hip joint is displaced
   C) The fracture is inside the capsule
   D) There is a tear in the hip capsule
   E) The blood supply to the femoral head has been disrupted

3. What is the classification system for this type of fracture?
   A) Garden's classification
   B) Gartland's classification
   C) Pauwel's classification
   D) Classified into 2 to 4 parts
   E) The AO (Arbeitsgemeinschaft für Osteosynthesefragen) classification

4. What is the best definitive management for an extracapsular fracture?
   A) 6 weeks of bed rest
   B) Early mobilisation as pain allows
   C) A DHS
   D) A THR
   E) An intramedullary nail

5. What is the expected mortality rate for this fracture?
   A) 1% at 1 month
   B) 2% at 1 month
   C) 5% at 3 months
   D) 30% at 6 months
   E) 5% at 1 month

Continue

CASE 4.14 *Contd.*

ANSWERS TO QUESTIONS

1. Why is it important to know the mechanism of injury in patients with neck of femur fractures?

   The correct answers are **A) To help exclude any other injury, B) To ensure the mechanism fits the injury, C) To ensure this was a mechanical fall and no underlying medical problems led to the fall, D) To make sure the patient is not a vulnerable adult and E) To help prevent further falls**.

   For all patients with a neck of femur fracture, it is crucial to take a full history and examination. There are multiple issues to consider in the history but it is important that the mechanism of injury be considered fully. Often patients have other injuries or an underlying medical problem. Missing these problems can lead to increased morbidity and mortality.

   A) To help exclude any other injury – Correct. A patient at the age of 99 may have simply slipped and fell, but it is important to ensure there are no other injuries. Common associated injuries from falls include proximal humeral or wrist fractures on the same side. Head injuries are also common and these patients may be taking anticoagulants such as warfarin, increasing the risk of an intracranial haemorrhage. In younger patients, this injury requires significant force and there may be significant head, chest or abdominal trauma which needs attention first.

   B) To ensure the mechanism fits the injury – Correct. If the patient sustained the fracture without a fall, then it is important to consider the possibility of a pathological fracture. Ask about any previous history of malignancy or pain in the hip prior to the fall. Examine the patient for masses, including masses in the breasts. In patients with a pathological fracture, it is necessary to X-ray the whole of the femur to look for further pathological lesions as this may change management. If there is cause for concern, a CT or an MRI scan will provide greater detail to delineate any pathological lesion.

   C) To ensure this was a mechanical fall and no underlying medical problems led to the fall – Correct. Although it is often said that the patient presented following a mechanical fall, there may well be an underlying problem that led to the fall. Therefore, it is important to ask about preceding symptoms. Did the patient black out? Have they had previous episodes/falls? Sepsis can also lead to falls, so assess for urinary tract infections and pneumonia in these patients with a urine dipstick and chest X-ray, respectively. An ECG may also demonstrate arrhythmias that could lead to falls.

   D) To make sure the patient is not a vulnerable adult – Correct. Sadly, patients with dementia or in nursing homes can occasionally be mistreated. Although it is often highlighted to clinicians that children can be the victims of abuse presenting with nonaccidental injuries, the same can happen in the elderly too, so consider this if the history of the fracture does not fit. More often there is neglect rather than abuse.

   E) To help prevent further falls – Correct. There may be a reversible cause to the patient's cause, such as postural hypotension or poor visibility. By taking a thorough history and performing a full examination, it should be possible to identify such factors which can then be managed appropriately to help prevent further falls and injuries.

> **❗ KEY POINTS**
>
> 1. Ensure that you are aware of what preceded a fall. There may have been an underlying medical problem explaining preceding symptoms.
> 2. Falls often result in multiple injuries, so it is important to thoroughly look for other potential injury.

2. In relation to hip fractures, what does the term extracapsular mean?

   The correct answer is **A) The fracture is outside of the capsule of the joint**.

   It is a very important concept to understand the difference between an extracapsular and intracapsular fracture of the femoral neck. This is important because the head of the femur gains its main blood supply from vessels that pass through the capsule of the hip joint. These vessels are branches of the profunda femoris, a branch of the common femoral artery, and are called the medial and lateral circumflex arteries. Fractures which are intracapsular usually disrupt the capsule and therefore the arteries within it. If the head of the femur loses its blood supply, it cannot survive and will undergo AVN. This will subsequently cause pain in the hip, with loss of mobility. Fractures that are extracapsular do not usually disrupt the femoral head's blood supply. Therefore, the two types of fracture are managed differently.

   A) The fracture is outside of the capsule of the joint – Correct. This is the case for extracapsular fractures. The blood supply to the head of the femur is intact and the fracture can be treated with surgical fixation. The femoral head is not at risk of AVN.

   B) The capsule of the hip joint is displaced – Incorrect. This is what occurs in intracapsular fractures. The blood supply to the head of the femur is compromised and there is risk of AVN. These fractures are most often best treated with a joint replacement. The head of the femur is removed and either a half (hemiarthroplasty) or THR is performed.

   C) The fracture is inside the capsule – Incorrect. This is an intracapsular fracture.

   D) There is a tear in the hip capsule – Incorrect. This is the same as B.

   E) The blood supply to the femoral head has been disrupted – Incorrect. This is what happens in intracapsular fractures.

❗ KEY POINTS

1. Intracapsular fractures are at risk of AVN of the femoral head and are therefore usually treated with a THR. Extracapsular fractures are not associated with AVN and can therefore be fixed surgically with a DHS or intramedullary nail.
2. By dividing neck of femur fractures into intracapsular and extracapsular, it is possible to come to the correct management option very quickly. Get this right and the patient will get the right operation. Getting this wrong may lead to the patient having the wrong operation, delaying mobilisation and leading to increased morbidity and mortality.
3. There are a few crucial points to make when assessing an X-ray of a neck of femur fracture:
   - Is the fracture intracapsular or extracapsular?
   - Is the fracture displaced or undisplaced?
   - Is there any suggestion the fracture is pathological?

3. What is the classification system for this type of fracture?
   The correct answer is **D) Classified into 2 to 4 parts**.
   Although there is no formal named classification for extracapsular fractures, these fractures can be classified into the number of parts of the fracture. Describing the number of parts of the fracture helps to predict how unstable the fracture is and gives the surgeon an idea of how difficult the fracture may be to fix. It is also important to comment on the degree of displacement: fractures with 3 or 4 parts are likely to be more displaced than 2-part fractures, which can be undisplaced.
   A) Garden's classification – Incorrect. This is the classification system used for intracapsular fractures (Table 4.3). It refers to the degree of displacement in intracapsular fractures.
   B) Gartland's classification – Incorrect. This is used for supracondylar fractures of the elbow in children (Table 4.1).
   C) Pauwel's classification – Incorrect. This classification again relates to intracapsular fractures. The classification system suggests that the more vertical the fracture the more likely fixation of the intracapsular fracture is going to fail.
   D) Classified into 2 to 4 parts – Correct. The fracture is classified into 2 to 4 parts. If there is a single fracture line between the neck and the shaft of the femur, this is a 2-part fracture. If the lesser trochanter is also fractured, then this becomes a 3-part fracture. If the greater trochanter is also fractured, then the fracture is in 4 parts. The more parts there are, the more unstable the fracture is likely to be.
   E) The AO classification – Incorrect. The AO classification system is a very complex general classification system for fractures. It is primarily used as a research tool.
4. What is the best definitive management for an extracapsular fracture?
   The correct answer is **C) A DHS and E) Intramedullary nail**.
   A neck of femur fracture is common and it is therefore one of the first fractures medical students and junior doctors learn the surgical treatment options for. These patients are often frail and the fracture is very painful. If the patient remains in bed, they will develop pressure sores and other complications such as pneumonia or venous thromboembolism. Operating early allows the patient to mobilise and reduces these risks. This helps to reduce the mortality associated with this type of fracture.
   A) 6 weeks of bed rest – Incorrect. As stated earlier, this is not the definitive treatment option. However, some patients are too unfit for surgery. This is uncommon, but in such patients, the use of bed rest and traction can heal the fracture.
   B) Early mobilisation as pain allows – Incorrect. Although this is possible following surgery, if the fracture has not been stabilised surgically, this will be extremely painful for the patient.
   C) A DHS – Correct. The DHS involves a large screw being placed into the head of the femur and a plate down the lateral side of the femur, normally with four screws into the shaft of the femur. This implant has been in use for many years, with excellent results for most extracapsular fractures of the femur. As the patient mobilises, the screw slides down the barrel of the plate, allowing compression of the fracture. This stabilises the fracture and allows the patient to weight bear early.
   D) A THR – Incorrect. This is a treatment option for intracapsular fractures. It is not possible to perform this operation for this fracture, as most hip replacements need the intertrochanteric region to be intact. In this fracture, the intertrochanteric region is broken and the hip replacement will fail.
   E) An intramedullary nail – Correct. The use of intramedullary nailing for the management of neck of femur fractures is increasing. The operation involves passing a large metal rod down the centre of the femur with one or two screws into the head of the femur. The implants cost more than a DHS and are not always necessary; hence, this is why a DHS is used more commonly. There are two situations with extracapsular fractures where a nail would be better: (1) when the fracture line runs from above the lesser trochanter to below the greater trochanter (reverse oblique fracture) and (2) where the fracture extends below the lesser trochanter (subtrochanteric).

❗ KEY POINT

Extracapsular neck of femur fractures occur in the elderly and carry a significant mortality rate. They are common and must be managed appropriately. Early operative intervention with the appropriate surgical implant will reduce morbidity and mortality.

5. What is the expected mortality rate for this fracture?
   The correct answer is **E) 5% at 1 month**.
   It is important to know the mortality rate for this fracture as it affects many elderly patients. These patients are often frail and although, as described earlier, an operation is usually the best treatment option, there is a significant postoperative mortality. This has led to significant

Continue

CASE **4.14** *Contd.*

investment across the country to minimise the risk of death. NICE guidelines have also been introduced which include in their recommendations involving a multidisciplinary team in the care of the patient and operating within 36 hours of admission.

The overall 1-year mortality rate for this fracture is 30%, although often the deaths are not directly related to the fracture or the surgery but rather to the patients' comorbid conditions and limited life expectancy.

With good management from the multidisciplinary team, it should be possible to achieve a 1-month mortality rate of 5% or less. This team should include preoperative assessment from an orthogeriatrician and careful anaesthetic assessment. Patients with potential medical problems should be discussed early with the medical team (including the medical registrar out of hours if necessary) to ensure there is no avoidable delay in time to surgery. Some hospitals also use scores to identify the high-risk patients. The most well known is the Nottingham Hip Fracture Score.

● KEY POINT

Femoral neck fractures and their associated surgical management carry a significant mortality, much of which is related to the fact that patients usually present with multiple comorbidities. A multidisciplinary team approach with specialist orthogeriatrician input helps reduce the mortality rate.

IMPORTANT LEARNING POINTS

- Hip fractures can be categorised into intra- or extracapsular.
- Extracapsular femoral neck fractures are common fractures that carry a 5% 1-month mortality.
- Extracapsular fractures are usually treated with a DHS although an intramedullary nail is sometimes better.
- Intracapsular fractures increase the risk of AVN of the femoral head and are often treated with a hip replacement.

A 14-year-old boy has presented to A&E following a football injury. He went in for a tackle and twisted his left knee. He has tenderness around his knee and proximal tibia. He is otherwise well. X-rays have been performed for further assessment.

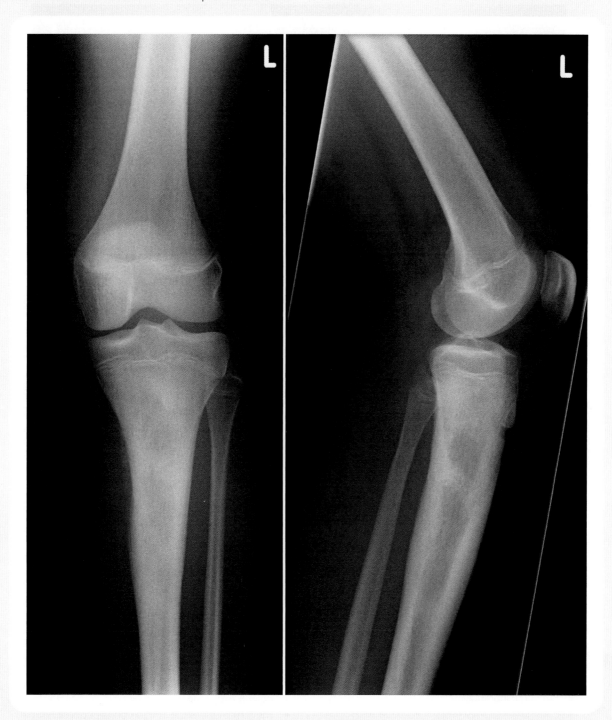

Continue

CASE **4.15**   *Contd.*

ANNOTATED X-RAY

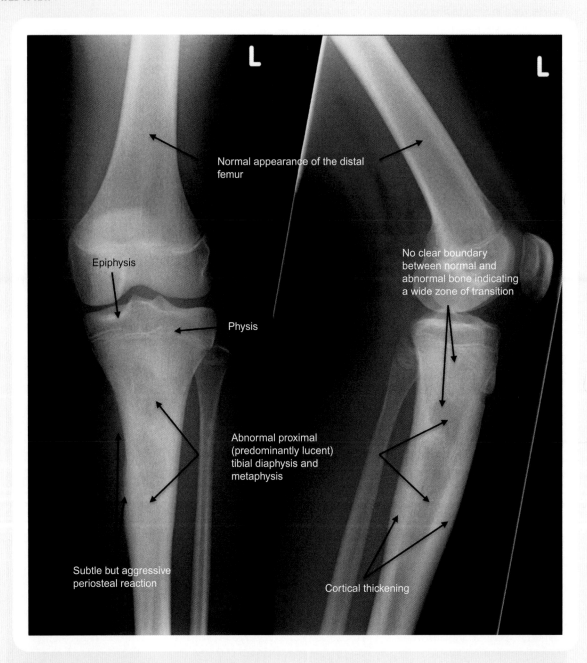

Normal appearance of the distal femur

Epiphysis

Physis

No clear boundary between normal and abnormal bone indicating a wide zone of transition

Abnormal proximal (predominantly lucent) tibial diaphysis and metaphysis

Subtle but aggressive periosteal reaction

Cortical thickening

PRESENT YOUR FINDINGS

- These are AP and lateral X-rays of the left knee in a skeletally immature individual.
- They have been anonymised and the timing of the examination is not available. I would like to confirm the patient's details and timing of the examination before I make any further assessment.
- The X-rays are adequately exposed, with no important areas cut off.
- Within the proximal tibia there is a large, ill-defined abnormal area in the proximal tibial diaphysis and metaphysis, which consists of a predominantly lytic lesion. It has a moth-eaten appearance and its margins

are difficult to clearly identify, in keeping with a wide zone of transition. There is associated cortical thickening and an aggressive appearing periosteal reaction.
- No soft tissue mass is visible.
- The remainder of the imaged bones appear normal, with no fracture or joint effusion visible.

IN SUMMARY – These X-rays show an aggressive bone lesion within the proximal tibia. Given its appearance, its location and the patient's age, the differential diagnosis includes primary bone tumours, such as osteosarcoma and Ewing's sarcoma, bone metastases (although these are uncommon in this age group) and infection.

QUESTIONS

1. Which of the following X-ray features is/are in keeping with an aggressive bone lesion?
   A) Narrow zone of transition
   B) Moth-eaten pattern of bone destruction
   C) Permeative pattern of bone destruction
   D) Spiculated periosteal reaction
   E) Soft tissue mass

2. The differential diagnosis for this patient includes which of the following?
   A) Osteomyelitis
   B) Ewing's sarcoma
   C) Giant cell tumour
   D) Multiple myeloma
   E) Osteochondroma

3. The initial assessment of this child should include which of the following?
   A) An ATLS assessment
   B) Full history and examination
   C) Routine bloods including inflammatory markers
   D) MRI of the knee
   E) A full skeletal survey

4. Following initial assessment, the patient is suspected of having a primary bone tumour. Which of these further investigations are likely to be required?
   A) Skeletal survey
   B) Ultrasound of the knee
   C) MRI of the knee
   D) CT of the chest
   E) Bone biopsy

5. Which of these bone tumours are correctly matched with their typical location and age?
   A) Ewing's sarcoma, diametaphysis of long bones, 5 to15 years
   B) Ewing's sarcoma, epiphysis of long bones, 5 to 15 years
   C) Enchondroma, phalanges, 10 to 30 years
   D) Multiple myeloma, appendicular skeleton, >40 years
   E) Osteosarcoma, metaphysis of long bones, 10 to 30 years

Continue

CASE **4.15** *Contd.*

ANSWERS TO QUESTIONS

1. Which of the following X-ray features is/are in keeping with an aggressive bone lesion?
   The correct answers are **B) Moth-eaten pattern of bone destruction, C) Permeative pattern of bone destruction, D) Spiculated periosteal reaction and E) Soft tissue mass**.
   It is difficult (and often impossible) to accurately diagnose a bone lesion/tumour on an X-ray. When presented with a bone lesion on an X-ray, you should be able to determine whether the appearances are in keeping with an aggressive or benign lesion. Note: the term aggressive not malignant is used as some nonmalignant conditions can give similar appearances. Further imaging and often biopsy are likely to be required to reach a precise diagnosis.
   A) Narrow zone of transition – Incorrect. The zone of transition is probably the most reliable indicator when assessing the aggression of a bone lesion. It consists of the area between the abnormal bone lesion and normal bone. If you can easily draw around the bone lesion, or the lesion has a sclerotic border, then it is said to have a narrow zone of transition and will (almost always) be benign. If the bone lesion is ill defined and it is difficult to clearly see where it ends and the normal bone begins, it has a wide zone of transition. A wide zone of transition indicates a fast-growing lesion and is consistent with an aggressive abnormality. Zone of transition can only be used for assessing lytic/predominantly lytic lesions with X-rays. Sclerotic lesions will always have a narrow zone of transition, even if malignant, and most lesions will appear to have a narrow zone of transition on MRI.
   B) Moth-eaten pattern of bone destruction – Correct. The pattern of bone destruction can give an indication of the aggressiveness of the lesion. Lesions with a well-defined lucency are likely slow growing and benign, particularly if there is a sclerotic rim. This pattern is known as geographic lucency. Lesions which consist of multiple small holes of varying size are known as moth-eaten. Both the trabecular and cortical bone may be affected. Moth-eaten lytic lesions are aggressive in nature.
   C) Permeative pattern of bone destruction – Correct. This refers to elongated holes within the cortex rather than defined circular holes and again reflects an aggressive process, such as myeloma, lymphoma or Ewing's sarcoma.
   D) Spiculated periosteal reaction – Correct. There may be new bone formation in the form of a periosteal reaction in response to bone destruction. A thick, single layered periosteal reaction indicates slow growth and is thus associated with benign lesions.
   Periosteal reactions in fast-growing aggressive lesions can:
   - Consist of multiple layers and look like an onion skin
   - Have a spiculated pattern that looks like a sunburst
   - Have an appearance like hair standing on end
   - Look incomplete

   E) Soft tissue mass – Correct. Soft tissue masses associated with a bone lesion usually indicate an aggressive process. They are often an extension of the primary bone abnormality. They can be difficult to appreciate on X-rays, due to the similar attenuation to the surrounding normal soft tissues, but are readily apparent on MRI.

❶ KEY POINT

The age of the patient and location of the lesion, along with whether a bone abnormality appears aggressive or not, are often the most helpful factors for diagnosing a specific type of bone lesion.

2. The differential diagnosis for this patient includes which of the following?
   The correct answer is **A) Osteomyelitis and B) Ewing's sarcoma**.
   The differential diagnosis of a bone lesion depends on its appearance (e.g. aggressive versus benign), the location of the lesion (which bone and which part of the bone) and the age of the patient. This an aggressive bone lesion in the proximal tibia of a 14-year old.
   A) Osteomyelitis – Correct. Osteomyelitis should be considered in the differential diagnosis of any aggressive bone lesion, regardless of the patient's age. Growing bones have a rich blood supply, especially the tubular bones, making them prone to osteomyelitis. Osteomyelitis in children tends to spread by the haematogenous route from other sources of infection and typically involves the distal femur, proximal or distal tibia, distal humerus or distal radius. Infants have blood vessels which cross the physis from the metaphysis to the epiphysis, whereas in older children (>1 year), the physis acts as a barrier. As a result, infants can have metaphyseal or epiphyseal osteomyelitis, whereas older children usually have metaphyseal osteomyelitis. In contrast, osteomyelitis in adults tends to affect the spine (vertebral bodies and discs) or is due to direct spread of infection (e.g. penetrating trauma, surgery) or surgical metalwork. Eosinophilic granuloma, a type of Langerhans cell histiocytosis, is another nonmalignant condition which can result in an aggressive bone lesion in a child.
   B) Ewing's sarcoma – Correct. Ewing's sarcoma is a relatively common malignant primary bone tumour. It typically affects children aged between 5 and 15 years. It can present with pain, fever, a mass or incidentally. Ewing's sarcoma is an aggressive tumour which results in a moth-eaten or permeative pattern of bone destruction, an aggressive periosteal reaction, and often a soft tissue mass. The metadiaphysis of the femur or tibia is most commonly involved. Other malignant processes to consider in this age group include osteosarcoma, lymphoma and leukaemia. Osteosarcoma typically affects patients aged 10 to 30, is usually centred in the metaphysis of long tubular

bones, such as the femur or tibia, and has aggressive features on X-ray.

C) Giant cell tumour – Incorrect. This is an uncommon tumour which arises in the epiphysis, abutting the articular surface. They are expansive lytic lesions with a narrow zone of transition. They only develop after physeal fusion and most occur around the knee. These are benign but aggressive lesions.

D) Multiple myeloma – Incorrect. Multiple myeloma is the most common primary bone tumour. It typically affects the vertebral bodies, ribs and skull, and almost always occurs in patients over the age of 40. It usually results in well-defined lytic lesions but can cause generalised osteopaenia (due to marrow infiltration) and wedge compression fractures. MRI is the most sensitive imaging modality for detecting myeloma. Other investigations, such as Bence Jones proteins and serum electrophoresis, are also helpful.

E) Osteochondroma – Incorrect. As the name suggests, osteochondromas are composed of bone (osteo) and cartilage (chondro). They appear as bony outgrowths from the metaphysis of long bones and can either be pedunculated or sessile (on a stalk or flat). The cartilage cap is not visible on X-ray, but is readily demonstrated on MRI. Osteochondromas can be asymptomatic or can result in pressure symptoms (e.g. due to effects on adjacent nerves, blood vessels or bones). They are almost always benign but <1% can become malignant.

❶ KEY POINT

The differential diagnosis of an aggressive bone lesion varies by age in children, Ewing's sarcoma, osteosarcoma, lymphoma/leukaemia and eosinophilic granuloma should be considered. In adults, metastases and primary bone tumours such as chondrosarcomas are possibilities. Infection can occur at any age.

3. The initial assessment of this child should include which of the following?
   The correct answers are **B) Full history and examination and C) Routine bloods including inflammatory markers**.
   Clinical assessment of the patient and simple blood tests are useful to try to narrow down the differential diagnosis of an aggressive bone lesion. Further investigations will be required (see question 4); however, these are not part of the initial assessment.
   A) An ATLS assessment – Incorrect. Whilst a thorough clinical assessment is required, ATLS is not indicated as the patient has not suffered significant trauma. However, it is important to assess for other injuries.
   B) Full history and examination – Correct. It is important to ask about systemic symptoms. Has there been any fever, weight loss or fatigue? Has the child previously had a malignancy or are they immunocompromised? Enquire about the nature of the pain. Be worried

about the child who describes a deep boring pain which is constant and getting worse, as this is suspicious of malignancy. Is there any clinical evidence of other bones or organs being affected? Examination, including assessment of the neurological system, is also important.

C) Routine bloods including inflammatory markers – Correct. Inflammatory markers are helpful for ruling out infection as the underlying cause. However, it should be noted that approximately one-third of children with Ewing's sarcoma present with a fever and raised inflammatory markers. Therefore, elevated white cell count, CRP and ESR are not specific for infection. Blood cultures are also useful for identifying infection but false negatives can occur, particularly in cases of osteomyelitis. Other routine bloods are useful to assess renal function, liver function and bone profile.

D) MRI of the knee – Incorrect. Urgent MRI is an important investigation (see question 4); however, it does not form part of the initial investigations.

E) A full skeletal survey – Incorrect. A skeletal survey may be indicated if there is a suspicion of NAI. This is a specialist investigation which should only be requested by a consultant paediatrician and not by the on-call junior doctor. Additionally, the imaging features and clinical scenario are not in keeping with NAI.

4. Following initial assessment, the patient is suspected of having a primary bone tumour. Which of these further investigations are likely to be required?
   The correct answers are **C) MRI of the knee, D) CT of the chest and E) Bone biopsy**.
   Further investigations are required to diagnose the type of tumour, assess its local extent and determine whether there is any distant disease. Treatment usually involves management of the primary site with surgery and/or radiotherapy, complimented by chemotherapy.
   A) Skeletal survey – Incorrect. A skeletal survey consists of a series of X-rays assessing most of the skeleton. In children, they are performed in cases of suspected NAI to identify fractures which may help confirm the clinical concern. It is a specialised investigation which should only be requested by a consultant paediatrician. It has no role in the assessment or staging of primary bone tumours.
   B) Ultrasound of the knee – Incorrect. Ultrasound allows an assessment of the soft tissues to be made. It can identify a knee joint effusion and will be able to demonstrate a soft tissue mass. Its usefulness for assessing bones is very limited and therefore it is not indicated in the assessment of primary bone tumours.
   C) MRI of the knee – Correct. MRI with IV contrast (gadolinium) is the best imaging investigation for assessing the local extent of the tumour, including any soft tissue component. It is very useful in determining its relationship with any adjacent neurovascular structures. CT can be used to show the bony

Continue

CASE 4.15 *Contd.*

characteristics of the tumour but MRI is superior for showing the extent of marrow involvement.

D) CT of the chest – Correct. Identifying any distant sites of tumour involvement (staging) is an important part of the investigations. The lung is one of the most common sites for metastases and is best assessed using CT. Whole body MRI or PET-CT are useful for detecting any other sites of disease involvement.

E) Bone biopsy – Correct. The age of the patient, the location of the tumour and its appearance on X-ray are helpful for narrowing the differential diagnosis; however, a tissue sample is ultimately required for confirmation. The biopsy should be planned after discussion with a paediatric oncologist and an orthopaedic surgeon to ensure the optimal approach is used (there is a risk of tumour seeding with percutaneous biopsy and therefore the biopsy track must be excised at surgery).

❗ KEY POINT

Investigations of a suspected primary bone tumour, aim to confirm the diagnosis (biopsy), assess its local extent (MRI) and identify any metastatic disease (CT, MRI and/ or PET-CT).

5. Which of these bone tumours are correctly matched with their typical location and age?
   The correct answers are **A) Ewing's sarcoma, diametaphysis of long bones, 5 to 15 years, C) Enchondroma, phalanges, 10 to 30 years and E) Osteosarcoma, metaphysis of long bones, 10 to 30 years**.
   Whilst a detailed knowledge of bone tumours in not required for junior doctors, the location of a bone tumour and the age of the patient give a big clue to the likely underlying diagnosis. Additionally, this sort of information often appears in exams.
   A) Ewing's sarcoma, diametaphysis of long bones, 5 to 15 years – Correct. Ewing's sarcoma is one of the commonest primary bone tumours in children. It usually affects the diaphysis and/or metaphysis of long bones, with the majority arising around the knee in the distal femur and proximal tibia. It most

commonly affects children aged between 5 and 15 years.

B) Ewing's sarcoma, epiphysis of long bones, 5 to 15 years – Incorrect. The metadiaphysis is typically affected. Only in 1% to 2% of cases is the epiphysis involved.

C) Enchondroma, phalanges, 10 to 30 years – Correct. Enchondromas are benign, lytic and often expansile lesions. They typically involve the phalanges and occur in patients aged 10 to 30 years.

D) Multiple myeloma, appendicular skeleton, >40 years – Incorrect. Multiple myeloma is the commonest primary bone tumour. It almost always occurs in patients over the age of 40. It typically causes multiple lytic lesions which are most commonly found in the axial skeleton (spine, skull, ribs and pelvis).

E) Osteosarcoma, metaphysis of long bones, 10 to 30 years – Correct. Osteosarcomas are the second commonest primary bone tumours. They are malignant tumours with aggressive features on X-ray. They usually occur in adolescents and young adults and typically involve the metaphysis of long bones, especially the lower limb. They can be very difficult to differentiate from Ewing's sarcoma on imaging.

👥 IMPORTANT LEARNING POINTS

- Bone lesions are uncommon and can be daunting.
- You should try to decide whether a lesion has an aggressive or benign appearance by assessing the pattern of bone destruction, the zone of transition, any periosteal reaction and the presence of a soft tissue mass.
- The age of the patient and location of the abnormality help to determine the differential diagnosis.
- Aggressive bone lesions in children include Ewing's sarcoma, osteosarcoma, infection and eosinophilic granuloma. In adults, metastases and chondrosarcomas should be considered. Osteomyelitis can affect patients of any age.
- Clinical assessment and blood tests are helpful for narrowing the differential diagnosis.
- Investigations in suspected primary bone tumours aim to confirm the diagnosis, assess the local extent of the tumour and identify any metastases.

CASE **4.16**

A 25-year-old motorcycle enthusiast has come off her bike at high speed and injured her right knee. Her knee is swollen and tender and she is unable to flex it. These are her X-rays.

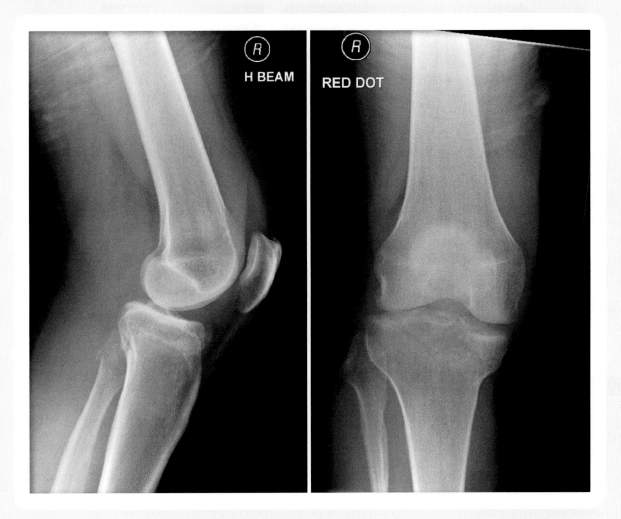

Continue

CASE **4.16**   *Contd.*

ANNOTATED X-RAY

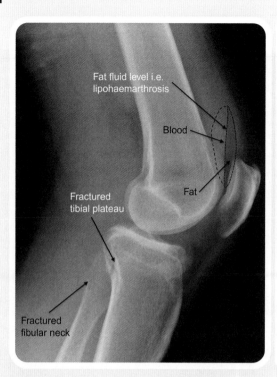

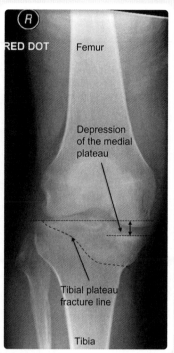

PRESENT YOUR FINDINGS

- These are AP and lateral X-rays of the right knee of a skeletally mature patient.
- They have been anonymised and the timing of the examination is not available. I would like to confirm the patient's details and timing of the examination before I make any further assessment.
- The X-rays are adequately exposed, with no important areas cut off.
- The most striking abnormality is the presence of a knee joint effusion of two densities (less dense material lying above the more dense material) separated by a horizontal line. This finding is consistent with a fat–fluid level, and signifies a lipohaemarthrosis.

- There is a displaced fracture of the tibial plateau with depression of the medial tibial plateau. There is an associated fibular neck fracture which is undisplaced.
- Soft tissue swelling is present.
- There is no evidence on the X-rays that this is an open fracture.
- Normal bone density with no lytic or sclerotic lesions.

IN SUMMARY – These X-rays demonstrate a lipohaem-arthrosis secondary to a tibial plateau fracture. There is an associated fracture of the fibular neck.

QUESTIONS

1. What is the significance of a lipohaemarthrosis?
   A) Signifies the presence of a simple joint effusion
   B) Signifies the presence of a significant injury in the joint
   C) Signifies the presence of a fracture communicating with the joint
   D) The patient is on warfarin or another anticoagulant
   E) Signifies the joint needs aspirating

2. What is the underlying injury this patient has sustained that has caused the lipohaemarthrosis?
   A) Fracture of the patella
   B) Fracture of the fibular neck
   C) Anterior cruciate ligament injury
   D) Tibial plateau fracture
   E) Meniscal tear

3. What complication may occur acutely as a result of a tibial plateau fracture?
   A) Head injury
   B) Arthritis
   C) Septic arthritis
   D) Osteomyelitis
   E) Compartment syndrome

4. What is the most common site for aspirating a knee joint?
   A) Lateral and slightly superior to the patella
   B) Anterior aspect medial to patella tendon
   C) Anterior aspect lateral to the patella tendon
   D) Medial and slightly superior to the patella
   E) Through the patella tendon

5. In this scenario, what imaging modality will be needed prior to operative intervention of this fracture?
   A) PET scan
   B) CT scan
   C) Bone scan
   D) MRI
   E) Further X-rays

Continue

CASE **4.16**   *Contd.*

ANSWERS TO QUESTIONS

1. What is the significance of a lipohaemarthrosis?
   The correct answer is **C) Signifies the presence of a fracture communicating with the joint**.
   Lipohaemarthrosis is a joint effusion which contains both fat (lipo) and blood (haem). It is an important radiological finding and should be looked for routinely. It is most commonly seen in the knee. Fat and blood have different densities, which can be identified on the lateral X-ray as a fat–fluid level.
   A) Signifies the presence of a simple joint effusion – Incorrect. A simple knee joint effusion can be identified on the lateral X-ray by the presence of soft tissue density within the suprapatellar pouch. A joint effusion may be caused by haemorrhage (after trauma or in haemophilia), infection (septic arthritis), inflammation (rheumatoid arthritis) or metabolic derangements (gout or pseudogout).
   B) Signifies the presence of a significant injury in the joint – Incorrect. A lipohaemarthrosis does suggest that there is some form of internal derangement to the knee. However, significant soft tissue injuries, such as meniscal or ligament tears, in the knee will not necessarily cause a lipohaemarthrosis.
   C) Signifies the presence of a fracture communicating with the joint – Correct. The specific importance of this finding is that fat in the joint suggests a communication between the inside of the bone and the joint. This essentially means there is an intraarticular fracture or an osteochondral defect (a defect in the cartilage of the joint) which allows fat from within the bone (intramedullary fat) to enter the joint. There is also haemorrhage within the joint due to injuries to vascularised structures. Because fat is less dense than blood, it will form a layer on top of the haemorrhage and this will be seen as a fat–fluid level on the horizontal beam lateral X-ray.
   D) The patient is on warfarin or another anticoagulant – Incorrect. Patients on warfarin can present with a spontaneous haemarthrosis of the joint (without an intraarticular fracture). This can be very painful but appears as a homogenous soft tissue density in the suprapatellar pouch. Patients with haemophilia are also at risk of spontaneous haemarthroses.
   E) Signifies the joint needs aspirating – Incorrect. The presence of a lipohaemarthrosis on X-ray does not mean that the joint needs to be aspirated. However, if a patient presents with a painful swollen knee following injury, some orthopaedic textbooks recommend aspirating the joint to reduce pain. Occasionally, a lipohaemarthrosis may only become apparent when aspirated fluid is analysed, but this is not a diagnostic test to perform routinely.

❗ KEY POINTS

1. A mnemonic for remembering the causes of a swollen joint is 'CHRIST'. It stands from Crystals (gout, pseudogout), Haemophilia, Rheumatoid arthritis and other inflammatory arthropathies, Infection, Synovial pathology (such as pigmented villonodular synovitis) and Trauma.
2. A lipohaemarthrosis is a particular type of joint effusion in which a fat–fluid level is visible. It is indicative of an intraarticular fracture, so if one is present on the X-rays, then referral to orthopaedics and consideration of further imaging, such as CT, are required.

2. What is the underlying injury this patient has sustained that has caused the lipohaemarthrosis?
   The correct answer is **D) Tibial plateau fracture**.
   The X-rays shown earlier demonstrate a complex fracture of the tibial plateau and fibular head. This is minimally displaced but visible. Occasionally, the tibial plateau fracture can be undisplaced and therefore the lipohaemarthrosis gives the only clue on X-ray that there is an underlying intraarticular fracture.
   A) Fracture of the patella – Incorrect. There is no fracture of the patella visible on this X-ray but this fracture would create a lipohaemarthrosis.
   B) Fracture of the fibular neck – Incorrect. There is a fracture of the fibular neck; however, this would not account for the lipohaemarthrosis as the fibula is outside of the joint capsule.
   C) Anterior cruciate ligament injury – Incorrect. An anterior cruciate ligament injury generally does not cause lipohaemarthrosis and the injury itself is not seen on a plain X-ray. However, if the bony insertion site of the anterior cruciate ligament has been fractured/avulsed, this may produce a lipohaemarthrosis. A Segond fracture (avulsion fracture of the lateral tibial plateau) is associated with a tear of the anterior cruciate ligament in 75% of cases and can be seen on the plain X-ray. However, it should be noted that most patients with a torn anterior cruciate ligament will only have the nonspecific finding of a knee joint effusion on X-ray.
   D) Tibial plateau fracture – Correct. This is a potentially significant injury which is often associated with high-energy trauma. Often the fracture is treated operatively and thus should be referred early to orthopaedics. The fracture is typically complex and patients will usually have a CT prior to surgery to characterise the fracture more clearly.
   E) Meniscal tear – Incorrect. Meniscal tears are not associated with a lipohaemarthrosis. In fact, the meniscus is a relatively avascular structure and often the effusions produced in response to this injury are synovial rather than blood.

❶ KEY POINT

Tibial plateau fractures are often complex and require accurate surgical fixation to reduce the chance of premature knee joint degenerative changes.

3. What complication may occur acutely as a result of a tibial plateau fracture?
The correct answer is **E) Compartment syndrome**.
In this scenario, the patient has come off her bike at high speed. It is important therefore to consider life-threatening injuries, such as head, chest or abdominal injuries first, before thinking about the fracture. However, this fracture, in particular, is associated with compartment syndrome.
A) Head injury – Incorrect. This patient may have more important life-threatening injuries, such as a head injury, which needs to be addressed before the fracture. However, this is not a direct complication of the fracture. The patient should be assessed using the ABCDE ATLS approach to allow such life-threatening injuries to be identified and managed in a timely manner. Always remember to also complete a secondary survey of the whole body to identify any other injuries.
B) Arthritis – Incorrect. The injury affects the knee joint and will disrupt the articular cartilage. Therefore, arthritis is an important long-term complication of this fracture, but it does not occur in the acute setting. The patient nevertheless needs to understand they may require a total knee replacement in the future.
C) Septic arthritis – Incorrect. Septic arthritis may become an issue in patients who have surgical fixation of this fracture or have an open fracture but it is not something that will occur acutely at the time of the fracture.
D) Osteomyelitis – Incorrect. Osteomyelitis is not associated in the acute phase with this injury. If there is an open fracture or surgical fixation, then a chronic osteomyelitis may develop if initial infection is not identified and treated.
E) Compartment syndrome – Correct. Compartment syndrome is a very important diagnosis which is mentioned more than once in the chapter. The patient will present with severe unremitting pain with a tense leg. There will be extreme pain on dorsi or plantar flexion of the toes or ankle. The diagnosis is often clinical, although pressure monitors can be used to monitor and confirm compartment syndrome. If suspicion is high, then the patient should have an urgent fasciotomy (the fascial compartments of the leg are opened) to relieve the pressure.

❶ KEY POINT

Compartment syndrome is defined as increased pressure in an osseofascial compartment, which leads to ischaemia. It can occur in the hands, forearms, arms, thighs, legs, feet and even the abdomen and can lead to significant morbidity from muscle necrosis. The key clinical finding is severe unremitting pain. The patient will also have severe pain on passive movement – the other typical symptoms of ischaemia (pallor, paraesthesia, pulseless and paralysis) occur late. Therefore, in an at-risk patient, you should not wait until these later clinical findings are present. If you are concerned, contact your senior for an urgent review. They may decide to measure the compartment pressure, or alternatively they may elect to perform emergency fasciotomies.

4. What is the most common site for aspirating a knee joint?
The correct answer is **A) Lateral and slightly superior to the patella**.
This is the first orthopaedic procedure most students or trainees get to do. The patient must be informed about the fact that the procedure is not without pain and that there is a small risk of introducing infection into the joint. It is important to check there is no metalwork in the knee, as it is not safe to aspirate a total knee replacement outside of the operating theatre.
The skin must be cleaned and draped. Sterile gloves and instruments should be used. Local anaesthetic is used to numb the skin. A large needle is then introduced into the joint with a syringe attached to aspirate any fluid. This is sent to the lab for microscopy to look for organisms and crystals (gout or pseudogout) and for culture and sensitivities.
A) Lateral and slightly superior to the patella – Correct. This is the commonest site to aspirate a knee. The lateral side is easily exposed and easy to access with a needle. In addition, the bulge of a tense effusion is easily palpable at this point. Identify the lateral border of the patella and identify a point just superior to the superior pole of the patella. Aim the needle along the under surface of the patella, slightly inferiorly. This should provide access to the suprapatellar pouch which is part of the joint.
B) Anterior aspect medial to patella tendon – Incorrect. This site is more commonly used as an entry point for arthroscopy of the knee.
C) Anterior aspect lateral to the patella tendon – Incorrect. This site is more commonly used as an entry point for arthroscopy of the knee.
D) Medial and slightly superior to the patella – Incorrect. This is an appropriate alternative, but is done less commonly (since this position is harder to access

Continue

with a needle, more difficult to expose and the bulge of an effusion may be less easy to palpate at this position). A knee should not be aspirated through cellulitis as this can introduce infection into the joint, so it may be safer to approach the aspiration from the medial side in some circumstances.
E) Through the patella tendon – Incorrect. This is not used for the aspiration of the knee joint.

❗ KEY POINT

Ensure informed consent is obtained before performing this procedure. Use sterile equipment and ensure samples are labelled correctly when sent to the lab. You do not want to have to aspirate the knee twice!

5. In this scenario, what imaging modality will be needed prior to operative intervention of this fracture?
The correct answer is **B) CT scan**.
Tibial plateau fractures can be difficult to see on X-ray. Furthermore, even if one is visible on X-ray, there may not be enough information to allow an operative plan to be made. Further imaging is used to accurately characterise the fracture.
A) PET scan – Incorrect. A PET scan is a form of radionuclide imaging that is primarily used in assessing cancer patients. It is not used for characterising tibial plateau fractures.
B) CT scan – Correct. The CT scan allows an excellent assessment of the bones and will be able to give the precise morphology of the fracture. It will show the fracture fragments and their relative positions. It is also possible to create 3D reconstructions with CT, which can provide further useful information for operative planning.
C) Bone scan – Incorrect. Bone scans are radionuclide tests which identify areas of increased osteoblastic activity. One of their uses is to diagnose occult fractures. However, their spatial resolution is relatively poor, and therefore, they would not provide any detailed morphological information regarding this fracture.
D) MRI – Incorrect. It may be necessary to assess the soft tissue structures of the knee, in addition to the fracture. Therefore, an MRI, which allows superior assessment of ligaments, tendons, menisci and other soft tissues than CT, may be required preoperatively. However, CT is better for assessing a tibial plateau fracture.
E) Further X-rays – Incorrect. Further X-rays are unlikely to provide a reliable assessment of the exact morphology of the tibial plateau which is needed by the surgeon for planning.

👥 IMPORTANT LEARNING POINTS

- A lipohaemarthrosis is an important X-ray sign which implies an underlying intraarticular fracture.
- Further imaging of a lipohaemarthrosis is usually required, either because the fracture is not visible on X-rays or to further characterise a visible fracture.
- Tibial plateau fractures commonly lead to a lipohaemarthrosis. They are often associated with high-energy trauma and need careful assessment with CT to guide orthopaedic management.
- Compartment syndrome is a potential acute complication of tibial plateau fractures. Its diagnosis requires a high index of suspicion to allow early appropriate management.
- Arthritis is a potential long-term complication of a tibial plateau fracture.

CASE **4.17**

A 59-year-old retired football player is referred to the elective orthopaedic clinic with a 1-year history of worsening knee pain. His X-rays are shown next.

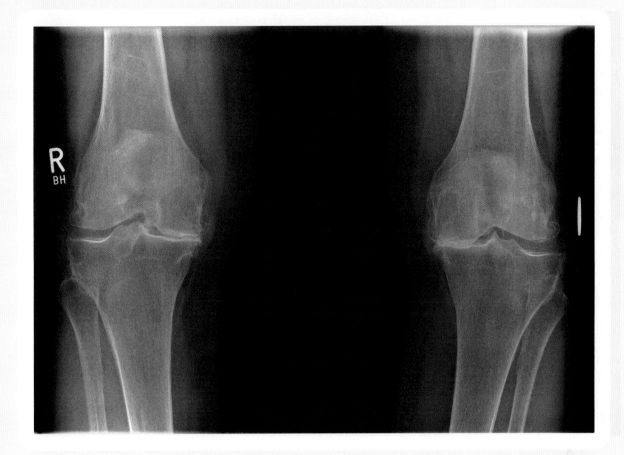

Continue

CASE **4.17**   *Contd.*

ANNOTATED X-RAY

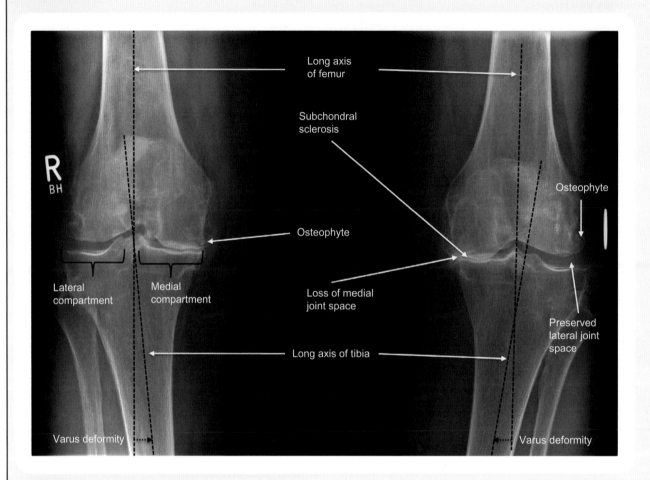

Long axis
of femur

Subchondral
sclerosis

Osteophyte

R
BH

Osteophyte

Lateral
compartment

Medial
compartment

Loss of medial
joint space

Preserved
lateral joint
space

Long axis of tibia

Varus deformity

Varus deformity

PRESENT YOUR FINDINGS

- This is an AP X-ray of both knees of a skeletally mature patient.
- It has been anonymised and the timing of the examination is not available. I would like to confirm the patient's details and timing of the examination before I make any further assessment.
- The X-ray is adequately exposed, with no important areas cut off.
- Within the medial compartments of both knees, there is marked loss of joint space, subchondral sclerosis and osteophyte formation. There is a resultant varus deformity of both knees.

- The lateral compartment joint spaces are well preserved. A lateral osteophyte is visible on the left knee.
- Bone density is normal, with no areas of lucency or sclerosis.
- No fracture is visible.
- The soft tissues appear normal.

IN SUMMARY – This X-ray shows moderate-to-severe osteoarthritis within the medial compartments of both knees. I would want to see lateral X-rays of the knees to complete my radiographic assessment.

QUESTIONS

1. Which of these is important when taking a history from this patient?
   A) History of previous trauma
   B) Severity of symptoms including effect on quality of life
   C) Previous interventions or surgery
   D) Symptoms of clicking or instability
   E) All of the above

2. Over which part of the knee will a patient with medial osteoarthritis typically have pain?
   A) At the back of the knee
   B) All over the knee
   C) At the tibial tuberosity
   D) Over the medial joint line
   E) Over the lateral joint line

3. What imaging is most commonly used when assessing osteoarthritis of the knee?
   A) MRI
   B) Bone scan
   C) CT
   D) Weight-bearing X-rays of the knee (AP and lateral)
   E) Skyline X-rays of the patella

4. Which of these is/are features of osteoarthritis on X-ray?
   A) Osteophytes
   B) Subchondral sclerosis
   C) Periarticular erosions
   D) Loss of joint space
   E) Subchondral cysts

5. Which is the best operation for a patient with severe osteoarthritis in all compartments of the knee?
   A) Total knee replacement
   B) Unicompartmental knee replacement
   C) Patellofemoral joint replacement
   D) Tibial osteotomy
   E) Arthroscopic washout

Continue

CASE 4.17   *Contd.*

ANSWERS TO QUESTIONS

1. Which of these is important when taking a history from this patient?
   The correct answer is **E) All of the above**.
   A thorough history from a patient with osteoarthritis is very important. There may have been multiple factors that have contributed to the development of osteoarthritis. It is also very important to assess the impact of arthritis on the patient's quality of life to help determine the most suitable management option.

   A) History of previous trauma – Incorrect. A history of previous trauma is important to ask about, but there are other features which should be considered in the history (see other answers). Many patients who present with osteoarthritis in the knee have had a previous injury or describe a period of overuse such as playing football. They may have previously had a meniscal injury treated with open meniscectomy (this procedure is a risk factor for developing osteoarthritis and is no longer performed). Fractures of the tibial plateau are also associated with development of osteoarthritis.

   B) Severity of symptoms including effect on quality of life – Incorrect. It is important to assess how the arthritis is affecting the patient to help determine the most appropriate treatment; however, there are other features which should be considered in the history (see other answers). The severity of symptoms and restrictions on the patient's daily activities help to determine if and when surgery is required.

   C) Previous interventions or surgery – Incorrect. We have already mentioned how an open meniscectomy is now known to be associated with the development of osteoarthritis. It is important to ask whether the patient has had any surgery on the knee, including arthroscopies, and what was found. It is also important to consider whether physiotherapy has been performed or whether steroid injections have worked previously. There are other features which should be considered in the history (see other answers).

   D) Symptoms of clicking or instability – Incorrect. Patients with mechanical symptoms of clicking, giving way or intermittent locking may have a degenerative tear of the meniscus or a loose body which is causing a lot of their symptoms. An arthroscopy may treat this problem and prevent an unnecessary joint replacement.

   E) All of the above – Correct. A thorough history together with an examination of the knee will identify the problem in most patients. Imaging is an adjunct to a good history and examination.

> **! KEY POINT**
>
> Important history points also include:
> - Age – most surgeons will try to avoid a knee replacement in patients under 65, if possible
> - The timing of pain – worse at night or following exercise
> - Cardiac and respiratory illness and other significant past medical histories which may preclude surgery
> - Medication

2. Over which part of the knee will a patient with medial osteoarthritis typically have pain?
   The correct answer is **D) Over the medial joint line**
   A good examination will often elucidate the cause of pain. Use the look, feel, move and special test approach when examining any joint. The site of pain on palpation may suggest the diagnosis. Tricompartmental osteoarthritis of the knee often causes pain all-round the knee rather than at a specific point; however, osteoarthritis in only one part/compartment of the knee may cause isolated pain to the affected part.

   A) At the back of the knee – Incorrect. Although not the most common complaint of patients with osteoarthritis of the knee, a Baker's cyst, which is a synovial cyst caused by excess joint fluid in response to osteoarthritis, may cause pain and tenderness at the back of the knee.

   B) All over the knee – Incorrect. Most people with osteoarthritis of the knee complain of a pain specific to the affected part of the knee. This pain is worse at night or comes on after little exercise. Standing up for long periods or lifting may exacerbate the pain. Occasionally patients complain of all over knee pain.

   C) At the tibial tuberosity – Incorrect. Pain and tenderness at the tibial tuberosity is a common complaint among children suffering from Osgood–Schlatter disease, which is irritation of the insertion of the patella tendon at the tibial tuberosity and typically affects athletic children and adolescents.

   D) Over the medial joint line – Correct. Patients with medial compartment osteoarthritis typically complain of pain on the medial side only.

   E) Over the lateral joint line – Incorrect. Similarly, patients may have lateral compartment osteoarthritis only and typically present with lateral joint line pain.

> **! KEY POINT**
>
> Osteoarthritis in the knee which is isolated to a specific compartment in the knee will produce pain in that compartment. Less typically patients complain of pain all over the knee.

3. What imaging is most commonly used when assessing osteoarthritis of the knee?

The correct answer is **D) Weight-bearing X-rays of the knee (AP and lateral)**.

Selecting the correct imaging modality for the correct knee pathology is important. Together with the history and examination, this will allow you to make the correct diagnosis and formulate an appropriate management plan.

A) MRI – Incorrect. An MRI scan is very useful for assessing soft tissue injuries. In young patients, this modality is frequently used to identify or exclude meniscal injuries, such as tears, as well as injuries to the ligaments, such as rupture of the anterior cruciate ligament. It is not commonly used in assessing an arthritic knee. If there is clinical suspicion of a meniscal tear, some surgeons would perform an arthroscopy of the knee rather than an MRI as the problem can be identified and treated at the same time.

B) Bone scan – Incorrect. Bone scans use a radiopharmaceutical to identify areas of increased osteoblastic activity. They are useful in patients where there is a suspicion of a fracture but no fracture is visible on X-rays. They are also helpful for assessing knee replacements to see whether they are loose and wearing out or for evidence infection. Bone scans are not used for assessing osteoarthritis.

C) CT – Incorrect. CT is good at assessing bone but less useful than MRI for demonstrating the soft tissue structures. CT would demonstrate the changes of osteoarthritis but compared with X-rays it is relatively costly and associated with significantly higher radiation doses. It is therefore not used for assessing osteoarthritis. Instead, it is useful for assessing complex fractures around the knee, such as tibial plateau fractures, to guide surgery. Occasionally, CT scans will be used in complex patients but only after discussion with a specialist.

D) Weight-bearing X-rays of the knee (AP and lateral) – Correct. Two X-rays with the patient standing are all that is needed to diagnose osteoarthritis of the knee in the majority of cases.

E) Skyline X-rays of the patella – Incorrect. A skyline view of the patella may be used as an adjunct to standard weight-bearing X-rays. This view is used to look specifically at the patellofemoral joint. Signs of osteoarthritis can be demonstrated, and an assessment of the alignment between the femur and the patella made, using this view. It is requested routinely by some surgeons, but usually it is only done if the patient has a lot of pain coming from the front of the knee.

❗ KEY POINT

There are three compartments of the knee joint – medial femorotibial, lateral femorotibial and patellofemoral compartments. The medial compartment is most frequently affected by the degenerative changes of osteoarthritis and can be adequately assessed on the AP view. This can result in a varus deformity of the knee (the distal part of the leg is angulated medially in relation to the knee). The lateral compartment is also clearly visible on the AP view of the knee. The patellofemoral compartment can be seen on the lateral view; however, the skyline view provides a better assessment of this compartment.

4. Which of these is/are features of osteoarthritis on X-ray?

The correct answers are **A) Osteophytes, B) Subchondral sclerosis, D) Loss of joint space and E) Subchondral cysts**.

The X-ray findings of arthritis is a very common exam question and cannot be emphasised enough! You will be expected to know how to differentiate between osteoarthritis and rheumatoid arthritis on X-ray, but also spend some time looking at the findings for psoriatic arthritis and gout.

A) Osteophytes – Correct. Osteophytes are a defining feature of osteoarthritis. You will not find osteophytes in other arthropathies. They are small abnormal bony growths best seen at the margin of the joint.

B) Subchondral sclerosis – Correct. Subchondral sclerosis is a common feature of early osteoarthritis. The subchondral bone is the bone next to the articular cartilage, and will appear whiter on X-ray if sclerosed.

C) Periarticular erosions – Incorrect. Periarticular erosions are a feature of erosive arthropathies such as rheumatoid and psoriatic arthritis. The inflammation from the arthritis essentially erodes the bone around the joint. There is an example of erosive arthropathy in the bonus chapter (p. 667).

D) Loss of joint space – Correct. Loss of joint space is probably the commonest but least specific finding in osteoarthritis. It is commonly found in other arthropathies.

E) Subchondral cysts – Correct. Subchondral cysts are a feature of osteoarthritis. They are also found in rheumatoid arthritis, AVN, gout and calcium pyrophosphate dehydrate disease (CPPD – pseudogout). Subchondral cysts are cysts seen just under the cartilage of the joint and are often quite small and numerous.

Continue

Table C4.17.1   Distribution and Radiological Findings of the Most Common Forms of Arthritis

FEATURE	OSTEOARTHRITIS	RHEUMATOID ARTHRITIS	PSORIATIC ARTHRITIS	GOUT
Joints affected	Hips, knees, spine, base of thumb, DIPJ and PIPJ	Proximal joints (MCPJ, MTPJ, PIPJ)	Distal joints (DIPJ, PIPJ)	1st MTPJ, hands and feet
Symmetry of involvement	Can be single joint or asymmetric	Symmetric	Asymmetric	Asymmetric
Joint space	Reduced	Reduced	Reduced	Preserved until late
Erosions	None	Juxta-articular erosions	Juxta-articular erosions	Well-defined articular and juxta-articular erosions with sclerotic margins
Bone density	Maintained	Reduced (periarticular osteopaenia)	Maintained	Maintained
Periosteal reaction	No	No	Yes	No
Deformity	Hands: Heberden's and Bouchard's nodes. Knee: varus or valgus deformity. Hip: fixed flexion deformity	Joint subluxation	Arthritis mutilans (severely deformed hands) in severe cases	Soft tissue swelling, joint effusions
Extraarticular findings	None	Rheumatoid nodules	Psoriasis, nail pitting	Tophi (classically the ear and olecranon bursa) are uncommon but pathognomonic

DIPJ, Distal interphalangeal joint; *MCPJ*, metacarpophalangeal joint; *MTPJ*, metatarsophalangeal joint; *PIPJ*, proximal interphalangeal joint.

❗ KEY POINT

The four features of osteoarthritis on X-ray are:
- Loss of joint space
- Osteophytes
- Subchondral sclerosis
- Subchondral cysts

Osteoarthritis typically affects the weight-bearing joints such as the knee, hip and ankle. The 1st carpometacarapal joint and DIPJ can also be affected.

Table C4.17.1 highlights the X-ray differences between osteoarthritis, rheumatoid arthritis, psoriatic arthritis and gout.

5. Which is the best operation for a patient with severe osteoarthritis in all compartments of the knee?
The correct answer is **A) Total knee replacement**.
A) Total knee replacement – Correct. Total knee replacement is the treatment of choice for severe osteoarthritis of the knee affecting all three compartments of the knee (medial femorotibial, lateral femorotibial and patellofemoral). It is important to council the patient on the risks of infection, stiffness, residual pain and the joint becoming loose or wearing out (loosening and wear). Overall, complications occur in up to 10% of patients. In addition, because of the risk of wear/loosening it is often best to delay the time to total knee replacement for as long as possible. Some hospitals will not offer total knee replacements for patients less than 65 years of age.
B) Unicompartmental knee replacement – Incorrect. Unicompartmental knee replacement is a useful operation for treating osteoarthritis of the knee specific to one compartment. The unaffected side of the knee is preserved. There is the potential for this unaffected side to develop osteoarthritis but this can be treated with a subsequent total knee replacement. The most common site for a unicompartmental knee replacement is the medial femorotibial joint.
C) Patellofemoral joint replacement – Incorrect. Patellofemoral joint replacement is a useful but contentious operation for treating osteoarthritis isolated to the patellofemoral joint. Resurfacing of the patella is also sometimes performed as part of a total knee replacement.

D) Tibial osteotomy – Incorrect. An osteotomy is where the bone is broken and the shape/alignment of the bone is changed. If one compartment of the knee is affected alone by osteoarthritis, an osteotomy can change how the mechanical forces are transmitted through the knee, reducing the strain on the affected compartment. This operation can be used to delay the need for a total knee replacement and is often used on younger patients. However, it does not work if the osteoarthritis is throughout the knee (rather than just one compartment).

E) Arthroscopic washout – Incorrect. Traditionally, arthroscopic washouts of the knee were performed to delay the need for surgery. However, this is not standard practice currently as patients do not get lasting pain relief. Arthroscopy can be used to treat many disorders of the knee including anterior cruciate ligament ruptures and meniscal tears but cannot treat advanced arthritis.

 IMPORTANT LEARNING POINTS

- Osteoarthritis of the knee is common.
- A thorough history and examination are more important than the X-ray findings.
- The X-ray changes are the same for osteoarthritis as any other joint and consist of loss of joint space, osteophyte formation, subchondral sclerosis and cysts.
- The routine X-rays performed for assessment are weight-bearing AP and lateral views.
- The treatment pathway for osteoarthritis of the knee should be as follows:
  - Simple analgesia, exercise, weight loss, physiotherapy and braces.
  - Joint injections with steroids.
  - Consider osteotomy if only one compartment of the knee is affected in young patients or if the arthritis is not yet bone on bone.
  - If symptoms persist and are severe, then proceed to total knee replacement (or unicompartmental knee replacement if only one compartment is affected).

CASE **4.18**

A 75-year-old woman is injured falling down the stairs. She noticed bleeding at the time of injury from her leg and is in severe pain. These are her X-rays.

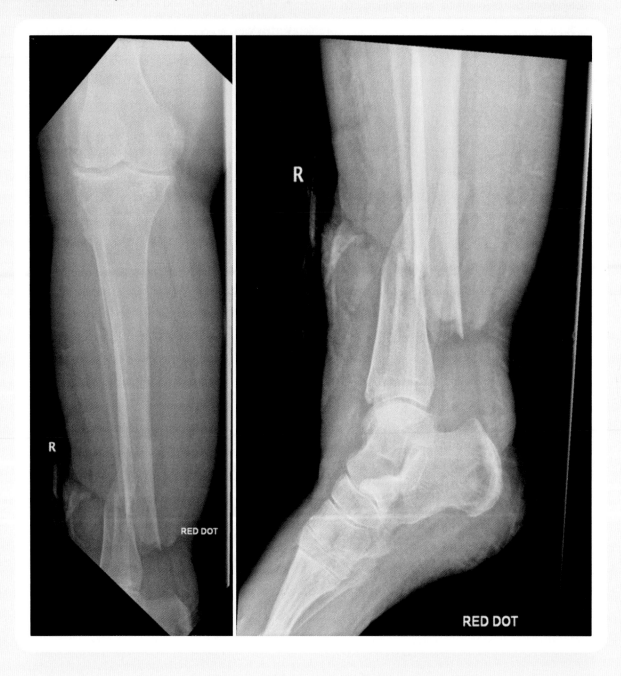

ANNOTATED X-RAY

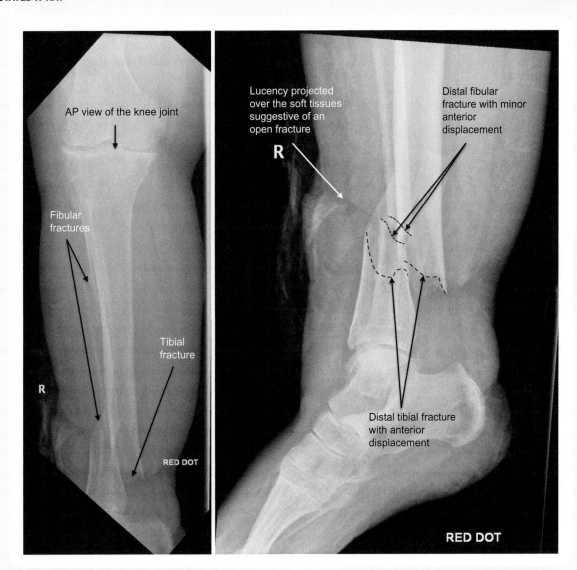

AP view of the knee joint

Fibular
fractures

Tibial
fracture

R

RED DOT

Lucency projected
over the soft tissues
suggestive of an
open fracture

R

Distal fibular
fracture with minor
anterior
displacement

Distal tibial fracture
with anterior
displacement

RED DOT

PRESENT YOUR FINDINGS

- These are AP X-rays of the right tibia and fibula of a skeletally mature patient.
- There are no patient identifiers on the X-rays. I would like to check the patient details and the time and date the examination was performed.
- The X-rays demonstrate the main abnormality but the X-ray on the right does not include the very proximal part of the tibia and the X-ray on the left does not include the distal tibia. Therefore, these X-rays are inadequate and repeat views including AP and lateral of the ankle joint and proximal tibia/knee joint are required.
- There is a displaced spiral shaft fracture of the distal third of the tibia with shortening, lateral displacement and external rotation of the distal fragment.
- There are two fractures of the fibular shaft, with shortening, lateral displacement and medial angulation at the proximal fracture site and lateral displacement,

angulation and external rotation at the distal fracture site.
- The ankle joint and proximal tibiofibular joint appear intact; however, I would like to see dedicated views of these joints.
- There is associated soft tissue swelling.
- There is change in the soft tissue density around the fracture site suggestive of an open fracture.
- The bones appear osteopaenic but there are no focal lytic or sclerotic areas to suggest an underlying pathological process.

IN SUMMARY – These X-rays show displaced tibial and fibular shaft fractures. The overlying soft tissues appear disrupted suggesting an open fracture may be present. I would like to review dedicated X-rays of the ankle and proximal tibiofibular joints, including a lateral film, to complete my radiological assessment.

Continue

CASE **4.18**   *Contd.*

QUESTIONS

1. Which of these is/are important when assessing this fracture?
   A) History
   B) Examination
   C) Assessment of the neurovascular status
   D) Complete X-rays
   E) Assessment of gait

2. What is the initial management of this fracture?
   A) Straight to theatre
   B) Wash out the wound, photograph it and dress it appropriately. IV antibiotics. Elevation and splinting of fracture. Theatre within 6 hours or first on next trauma list
   C) Wound washout out and closure in A&E. Patient can go home for discussion at trauma meeting
   D) Plaster below knee and discharge
   E) Admit for elevation and observation

3. What is the most appropriate definitive management option for this fracture?
   A) Nonoperative – above knee plaster
   B) Operative – intramedullary nail
   C) Operative – plate fixation
   D) Operative – intramedullary nail and washout debridement of the wound
   E) Operative – external fixation

4. The patient is day 1 postop and is having a lot of pain in the leg. What concerning diagnosis must be excluded?
   A) Pulmonary embolism
   B) Fat embolism
   C) Compartment syndrome
   D) Chest Infection
   E) Postoperative delirium

5. Which classification system is specifically used for open fractures?
   A) Gustilo classification
   B) Tscherne classification
   C) Gartland classification
   D) Schatzker classification
   E) Lauge-Hansen classification

ANSWERS TO QUESTIONS

1. Which of these is important when assessing this fracture?

   The correct answers are **A) History, B) Examination, C) Assessment of the neurovascular status and D) Complete X-rays**.

   This theme is repeated throughout this chapter, but too often the trauma patient does not get a full assessment, typically as the primary injury is usually clinically obvious. However, whilst a fracture is usually easy to spot, the management is often more complex. A thorough approach to these patients using the same format each time will ensure a careful assessment. The initial assessment of a trauma patient is centred on the ABCDE ATLS approach. This is aimed at identifying and managing life-threatening injuries first, before conducting a secondary survey to pick up other injuries.

   A) History – Correct. The history must include mechanism of injury – does it fit the injury in front of you? If the patient fell, it is important to elucidate whether it was a simple trip (mechanical fall) or whether there were preceding symptoms, such as breathlessness, chest pain or palpitations, which resulted in the fall. Such symptoms may signify serious underlying pathology which will need further assessment and management. Consider whether the patient is describing any symptoms of an impending compartment syndrome or neurovascular deficit. Ask what the patient saw as well; the leg may have been grossly deformed initially with bone protruding but this may no longer be the case. Does the patient have any other injuries? It is important to ask about allergies, past medical history and when the patient last ate – these are useful for the anaesthetist to know should the patient require surgery.

   B) Examination – Correct. Examination of a trauma patient initially consists of assessing the airway, breathing, circulation and disability, and managing these appropriately, as problems with these can be life-threatening. Once the patient is stabilised, the patient can be exposed and a secondary survey can be performed. In this case, the joint above and below should be assessed. Other coexisting injuries should be identified/excluded. For compartment syndrome, focus your examination on palpating the four compartments of the leg individually and assessing for pain on passive stretch of the ankle and toes. We will focus on this important diagnosis again in question 4.

   C) Assessment of the neurovascular status – Correct. Palpate the posterior tibial and dorsalis pedis pulses and check distal sensation. Assessing the neurovascular status should be performed on initial examination and after any manipulation/reduction is performed.

   D) Complete X-rays – Correct. The X-rays shown earlier are not sufficient for this patient. The whole tibia should be examined and so further X-rays of the knee and ankle are necessary. Also, for all limb X-rays you must have at least two views (usually AP and lateral views). For some bones/joints, such as the scaphoid or shoulder, you may need more views. It is important to assess the joint above and below any injury as there may be an associated injury, such as a fracture or dislocation.

   E) Assessment of gait – Incorrect. This patient will be in severe pain and unable to weight bear. Attempting to assess the patient's gait will cause further discomfort and displacement of the fracture.

2. What is the initial management of this fracture?

   The correct answer is **B) Wash out the wound, photograph it and dress it appropriately. IV antibiotics. Elevation and splinting of fracture. Theatre within 6 hours or first on next trauma list**.

   Having fully assessed this patient, you find that they are comfortable but there is a small wound at the fracture site making this an open fracture. There are several issues to address. These are: the management of the open fracture, controlling the fracture temporarily and then operating when it is safe and as soon as possible.

   A) Straight to theatre – Incorrect. There may be occasions where a trauma patient with this fracture needs to go straight to theatre. This is the case where there is a compartment syndrome or a neurovascular compromise. Patients with polytrauma may also need to go to theatre urgently for other conditions. In this case, this is not necessary.

   B) Wash out the wound, photograph it and dress it appropriately. IV antibiotics. Elevation and splinting of fracture. Theatre within 6 hours or first on next trauma list – Correct. To manage the open fracture, you must wash the wound thoroughly with sterile saline. The wound need not be debrided in A&E, as this can be performed in theatre. Once the wound is clean, take photos of it to stop the unnecessary repeated undressing of the wound which increases the risk of infection. Dress the wound with saline soaked gauze. The patient should have IV antibiotics as soon as possible, taking into account hospital policy, degree of wound contamination and allergies. Check the patient's tetanus status. By putting the patient in an above knee backslab and elevating the limb, you prevent further swelling which could lead to compartment syndrome. Finally, with open fractures, it is said that the patient should be operated on within 6 hours. However, this does not mean operating at 2 a.m., as operating in the middle of the night is associated with higher complications. Therefore, it may be more appropriate to wait longer than 6 hours (e.g. until the following morning) to operate.

   C) Wound washout out and closure in A&E. Patient can go home for discussion at the trauma meeting – Incorrect. Although the wound needs to be washed out, it should not be closed. This is an open fracture and the bone has come out of the skin and gone back in. This can often lead to clothing being dragged back down to the bone. If left, this is a potential source for

Continue

infection, which can cause serious complications, particularly if it occurs at a site with metalwork in situ.

D) Plaster below knee and discharge – Incorrect. This is not sufficient for open fractures and for tibial fractures in general. Some tibial fractures can be treated without surgery if there is minimal displacement or the patient is not fit for an operation, but if this is the case, the fracture will not be controlled with a plaster stopping below the knee. The plaster must include the joint above and below the injury to prevent displacement. Therefore, if a tibial fracture is to be treated nonoperatively, the patient should be in an above knee plaster cast.

E) Admit for elevation and observation – Incorrect. The patient needs elevation and observation for signs of compartment syndrome but there are other issues which need to be addressed as well, and therefore this is not the best answer.

❗ KEY POINT

Open fractures need to have the wound washed out in A&E, the fracture reduced, photos of the wound taken to prevent repeated wound exposure, dressing with a saline soaked gauze, antibiotic treatment and tetanus prophylaxis if indicated. Open reduction and internal fixation is usually required, ideally within 6 hours or first on the next trauma list.

3. What is the most appropriate definitive management option for this fracture?
   The correct answer is **D) Operative – intramedullary nail and washout debridement of the wound**.
   There are multiple surgical options available for tibial fractures. There will often be a debate over which option is best and although we have chosen the intramedullary nail, some surgeons would argue against this surgical option. The best approach to adopt when asked how to manage a fracture is to use the two categories of nonoperative and operative. Use this sieve, then consider the operative options and proceed from there.

A) Nonoperative – above knee plaster – Incorrect. Nonoperative management is only reserved for closed injuries with minimal displacement. With an operation, the patient can be free from plaster and return to walking sooner. There is therefore less chance of stiffness developing, as the joint above and below can potentially be mobilised earlier. Thus, the majority of these fractures are best treated surgically. If the nonoperative option is chosen, the patient must be followed up with weekly X-rays for the first 3 weeks to ensure the fracture does not displace.

B) Operative – intramedullary nail – Incorrect. This option is one of the most popular surgical options for closed tibial fractures; however, for an open fracture wound, washout and debridement is also necessary. A large metal rod/nail is inserted across the fracture in the medullary canal of the bone. Screws are then placed either side of the fracture percutaneously to secure the rod. There are risks to such a procedure. The most serious complication is related to the risk of infection, particularly with open fractures. Infection around surgical metalwork is usually difficult to treat with antibiotics alone and often requires the metalwork to be removed. Another potential complication is pain at the front of the knee (anterior knee pain). The nail is inserted from the top of the tibia via a small cut made at the front of the knee. Pain can occur if the nail is left sticking out beyond the cortex of the bone rubbing on the surrounding tissues. However, even if the nail is then removed, the pain may persist.

C) Operative – plate fixation – Incorrect. A plate fixation may be appropriate and is a more commonly used option in children (an intramedullary nail cannot be used in skeletally immature patients as it would disrupt the proximal tibial growth plate). As the tibia is quite superficial the plate tends to be easily palpable and sometimes requires removal. Plate fixation is generally avoided in adults and in open fractures as an intramedullary nail provides a better fixation. Fractures near the ankle or knee joint cannot be treated with a nail and a plate is a better option in these circumstances.

D) Operative – intramedullary nail and washout debridement of the wound – Correct. This is the best surgical option for this patient. It addresses the open fracture and also gives a stable fixation which can allow early mobilisation of the knee and ankle. Depending on the surgeon and the fracture, patients are often allowed to weight bear relatively early in the recovery period.

E) Operative – external fixation – Incorrect. An external fixator involves pins passing percutaneously into the bone on either side of the fracture. If there is a larger open wound or loss of skin and bone with gross contamination, then the risks of internal fixation (a plate or nail) including infection are too high. In such cases, an external fixator can be used to stabilise the fracture temporarily or for the duration of fracture healing. However, external fixation still carries an infection risk from the percutaneous pins and is only used in severe injuries.

❗ KEY POINT

Giving a structured answer will improve exam marks. When asked how to manage an orthopaedic condition, think of the initial assessment and management (e.g. ABCDE, assessing distal neurovascular status, specific management for open fractures). Then consider the definitive treatment (including both operative and nonoperative interventions). By following this structure, you are more likely to score well, even if you do not get the answer totally correct!

4. The patient is day 1 postop and is having a lot of pain in the leg. What concerning diagnosis must be excluded?
   The correct answer is **C) Compartment syndrome**.

Compartment syndrome is a very important diagnosis that all students and junior doctors should fully understand. Muscles and the neurovascular structures of the lower limb are contained in tight osseofascial compartments which do not permit much stretching. A small amount of swelling or bleeding in these compartments may therefore cause some pain. Further swelling may cause the pressure in the compartment to rise above venous blood pressure, resulting in venous congestion and ultimately ischaemia of the nerves and muscles. The four compartments in the lower limb are: anterior, lateral, deep posterior and superficial posterior. The classic symptoms of ischaemia are the six P's (Pain, Pallor, Pulselessness, Paralysis, Paraesthesia and Perishing cold). However, the only P of importance in compartment syndrome is pain as the other P's occur relatively late. Once there is no pulse, it is too late and the limb is lost. Patients commonly find that pain is exacerbated by testing the muscles which run in the affected compartment.

A) Pulmonary embolism – Incorrect. Although this patient is at risk of a deep vein thrombosis and pulmonary embolism, this is unlikely to occur 1 day postop. All patients who have lower limb surgery should be assessed for the risk of deep vein thrombosis and prescribed appropriate thromboprophylaxis if necessary.

B) Fat embolism – Incorrect. The fat embolism syndrome is less common and would present with respiratory distress rather than pain. Intramedullary fat can be forced into the blood stream by the fracture and surgical fixation. This can embolise to the lungs in a similar fashion to a pulmonary embolism but there is also a significant inflammatory reaction which can trigger an acute respiratory distress syndrome. This condition can be fatal and any patient with a long bone fracture with respiratory symptoms should be monitored closely.

C) Compartment syndrome – Correct. Confirming the diagnosis is usually through clinical judgement with the signs described earlier. However, if in doubt, you can check compartment pressures by placing a pressure transducer attached to a monitor into each of the leg compartments and monitoring the differential pressure. A differential pressure (the difference between diastolic pressure and compartment pressure) of <30 mmHg is an indicator of developing compartment syndrome and immediate treatment is required.

Initial management includes releasing the plaster cast, even if it is a back slab. This helps to reduce the external pressure placed on the leg and may be all that is required. If the pain is not settling or there is a low differential pressure, then urgent compartment decompression using a fasciotomy is required. This is a two-incision, four-compartment fasciotomy (i.e. two incisions are made to access all four compartments). Often as the incision is made, the muscles will bulge out, confirming the diagnosis.

D) Chest infection – Incorrect. A chest infection may develop, especially in an elderly patient or a patient with a preexisting respiratory condition. However, it is less likely in this patient, usually does not occur until a few days postop, and would not present with leg pain.

E) Postoperative delirium – Incorrect. This is common, particularly in the elderly and those with sensory impairment and/or dementia. However, it is unlikely to present with leg pain. Precipitating factors include infection, metabolic abnormalities, medication such as opioid analgesics and alcohol withdrawal. Additionally, pain may precipitate delirium. Management involves identifying and managing reversible causes and reorientating the patient.

---

❶ KEY POINT

Compartment syndrome is an important diagnosis not to miss. Do not be reassured by the presence of a pulse, and if worried, seek senior advice immediately.

---

5. Which classification system is specifically used for open fractures?
    The correct answer is **A) Gustilo classification**.
    The Gustilo classification is an important classification system for open fractures. It is divided into 1, 2 and 3:
    *   Type 1 – is the least serious, with a wound <1 cm in length and no vascular compromise.
    *   Type 2 – the wound is greater than 1 cm but is not a high-energy injury and can be closed.
    *   Type 3 – fractures are the most serious and are subdivided into A, B and C:
        *   3 A fractures – there is a large wound from a significant trauma but it can be closed. This group also includes fractures where there has been particularly bad contamination from either farmyard injuries or exposure to sewage or seawater.
        *   3 B fractures – they are large, involve high energy and require plastic surgery for wound closure.
        *   3 C fractures – they are associated with a vascular injury regardless of the size of the wound.

    A) Gustilo classification – Correct. Using the classification system described earlier we can say that the fracture in this case is a Gustilo 1 open fracture.

    B) Tscherne classification – Incorrect. The Tscherne classification is also a useful classification system but focuses on the degree of soft tissue injury associated with a fracture. This runs from 0 to 3 with 3 being the most severe. This group includes patients with a compartment syndrome. A fracture is not just an isolated injury to bone, but also affects the surrounding tissues. It is useful to use the Tscherne classification to decide the degree of soft tissue injury associated with an open fracture, but it can also be used for closed fractures.

    C) Gartland classification – Incorrect. The Gartland classification is used for supracondylar fractures of the elbow.

    D) Schatzker classification – Incorrect. The Schatzker classification is used for fractures of the tibial

Continue

CASE 4.18 *Contd.*

plateau. It goes from 1 to 6 with increasing severity. Each pattern needs a slightly different surgical approach.

E) Lauge-Hansen classification – Incorrect. The Lauge-Hansen classification is an interesting classification system for ankle fractures. It is quite complex but is very useful for considering the sequence of how an ankle breaks. By understanding this classification system, it is possible to work out which ankle fractures are stable or unstable and therefore which require surgical intervention.

 IMPORTANT LEARNING POINTS

- The initial management of open fractures is the same regardless of the bones involved. It includes starting with ABCs, irrigating the wound, covering it with a sterile dressing, reducing the fracture, administering IV antibiotics and tetanus prophylaxis if required.
- Operative management of tibial shaft fractures can involve internal fixation (intramedullary nail or plate and screws) or external fixation.
- Compartment syndrome is a serious complication of fractures, particularly tibial fractures. It is diagnosed clinically by pain or with the use of compartment pressure monitors. It can occur pre- and postoperatively. The definitive management involves decompressive fasciotomies.
- The Gustilo classification is useful for assessing open fractures.

CASE **4.19**

A 5-year-old girl presents to the ED with a 48-hour history of a painful swollen right shin and ankle. She is unable to weight bear, has a limited range of movement and pyrexia. There has been no trauma. Her X-ray is shown here.

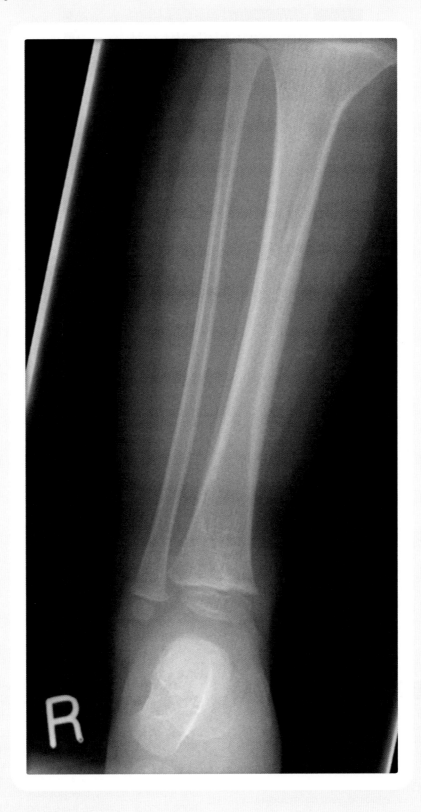

Continue

CASE **4.19**   *Contd.*

ANNOTATED X-RAY

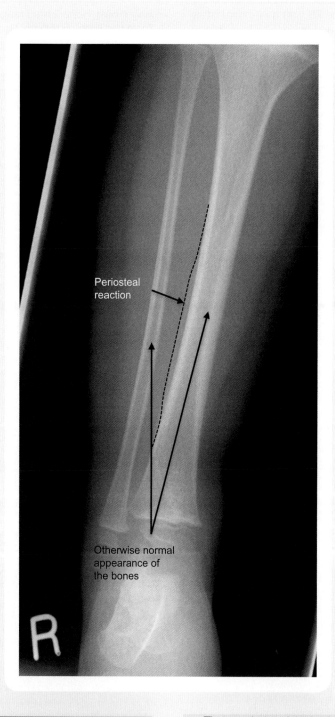

Periosteal reaction

Otherwise normal appearance of the bones

R

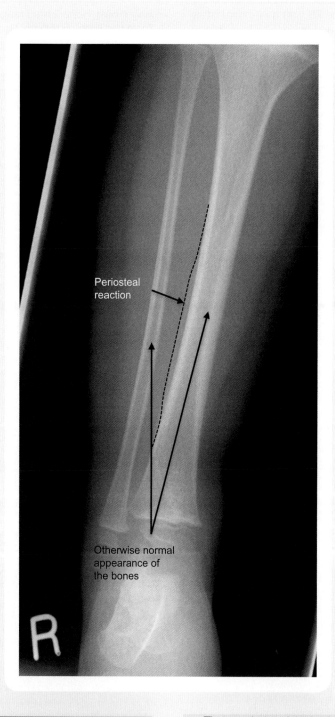

🔍 PRESENT YOUR FINDINGS

- This is an AP X-ray of the right tibia and fibula of a skeletally immature patient.
- It has been anonymised and the timing of the examination is not available. I would like to confirm the patient's details and timing of the examination before I make any further assessment.
- The X-ray is adequately exposed, with no important areas cut off.
- There is evidence of periosteal reaction along the lateral border of the tibia. No fracture is visible and the bone texture appears normal with no areas of lucency or sclerosis.

- The remainder of the bones appear normal.
- There is no soft tissue abnormality.

IN SUMMARY – This X-ray shows evidence of a periosteal reaction. The differential diagnosis includes early osteomyelitis, especially given the patient's temperature and lack of any recent trauma. Other possible causes are a fracture or bone tumour; however, there is no history of trauma and no abnormality of the bone texture. I would like to review the lateral X-ray, examine the patient and perform routine blood tests, including inflammatory markers.

QUESTIONS

1. What other clinical findings is/are important to identify?
   A) Temperature of the joint
   B) Surrounding cellulitis
   C) History of trauma
   D) History of fever
   E) History of malignancy

2. Which organism is most likely to cause osteomyelitis?
   A) *Staphylococcus aureus*
   B) *Streptococcus pneumoniae*
   C) *Neisseria gonorrhoeae*
   D) *Escherichia coli*
   E) *Haemophilus influenzae*

3. Which imaging modality is most useful in identifying early osteomyelitis?
   A) X-ray
   B) Bone scan
   C) MRI
   D) PET scan
   E) Ultrasound

4. Which of these is/are important in the management of acute osteomyelitis?
   A) Infliximab
   B) Splinting the affected limb
   C) Surgical drainage
   D) Analgesia
   E) Antibiotics

5. Which of these is/are useful when differentiating between irritable hip and septic arthritis?
   A) History of trauma
   B) Raised urea
   C) Weight-bearing status
   D) ESR and CRP
   E) Evidence of an effusion on X-ray

Continue

CASE 4.19 *Contd.*

ANSWERS TO QUESTIONS

1. What other clinical findings is/are important to identify?
   The correct answers are **A) Temperature of the joint, B) Surrounding cellulitis, C) History of trauma, D) History of fever and E) History of malignancy**.
   It is important that all children presenting with a painful joint or limb are fully assessed with a complete history and examination. The history should be comprehensive and the examination should include an examination of the joint above and below. X-rays cannot replace a good clinical assessment.

   A) Temperature of the joint – Correct. It is important to feel the temperature of the joint. A warm joint is suggestive of an inflammatory process, such as osteomyelitis or septic arthritis. Depending on the joint/limb it may be possible to also examine for an effusion at the same time.

   B) Surrounding cellulitis – Correct. Cellulitis surrounding a joint can cause significant pain when moving the joint and is an important differential in a patient presenting with a painful joint. It is important to consider osteomyelitis and septic arthritis in patients with surrounding cellulitis. These entities are serious conditions which need early and appropriate management. However, they are relatively rare and most often overlying erythema and warmth are due to uncomplicated cellulitis rather than a deeper infection of the bone or joint.

   C) History of trauma – Correct. Injuries to a bone or joint can present with a warm swollen part of the body. Additionally, a healing fracture will often result in a periosteal reaction. Minor trauma can also be the trigger for an osteomyelitis or septic arthritis and sometimes a retained foreign body following trauma may cause an infection.

   D) History of fever – Correct. Children with osteomyelitis or septic arthritis can present with systemic signs of infection. It is important to check whether the patient has a temperature and record the other observations, such as pulse rate, blood pressure and oxygen saturations.

   E) History of malignancy – Correct. Tumours are rare in children but bony involvement can present with a painful limb and result in a periosteal reaction. The commonest primary paediatric bone tumours include Ewing's sarcoma and osteosarcoma. Such tumours can present with mildly raised inflammatory markers, thus mimicking osteomyelitis. Lymphoma, leukaemia and neuroblastoma are the most common secondary bone tumours in children.

❗ KEY POINTS

1. Septic arthritis and osteomyelitis are potential emergency diagnoses which need to be identified early and managed appropriately. Rapidly assess the patient as discussed above but do not delay calling your senior.
2. Sepsis can occur when there is systemic spread of infection. It is a term which is often used loosely in clinical practice, although it has a strict definition. It is defined as the presence of two or more of the following: (1) pulse >90 bpm, (2) respiratory rate >20 or $PaCO_2$ <4.3 kPa, (3) white cell count >12 × 10^9/L or <4 × 10^9/L and d) temperature >38°C or <36°C, with confirmed or suspected infection. Patients who are septic have an increased morbidity and mortality, and require closer monitoring and often cardiovascular system support.
3. The likely location of osteomyelitis within a bone varies by age. In children, the metaphysis of tubular bones with rapid growth, such as the tibia and femur, are most likely to be involved. In adults, the flat bones, such as vertebral bodies, feet (in diabetics) and any bone with surgical metalwork in are most frequently involved.

---

2. Which organism is most likely to cause osteomyelitis?
   The correct answer is **A) S. aureus**.
   Osteomyelitis can be acute or chronic. Acute osteomyelitis occurs almost exclusively in children. It is important to know which organisms are commonly implicated as this will guide appropriate antibiotic therapy.

   A) *S. aureus* – Correct. *S. aureus* is the most common organism to cause osteomyelitis, regardless of age group or presentation. It is a gram-positive organism and accounts for 80% to 90% of cases of osteomyelitis.

   B) *S. pneumoniae* – Incorrect. *S. pneumoniae* is a gram-positive organism. Although it is most commonly associated with causing pneumonia, it can cause osteomyelitis.

   C) *N. gonorrhoeae* – Incorrect. *N. gonorrhoeae* is a gram-negative organism which is not commonly associated with osteomyelitis. However, it is the commonest cause of septic arthritis in sexually active adults.

   D) *E. coli* – Incorrect. *E. coli* is a gram-negative anaerobic organism which is found in the gastrointestinal tract. It is commonly associated with urinary tract infections but not with osteomyelitis.

   E) *H. influenzae* – Incorrect. *H. influenzae* is a gram-negative bacillus which is most often associated with epiglottitis. It is a known causative organism of osteomyelitis in children, although it is not the most common cause. Vaccination against *H. influenzae* B has reduced infection from this subgroup.

❗ KEY POINTS

1. Any patient presenting with a possible septic arthritis or osteomyelitis needs to have blood cultures sent prior to starting antibiotics. It is also important to contact your senior as they may want to aspirate a joint or obtain a biopsy before antibiotics are started.
2. No organism is identified in 50% of cases.
3. The choice of antibiotics is guided by the likely organism, local sensitivities and hospital policy.

---

3. Which imaging modality is most useful in identifying early osteomyelitis?
   The correct answer is **C) MRI**.
   Making the diagnosis of acute osteomyelitis in a child can be difficult. It can take up to 2 weeks for an X-ray of the affected bone to demonstrate any changes. Any early changes may be very subtle and can be easily missed.

If the suspicion is there, then further imaging is advised. There are different imaging modalities which have their uses. CT is superior to X-rays and MRI for assessing bony changes overall, such as the formation of a sequestrum or involucrum. However, MRI is the more sensitive and specific than CT at identifying the subtle early changes of osteomyelitis.

A) X-ray – Incorrect. X-rays have very limited sensitivity for early osteomyelitis. Often the X-rays are initially normal, although there may be a visible periosteal reaction. This correlates to a collection of pus under the periosteum which is very painful. Later changes include bone destruction and formation of a sequestrum or involucrum.

B) Bone scan – Incorrect. Bone scans detect areas of increased osteoblastic activity, such as areas of infection. However, fractures, neoplastic processes and other conditions, such as Paget's disease, cause increased osteoblastic activity. Therefore, whilst bone scans are sensitive for early osteomyelitis, their findings are not specific.

C) MRI – Correct. MRI is the most sensitive and specific imaging modality for osteomyelitis. It is noninvasive and does not use ionising radiation (unlike X-rays, CT and bone scans). Changes due to osteomyelitis include bone marrow oedema with enhancement following administration of contrast (gadolinium). MRI is also useful for assessing the surrounding soft tissues around bones and adjacent joints.

D) PET scan – Incorrect. PET scanning is an imaging modality which uses radionuclides to identify areas of increased metabolism. It is a specialist investigation with limited indications. It is most commonly used in the investigation of specific types of cancer. It is not used in the assessment of osteomyelitis.

E) Ultrasound – Incorrect. Ultrasound is a useful imaging modality which is cheap and does not involve ionising radiation. Ultrasound can demonstrate a subperiosteal collection but cannot be used to assess the bone. It is useful for assessing the soft tissues and joints, looking for abscesses, cellulitis and joint effusions.

KEY POINTS

1. There are various different imaging modalities for diagnosing osteomyelitis. Each has its strengths and weaknesses. MRI is currently the primary imaging investigation.
2. As with all infections, the only way to be 100% sure of the diagnosis is to isolate an organism. Therefore, it is often necessary to aspirate the subperiosteal collection, usually under ultrasound guidance, to obtain a sample.
3. Involucrum and sequestrum are specific terms related to osteomyelitis. An involucrum is a thick sheath of new bone which forms around and encloses a sequestrum. A sequestrum occurs when there is devascularisation (as a result of raised intraosseous pressure) and necrosis of the surrounding bone, leaving a fragment within a cavity. This can act as a source of infection and usually needs to be removed.

4. Which of these is/are important in the management of acute osteomyelitis?
The correct answers are **B) Splinting the affected limb, C) Surgical drainage, D) Analgesia and E) Antibiotics**.

A) Infliximab – Incorrect. Infliximab is a monoclonal antibody against TNF-alpha. It is used in a variety of autoimmune conditions, such as inflammatory bowel disease and psoriasis. As an immunosuppressant, an important side effect to be aware of is an increased risk of infections.

B) Splinting the affected limb – Correct. Splinting the affected limb is an important part of management of any orthopaedic problem. It can provide pain relief as well as preventing other complications such as joint contractures.

C) Surgical drainage – Correct. If treated early, then antibiotics may be sufficient to manage the infection but if a large periosteal collection develops this will need to be drained. If left untreated, the collection under the periosteum can increase the pressure and cause periosteal stripping. This devitalises the bone which will lead to necrosis. Drainage of the periosteal collection will reduce the risk of this complication.

D) Analgesia – Correct. This patient will have severe pain and will therefore require analgesia. They may also present with sepsis, so it is also worth considering the use of intravenous fluids/other supportive measures.

E) Antibiotics – Correct. Obviously antibiotic treatment is important and in osteomyelitis the patient usually requires a prolonged course. Choice of antibiotics is determined by the likely organism and local sensitivities. Early discussion with a microbiologist is important. It is important to adjust the antibiotics once the results of the cultures are available.

KEY POINT

The management of osteomyelitis in children is complex and requires specialist input from an early stage. A multidisciplinary approach will be needed including radiologists, orthopaedic surgeons, paediatricians and microbiologists. Treatment usually involves an extended course of antibiotics with the drainage of any subperiosteal abscess and potentially excision of the sequestrum or drilling of the bone cortex to allow the drainage of intraosseous pus.

5. Which of these is/are useful when differentiating between irritable hip and septic arthritis?
The correct answers are **C) Weight-bearing status and D) ESR and CRP**.
This is a very common problem encountered in orthopaedics. A child presents with a limp which is atraumatic and acute in onset. How do you differentiate between an irritable hip and septic arthritis? This is important as septic arthritis requires emergency surgical intervention with drainage of pus from the joint whilst an irritable hip requires supportive measures only. Fortunately, there are a lot of clues in the history. Irritable hip is a reactive

type of problem and the child will likely have symptoms of a viral infection elsewhere. Other people in the family may have also been unwell with a viral illness. A fever of >38°C is more suggestive of septic arthritis.

A) History of trauma – Incorrect. This is important to consider for any limping child and especially important to always exclude NAI, but trauma is not relevant in differentiating these two diagnoses.

B) Raised urea – Incorrect. Urea has little value when diagnosing these conditions but can be raised in cases where septic arthritis has led to septicaemia and should be included in the blood tests performed.

C) Weight-bearing status – Correct. This is a very important consideration. A child with septic arthritis of the hip will struggle/be unable to walk on the hip. A child with an irritable hip may have pain in the hip but will often be able to walk on it.

D) ESR and CRP – Correct. Raised inflammatory markers are useful and tend to be significantly raised in septic arthritis. It is especially important to include a full blood count, CRP and ESR.

E) Evidence of an effusion on X-ray – Incorrect. An effusion may be visible on hip X-rays with a limping child but both irritable hip and septic arthritis of the hip can produce an effusion. Furthermore, ultrasound is a more accurate modality for identifying hip joint effusions.

IMPORTANT LEARNING POINTS

- Acute osteomyelitis most commonly occurs in children, where the metaphysis is most often involved. In adults, the vertebrae are commonly affected and the feet in diabetics (the diabetic foot).
- The most common organism is *S. aureus*.
- A thorough clinical assessment and X-rays are the first steps in the management. However, if there is doubt, MRI is indicated to help confirm the diagnosis.
- Early referral for a suspected osteomyelitis is required and the patient may need surgical drainage of a subperiosteal collection.

CASE **4.20**

A 55-year-old man presents after falling over on the ice. He remembers his ankle twisting sharply, followed by pain in the ankle and an obvious deformity. He has been admitted to A&E and X-rays have been taken. As the orthopaedic SHO you are asked to assess the patient and his X-rays.

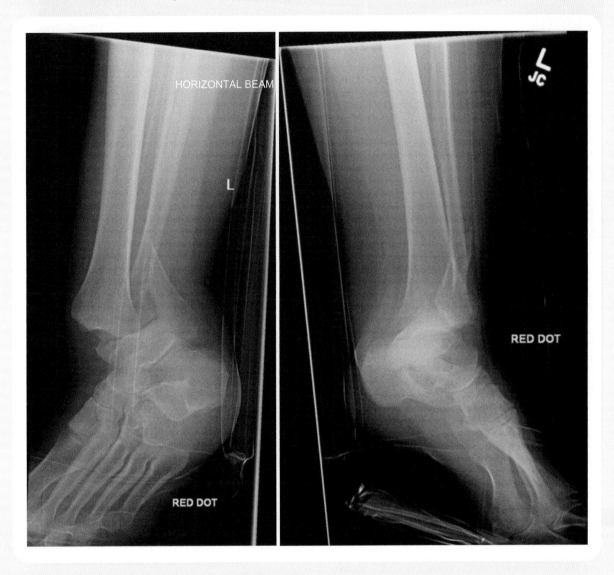

Continue

CASE **4.20** *Contd.*

ANNOTATED X-RAY

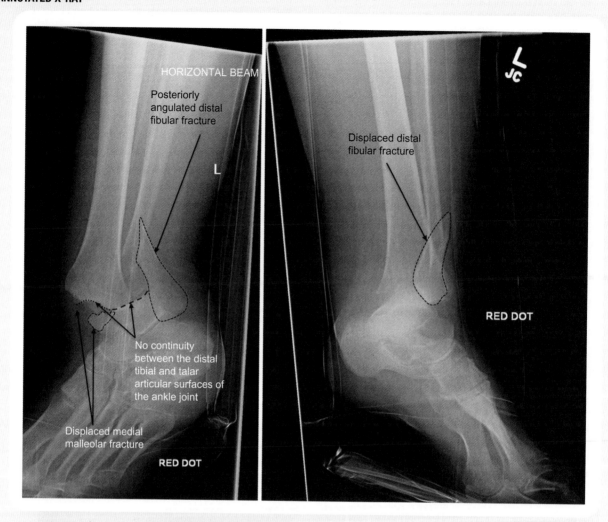

HORIZONTAL BEAM

Posteriorly
angulated distal
fibular fracture

L

No continuity
between the distal
tibial and talar
articular surfaces of
the ankle joint

Displaced medial
malleolar fracture

RED DOT

Displaced distal
fibular fracture

RED DOT

PRESENT YOUR FINDINGS

- This is an AP and lateral X-ray of the left ankle of a skeletally mature patient.
- There are no identifying marks on the X-ray but I would check this was the correct patient, and the date and time the examination was performed.
- The X-ray is adequately exposed, with no important areas cut off.
- The ankle joint is dislocated and there are multiple fractures of the ankle joint. There is an oblique fracture through the fibula and a fracture of the medial malleolus. The distal fibular fracture is at the level of the syndesmosis, and is posteriorly angulated. There is shortening of the fibula. The displacement of the medial malleolar fracture is difficult to determine on these X-rays.

- There is soft tissue swelling associated with the fracture.
- There is no evidence on the X-rays that this is an open fracture.
- The other bony structures X-rayed appear intact.
- There are no cystic changes or areas of lucency to suggest a pathological fracture.

IN SUMMARY – These X-rays show a markedly displaced bimalleolar fracture with dislocation of the ankle joint. The neurovascular integrity of the foot should be immediately assessed and an attempt to reduce the fractures and relocate the ankle joint under sedation should be made as soon as possible.

QUESTIONS

1. Which of these fits the Ottawa ankle rules for X-raying an ankle or a foot?
   A) Patient complaining of pain over heel and tenderness over the big toe
   B) Patient complaining of pain in the malleolar region with bony tenderness along the distal 6 cm of the fibula
   C) Patient complaining of pain in the mid-foot with tenderness over the navicular bone
   D) Patient complaining of pain in the foot, able to weight bear and no tenderness
   E) Patient complaining of pain in the Achilles tendon starting as a sudden onset pain whilst playing squash

2. How would you classify this fracture using the Weber classification?
   A) Weber B
   B) Weber A
   C) Weber 1
   D) Weber 3
   E) Weber C

3. What is the medial clear space?
   A) The space between the talus and the medial malleolus
   B) The space between the medial and lateral malleoli
   C) The space between the talus and the lateral malleolus
   D) The space between the fibula and tibia
   E) The space between the medial malleolus and the skin

4. Which of these defines talar shift?
   A) The medial malleolus is displaced medially in comparison to the talus
   B) The talus is displaced medially
   C) The talus is displaced laterally in relation to the tibia
   D) The fibula is displaced away from the tibia
   E) The talus is dislocated

5. Which is the best option for the acute management of this fracture?
   A) Discharge to fracture clinic
   B) Elevation with operation on next available trauma list
   C) Wait 10 days for swelling to go down, then operate
   D) Repeated manipulation to reduce the joint, check neurovascular status, elevate and operate
   E) Take immediately to theatre; this is a limb-threatening emergency

Continue

CASE 4.20   *Contd.*

ANSWERS TO QUESTIONS

1. Which of these fits the Ottawa ankle rules for X-raying an ankle or a foot?

   The correct answers are **B) Patient complaining of pain in the malleolar region with bony tenderness along the distal 6 cm of the fibula and C) Patient complaining of pain in the midfoot with tenderness over the navicular bone**.

   The Ottawa ankle rules have been developed by clinicians to aid in the management of patients attending A&E. The rules allow clinicians to decide which patients require an X-ray of the ankle or foot and which patients have less serious injuries and do not need an X-ray. However, remember that the Ottawa ankle rules are for guidance and X-rays should be considered if there is clinical suspicion of a fracture, even if the patient does not fit into the 'correct' category in the guidelines.

   An ankle X-ray is required if there is pain in the malleolar zone plus one of:
   - Bone tenderness at the posterior tip/lateral edge of lateral malleolus
   - Bone tenderness over the distal 6 cm of the posterior edge of the fibula
   - Bone tenderness at the posterior tip/lateral edge of medial malleolus
   - Bone tenderness over the distal 6 cm of the posterior edge of the tibia
   - Inability to weight bear both immediately AND in A&E.

   A foot X-ray is required if there is pain in the mid-foot plus one of:
   - Bone tenderness at the base of the 5th metatarsal
   - Bone tenderness over the navicular bone
   - Inability to weight bear both immediately AND in A&E

   A) Patient complaining of pain over heel and tenderness over the big toe – Incorrect. This does not follow the patterns described in the Ottawa rules but if the patient has fallen from a significant height, they may have a calcaneal fracture and need an X-ray and further assessment.

   B) Patient complaining of pain in the malleolar region with bony tenderness along the distal 6 cm of the fibula – Correct. This meets the criteria as outlined earlier.

   C) Patient complaining of pain in the mid-foot with tenderness over the navicular – Correct. These meet the criteria as outlined earlier.

   D) Patient complaining of pain in the foot, able to weight bear and no tenderness – Incorrect. It is unlikely this walking injured patient has a fracture but beware. Examine the patient thoroughly, including the joint above and below, and make sure there is not a missed injury.

   E) Patient complaining of pain in the Achilles starting as a sudden onset pain whilst playing squash – Incorrect. This patient likely has a significant injury not picked up on X-ray. This presentation is classical for a rupture of the Achilles tendon. Use Simmonds' squeeze test to confirm the diagnosis.

This involves squeezing the calf whilst the patient lies face down with feet hanging off the edge of the bed. In a positive test (implying likely rupture of the Achilles tendon), there is no plantar flexion in response to calf squeezing. The patient may benefit from an operation and therefore needs referral to orthopaedics.

> **❶ KEY POINT**
>
> Achilles tendon ruptures tend to occur in the 'weekend athlete'. Nonoperative treatment is in an equinus cast/or boot with the foot fully plantar flexed to oppose the two ends of the tendon. This inactivates the calf pump and these patients are at high risk for a deep vein thrombosis. With an operation, the risk of rerupture is slightly lower and therefore a select few are operated on.

2. How would you classify this fracture using the Weber classification?

   The correct answer is **A) Weber B**.

   The Weber classification classifies the fractures of the lateral malleolus (fibula) into A (below the level of the syndesmosis – usually stable), B (at the level of the syndesmosis – can be either stable or unstable) and C (above the level of the syndesmosis – usually unstable). It does not take into account fractures of the medial or posterior malleolus, but provides an idea of the stability of the ankle joint, which can guide management. As a rule, stable fractures can be treated without operation whereas unstable fractures require internal fixation.

   A) Weber B – Correct. Weber B fractures occur at the level of the syndesmosis. This is the name given to the ligamentous structures which surround the distal tibiofibular joint. The syndesmosis is an important stabilising structure of the ankle that holds the tibia and fibula together. Therefore, the position of the fracture in relation to it provides an idea about whether the fracture is stable or unstable. Weber B fracture can be either stable or unstable. It depends on whether the medial structures of the ankle have been injured (medial malleolus or deltoid ligament). Therefore always examine the patient to find out exactly where they are tender. Pain on both sides of the ankle may suggest an unstable ankle fracture.

   B) Weber A – Incorrect. Weber A fractures occur below the level of the syndesmosis. Generally, these are avulsion fractures and the ankle joint itself is stable. These fractures, if there is no displacement of the ankle on X-ray, can be treated conservatively with weight bearing and early mobilisation. They must be followed up, however, as there is a small chance of nonunion.

   C) Weber 1 – Incorrect. The classification is A to C not 1 to 3.

   D) Weber 3 – Incorrect. The classification is A to C not 1 to 3.

   E) Weber C – Incorrect. Weber C fractures occur above the level of the syndesmosis. These fractures are rarely stable (but sometimes are when caused by a direct blow). They are generally part of a more significant injury to the ankle and are unstable injuries. The energy that has gone through the ankle at the time of the injury will have gone through the syndesmosis causing it to rupture. Sometimes, the fracture of the fibula is very proximal to the knee and this is called a Maisonneuve fracture. If a patient presents with a dislocated ankle or an ankle joint with displacement and no fracture can be seen, it is important to check the fibula higher up the leg with examination and X-rays. This follows the important rule of examining the joint above and below!

3. What is the medial clear space?

The correct answer is **A) The space between the talus and the medial malleolus**.

This is a very useful measurement to make when assessing an X-ray of the ankle for talar shift. The medial clear space is the space between the talus and the medial malleolus when looking at the ankle mortice view (which is an AP X-ray with 15 degrees of internal rotation), though it can also be assessed on standard AP X-rays. A space greater than 4 mm suggests a talar shift.

A) The space between the talus and the medial malleolus – Correct. By looking for this each time you assess an X-ray you will identify the subtle talar shift which may otherwise have been missed. This will ensure your patients are managed properly and those that require operative intervention are identified.

B) The space between the medial and lateral malleoli – Incorrect. This is the ankle mortice. It is in here that the talus sits and this forms the ankle joint. The only movements that can occur at the ankle joint are flexion and extension.

C) The space between the talus and the lateral malleolus – Incorrect. This is the lateral clear space, which is not as important when assessing ankle X-rays.

D) The space between the fibula and tibia – Incorrect. Distally, this represents the syndesmosis. If this area is widened, then there is diastasis (separation of the syndesmosis), which may need operative intervention.

E) The space between the medial malleolus and the skin – Incorrect. This is not a radiological measurement. This distance, however, is very small in some people, as the bone is very superficial. Swelling will be easy to identify if visible at this point.

4. Which of these defines talar shift?

The correct answer is **C) The talus is displaced laterally in relation to the tibia**.

It is always important to describe the displacement of a fracture by describing the distal fragment. Similarly, the position of the distal part of the joint is used to describe the displacement of a joint. In the ankle, this is the talus. Talar shift describes how the talus displaces in unstable fractures of the ankle on the AP X-ray. In Weber B fractures, this can be the difference between operative and nonoperative management. Generally, talar shift needs correction by fixing the fractured fibula and restoring the bone and ankle joint to their normal anatomical positions.

A) The medial malleolus is displaced medially in comparison to the talus – Incorrect. This is often thought to be the case. If the doctor then tries to reduce the fracture by pushing on the medial side, this will displace the talus further laterally, making things worse. It is important to understand this concept not only when assessing whether the fractures needs fixing but also when reducing the fracture in plaster.

B) The talus is displaced medially – Incorrect. It is correct to consider the position of the talus in relation to the ankle joint but talar shift relates to lateral displacement of the talus.

C) The talus is displaced laterally in relation to the tibia – Correct. This is the correct definition. If present, the ankle joint is not congruent and the patient will need surgical intervention. This case is an example of an unstable Weber B fracture. The lateral malleolus is fractured and the medial ligament (deltoid ligament) is injured allowing the talus to displace laterally with the fibula. It is important to assess for medial tenderness, therefore, when assessing a Weber B fracture as this may indicate a deltoid ligament injury and an unstable fracture pattern which needs fixation or close observation.

D) The fibula is displaced away from the tibia – Incorrect. If the fibula is displaced from the tibia at the level of the ankle joint, there is diastasis (abnormal separation of parts normally joined together). This suggests the syndesmosis has been injured, as is commonly seen in Weber C fractures. These fractures can occur high up the fibula so if you see diastasis with no fracture make sure you get X-rays of the whole fibula. If there is a diastasis, this needs accurate reduction to prevent future ankle arthritis.

E) The talus is dislocated – Incorrect. A talar dislocation is a rare but very serious injury which is seen in high-energy injuries such as road traffic accidents. A talar dislocation needs careful assessment in A&E with analgesia and reduction of the dislocation as an emergency. There may also be other fractures or internal injuries which need assessment and management.

5. What is the best option below for the acute management of this fracture?

The correct answer is **D) Manipulation to reduce the joint, check neurovascular status, elevate and operate**.

All fracture dislocations need acute management before deciding on a definitive plan. This includes analgesia, checking the neurovascular status of the limb, ensuring this is not an open fracture and reducing the dislocated joint. In the ankle, the dislocation is clinically obvious and it is often said that you should never see an X-ray of a dislocated ankle; the dislocation should be reduced before X-ray to save time and reduce the pressure on the tissues.

A) Discharge to fracture clinic – Incorrect. This would be negligent as the patient has a dislocated ankle. Without reduction, this patient will likely develop

Continue

ulceration where the soft tissues are stretched, requiring plastic surgical repair and potentially amputation.

B) Elevation with operation on next available trauma list – Incorrect. Although this patient will need an operation for this fracture and elevation will prevent swelling of the soft tissues in the interim, this patient first needs to have the fracture dislocation reduced and the neurovascular status checked. Without careful elevation, the soft tissues will remain swollen and blisters will develop. This increases the risks of wound problems postoperatively.

C) Wait 10 days for swelling to go down then operate – Incorrect. Operating on a very swollen ankle can be troublesome. If the soft tissues are very swollen and fragile, then there is the possibility of the wound breaking down. With the bony structures being superficial this can result in bone and surgical metalwork being exposed, which can lead to the requirement of skin flaps, removal of the metal and, in the most severe cases, amputation. It is recommended therefore to operate within 24 hours or after 10 days either before swelling has settled in or after it has gone. However, in this case, urgent manipulation is required before any surgical intervention.

D) Repeated manipulation to reduce the joint, check neurovascular status, elevate and operate – Correct. By reducing the fracture, the pressure is off the soft tissues, swelling is less and the risk of neurovascular compromise or skin breakdown is reduced. It is important to repeat X-rays following an attempted reduction to confirm an improved position and the neurovascular status must be rechecked as well. After manipulation the fracture needs to be assessed but as a general rule fracture dislocations are unstable and require fixation.

E) Take immediately to theatre; this is a limb-threatening emergency – Incorrect. Although this is unlikely to be the case here, there may be situations where it is appropriate to take this fracture straight to theatre. This includes open fractures or neurovascular compromise. In higher-energy injuries such as road traffic collisions, there may be dramatic swelling that can lead to compartment syndrome and this too is an emergency. There is no evidence of any of these indications in this case.

❶ KEY POINT

- Fracture dislocations of the ankle need immediate reduction and plaster application. Before and after this, the ankle should be assessed to make sure this is a closed injury and that the foot is distally neurovascularly intact; otherwise, emergency surgery may be required.
- Remember that this patient may have other injuries and make sure you examine for these.

IMPORTANT LEARNING POINTS

- The Ottawa ankle and foot rules provide a useful guide for clinically managing patients with ankle injuries.
- Ankle fractures can be stable or unstable.
- They can be unimalleolar, bimalleolar or trimalleolar (distal posterior aspect of the tibia is defined as the posterior malleolus).
- Fracture dislocation of the ankle requires immediate reduction to reduce the pressure on the soft tissues, or immediate surgery if neurovascular compromise, open fracture or suspected compartment syndrome.
- The Weber classification is useful in guiding decision-making.

CT Scans

5

Erin Visser and Bryan Dalton

Chapter Outline

WHAT IS CT?

A Computed Tomography Scanner (CT scanner) essentially consists of an X-ray tube which spins around the CT table (Fig. 5.1). The X-ray tube is housed in the gantry, which is the donut-shaped part of the scanner. The patient lies on the table (usually supine). The table travels through the centre of the gantry as the X-ray tube spins around the patient, taking hundreds of X-rays from different angles. The data are then processed by a computer to produce images.

The hole in the gantry is relatively large and the scan is quite fast (lasting seconds), making CT suitable for, and well tolerated by, most patients, including those who are unwell. Patients need to be able to lie flat on their back and remain still, albeit for a short period of time. Depending on the scan, they may be required to hold their breath momentarily. Contrast agents (IV, oral or rectal) may be required to improve diagnostic accuracy of the scan (this will be decided by the radiologist). Indications for contrast will be considered within the text. IV contrast can cause a 'hot flushing' sensation and a metallic taste when administered – the contrast administrators will advise the patient about this.

CT produces images with much greater contrast between structures than is usually seen with X-rays, although MRI gives more detail than CT in most cases.

THE CT IMAGE

Looking through a CT scan allows you to view **axial, coronal** and **sagittal planes** of the body (Fig. 5.2). The standard CT image is the axial (transverse) image and on this, the left side of the image corresponds to the

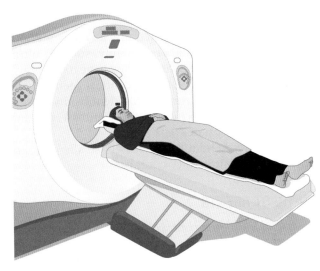

Fig. 5.1 Illustrative diagram of a CT scanner.

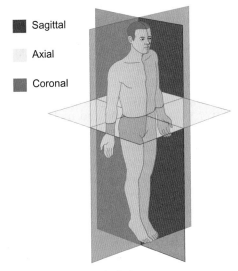

Sagittal

Axial

Coronal

Fig. 5.2 Axial, coronal and sagittal planes.

right side of the body (for example, later in Fig. 5.17, the heart, which is a left-sided structure, is on the right side of the image). This is because radiologists view images as if they are looking from the feet up (CT and MRI). Considering how we look at a frontal chest X-ray helps us understand why the CT images are displayed in this way.

When we look at a frontal chest X-ray, it is as if the patient is standing directly opposite and looking towards us (i.e. we are face to face). Therefore their left-hand side is in the right side of our field of view, and so the cardiac shadow and other left-sided structures appear on the right side of the X-ray, and vice versa. A coronal CT image is exactly the same – it is as if the patient is standing opposite and looking directly at us.

Now imagine the patient lies back onto a bed (or the CT table) so their feet are nearest us and their head is furthest away. As we look at them, their left side still remains in the right side of our field of view and vice versa. So, if we take an image in the axial (transverse) plane with the patient lying on their back and view it from their feet end, then we will see that their left-sided structures, such as the heart, will be on the right side of the image. When we look at axial CT images on a monitor, it is as if we are standing at the feet end of the patient and looking up towards their head.

The same principles apply to MRI images.

WINDOWING

Each pixel in the CT image represents the average attenuation of the tissues within it.

The attenuation of tissues is similar to the density of the tissues and can be represented as the CT number or **Hounsfield unit (HU)**. The pixel data are displayed using a grey scale, with black representing the lowest HU and white the highest.
- Water has a HU of 0.
- Tissues and substances which are less dense than water have a negative HU (fat is approximately −100 HU, lung (which is mainly composed of air) is approximately −600 HU and air is approximately −1000 HU). Tissues which are denser than water have a positive HU (bone ranges from +700 (cancellous bone) to +3000 HU (dense bone).

There are several thousand possible HU within the image, ranging from large negative values for gas to large positive values for bone and metal. The human eye, however, can only identify 30 to 50 different shades of grey. If the image displayed all the data on the grey scale (gas as black and bone as white), it would be impossible to distinguish much of the detail as the relatively small differences in attenuation between soft tissues would be represented by very similar shades of grey, which would be unperceivable to the human eye.

This problem is overcome by windowing the CT image, which emphasises different tissues by restricting the range of HU which are displayed on the greyscale. For example, the soft tissues can be shown in detail by setting the window range from −120 to 240 HU. This means any pixel with a HU <−120 is displayed as black and any with a HU of >240 is displayed as white. The visible levels of grey are used to represent the pixels which fall within the window range. In contrast, the window range of −1400 to 200 HU would be useful for assessing the lungs, and −200 to 1800 HU for bone.

There are several different automatic windowing presets, such as lung, abdomen/soft tissue, bone and brain, which are optimised to identify abnormalities in the respective organs/tissues. There is also the option to manually alter the windows. The main windows are shown in Fig. 5.3.

The left-sided lung tumour is visible on all three window settings; however, note how an enlarged mediastinal lymph node is most visible on the soft tissue windows, the emphysema is most visible on the lung windows and the extent of bone destruction is most visible on the bone windows.

USE OF IONISING RADIATION

As CTs use hundreds of X-rays, they are associated with relatively high radiation doses. Advances in technology are continually reviewing methods to reduce the associated radiation dose; however, it still remains one of the biggest disadvantages of CT scanning (Table 5.1). In particular, care must be taken with young or pregnant patients and those undergoing multiple CT scans – in these cases, alternative imaging which does not involve ionising radiation, such as MRI and ultrasound, should be considered.

ALLERGY

- There is a risk of allergic reactions to contrast agents.
- Those with other allergies/atopy and cardiac disease are the highest risk and may need premedication (antihistamine or steroids) prior to any contrast administration.
- Alternatively, they may require imaging without contrast or with another modality, such as ultrasound or MRI, particularly if they have had a previous severe allergic reaction to contrast agents.
- The radiology department will identify any patient with a previous reaction, or those at high risk, and take the appropriate steps.
- Contrary to popular belief, a shellfish allergy is not a contraindication to IV contrast.

CONTRAST AGENTS

The use of iodinated contrast material (IV, oral or rectal) further enhances the contrast differences between structures and tissues, which helps with image

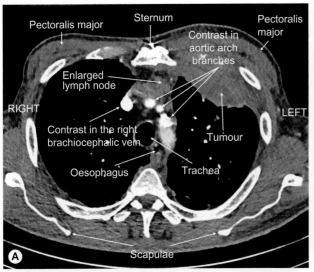

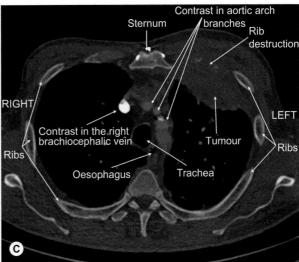

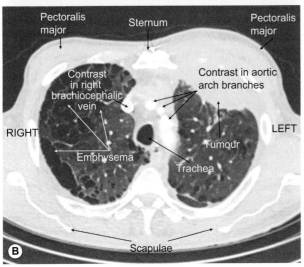

Fig. 5.3 These three images show the same axial slice through the chest but with different windows applied. **(A)** Demonstrates a soft tissue window, **(B)** demonstrates a lung window and **(C)** demonstrates a bone window.

TABLE 5.1	Approximate Effective Radiation Doses Associated with Selected X-rays and CT Scans	
EXAMINATION	**APPROXIMATE EFFECTIVE DOSE (mSv)**	**EQUIVALENT DOSE AS CHEST X-RAYS**
Chest X-ray	0.02	1
Abdominal X-ray	0.7	35
CT brain	1.5	75
CT chest	7	350
CT abdomen/pelvis	10	500

interpretation. The main issues associated with contrast agents which medical students and doctors need to be aware of revolve around the use of IV contrast. Remember: the radiology department will advise on issues relating to scanning, including contrast agents.

IV contrast agents are frequently used for imaging of the chest, abdomen or pelvis. They are therefore commonly prescribed medications and it is important to be aware of their side effects and contraindications.

CONTRAST-INDUCED NEPHROPATHY

- IV contrast has the potential to cause acute tubular necrosis, leading to contrast-induced nephropathy.
- Most episodes are self-limiting; however, patients at highest risk should be identified and managed appropriately prior to administration of IV contrast.
- Risk factors for developing contrast-induced nephropathy include acute or chronic renal failure, diabetes and myeloma.
- Patients with any of these risk factors may be given prophylactic measures, such as prehydration with IV fluids, to attempt to reduce the risk of contrast-induced nephropathy.
- Another prophylactic measure is to administer bicarbonate. Bicarbonate acts by alkalinising the renal tubular fluid which prevents free radical injury.
- The lower the renal function, the more likely contrast-induced nephropathy is to occur and the more significant its effects are likely to be. Hospitals generally use an arbitrary cut-off (e.g. **eGFR <30 mL/ minute**), below which CT scanning with IV contrast is a relative contraindication.

- In such patients, there are four options:
  1. If clinically acceptable, the contrast-enhanced scan could be postponed until the renal function has improved to an acceptable level.
  2. A noncontrast CT can be considered if it would still give enough information to be clinically beneficial. For example, a noncontrast CT of the abdomen and pelvis would be sufficient to identify a collection and any free intraperitoneal gas in a patient suspected of having a diverticulitis/abscess; however, it would not permit an accurate assessment of the solid abdominal organs and vascular tree.
  3. An alternative imaging technique, such as ultrasound or MRI, may be an option.
  4. Finally, if the earlier options are not appropriate, and the benefits of making a diagnosis using a contrast-enhanced CT outweigh the risks of contrast-induced nephropathy, then the CT can be performed, and any resultant renal impairment managed (e.g. with IV fluids or renal replacement therapy). This final option should not be taken lightly and should involve a discussion between the senior clinicians and radiology department.

METFORMIN

- Patients taking metformin for diabetes are at risk of developing a potentially lethal lactic acidosis following IV contrast, particularly if they have renal or hepatic failure.
- Patients should have their renal function checked prior to contrast administration. In the context of this, and local guidelines, metformin may be stopped pre- and postprocedure.
- If an emergency contrast-enhanced CT is required, the patient should ideally have their renal function checked first.
  - If normal, the CT can be performed and the metformin withheld for 48 hours following the scan. The patient should be well hydrated before the scan.
  - If abnormal, the metformin should be stopped for 48 hours prior to scanning (the CT scan may have to be postponed) as well as for 48 hours after the CT.
- There will be situations when the clinical condition of these patients necessitates an urgent scan before the blood results are available. Such cases must be assessed on an individual basis by the clinical and radiology teams. If the perceived benefits of a contrast-enhanced scan (e.g. identifying a surgical problem which requires an urgent operation) outweigh the risks of lactic acidosis and contrast-induced nephropathy, then the scan can be performed, and any side effects managed as they occur.

INDICATIONS

There is a large range of indications for CT scanning. Broad indications include cancer staging (CT thorax, abdomen +/− pelvis +/− neck with IV contrast), trauma (noncontrast CT brain +/− neck +/− CT thorax, abdomen and pelvis with IV contrast) and suspected intracranial pathology, such as strokes or intracranial haemorrhage.

CONTRAINDICATIONS

The main absolute contraindication to CT scanning is previous anaphylactic reaction to the iodinated contrast which is often used. In such cases, a noncontrast CT scan may be able to provide sufficient information to answer the clinical question. Alternatively, other imaging techniques may be an option. The other absolute contraindications are if the patient is unable to lie flat for the scan, or the patient is too large/heavy for the scanner (the weight limit varies from scanner to scanner but is usually over 200 kg).

In the past, CT scanning was considered to be contraindicated in an **unstable patient** due to the risk of death (CT was referred to as the 'donut of death'), and this is still advocated in ATLS guidelines. However, there is now a move towards early CT scanning in unstable patients to provide a quick and accurate diagnosis, particularly in trauma patients. Remember that such patients should still be resuscitated as much as possible without delaying the CT and require an appropriate medical/surgical/anaesthetic escort to and from the CT scanner.

Relative contraindications again revolve around the use of IV contrast, as discussed above. The other main relative contraindication is related to **radiation dose** and is particularly relevant to children, young adults, pregnant women and those undergoing multiple CTs. Again, however, a CT may be performed if the benefits of making a diagnosis outweigh the risks of exposure to ionising radiation. If not, an alternative imaging technique such as MRI or ultrasound should be considered.

BRAIN

- One of the most commonly requested CT scans.
- They are very quick to perform but sensitive to patient movement; therefore the patient must be able to lie still.
- Common indications include:
  - Acute stroke (to identify haemorrhagic and ischaemic stroke (less sensitive than MRI for ischaemic stroke) or other pathology such as a space-occupying lesion).
  - Trauma (to identify intracranial haemorrhage – extradural, subdural, subarachnoid and parenchymal haemorrhages – and fractures).

- Abnormal neurological signs/symptoms (to identify space-occupying lesions, e.g. metastases, primary tumours, abscesses).

HAEMORRHAGE

- Acute haemorrhage is hyperdense when compared to brain parenchyma (i.e. increased attenuation/bright).
- As blood ages it becomes less dense and its attenuation drops; for example, a chronic subdural haemorrhage will have a similar density/attenuation as the CSF.
- Haemorrhage can be intraaxial (i.e. within the brain parenchyma), extraaxial (i.e. within the space between the brain and the skull) or both (Table 5.2).
- Intraaxial haemorrhage (Fig. 5.4) may be the result of several different disease processes such as a haemorrhagic stroke, a bleed into an underlying lesion, such as a tumour, vascular malformation, trauma or venous sinus thrombosis. Further imaging, such as CT angiogram or venogram or MRI, may often be required to clarify its aetiology.
- Extraaxial haemorrhage includes subarachnoid, subdural and extra/epidural haemorrhages (Figs 5.5–5.7).

❶ KEY POINT

The foremost but not sole role of CT in acute stroke is to identify haemorrhage or an alternative cause for the clinical findings, such as a space-occupying lesion. It is less useful for diagnosing an acute ischaemic stroke as the CT findings of an ischaemic stroke are usually only visible at least 6 hours after the stroke started. An ischaemic stroke is usually diagnosed on clinical grounds once CT has deemed a haemorrhagic stroke or alternative causes such as space-occupying lesion less likely.

SPACE-OCCUPYING LESIONS

- Masses can arise within the brain parenchyma (Fig. 5.8) or the surrounding space between the brain and the skull.
- The most common parenchymal masses are metastases (primary tumours which commonly metastasise to the brain include lung cancer, breast cancer, genitourinary tract tumours and melanoma).
- There are a variety of primary brain tumours which are much less common than metastases. Differentiating them is difficult on CT (and beyond what is expected of medical students/junior doctors).

Table 5.2   Types of Haemorrhages on CT Imaging

TYPE OF HAEMORRHAGE	SITE OF BLEEDING	CLINICAL PRESENTATION	CAUSES	CT FEATURES
Intraaxial (Fig. 5.4)	Within the brain parenchyma	Headache, loss of consciousness, features of space-occupying lesion such as seizures/vomiting/focal neurological deficit	Haemorrhagic stroke, bleed into underlying lesion (e.g. tumour), trauma	High attenuation in the brain Parenchyma
Acute sub-arachnoid (Fig. 5.5)	Between pia mater and arachnoid mater	Sudden onset, severe (thunder-clap) headache, seizures, focal neurology, vomiting, neck stiffness (meningism)	Ruptured aneurysm (90%), trauma, vascular malformation, extension of intraparenchymal haemorrhage, idiopathic	1. High attenuation in the sub-arachnoid space (CSF spaces and cisterns around the circle of Willis/brainstem, Sylvian fissure, cortical sulci and ventricles) 2. Resultant hydrocephalus 3. CT angiogram will often demonstrate an aneurysm
Acute subdural (Fig. 5.6)	Between arachnoid mater and dura mater	Gradual onset, headache, confusion, seizures, focal neurology	Traumatic rupture of bridging veins. Commonest in neonates, infants and elderly	1. High-attenuation crescent-shaped collection over brain surface (usually cerebral hemispheres) 2. Resultant mass effect (midline shift, effacement of adjacent ventricle/CSF space, herniation)
Acute extradural (Fig. 5.7)	Between dura mater and skull	Headache, focal neurology, loss of consciousness. Initial lucent period is typical	Traumatic arterial bleeding (most commonly the middle meningeal artery in the temporal region)	1. High-attenuation biconvex collection (lens-shaped) overlying the brain 2. Frequently associated with skull fractures 3. Resultant mass effect

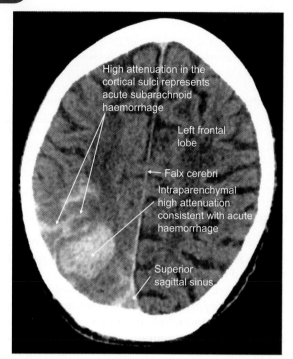

Fig. 5.4 Axial slice from a noncontrast CT brain demonstrating an intraparenchymal acute haematoma (with some acute blood within the adjacent subarachnoid space). The cause of the haemorrhage is unclear in this image – it may be due to an underlying tumour or vascular malformation; however, these can only be identified on imaging once the haematoma has resolved (usually a delayed MRI scan (waiting for at least 6 weeks) is required).

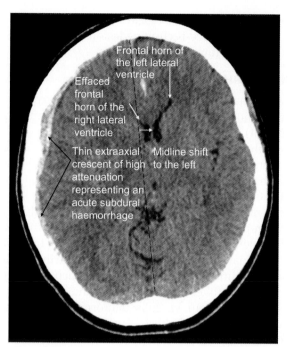

Fig. 5.6 Axial slice from a noncontrast CT brain demonstrating a thin crescent-shaped collection overlying the right cerebral hemisphere, consistent with an acute subdural haemorrhage. Despite its relatively small size, there is evidence of mass effect, with a shift of the midline to the opposite side.

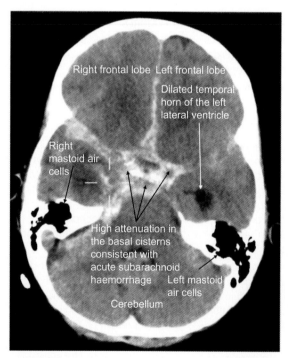

Fig. 5.5 Axial slice from a noncontrast CT brain demonstrating high attenuation in the basal cisterns and surrounding CSF spaces, consistent with an acute subarachnoid haemorrhage. The dilated temporal horn of the left lateral ventricles is just visible, in keeping with hydrocephalus.

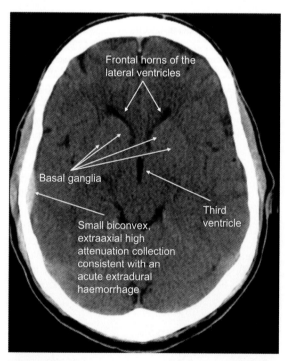

Fig. 5.7 Axial slice from a noncontrast CT brain demonstrating a small biconvex high-attenuation collection overlying the right temporal lobe, in keeping with an acute extradural haemorrhage.

- There is often associated oedema (low attenuation) in the white matter surrounding brain tumours, which can lead to mass effect.
- Contrast-enhanced CT and MRI are often helpful for further assessment.

MASS EFFECT

- Mass effect can result from space-occupying lesions (see Fig. 5.8), areas of haemorrhage, localised oedema or generalised cerebral oedema (which can occur after prolonged hypoxia).
- There may be effacement of the normal CSF spaces, such as the ventricles or sulci, midline shift to the opposite side (see Fig. 5.6) and herniation, such as cerebellar tonsillar herniation.

> ❗ KEY POINT
>
> Criteria for immediate request for CT brain following a head injury in adults: NICE guidelines 2019
> - GCS less than 13 on initial assessment in the emergency department.
> - GCS less than 15 at 2 hours after the injury on assessment in the emergency department.
> - Suspected open or depressed skull fracture.
> - Any sign of basal skull fracture (haemotympanum, 'panda' eyes, CSF leakage from the ear or nose, Battle's sign).
> - Posttraumatic seizure.
> - Focal neurological deficit.
> - More than one episode of vomiting.
> - Amnesia for events more than 30 minutes before impact.
> - In 2019, NICE updated their guidelines to indicate that adults and children who are on any anticoagulant (including warfarin) should have a CT scan within 8 hours of head injury.

HYDROCEPHALUS

- Hydrocephalus is dilatation of the ventricular system. It can be obstructive or communicating.
- **Obstructive hydrocephalus** is caused by a *blockage* to the flow of CSF between the ventricles. This is usually a mass but can occur with subarachnoid haemorrhage and meningitis. There will only be dilatation of the ventricles upstream of the blockage.
- **Communicating hydrocephalus** is the result of a problem with *reabsorption* of CSF by the arachnoid granulations, usually caused by a subarachnoid haemorrhage or meningitis. There is dilatation of the entire ventricular system.

Note: Dilatation of the temporal horn of the lateral ventricle is usually the earliest sign of hydrocephalus (see Fig. 5.5).

LOSS OF THE NORMAL GREY-WHITE MATTER DIFFERENTIATION

- The myelinated sheaths of normal white matter make it less attenuating than grey matter (cortex), and it therefore is darker in appearance. The boundary between normal grey and white matter should be visible on CT.
- If there is oedema affecting the grey and white matter, this normal boundary becomes obscured (Fig. 5.9). This is known as **loss of grey-white matter differentiation**. It can occur as an early sign of an ischaemic stroke.

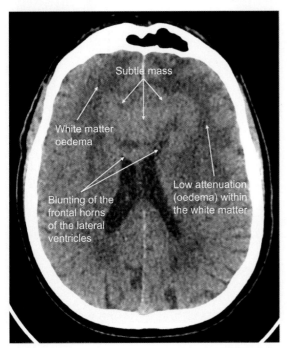

Fig. 5.8 Axial slice of a noncontrast CT brain which shows a subtle mass in bilateral frontal lobes. There is surrounding white matter oedema and blunting of the anterior horns of the lateral ventricles due to mass effect.

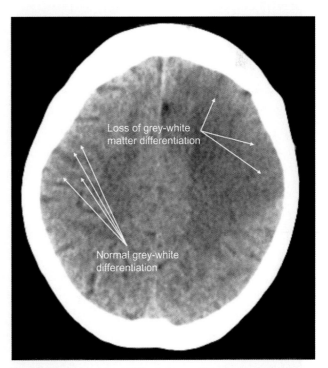

Fig. 5.9 Axial noncontrast CT brain image. This shows a subtle abnormality of an acute ischaemic stroke. The difference between the grey matter of the cortex (higher attenuation = lighter) and the white matter (lower attenuation = darker) is visible in the right cerebral hemisphere. This is not the case in the anterior and midportion of the left hemisphere. Such a finding represents loss of the grey-white matter differentiation and is caused by grey and white matter oedema. The commonest cause of this is an acute ischaemic infarct.

CONTRAST-ENHANCED CT BRAIN

- Most CT brain scans are performed without IV contrast.
- The use of IV contrast is usually decided by the radiologist.
- There are three types (phases) of contrast-enhanced CT brain scans, depending on the delay between administering the IV contrast and acquiring the CT scan.
    - **Arterial phase scan (angiogram)** (Fig. 5.10)
        - CT acquired when the majority of the IV contrast is within the arterial system.
        - Usually performed to *look for an aneurysm* in cases of subarachnoid haemorrhage.
    - **Venous phase scan (venogram)** (Fig. 5.11)
        - CT acquired when the majority of the IV contrast is within the venous system.
        - Usually performed to *look for thrombosis of the venous sinuses*, which can cause haemorrhage in unusual areas and headaches.
    - **Delayed phase** (Fig. 5.12)
        - CT acquired 5 to 10 minutes after the IV contrast is administered. By this time, the contrast is 'within' the brain parenchyma.
        - Used to identify *abnormal areas of enhancement*, such as primary and secondary tumours and abscesses.

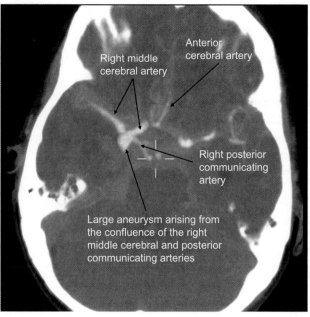

Fig. 5.10 Axial slice from a CT angiogram performed in the same patient with the acute subarachnoid haemorrhage shown in Fig. 5.5. It shows a large aneurysm arising at the right-side middle cerebral artery of the circle of Willis.

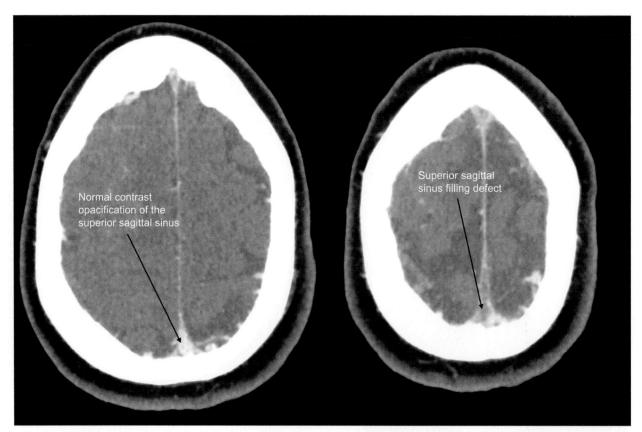

Fig. 5.11 Axial slices from a CT venogram showing abnormal areas in the superior sagittal sinus which are not opacified by contrast (filling defects), in keeping with dural venous sinus thrombosis.

CERVICAL SPINE

- Provides a very detailed assessment of the bony structures within the cervical spine (Fig. 5.13).

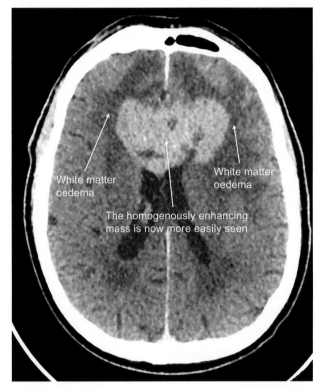

Fig. 5.12 Axial slice of a delayed phase contrast-enhanced CT. This CT is from the same patient as shown in Fig. 5.8. The extent of the tumour is much more easily assessed on the contrast-enhanced scan, and any other tumour deposits will also be more easily seen.

- The images can be reformatted, allowing review of the cervical spine in any plane.
- It is a noncontrast scan.
- Common indications include:
  - Trauma patients with inadequate X-rays (i.e. they do not cover the entire cervical spine)
  - Trauma patients requiring further assessment/imaging (e.g. if there is evidence of a fracture or ongoing clinical concern despite 'normal' X-rays)

CT IN ORTHOPAEDICS

CT can be used to investigate potential fractures at sites other than the cervical spine:

- CT is extremely useful for assessing and characterising fractures of the thoracic and/or lumbar spine. Accurate assessment is needed to determine whether a spinal fracture is potentially stable or unstable.
- CT is very helpful in the assessment of facial fractures, which can be complex and are often difficult to identify fully on facial X-rays. CT also has the advantage in this setting of identifying any associated intracranial abnormality, such as intracranial haemorrhage.
- Other examples where CT is commonly used include the further evaluation of tibial plateau fractures of the knee (Fig. 5.14) and Lisfranc fractures of the foot. Both of these types of injury require accurate assessment prior to surgical fixation; however, this is usually not possible using X-rays alone.

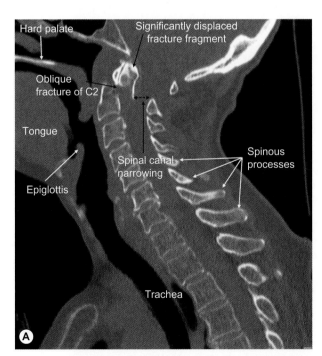

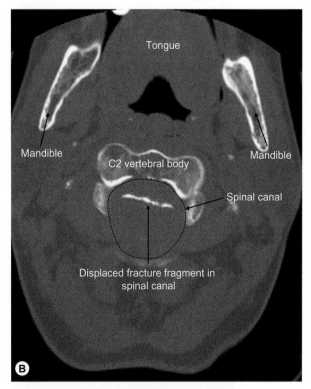

Fig. 5.13 Cervical spine CT in a trauma patient. **(A)** Sagittal image clearly showing an oblique fracture through the base of the odontoid peg *(C2)*. There is significant posterior displacement of the superior fracture fragment and resultant spinal canal narrowing. **(B)** Axial image showing the significant encroachment of the fracture fragment into the spinal canal. Note how the spinal canal and other soft tissue structures (intervertebral discs and ligaments) cannot be clearly seen.

⚠ KEY POINT

CT provides very limited assessment of the intervertebral discs, ligaments and spinal cord. Therefore a normal CT does not exclude significant injury and an MRI may be required.

- CT can be used for any bone or joint where there is ongoing clinical suspicion of a fracture despite normal

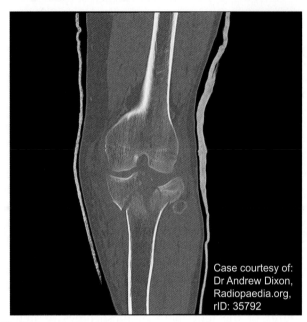

Case courtesy of:
Dr Andrew Dixon,
Radiopaedia.org,
rID: 35792

Fig. 5.14 Comminuted bicondylar intraarticular tibial plateau fracture which extends across the metadiaphysis (Schatzker VI). (Courtesy Dr Andrew Dixon, Radiopaedia.org, rID: 35792.)

X-rays. This is most commonly required for potential femoral neck fractures. It should be noted that MRI can also be used for this purpose with the added advantage of being able to demonstrate soft tissue injuries, such as muscle tears or tendinopathies, which may mimic a fracture. MRI is preferred to CT in cases of suspected scaphoid fractures with normal X-rays.

THORAX

- CT Thorax is performed with the patient holding their breath in *full inspiration* (to prevent respiratory motion artefact degrading the images of the lungs and other tissues).
- It can be performed as a noncontrast scan or with IV contrast depending on the indication.
- Common indications include:
  - Suspected pulmonary embolism (specifically a CT pulmonary angiogram)
  - Suspected malignancy (diagnosis/staging)
  - Assessment of lung parenchymal abnormalities (high-resolution CT is a type of CT that uses specific techniques to enhance image resolution which is useful in assessing pathology of lung parenchyma)
  - Trauma
  - Suspected aortic dissection

PULMONARY EMBOLISM

- A CTPA is performed. The patient is given a bolus of IV contrast and scanned when most of the contrast is within the pulmonary arterial tree (Fig. 5.15).

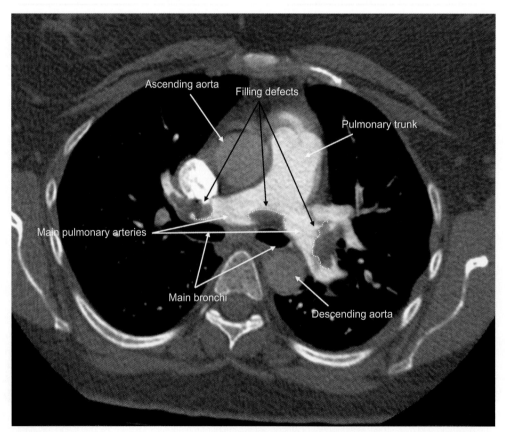

Fig. 5.15 An axial slice from a CTPA at the level of the pulmonary trunk and main pulmonary arteries. There are several filling defects in the contrast-opacified main pulmonary arteries, indicating multiple pulmonary emboli.

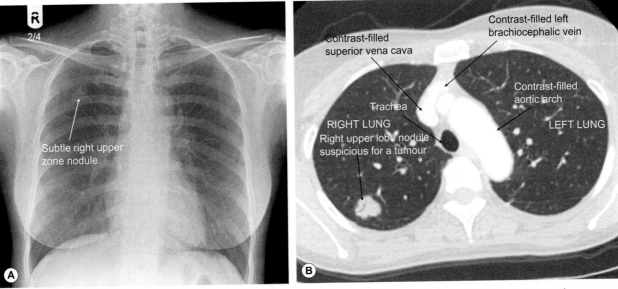

Fig. 5.16 (A) The chest X-ray shows a subtle right upper zone nodule. **(B)** Contrast-enhanced CT shows a mass of the right upper lobe.

- Pulmonary emboli appear as nonopacified regions within the contrast-filled pulmonary arteries.
- There may be evidence of right heart strain (straightening of the interventricular septum or reflux of contrast into the IVC) if there is a significant volume of embolus.

PULMONARY NODULE/MASS/LOBAR COLLAPSE

- These may have been identified on chest X-ray and may require further evaluation (Fig. 5.16).
- In addition, CT can identify any pulmonary masses which are not visible on X-ray and is used as part of the staging of many cancers.
- These scans are often performed with IV contrast.
- The size and appearance of any mass, along with other findings such as lymph node enlargement, are used to help determine whether the lesion is benign or malignant.
- Large, spiculated masses are suspicious for malignancy; however, a biopsy (CT-guided or via bronchoscopy) is required for a definitive diagnosis in most cases.

ASSESSMENT OF THE LUNG PARENCHYMA

- To further assess abnormalities of the lung parenchyma identified on X-ray, a **noncontrast HRCT** is often performed.
- Pathologies such as pulmonary fibrosis, bronchiectasis, sarcoidosis or occupational lung disease (such as silicosis, asbestos exposure, etc.) can be demonstrated.
- Differentiating these pathologies on CT can be difficult and their specific CT features are beyond the

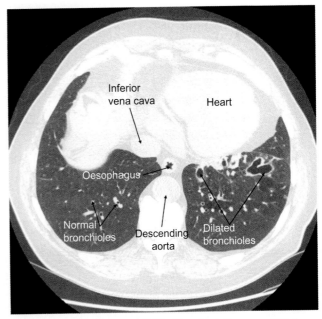

Fig. 5.17 Axial slice from an HRCT of the chest. There are dilated bronchioles in the left lower lobe (the diameter of the bronchus/bronchiole should not be greater than the adjacent pulmonary artery) indicating bronchiectasis. This has various causes and the clinical assessment will be important for narrowing the differential diagnosis.

scope of this book. One example (bronchiectasis) is shown in Fig. 5.17.

TRAUMA

- Contrast-enhanced CTs are used as part of the trauma CT to identify thoracic injuries (Fig. 5.18).
- Pneumothoraces appear as gas within the pleural spaces. Look for associated rib fractures, evidence of tension (a mediastinal shift to the opposite side) and subcutaneous emphysema.

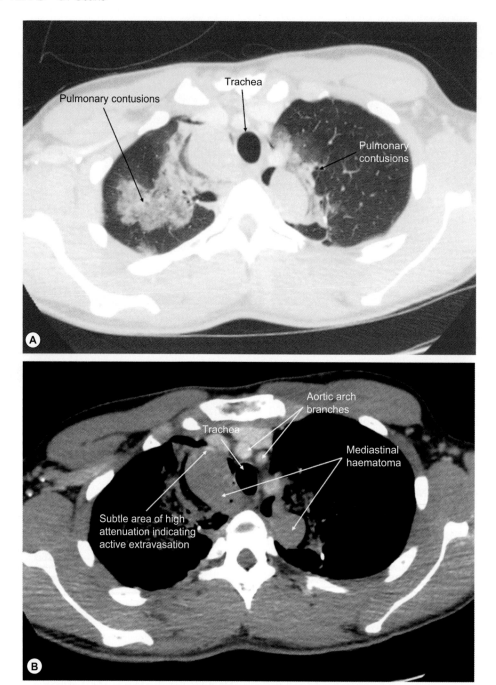

Fig. 5.18 Axial slices from a contrast-enhanced CT of the chest in a trauma patient. **(A)** Shows bilateral pulmonary contusions. **(B)** Shows bilateral superior mediastinal acute haematomas, with evidence of active extravasation into the right-sided haematoma. Other slices of the CT showed further pulmonary contusions, bilateral pneumothoraces and rib fractures.

- Lung contusions usually occur with blunt trauma. They are caused by haemorrhage within the lung parenchyma and appear as areas of consolidation within the lung. They are often multifocal.
- Mediastinal haemorrhage appears as abnormal areas of soft tissue density within the mediastinum. There may be evidence of active bleeding (high attenuation extending from a blood vessel). The haemorrhage may compress structures within the

mediastinum, such as the airway, oesophagus, vena cava or aorta.
- Fractures of the ribs, clavicles, spine and sternum are common. The bones are best assessed in all three planes.

SUSPECTED AORTIC DISSECTION

- A CT of the entire aorta is usually performed (ascending aorta, aortic arch and descending aorta

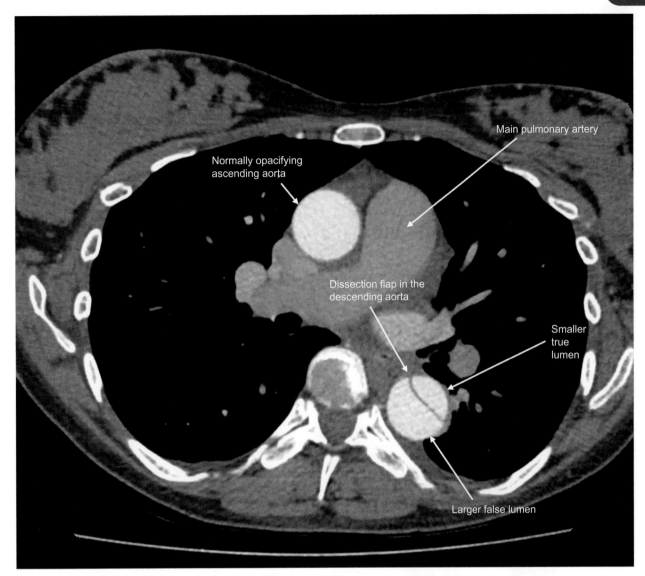

Fig. 5.19 Axial slice from an arterial phase CT of the chest. There is a dissection flap in the descending aorta. The true lumen is smaller and lies anterolaterally and the larger false lumen posteromedially. The ascending aorta appears normal.

down to its bifurcation at approximately the level of L4/L5, Fig. 5.19).

- A **dissection** is blood between the intima and media layers of the arterial wall. A dissection flap is created: this is the elevated intimal layer as a result of the blood underneath it.
- Both noncontrast and arterial phases are acquired.
- The noncontrast phase is used to look for evidence of an intramural haematoma (this is an atypical form of dissection in which there is bleeding into the aortic wall but no dissection flap).
- The arterial phase will show blood between the intimal and medial layers, plus the dissection flap.
- A dissection will result in a 'true' lumen – this is the normal lumen of the aorta – and a 'false' lumen – this is caused by the blood within the aortic

wall between the intimal and medial layers. The false lumen is larger as the blood in this lumen is under higher pressure.

- Two common classification systems are used based on the involvement of the ascending aorta. These are the Stanford and DeBakey classifications. In our following descriptions, we describe the Stanford type A and B classifications.
- A dissection which involves the ascending aorta (+/− the aortic arch and descending aorta) is classed as a **type A dissection** (Fig. 5.20) and usually requires surgical management.
- A dissection of the descending aorta (distal to the left subclavian artery) is classed as a **type B dissection** (Fig. 5.21) and is usually managed medically.

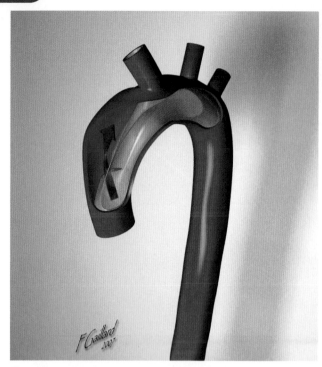

Fig. 5.20 Illustrative graphic depicting Stanford type A – proximal aortic dissection. (Courtesy Associate Professor Frank Gaillard, Radiopaedia.org, rID: 7640.)

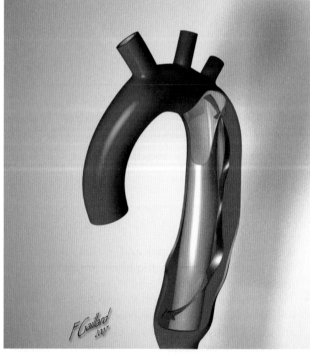

Fig. 5.21 Illustrative graphic depicting Stanford type B – distal aortic dissection. (Courtesy Associate Professor Frank Gaillard, Radiopaedia.org, rID: 7640.)

ABDOMEN AND PELVIS

- CT of the abdomen and pelvis usually requires IV contrast.
- The commonest phase of imaging is the portal venous phase (the CT is performed when the contrast is within the portal venous system), as this gives the best images of the abdominal viscera.

- Oral or rectal contrast may also be used, but this decision is usually made by the radiologist depending on the clinical scenario. In general, oral contrast is used to opacify the small bowel, helping to highlight any pathology. Rectal contrast is used to assess the integrity of surgical anastomoses in the lower GI tract and determine whether a stricture is causing complete or partial obstruction.
- Common indications include:
  - Trauma
  - Acute surgical abdomen
  - Acute gastrointestinal haemorrhage (oesophago-gastro-duodenoscopy (OGD) is the first-line investigation of most cases of acute upper GI haemorrhage)
  - Suspected malignancy (diagnosis/staging)
  - Haematuria or suspected renal stones
  - Assessment of vascular disease

TRAUMA

- Contrast-enhanced CT is part of the trauma CT (Fig. 5.22).
- A **dual phase scan** is performed where the IV contrast is given in two boluses and a single CT is performed, which has contrast in both the arterial and portal venous systems. This permits identification of sites of active bleeding as well as allowing an accurate assessment of the solid abdominal organs.
- It is used to identify injuries to the abdominal or pelvic viscera, such as liver, splenic or renal lacerations, vasculature, such as aortic dissection/transection, and lumbar spine/pelvis.
- There may be perforation of a viscus and a haemoperitoneum (relatively high-attenuation free fluid representing acute blood).
- Sites of active bleeding are indicated by extravasation of contrast, which permits surgical/interventional radiology planning.

ACUTE SURGICAL ABDOMEN/ABDOMINAL SEPSIS

- Portal venous phase CT is extremely useful for assessing these patients, although it does not replace thorough clinical assessment (Fig. 5.23).
- It is often used to make or confirm the diagnosis and if surgery is subsequently required, up-to-date imaging is useful.
- Inflammatory pathologies, such as diverticulitis and colitis, are associated with inflammatory stranding (white lines) in the surrounding fat (usually the fat is a 'clean', uniform black) and free fluid, which usually collects around the inflamed structure and in the pelvis.
- Free fluid may become 'walled-off' into a more discrete collection/abscess.
- Gas outside the GI tract is always abnormal and is commonly a result of a perforated viscus. The location of the gas and evidence of localised inflammation can often indicate the likely site of a perforation. Recent surgery is another common cause of free intraabdominal gas.

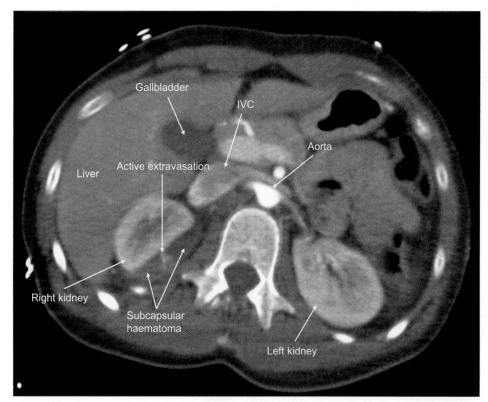

Fig. 5.22 Axial slice from a trauma CT abdomen and pelvis with IV contrast (split bolus resulting in both arterial and portal venous enhancement). Notice how there is contrast within the arterial system (e.g. aorta) and enhancement of the abdominal organs (e.g. kidneys). There is a fluid collection around the medial aspect of the right kidney, in keeping with a subcapsular haematoma. A small area of high attenuation in this region indicates active extravasation.

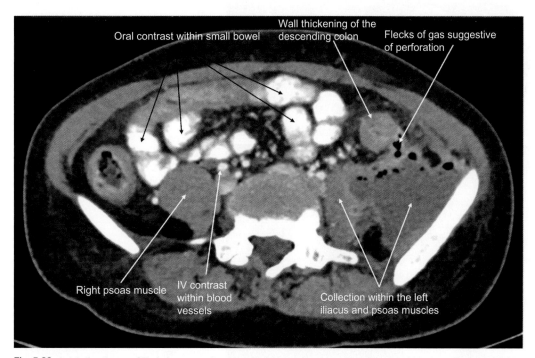

Fig. 5.23 Axial slice from a CT abdomen and pelvis with IV (portal venous phase) and oral contrast. There is thickening of the descending colon with surrounding flecks of gas. A large adjacent fluid and gas containing collection is present within the left iliacus muscle and extending into the left psoas muscle. The findings are in keeping with perforated colitis and abscess formation.

- A dilated small and/or large bowel can be easily identified. Tracing the dilated bowel distally will often allow identification of the cause. There may be an abrupt point where the calibre changes from dilated to collapsed (transition point) due to an intrinsic mass, extrinsic compression (e.g. adhesion), a hernia or volvulus. If there is no discrete transition point, it may be a functional obstruction, such as an ileus.

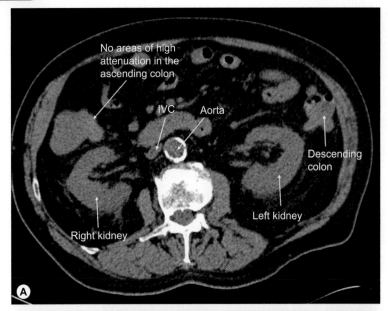

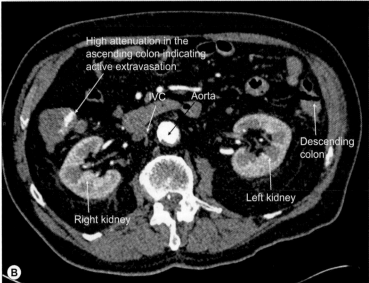

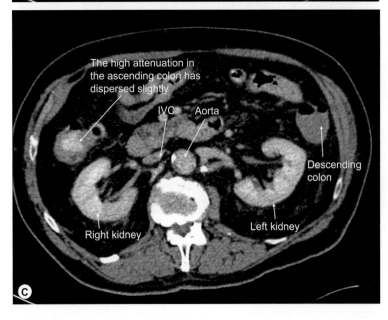

Fig. 5.24 Axial slices from a CT of the abdomen and pelvis to investigate an acute GI haemorrhage. **(A)** Noncontrast CT shows no high attenuation in relation to the ascending colon. **(B)** The arterial phase CT shows an area of high attenuation arising from the medial aspect of the ascending colon, indicating active extravasation. **(C)** The high attenuation has dispersed slightly on the portal venous phase CT. The arterial phase CT can be used to help identify the arterial branch responsible, which can be treated using embolisation (interventional radiology) or surgery.

- CT has an important role in identifying complications of the primary pathology, such as peripancreatic fluid collections and pancreatic necrosis in pancreatitis, and complications related to any surgery, such as anastomotic leaks.

! KEY POINTS

1. CT is not required in a large proportion of general surgical patients. For example, appendicitis is usually a clinical diagnosis and gallstone pathology is better diagnosed using ultrasound.
2. The role of CT in acute pancreatitis is to identify any complications (not to make the diagnosis). CT is therefore usually performed 48 to 72 hours after the onset of acute pancreatitis in those patients who are suspected to have developed complications (usually patients with severe pancreatitis as determined by clinical scoring systems).

ACUTE GASTROINTESTINAL HAEMORRHAGE

- CT angiography can be used as a noninvasive method fvor identifying an active bleeding point, especially within the colon (Fig. 5.24).
- Usually, noncontrast, arterial and portal venous phase CTs are required for a comprehensive assessment.
- Active haemorrhage appears as an area of high attenuation within the lumen of the gastrointestinal tract on the arterial phase (the noncontrast phase scan is used as a baseline to compare with as there may be artefact and other reasons for high attenuation).
  (Note: To be detectable, active haemorrhage must be occurring at the time of the CT, at a rate of >0.5 mL/minute.)
- The portal venous phase allows accurate assessment of the abdominal organs.
- Identification of a bleeding point can help guide further management (either interventional radiological embolisation or surgery).

TUMOUR/STAGING

- Portal venous phase CT of the abdomen +/− pelvis is needed for diagnosing and staging many tumours, such as lung, oesophageal, bowel, renal and ovarian cancers (Fig. 5.25).
- Abnormal masses within the solid abdominal organs (liver, kidneys, spleen, pancreas and adrenals) are usually easily identified.
- Masses within the bowel can be more difficult to detect as the GI tract is often collapsed in places and contains food and faecal material. CT colonoscopy is the best type of CT for identifying large bowel tumours.
- CT is used in staging to identify any lymph node enlargement, solid organ metastases such as the liver or adrenals, peritoneal nodules and bone metastases. Each type of cancer has its own specific

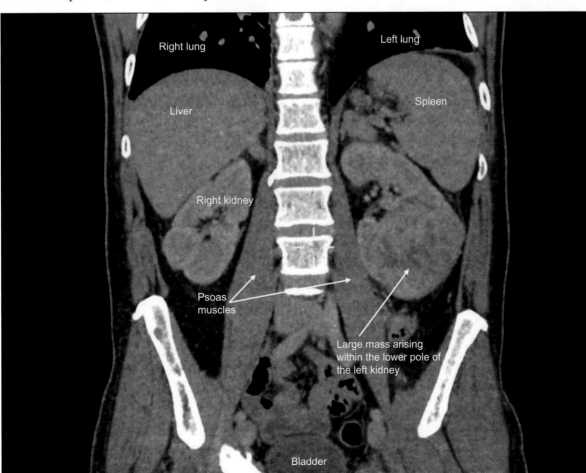

Fig. 5.25 Coronal image from a CT abdomen and pelvis with IV contrast (portal venous phase). A large mass within the lower pole of the left kidney is clearly visible, in keeping with a primary renal tumour. Assessment of the rest of the CT abdomen and pelvis and a CT chest is required for staging this malignancy.

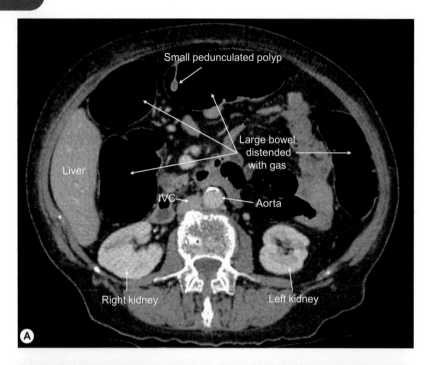

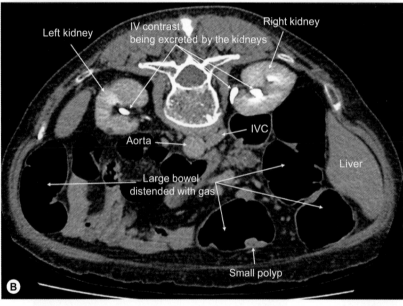

Fig. 5.26 Axial images from CT colonoscopy with IV contrast. **(A)** Axial slice from the supine CT. The bowel preparation and distension with carbon dioxide permits accurate assessment of the colon and a small pedunculated polyp is visible within the transverse colon. **(B)** Axial slice from the prone CT showing the same colonic polyp. Because the polyp is on a stalk, it is now lying dependently against the bowel wall but it is in the same location. This scan has been acquired after the supine CT and the IV contrast is starting to be excreted into the urinary collecting system by the kidneys.

staging criteria (American Joint Committee on Cancer Staging Manual), the details of which are beyond the scope of this book.

- CT is used to follow up patients after treatment to help assess their response.

CT COLONOSCOPY

- This provides a noninvasive alternative to colonoscopy for assessing the bowel. It is as accurate as colonoscopy at detecting polyps and tumours >1 cm and allows assessment of the extracolonic structures in the abdomen and pelvis (Fig. 5.26). However, unlike the case with colonoscopies, biopsies cannot be taken.
- It is usually performed in patients who are unable or unlikely to tolerate colonoscopy or in a screening setting and it has largely replaced barium enema.

- Patient preparation is not trivial and includes 2 to 3 days of bowel preparation prior to the CT.
- Just prior to the scan, a catheter is inserted into the patient's rectum and the colon insufflated with carbon dioxide. This can cause temporary discomfort, like trapped wind.
- Two CT scans are then performed – one with the patient supine and another with the patient prone – this helps differentiate between a tumour/polyp, which will remain in roughly the same position, and faecal residue, which will usually lie dependently.
- IV contrast may also be given during the CT to allow more accurate assessment of the other abdominal organs.

RENAL TRACT CALCULI

- CT is the most accurate imaging test for diagnosing renal calculi (Fig. 5.27).

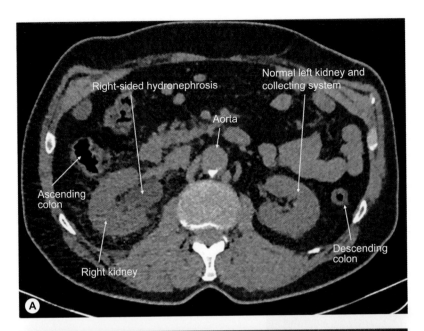

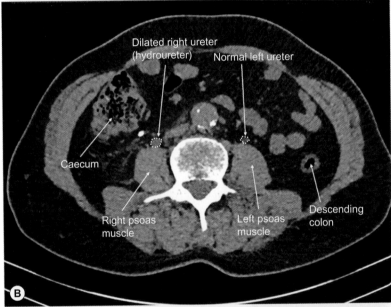

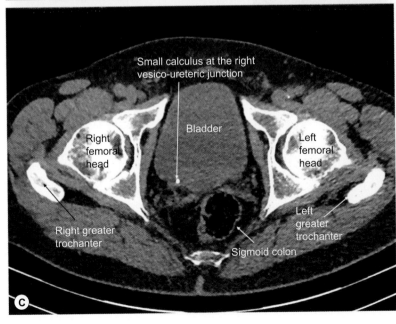

Fig. 5.27 Selected axial images from a low-dose, noncontrast CT KUB. **(A)** and **(B)** Right-sided hydronephrosis and hydroureter (compared to the normal left side). **(C)** Small calculus impacted at the right vesico-ureteric junction.

- A noncontrast, low-dose CT can be performed, known as a CT KUB.
- Almost all renal calculi are radio-opaque on CT and therefore easily identified. Other causes of calcification, such as phleboliths, can sometimes mimic renal tract calculi.
- Complications such as dilatation of the ureter and pelvicalyceal system (hydroureter and hydronephrosis, respectively) caused by an obstructing calculus can be detected.
- Additionally, alternative pathology, such as appendicitis or diverticulitis, can be diagnosed, although the low-dose and noncontrast nature of the CT limits the possible assessment of the abdominal viscera.

❗ KEY POINT

CT KUB has superseded X-ray KUB for diagnosing urinary tract calculi. X-ray KUBs are now usually only performed in patients who have a calculus identified on CT – if the stone is radio-opaque on X-ray then the patient can be followed up with X-rays rather than CT following treatment.

HAEMATURIA

- A CT urogram is a useful test in some patients with haematuria (Fig. 5.28).
- IV contrast and furosemide are given and the CT timed to scan the patient when the contrast is within the urinary tract (remember: IV contrast is renally excreted).

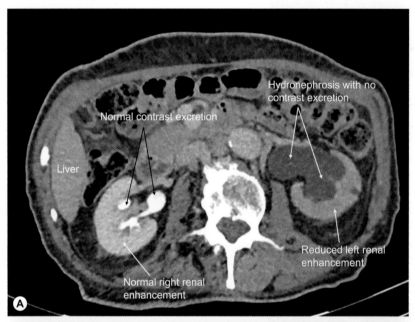

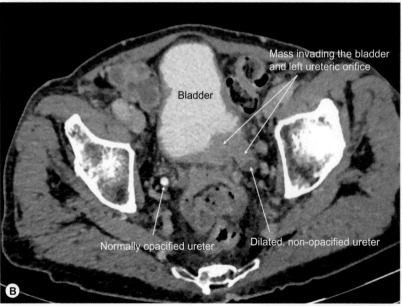

Fig. 5.28 Axial slices from a split bolus CT urogram. **(A)** There is normal enhancement of the right kidney. Contrast is excreted into a nondilated, normal-appearing right renal pelvicalyceal system. There is less enhancement of the left kidney and no excretion of contrast on this side. The left pelvicalyceal system is dilated (i.e. hydronephrosis as labelled). These findings indicate a left-sided obstructive uropathy which is compromising the function of the left kidney. **(B)** There is a mass invading the left side of the trigone of the bladder and the left ureteric orifice, causing the obstruction. Other images from the CT revealed this to be a locally advanced prostate tumour.

- Often, the contrast is given as a split bolus to allow some of it to be within the portal venous system, which improves the imaging of the abdominal viscera, whilst the rest is opacifying the renal tracts.
- CT urograms are useful for detecting urinary tract calculi, especially for radiolucent stones which are not visible on CT KUB but appear as filling defects on CT urography. Tumours and masses of the renal tracts and bladder are also readily detectable.
- A non- or poorly functioning kidney will show reduced/no enhancement of the renal parenchyma and reduced/no excretion of the IV contrast into the renal tract.

VASCULAR DISEASE

- CT angiograms can be used to assess the arterial system for vascular disease, such as aneurysms and atherosclerosis (Fig. 5.29). The CT is acquired once the IV contrast is within the arterial system.
- It is a specialist test which provides detailed images that can be used to determine and plan the most appropriate further management, considering the options of angioplasty, EVAR or surgery.
- MRA can also be performed to assess the vascular tree.
- Patients with a suspected ruptured AAA usually initially undergo a noncontrast CT of the abdomen and pelvis. This will demonstrate whether the abdominal aorta is aneurysmal, whether there has been a rupture of an aneurysm or if there are any signs of an impending rupture (such as high attenuation within the aortic wall indicating acute intramural haematoma). (Note: Patients with a suspected AAA in emergency departments can undergo point of care ultrasound (POCUS) to estimate size, shape and location, which can then be escalated to further imaging (see Chapter 7).)
- CT angiogram will allow the size, shape and location of an aneurysm to be accurately characterised. The relation of the aneurysm to any aortic branches, such as the renal or mesenteric arteries, can be identified. These features are useful for determining the most appropriate management (e.g. surgery versus EVAR).

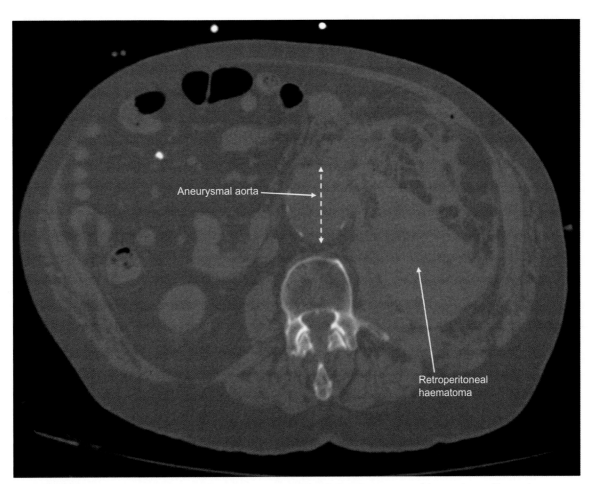

Fig. 5.29 Axial noncontrast CT slice showing a ruptured abdominal aortic aneurysm. A large volume of haematoma is evident surrounding the aneurysmal aorta. No further imaging was performed as the patient proceeded to urgent surgery.

- Additionally, the CT angiogram can show whether there is continued haemorrhage from a ruptured aneurysm.
- Many centres (those without EVAR services) will not perform a CT angiogram if a ruptured aneurysm is demonstrated on the noncontrast scan, as the patient will usually require emergency surgery regardless of what the CT angiogram shows. If there is an EVAR emergency service, then having an arterial scan is useful to allow them to quickly plan the procedure (e.g. one of the iliac vessels may be occluded and would mean you have to use the other side for gaining access to the aorta).

MRI Scans

Erin Visser and Bryan Dalton

WHAT IS MRI?

The physics behind MRI is complicated. It is not necessary to fully understand how MR images are produced (in the same way you can drive a car without knowing exactly how the engine works!); however, a basic understanding is helpful.

In simple terms, MRI uses a magnetic field and radiowaves to produce images. The patient lies inside the magnet which is enveloped by a covering. This causes hydrogen ions (protons) within the body to align (either with or against the magnetic field). A radiofrequency pulse of a specific magnitude and duration is then sent through the patient. This transfers energy to the protons (excitation) and changes their direction of alignment. Over time, the energy from these excited protons is lost (decays) and the protons realign with the magnetic field (relaxation). This process emits radiofrequencies which are detected by the MRI scanner and result in the image. The speed of the relaxation process depends on the size and duration of the initial radiofrequency pulse, the structure of the substance in which the hydrogen ions/protons are in and the influence of surrounding hydrogen ions/protons. Thus the different tissues and substances result in different signals which are detected by the MRI scanner and influence the image produced. The strength of a magnet in an MRI is measured using the unit of measure Tesla (T). For clinical and research scans, 1.5T and 3T are the most common magnet strengths used today, and 7T MRI is also increasing in use but remains in very limited availability.

In contrast to CT, the space for the patient in the MRI scanner where the patient lies is small (but there have been concerted efforts to increase the diameter to allow for larger subjects), acquisition time of images is longer and the scanner is loud. Patients who are claustrophobic or unable to lie still for prolonged periods may not be able to tolerate an MRI (Fig. 6.1).

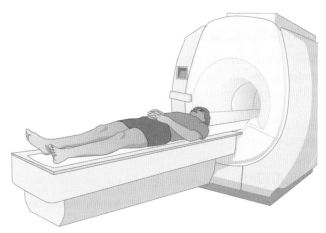

Fig. 6.1 Diagram of an MRI scanner.

Various different types of sequences can be acquired which provide different types of information. The science behind the different types of sequence is complex and does not need to be understood by nonspecialists. T1-weighted images are useful for demonstrating anatomy and lymph nodes, whereas T2-weighted sequences are useful for showing fluid and therefore areas of oedema.

Images can be acquired in various planes. However, unlike CT, the images usually cannot be reformatted into different planes once they have been acquired.

USE OF IONISING RADIATION

One of the benefits of MRI over CT is that ionising radiation is not used. Instead, as described earlier, MRI uses a magnetic field and radiowaves to produce the images. However, MRI scanning has other hazards associated with it.

MAGNETIC FIELDS

- The strong magnetic field of the MRI scanner can turn ferromagnetic objects, such as coins, scissors, earrings and non-MRI-compatible oxygen cylinders, into projectiles, with the potential to cause serious injury or death to patients or staff. The MRI magnet is essentially always on; therefore only MRI-compatible metallic objects should be taken into the MRI scanner room.
- The magnetic fields can interfere with some electronic devices, such as certain pacemakers and cochlear implants. Such devices must be checked to see whether they are MR safe before a patient or staff member with one of them can enter the MRI room. MRI safety is of paramount importance.

RADIOFREQUENCY FIELDS

These can result in heating of tissues and structures. Usually, the body can dissipate the heat with vasodilation. However, the potential for burns exists if non-MRI-compatible monitoring leads and electrodes are used.

CONTRAST AGENTS

The most commonly used MRI contrast agent is **gadolinium**. It has been linked to a rare condition called nephrogenic systemic fibrosis, although this tends to only occur in patients with renal dysfunction. Gadolinium should therefore generally be avoided in patients with an eGFR <30 mL/minute.

INDICATIONS

MRI scanning has a wide range of indications; some specific indications are discussed next.

MRI tends to be a specialised examination which is requested by senior clinicians, often following discussion with radiology. Further details can be found in the Royal College of Radiologist's guidelines (making the best use of clinical radiology services/iRefer).

In general, MRI provides superior assessment of the soft tissues compared to CT, making it very useful for neurological (brain, spinal cord and spinal nerve roots) and musculoskeletal (muscles, tendons, ligaments and bone marrow) imaging. However, it is a relatively slow imaging technique which requires the patient to lie still for prolonged periods. It is therefore not commonly used for acutely unwell patients.

CONTRAINDICATIONS

Patients who have non-MRI-compatible implanted devices, such as pacemakers, those who are claustrophobic, unable to lie flat or too large for the scanner are unable to undergo MRI. Most current-day devices are MRI-compatible but this compatibility always needs to be double checked by MR radiographers. Additionally, patients who have had a history of working with metal and potential metallic foreign bodies in their orbits should not enter the MRI scanner as they may move and cause serious harm. An orbital X-ray should be carried out to assess for any residual metallic fragments. As mentioned, those with renal failure should not have gadolinium.

The patient will have to complete an MRI safety checklist prior to scanning to ensure there are no contraindications.

> ❗ KEY POINT
>
> You should always discuss with the radiology department if you are unsure whether a patient's metallic implant, such as a pacemaker, is MRI compatible.

SEQUENCES

Multiple different MRI sequences are usually acquired for each scan. Each sequence is used to identify specific abnormalities, and accurate interpretation requires interrogation of all the sequences performed. We will look at the two fundamental sequences, T1- and T2-weighted sequences, in more detail.

T1- and T2-weighted sequences are often the main sequences performed (Fig. 6.2). The key difference between the two is that fluid appears dark (low signal) on T1-weighted images but bright (high signal) on T2. Fat is bright (high signal) on both T1 and T2. T1 provides a good assessment of anatomical structure and lymph nodes. Most pathology causes localised oedema and therefore T2-weighted sequences are better for identifying pathology.

MRI scans are described in terms of signal intensity. Hyperintense (high signal) refers to 'bright' structures. Isointense means the object of interest has the same brightness as its comparator. Hypointense (low signal) refers to 'dark' structures.

HEAD/BRAIN

- Commonly requested MRI examination.
- As with all MRIs, it is sensitive to movement so the patient must be able to lie still.
- The sequences performed vary depending on the differential diagnosis but almost always include a T1 and T2 sequence.
- Common indications include:
  - Acute stroke (can diagnose acute ischaemic stroke much earlier than CT)
  - Suspected demyelinating diseases (e.g. multiple sclerosis)
  - Further assessment of space-occupying lesions (superior to CT for identifying early tumours and determining the exact size of a lesion) and post-operative follow-up after tumour surgery
  - Assessing the pituitary gland
  - Investigation of epilepsy (to identify an underlying structural cause)
  - Assessment of congenital abnormalities
  - Assessment of vascular abnormalities

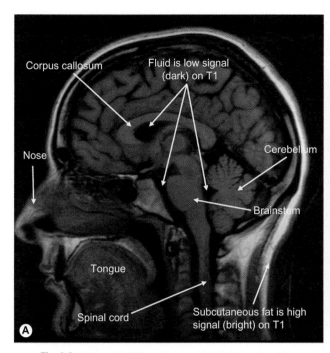

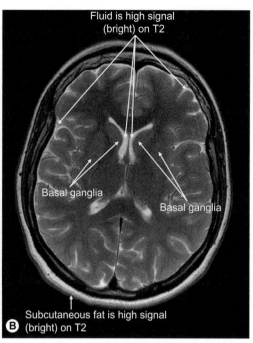

Fig. 6.2 Selected MRI head images highlighting the difference between T1- and T2-weighted images. **(A)** Sagittal T1-weighted image showing fluid (in this case, the CSF in the third and fourth ventricles and the basal cisterns) is low signal. **(B)** Axial T2-weighted image demonstrating fluid (CSF in the lateral ventricles and CSF spaces) is high signal. The subcutaneous fat is high signal on both sequences.

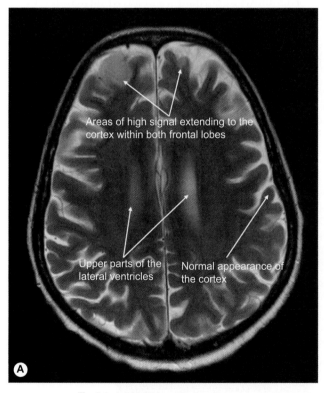

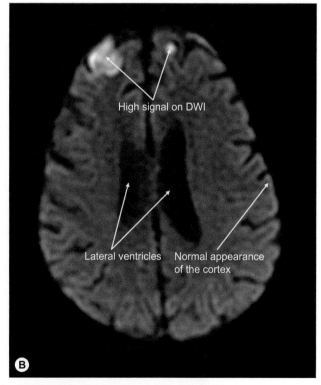

Fig. 6.3 Axial MRI head images in a patient with an acute stroke. **(A)** T2-weighted image showing high signal within both frontal lobes, which extends to the cortex, in keeping with oedema. **(B)** These areas are high signal on DWI. This is in keeping with acute ischaemic infarcts.

ACUTE STROKE

- Acute ischaemic strokes appear as areas of oedema, which usually involve both grey and white matter and show restricted diffusion on diffusion-weighted images (Fig. 6.3).

- DWI measures the rate of water diffusion in the extracellular space and allows diagnosis of an acute ischaemic stroke much earlier than CT. Faster water diffusion rates result in low signal (dark), slower diffusion rates result in high signal (bright).

- Because diffusion of water is strongly influenced by the surrounding cellular environment, changes in its rate of diffusion can indicate early pathological abnormalities.
- Normally, water molecules freely move/diffuse throughout the extracellular space.
- Ischaemia, including ischaemic infarcts, results in dysfunction of the ATP-dependent ion pumps in cells. This results in accumulation of intracellular sodium. Water subsequently diffuses into cells, leading to swelling (cytotoxic oedema). The swollen brain cells compress the surrounding extracellular space, restricting the movement/diffusion of extracellular water, leading to a high signal on DWI.
- Other pathologies, such as abscesses and some tumours, also show restricted diffusion; therefore clinical and radiological correlation is important.
- MRI is a specialised investigation and not routine for imaging all patients with a potential stroke (even though with increasing MRI availability, it is becoming more standard). Instead, it should be considered in young patients who have had a stroke and those with suspected posterior fossa and brainstem infarcts (as CT is less accurate at assessing these regions).

> **❶ KEY POINT**
>
> The terms acute, subacute and chronic are commonly used to indicate an age of a stroke or intracranial haemorrhage. Acute refers to <3 days old, subacute 3 to 14 days and chronic >14 days.

DEMYELINATION

- In conjunction with the clinical assessment, MRI plays an important role in establishing the diagnosis of multiple sclerosis and other demyelinating disorders (Fig. 6.4).
- It is the most sensitive and specific investigation for such conditions and can show dissemination of demyelinated plaques in time and space (i.e. plaques of different ages and in different locations), which is required for the diagnosis of multiple sclerosis as per the McDonald criteria.
- Imaging features include high T2 signal lesions within the deep white matter, which are typically elliptical in shape and often radiate from the corpus callosum.
- FLAIR MRI sequences are often used. FLAIR sequences are similar to T2-weighted sequences except the signal from the free fluid (CSF in the ventriculosulcal system) is nulled and appears black. This allows abnormalities in the white matter around the ventricles to be more easily seen.

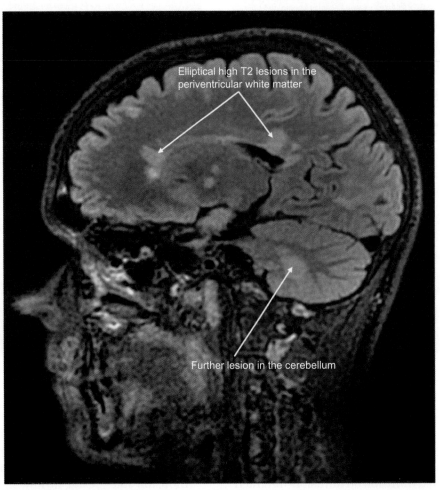

Fig. 6.4 Sagittal FLAIR (fluid attenuation inversion recovery) MRI sequence of the head. Typical high-signal plaques within the periventricular and cerebellar white matter are suggestive of demyelination, such as multiple sclerosis.

- Contrast enhancement can demonstrate dissemination in time (acute demyelination enhances whereas chronic lesions do not).
- The spine should also be imaged as it can be affected by demyelination.

SPACE-OCCUPYING LESIONS

- MRI is usually more sensitive than CT at identifying tumours and better at characterising them (Fig. 6.5).
- It is particularly useful for small tumours, posterior fossa lesions and tumours which involve the meninges.
- MRI is also very helpful for identifying the macroscopic extent of a tumour. The site, relationship to other structures, imaging characteristics and age of the patient are all helpful for narrowing the differential diagnosis.
- MRI is used in the postoperative follow-up of patients with brain tumours to look for recurrence.

PITUITARY ASSESSMENT

- MRI is significantly better than CT for assessing the pituitary gland.
- It is particularly helpful for demonstrating the relationship between a pituitary mass and the optic nerves, chiasm and tracts, which run just above the pituitary gland. IV gadolinium is almost always used for MRIs of the pituitary.

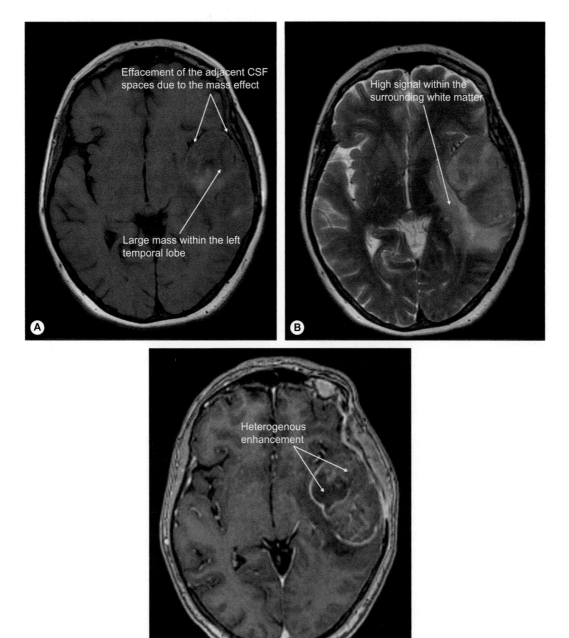

Fig. 6.5 Selected axial MRI images of a left temporal lobe tumour. **(A)** Noncontrast T1-weighted image. The mass can be appreciated but it is difficult to clearly identify its boundaries. Effacement of the adjacent CSF spaces and midline shift is apparent. **(B)** Noncontrast T2-weighted image. Oedema within the white matter surrounding the mass is visible. **(C)** T1-weighted image post IV gadolinium. The mass shows heterogeneous enhancement and its margins are clearly visible.

- MRI is again useful in the postoperative follow-up of patients following pituitary tumour surgery.

EPILEPSY

- MRI provides an accurate assessment of the brain parenchyma in patients with epilepsy.
- It permits the identification of any structural abnormalities, such as tumours or cortical malformations, which may be the underlying cause for seizures.

CONGENITAL ABNORMALITIES

- MRI provides the most accurate assessment of the brain parenchyma. It is very useful in the assessment of neonates and children with suspected congenital cranial abnormalities.
- Such abnormalities are uncommon but include Chiari malformations, Dandy–Walker malformations and migration anomalies.

VASCULAR ABNORMALITIES

- MRI can be used to investigate intracranial aneurysms, vascular malformations and venous sinus thromboses.
- MRA is a group of techniques utilised to visualise intracranial vessels, eliminating the need for an iodinated contrast medium and no contrast media at all is required for certain sequences.

SPINE

- The advantage of MRI over CT is its ability to accurately depict the soft tissue structures of the spine, such as the intervertebral discs, the thecal sac, CSF, spinal cord and nerve roots (Fig. 6.6).
- It also shows the bone marrow and any areas of abnormal marrow infiltration, for example with bony metastatic disease, can be easily identified.

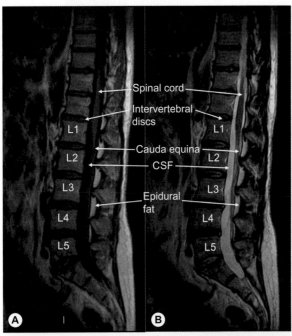

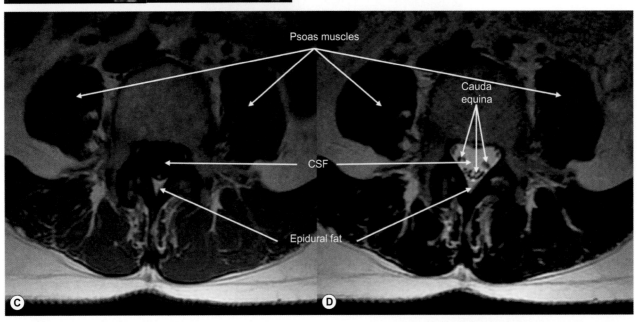

Fig. 6.6 Sagittal and axial MRI images of a lumbar spine. **(A)** T1- and **(B)** T2-weighted sagittal images showing the vertebrae, intervertebral discs, spinal cord, cauda equina and CSF. Normal, uniform bone marrow signal. **(C)** T1- and **(D)** T2-weighted axial images showing the normal appearance of the cauda equina and surrounding CSF.

- The standard sequences are sagittal T1 and T2 images with axial T1 and T2 images at any level where there is particular concern.
- Common indications include:
  - Suspected cauda equina compression
  - Suspected spinal cord compression
  - Spinal canal stenosis
  - Assessing the spinal cord (e.g. for contusions following trauma, for evidence of demyelination or for cord tumours or infarcts)

CAUDA EQUINA COMPRESSION

- This is a medical emergency which must be treated as soon as possible to minimise the risk of permanent disability (Fig. 6.7). It is important to remember that cauda equina syndrome is diagnosed clinically; imaging is used to assess the cause but not necessary for diagnosis.
- It is commonly the result of intervertebral disc herniations compressing the cauda equina.
- Other causes include epidural collections (infection, haematoma), which commonly occur postoperatively, trauma and compression from bony metastatic disease.
- As discussed, MRI is an excellent modality for diagnosing such abnormalities by permitting an assessment of the cauda equina and the exiting nerve roots.

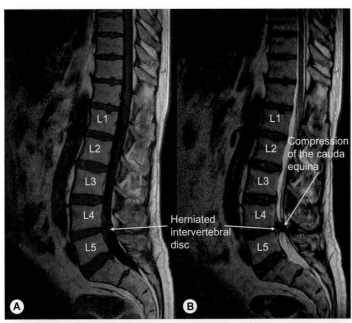

Fig. 6.7 Sagittal and axial MRI images of a lumbar spine. **(A)** Sagittal T1 and **(B)** T2 images showing a herniated L4/5 disc which is compressing the cauda equina. **(C)** Axial T1 and **(D)** T2 images at the L4/5 level showing the herniated disc compressing the cauda equina, with no CSF visible around the nerve roots at this level.

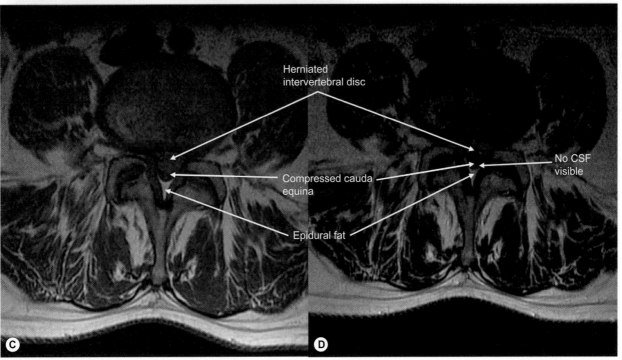

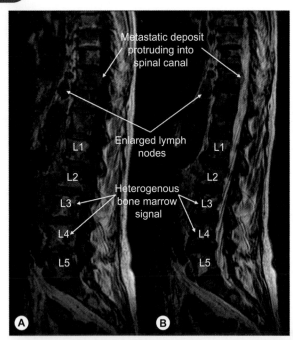

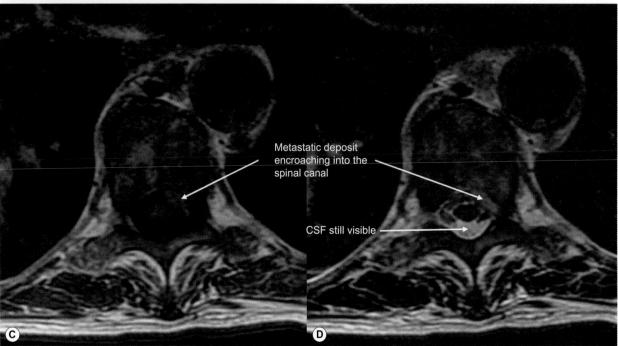

Fig. 6.8 Sagittal and axial MRI images of a lumbar spine. **(A)** Sagittal T1 and **(B)** T2 images showing diffusely heterogeneous and abnormal bone marrow signal, in keeping with bone metastases. A metastatic deposit protrudes into the spinal canal from the posterior aspect of the T10 vertebral body. **(C)** Axial T1 and **(D)** T2 images at the T10 level, showing the metastatic deposit encroaching into the left side of the spinal canal. It currently touches the spinal cord but CSF is still visible, indicating there is no compression. However, if it enlarges, it could result in spinal cord compression.

SPINAL CORD COMPRESSION

- Narrowing of the spinal canal above the level of the cauda equina (roughly L1 level) can cause compression of the spinal cord (Fig. 6.8).
- The causes are similar for cauda equina compression although it is more commonly seen with bony metastatic disease rather than disc herniations.
- If bony metastatic disease is suspected, the entire spine should be imaged as there may be multiple sites of bone metastases which could benefit from treatment (usually radiotherapy).

❗ KEY POINTS

Compression of the spinal cord and cauda equina may seem similar but they are different clinical entities.
1. The cause of spinal cord compression is more commonly bony metastatic disease, whereas cauda equina compression is usually the result of intervertebral disc herniations.
2. The spinal cord is part of the central nervous system and therefore its compression results in upper motor neurone findings, such as hyperreflexia and an extensor plantar response. The cauda equina is part of the peripheral nervous system and its compression causes a range of different signs such as urinary/bowel dysfunction, saddle anaesthesia and decreased rectal tone.

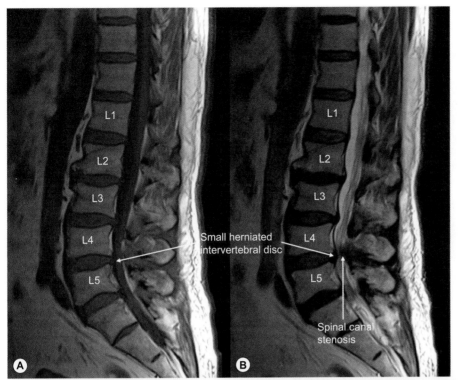

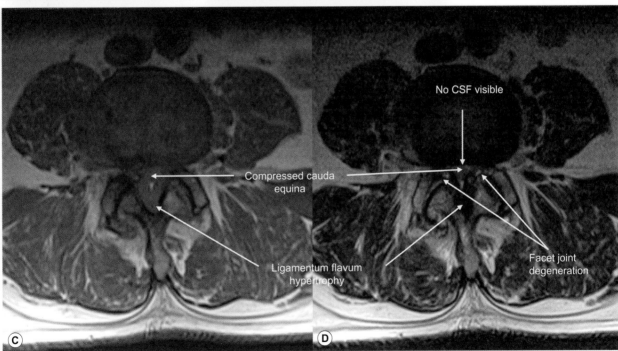

Fig. 6.9 Sagittal and axial MRI images of a lumbar spine. **(A)** Sagittal T1 and **(B)** T2 images showing a severe stenosis of the spinal canal at the L4/5 level with compression of the cauda equina. **(C)** Axial T1 and **(D)** T2 images at the L4/5 level showing the stenosis is largely due to degenerative changes (ligamentum flavum hypertrophy and facet joint degeneration). There is compression of the cauda equina, with no CSF visible around the nerve roots at this level.

SPINAL CANAL STENOSIS

- Degenerative changes in the spine can result in a gradual narrowing of the spinal canal, which over time can result in compression of the spinal cord or cauda equina (Fig. 6.9).

- The clinical findings associated with canal stenosis are usually chronic in nature, reflecting the slow progression of the degenerative disease.
- The sequences performed are the same as those for suspected spinal cord or cauda equina compression.

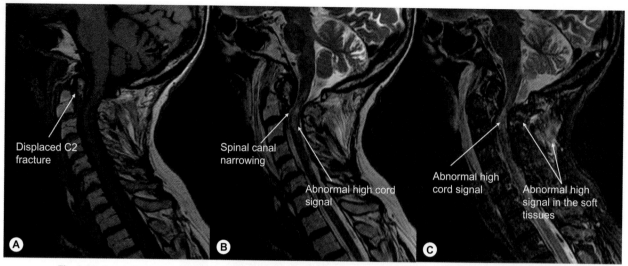

Fig. 6.10 Sagittal MRI images of a patient who has sustained a traumatic neck injury. **(A)** T1 image shows the displaced fracture clearly. **(B)** T2 image shows the resultant narrowing of the spinal canal, with almost complete loss of CSF surrounding the cord at this level. There is also an abnormally high internal cord signal. **(C)** Fat-suppressed T2-weighted image again shows an abnormal intrinsic cord signal. In addition, oedema is evident within the posterior soft tissues and ligaments. The findings are consistent with an acute contusional spinal cord injury.

ASSESSMENT OF THE SPINAL CORD

- MRI is the best method for assessing the spinal cord (Fig. 6.10).
- Traumatic cord contusions or spinal cord ischaemia can result in specific constellations of clinical findings, which point to a spinal cord injury.
- As mentioned earlier, demyelinating processes, such as multiple sclerosis or neuromyelitis optica (NMO), can affect the spinal cord as well as the brain.
- Some tumours can also affect the spinal cord and MRI is integral to their detection.

MAGNETIC RESONANCE CHOLANGIOPANCREATOGRAPHY

- MRCP provides a noninvasive technique for assessing the biliary tree and pancreatic duct (Fig. 6.11).
- It has replaced ERCP for diagnosis. ERCP is still used for therapeutic purposes, such as removing ductal stones and placing ductal stents.
- The main MRCP sequences are heavily T2-weighted, and therefore the bile appears hyperintense/bright.
- MRCP can demonstrate the site and extent of biliary dilatation, intraductal calculi (rounded filling defects in the bright bile) and extrinsic compression of the biliary tree.
- The main indication is the investigation of obstructive jaundice, which may be caused by an intraductal calculus, cholangiocarcinoma or extrinsic compression by a pancreatic mass or enlarged lymph nodes.

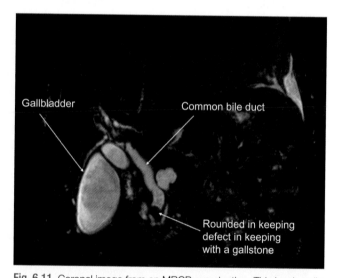

Fig. 6.11 Coronal image from an MRCP examination. This is a heavily T2-weighted sequence and so the bile appears bright. The gallbladder and biliary tree can be easily seen. There is a rounded filling defect in the distal common bile duct, in keeping with a ductal calculus. This could be removed by ERCP.

SMALL BOWEL

- MRI small bowel has superseded barium follow-through examinations for the assessment of small bowel pathology, particularly Crohn's disease (Fig. 6.12).
- This is a specialised examination which should be requested by the gastrointestinal team.
- It permits an assessment of the small bowel thickness and degree of wall enhancement to be made.

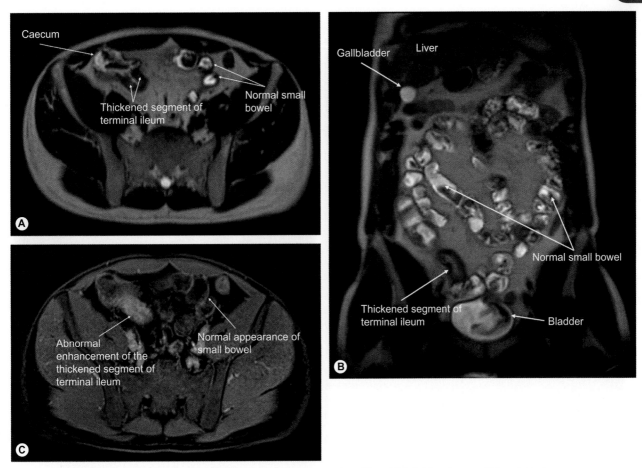

Fig. 6.12 Selected images from an MRI small bowel examination. **(A)** and **(B)** Axial and coronal T2-weighted images showing abnormal wall thickening of the terminal ileum. **(C)** Axial image following the administration of gadolinium showing abnormal enhancement of the thickened terminal ileum. These findings are in keeping with Crohn's disease.

In addition, abnormally enlarged lymph nodes, free fluid and fistulae can often be identified.
- It therefore allows the site, extent and activity of Crohn's disease to be characterised.

KNEE AND OTHER JOINTS

- MRI is very useful for assessing the knee and other joints (Fig. 6.13).

- It provides detailed images of the soft tissue structures, such as tendons, ligaments and cartilage, which are not clearly visible on X-ray or CT.
- In addition, the bone, including bone marrow, can be assessed.

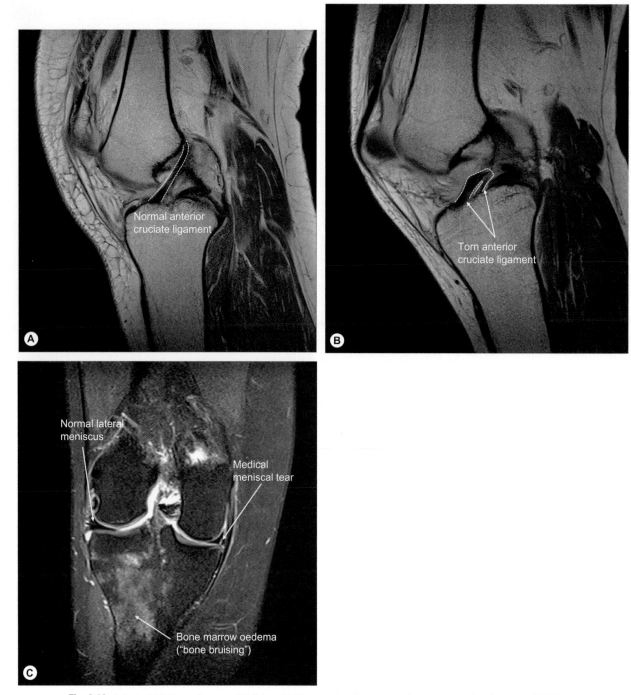

Fig. 6.13 Selected MRI knee images. **(A)** T1 sagittal image showing a normal anterior cruciate ligament. **(B)** T1 sagittal image showing a complete tear of the anterior cruciate ligament, which has flipped back on itself. **(C)** T2 fat-suppressed coronal image showing a medial meniscal tear and bone bruising in the proximal tibia.

7

Ultrasound Scans

Erin Visser and Bryan Dalton

Chapter Outline

WHAT IS ULTRASOUND?

Ultrasound (US) is a medical imaging technique that uses very high-frequency sound waves (which are inaudible to humans) to produce images. The high-frequency ultrasound waves are produced by the ultrasound transducer (hand-held probe) and travel as a beam through the body. In medical diagnostics the waves range from 1 to 15 MHz, although higher frequencies may be used in specific situations. When they come across a boundary between two different tissues, the waves can either be absorbed, reflected or refracted. The ultrasound waves which are reflected back are detected by the transducer and are used to make the images. The amplitude of the reflected waves, combined with the time they take to return to the transducer, are used to generate the image.

Ultrasound waves travel well through solid and liquid media. In contrast, the ultrasound waves are scattered by gases; essentially, air does not conduct ultrasound waves. Therefore a water-based gel is used as an interface between the transducer and the patient to improve the transmission of ultrasound waves between the transducer and the body.

There are a myriad of different ultrasound machines. Important facets include raising or lowering the monitor, recognising the probe marker and manipulating the machine to fit the ergonomics between the operator and the patient. It is important to be aware that there are different transducers one can select to optimise the image.

The linear probe is used for superficial structures. It has a high frequency (7–15 MHz) which creates a high resolution of vasculature, lungs and musculoskeletal structures close to the body surface. This probe is commonly used in ultrasound-guided peripheral vascular access and nerve blocks.

The phased-array (cardiac) probe is used for echocardiography predominantly. It has a lower varying frequency (1–3 MHz) and a small footprint, focussing the ultrasound waves to achieve high resolution and recognition of contractions of the heart. It can be manipulated to gain various cardiac windows which are beyond the scope of this chapter.

The curvilinear probe is used for imaging deep structures using a lower frequency (2–5 MHz) which is optimal for image resolution of abdominal structures and pelvic structures. The curvilinear probe is useful in emergency medicine for POCUS (point-of-care ultrasound) imaging such as FAST scans, which will be discussed later in this chapter.

Once an ultrasound transducer is selected, the type of image or mode must be selected, a few of which are discussed later. There are three main types of ultrasound imaging:

- **B-mode** (brightness mode) produces real-time two-dimensional images (see Fig. 7.6A). The amplitude of the echo for each pixel is represented using a greyscale. This is the standard ultrasound image. Pathology may be demonstrated by a change in the size or shape of a structure, or an alteration in its brightness (echogenicity).
- **Colour flow imaging** is used to show the direction of flow and provides an estimation of velocity (see Fig. 7.6B). The flow assessed is usually blood flow but can be any flowing or moving substance, such as a jet of urine entering the bladder from the ureter. The colour flow information is superimposed on the B-mode image. In general, red indicates flow towards the ultrasound transducer, blue away and yellow/green turbulent flow. Alterations in velocity

and/or the direction of flow can indicate pathology. It is important to note that each ultrasound machine can be set to different colour flow modes. Therefore, before commenting on direction of flow, one should take into account the machine settings.

- **Doppler imaging** can be used to calculate the velocity of flow (see Fig. 7.2). The change in frequency of the transmitted ultrasound waves compared with those received by the transducer allows the velocity to be calculated (the angle between the ultrasound beam and the direction of flow also needs to be measured). The velocity of flow can be used to determine the degree of a stenosis. Doppler also provides a tracing of the flow in terms of amplitude and direction (waveform) and the appearance of the waveform can be a useful indicator of pathology.

In ultrasound, the echogenicity of tissues is the tissue's ability to reflect ultrasound waves with respect to the surrounding tissues. Structures may be anechoic (black), hypoechoic (grey) or hyperechoic (white).

Ultrasound is usually a quick and well-tolerated examination. Ideally, it is performed in the radiology department using the departmental ultrasound machines. The patient can be scanned on the ultrasound couch or in a bed depending on their clinical condition. Portable ultrasounds can be used on patients who are clinically unstable, or who have poor mobility and are unable to attend the radiology department. However, portable ultrasound machines produce inferior images compared with the departmental machines, meaning the examination is usually less comprehensive.

The patient may have to move into different positions during the examination; therefore patient mobility and cooperation are important. The more tissue ultrasound waves have to travel through, the fewer that are returned and detected. Therefore it is easier to image superficial rather than deep structures. Additionally, the image quality in overweight and obese patients is often reduced and occasionally a diagnostic scan is not possible if the patient is too large.

IONISING RADIATION

Ultrasound does not use ionising radiation, it has no significant adverse effects and is safe to use in all patients (safe to use in pregnancy and in children).

INDICATIONS

Ultrasound travels well through solid and liquid. It is therefore most useful for imaging solid organs, such as the liver, kidneys and spleen, and fluid-filled structures, such as the bladder. However, ultrasound can be used to investigate a possible pneumothorax, by looking for absence of sliding lung pleura and B-lines for example. The main common indications are discussed later but further details can be found in the Royal College of Radiologist's guidelines (making the best use of clinical radiology services/iRefer).

CONTRAINDICATIONS

There are no absolute contraindications to ultrasound. The main reason for not performing ultrasound is if it is not clinically indicated and/or another imaging modality is more appropriate. As mentioned earlier, the diagnostic accuracy is reduced as the patient's size increases. Ultrasound may therefore not be useful in some very large patients. Patient cooperation is important and it may not be possible to scan a confused or otherwise uncooperative patient.

BASIC INTERPRETATION

Ultrasound is a dynamic investigation and the still images which are usually saved from the examination can be difficult to interpret alone, especially if you have not performed the scan yourself.

Fluid is anechoic (black) on ultrasound, and soft tissues can range in their echogenicity. Dense structures, such as gallstones or renal calculi, appear as hyperechoic (white/bright) foci with an area of 'posterior' acoustic shadowing (i.e. shadowing posterior to the structure). Most structures only reflect a proportion of ultrasound waves, allowing some sound waves to travel through them, which allows us to see structures which are beyond them. Acoustic shadowing refers to the shadow cast by things like gallstones. As no ultrasound waves can travel through them, the area behind them appears black (i.e. it looks like a shadow – exactly like the shadow cast by an opaque object). See Fig. 7.4B for an example.

HEAD AND NECK

- Ultrasound of the head and neck is a specialised test which can assess the thyroid and various structures including the parotid and submandibular salivary glands (Fig. 7.1). It is also useful for identifying enlarged cervical lymph nodes and can be used to guide biopsies of abnormal lesions.
- Carotid Doppler ultrasound can assess the velocity of blood flow in the carotid arteries and can indicate the degree of any stenosis (Fig. 7.2). It is essentially used to identify patients who would benefit from a carotid endarterectomy (i.e. those with a transient ischaemic attack or nondisabling stroke). It is therefore a specialised investigation which should only be requested in a small cohort of patients.
- Cranial ultrasound can be used in some instances to assess scalp pathologies; however, it is much more commonly used in premature infants to assess for hydrocephalus or other ventricular abnormalities.

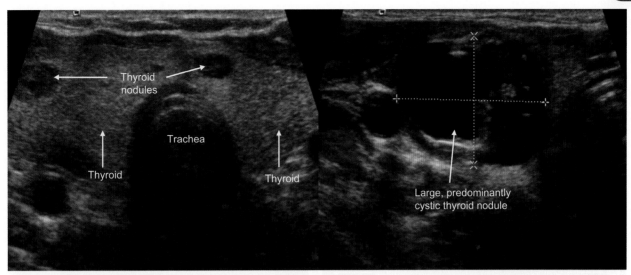

Fig. 7.1 Selected images from an ultrasound of the thyroid showing a multinodular goitre. The thyroid and other neck structures, such as the salivary glands (not in image), are easily imaged by ultrasound due to their superficial location.

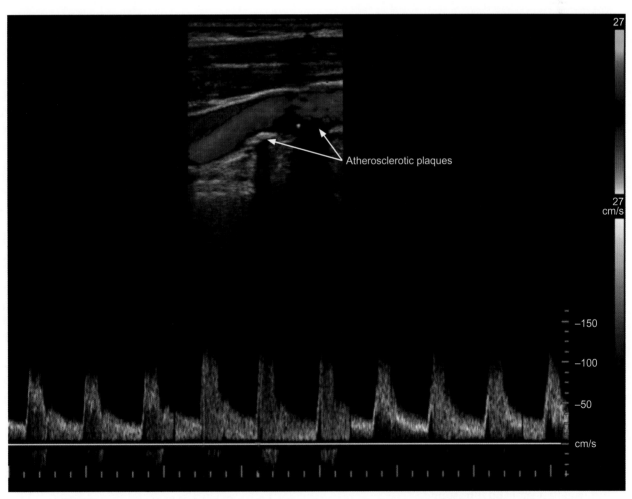

Fig. 7.2 Image from a carotid Doppler ultrasound. Two atherosclerotic plaques are visible. The velocity of the blood flow can be accurately calculated and the degree of any carotid stenosis estimated. The waveform displayed at the bottom of the image shows a typical arterial tracing. The y axis demonstrates the velocity of blood in cm/s and the x axis the time.

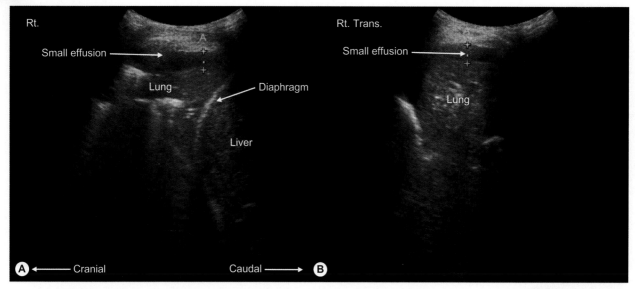

Fig. 7.3 Images from a chest ultrasound. **(A)** Longitudinal view of the right lung base showing a small pleural effusion. **(B)** Transverse view of the same small pleural effusion. Given its small size (the depth is measured by the ruler marked A (in *blue*) and proximity to the liver), it is not suitable for aspiration or drainage.

CHEST

- Ultrasound provides a limited assessment of the lungs as they are largely filled with gas; however, it is useful for detecting pneumothoraces (primary, secondary or tension), pleural effusions and assessing their size and characteristics (Fig. 7.3). It can be used to guide pleural aspiration or drainage.

ABDOMEN

- Assessment of the solid abdominal organs is one of the most common ultrasound requests (Fig. 7.4).
- Patients should be fasted for 6 hours (clear fluids are permitted) to allow the gallbladder to distend with bile (the gallbladder empties in response to food, hindering its assessment). The rules for fasting may vary between different institutions.
  - Ultrasound can identify liver lesions, such as metastases and primary tumours, and diffuse liver abnormalities, such as fatty infiltration. The appearance of the liver, in combination with other features on ultrasound, can indicate the presence of cirrhosis and portal hypertension.
  - The gallbladder can be assessed for gallstones. Focal tenderness over the gallbladder, along with gallbladder wall thickening and surrounding fluid (pericholecystic fluid), are suggestive of acute cholecystitis. Gallbladder tumours are rare but usually visible on ultrasound.
  - Dilatation of the intra- and/or extrahepatic biliary tree can be accurately assessed. The cause may also be visible (e.g. a mass at the liver hilum); however, a large part of the course of the common bile duct is often obscured by bowel

gas, precluding its assessment. Pathology of the common bile duct can be inferred by dilatation of the visible biliary tree.
  - The size, appearance and vascularity of the kidneys can be assessed. Common abnormalities include atrophic kidneys associated with chronic kidney disease, hydronephrosis and masses, such as renal cell carcinoma. Renal calculi are often not visible on ultrasound.
  - The size and appearance of the spleen can be assessed. There are multiple causes of splenomegaly, one of the commonest being portal hypertension.
  - The head and neck of the pancreas is often visible; however, its body and tail tend to be obscured by bowel gas. Pancreatic masses and duct dilatation can be detected on ultrasound.
  - Free fluid in the abdomen is commonly seen in trauma, portal hypertension, inflammation or malignancy. This is often easily identified by ultrasound, which can be used to guide aspiration or drainage of the fluid.
  - When comparing the abdominal organs a useful mnemonic to remember is PLiSK regarding the organs echogenicity. The pancreas is normally more echogenic (bright) than the liver, the liver is more echogenic than the spleen which is lastly more echogenic than the kidneys.

PELVIS

- Assessment of the female pelvic organs is the most common indication (Fig. 7.5).
- Common abnormalities include ovarian cysts and masses, uterine fibroids, endometrial thickening and pelvic free fluid.

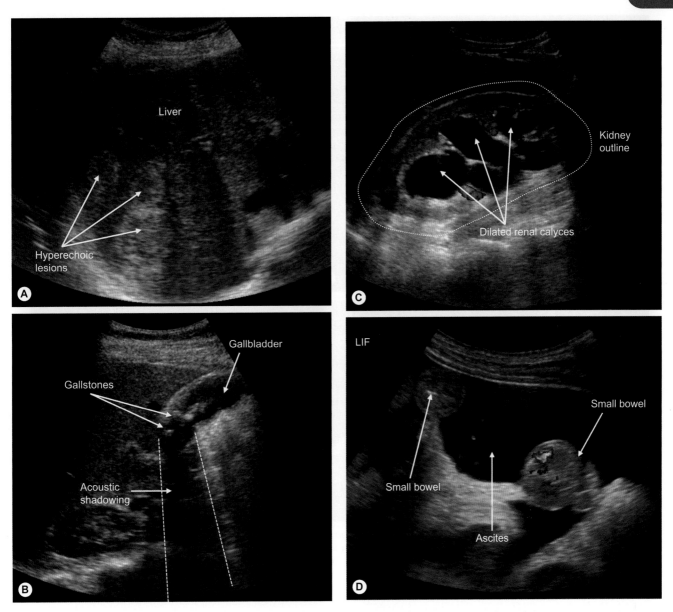

Fig. 7.4 Abdominal ultrasound images. **(A)** A view of the right lobe of the liver showing several rounded hyperechoic (bright) lesions. These are suspicious for liver metastases. Normal liver on ultrasound has a homogeneous appearance. **(B)** An image showing a gallbladder containing several small echogenic lesions which cast acoustic shadows (the black area in between the *white dotted lines* are where the lesions have completely blocked ultrasound waves. However, this strip is not entirely black because ultrasound waves can pass between the gaps between the gall stones). This is the typical appearance of gallstones. There is no gallbladder wall thickening or surrounding fluid to suggest acute cholecystitis. **(C)** This right kidney has several avascular, echo-poor areas within its medulla (these are labelled dilated renal calyces). These represent a dilated pelvicalyceal system, consistent with hydronephrosis. Colour flow represents blood flow within the renal vessels. The kidney outline is just inside the *white dotted line*. **(D)** This image of the left iliac fossa shows a large volume of free fluid (dark) surrounding small bowel loops. It is of a suitable depth to accommodate aspiration/drainage. Colour flow represents movement of the ascitic fluid.

- Ultrasound is also commonly used to assess foetuses and can identify ectopic pregnancies.
- For transabdominal pelvic ultrasound, the patient will need a full bladder. This helps to push bowel loops out of the pelvis and acts as a window through which ultrasound waves can pass (acoustic window) to permit assessment of the uterus and ovaries.

- Transvaginal ultrasound allows the ultrasound probe to lie closer to the uterus and ovaries, with no intervening bowel loops. This permits a more detailed assessment of these structures. For this examination, the patient needs an empty bladder.
- Often, the radiologist/sonographer will start with a transabdominal scan and only proceed to transvaginal scanning if further clarification is required.

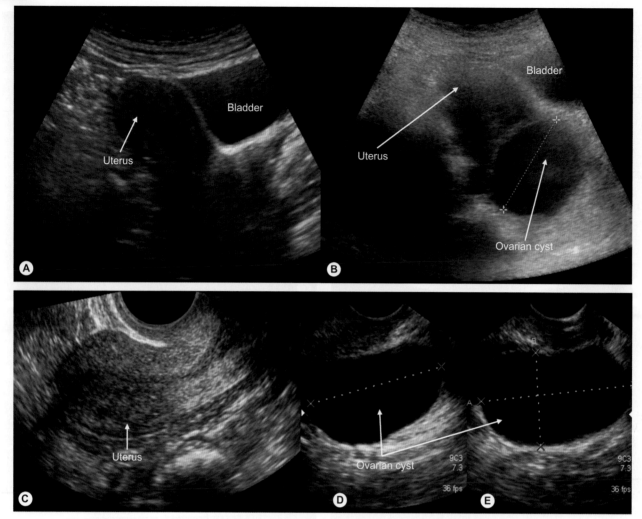

Fig. 7.5 Pelvic ultrasound images. **(A)** Transabdominal/longitudinal view of the uterus. **(B)** Transabdominal/longitudinal view of a left-sided, well-defined cyst in the same patient. **(C)** Transvaginal view of the uterus. **(D)** and **(E)** The transvaginal images (D: transverse view, E: longitudinal view) clearly show the left ovarian cyst.

- Free fluid in the pelvis in a female patient can be physiological/normal. It can accumulate in the menstrual cycle. If there is suspicion of internal bleeding, and the patient is stable, wait 15 minutes and scan again. If there is an increase in fluid, internal bleeding is likely.

FAST SCANNING

- FAST (Focused Assessment with Sonography in Trauma) scanning is used to survey trauma patients and guide decision making.
- It is used primarily to identify haemorrhage/large intraperitoneal free fluid, which appears as dark/black areas on ultrasound and may not be evident from clinical assessment alone.
- The main areas assessed are the pericardium and the area around the liver/spleen/pelvis.
- It can be rapidly performed at the bedside by emergency department physicians and trauma surgeons with a portable machine. It is usually performed after the primary survey.
- FAST scanning may not be as sensitive or specific as CT; however, unlike CT, it can be conducted quickly and simultaneously with resuscitation. The sensitivity will depend on the volume of fluid and its distribution.
- It is most useful in haemodynamically unstable patients to identify those who may require emergency surgery or further imaging with CT (e.g. those with large-volume intraabdominal haemorrhage or pericardial tamponade).
- The limitations of FAST scanning include:
  - Operator dependent (like all ultrasound).
  - Performed in suboptimal conditions (noisy, busy and bright resuscitation room), which can make accurate assessment difficult.
  - A negative FAST scan cannot exclude serious injury, and thus the patient may need a CT anyway.

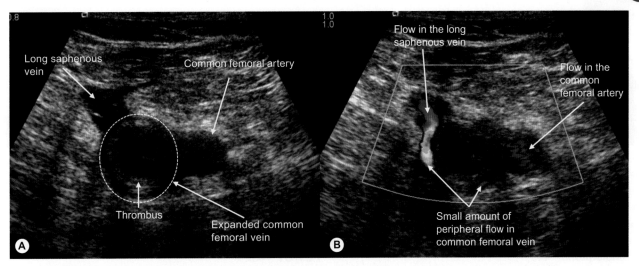

Fig. 7.6 Ultrasound images of the left common femoral vein. **(A)** The left common femoral vein is expanded with visible thrombus. It was incompressible (normal veins are easily compressible). **(B)** Colour flow imaging shows absent flow in most of the common femoral vein, with only a small amount of flow visible peripherally (*red*: flow towards the probe, *blue*: flow away from the probe. *Yellow/green* represents turbulent flow).

- Patients with a positive FAST scan often require a CT for more comprehensive assessment of their injuries.
- With the move towards early CT in trauma patients, FAST scanning may be most useful for triaging patients from a multitrauma. Those who are haemo-dynamically unstable and FAST positive (i.e. have evidence of haemorrhage) can be prioritised for either immediate CT or surgery depending on the clinical condition.

VASCULAR

- Exclusion of a deep vein thrombosis is a common indication for ultrasound (Fig. 7.6). The visible deep venous system can be assessed for compressibility and blood flow – an acute thrombus leads to an enlarged, noncompressible vein (cannot be compressed by the ultrasound probe), and if occlusive, there will be no demonstrable flow in that segment. Other causes of a painful swollen limb, such as a ruptured Baker's cyst or cellulitis, may be evident on ultrasound.
- Ultrasound can be used to assess the arterial system, looking for areas of stenosis or aneurysm. Measuring the velocity proximal and distal to a stenosis gives an indication of the degree of stenosis.

Asymptomatic AAA between 5 and 5.4 cm have surveillance scans every 6 months as per Society of Vascular Surgery guidelines, but other guidelines vary.

MUSCULOSKELETAL

There are various indications for musculoskeletal ultrasound. The more common ones include ultrasound of the shoulder to assess the rotator cuff, imaging of the Achilles and quadriceps tendons looking for partial or complete tears, assessing for tenosynovitis and trying to characterise soft tissue lumps.

ULTRASOUND-GUIDED PROCEDURES

Ultrasound is increasingly used to assist the placement of vascular lines and catheters, such as internal jugular and femoral vein lines (central lines). It allows the operator to assess the anatomy and location of the vessels and surrounding structures. Furthermore, it provides real-time images during the procedure to help ensure accurate line placement. The use of ultrasound in line placement is usually employed by critical care, anaesthetics and interventional radiology. It can also be used to guide biopsies (e.g. of the liver or a lymph node).

8

Nuclear Medicine

Erin Visser and Bryan Dalton

Chapter Outline

WHAT IS NUCLEAR MEDICINE?

Nuclear medicine (nuclear imaging/gamma imaging) uses radiopharmaceuticals to produce images. Radiopharmaceuticals are composed of two components: a radionuclide and a pharmaceutical. Radionuclides are unstable isotopes which undergo radioactive decay. The radiation emitted from certain radionuclides can be detected and measured, for example by a gamma camera. The pharmaceutical is used to localise the radionuclide to tissues of diagnostic interest. For example, Technetium 99 methylene diphosphonate (^{99m}Tc MDP) is a commonly used radiopharmaceutical in bone scanning. The methylene diphosphonate (pharmaceutical) is a bisphosphonate analogue and therefore localises to areas of osteoblastic activity. As ^{99m}Tc (a radionuclide) decays, it emits gamma rays which can be detected.

The exact combination of pharmaceutical and radionuclide depends on the indications for the scan. The main radiopharmaceuticals will be briefly mentioned later.

The methods of acquiring the images vary depending on the type of scan. In general, the radiopharmaceutical is delivered to the patient (IV, oral, inhaled) and after an appropriate amount of time, the patient lies in the gamma camera, which detects the location and amount of radiopharmaceutical in the body.

X-rays, CT, MRI, ultrasound and fluoroscopy provide anatomical imaging (i.e. they acquire images of anatomical structures and pathology is identified as changes in the normal anatomy). By contrast, nuclear medicine provides functional imaging: the pharmaceutical components take part in metabolic reactions and other processes in the body (e.g. bisphosphonate analogues used in bone imaging localise to areas of osteoblastic activity, fluorodeoxyglucose used in positron emission tomography (PET) scanning is metabolised like glucose and some radiopharmaceuticals used in renal imaging are filtered by kidneys).

The use of a pharmaceutical in the imaging process therefore means nuclear medicine can assess metabolic reactions and other functional processes in the body and hence provides functional rather than anatomical imaging. This has many advantages; it is particularly helpful as there may be significant functional changes before there is a resultant anatomical and hence consequential radiological change (e.g. the function of a kidney may significantly decrease before any obvious anatomical change occurs). Conversely, an anatomical abnormality may persist long after appropriate treatment even though it is no longer functionally active (e.g. fibrotic scarring at the site of a previous tumour deposit). Such changes may not be detectable by other imaging techniques, such as CT or MRI, but the functional changes may be picked up with nuclear medicine techniques.

The main limitation of nuclear imaging is the lack of spatial resolution and poor anatomical detail. Therefore functional and anatomical imaging are complementary and the two are increasingly used concomitantly.

PET is a specific type of nuclear medicine. Fluorine-18 (^{18}F) combined with deoxyglucose (FDG) is the most commonly used radiopharmaceutical. Deoxyglucose is a glucose analogue and therefore localises to sites of increased metabolic activity. The physics behind PET is different from other forms of nuclear imaging. As ^{18}F decays, it releases a positron (a positively charged electron), which travels only a few millimetres in the body before being annihilated by an electron. This reaction results in two high-energy photons being released simultaneously in opposite directions. A specific PET camera is used to detect the two annihilation photons and from this determine where the annihilation reaction occurred. PET is almost always combined with CT (PET-CT) to improve the quality of the data (the CT is used to permit attenuation corrections and it allows the data from PET to be fused onto a CT, which provides detailed anatomical information).

TABLE 8.1 Approximate Effective Dose of Radiation of Common Nuclear Medicine and CT Scans

TYPE OF SCAN	AGENT	APPROXIMATE EFFECTIVE DOSE (MSV)	EQUIVALENT DOSE AS CHEST X-RAYS
Bone scan	99mTc MDP	5	250
Lung perfusion scan[a]	99mTc albumin aggregated	1	50
PET/CT	18FDG	15	750
CT head	–	1.5	75
CT chest[a]	–	7	350
CT abdomen and pelvis	–	10	500

[a]A lung perfusion scan is associated with a lower overall effective dose than CTPA. This is useful in pregnant or breastfeeding mothers as it reduces the dose to the very radiosensitive breast tissue. Lung perfusion studies, however, are associated with a higher dose to the pelvic organs and therefore the foetus of pregnant patients. Due to the reduced harm to the mother's breast, lung perfusion scans are still preferred overall in pregnant patients. Mostly used in ventilation–perfusion scan combination.
18FDG, Fluorine-18 (18F) combined with deoxyglucose; MDP, methylene disphosphonate; PET/CT, positron emission tomography/computed tomography.

IONISING RADIATION

Nuclear imaging relies on radioactive decay of radionuclides and therefore is a source of ionising radiation. When the radionuclide is administered to the patient, it usually travels throughout the body and therefore results in a radiation dose to the entire body (in contrast, X-rays and CT only give a significant radiation dose to the areas being imaged). Table 8.1 gives the effective dose of some commonly performed nuclear medicine tests, along with some CT scans for comparison.

Many radiopharmaceuticals are renally excreted and therefore collect in the bladder. This can result in a high dose to the pelvic organs, including the uterus and (potentially) a foetus. Patients are instructed to frequently pass urine to reduce this.

It is important to appreciate the radiation dose delivered to the patient is unrelated to the number of images acquired. This is in contrast to X-rays and CT.

The patient is likely to remain radioactive for a few days after the examination (depending on the dose of radiopharmaceutical and its half-life). They should therefore avoid children during this period. Additionally, some radiation can be excreted into breast milk, and thus breastfeeding mothers should stop breastfeeding for a few days after the examination (exact details are available from the radiology/nuclear medicine department).

In many waiting areas, patients are isolated in individual rooms, or socially distanced by 6 feet. If they are inpatients, they are given identification markers, such as coloured wristbands, upon returning to their wards.

INDICATIONS

There are a variety of indications for nuclear medicine imaging. They are usually specialised investigations which are requested by senior clinicians. Some of the main indications are discussed later but further details can be found in the Royal College of Radiologist's guidelines (making the best use of clinical radiology services/iRefer).

CONTRAINDICATIONS

The radiation dose is the main issue to be aware of with nuclear imaging. Specific tests have specific contraindications, for example cardiac stress testing should not be performed in patients with acute myocardial infarction, unstable angina and aortic stenosis (there are other contraindications). Most other nuclear imaging tests are well tolerated.

LUNG VENTILATION–PERFUSION SCAN

- The main indication for ventilation–perfusion (V/Q) scans is to diagnose a potential pulmonary embolus.
- They are used predominantly in young patients, particularly pregnant or breastfeeding women, as the overall dose, and the dose to the breast tissue, is significantly less than a CTPA. The breast tissue in these patients is particularly radiosensitive and reducing the dose to this area reduces the risk of inducing breast cancer in the future.
- It should be noted that the radiation dose to the foetus is actually higher with a V/Q scan as the IV radiopharmaceutical is renally excreted and therefore collects in the bladder until voiding.
- The patient is given a radionuclide to inhale. Imaging with a gamma camera shows which parts of the lung are ventilated.
- A radiopharmaceutical is then given IV (usually 99mTc macroaggregated human serum albumin) to show which parts of the lung are perfused.
- Pulmonary embolism is suspected if there are areas of the lung which are ventilated but not perfused (V/Q mismatch).
- Areas in which there is both a ventilation and perfusion deficit indicate pulmonary disease.
- In reality, V/Q scans are often nonspecific and may require a further examination (e.g. CTPA) to provide the final diagnosis.
- Some centres only perform the perfusion part of the scan (Fig. 8.1) and if this raises the possibility of a PE, then a CTPA will be performed for confirmation.

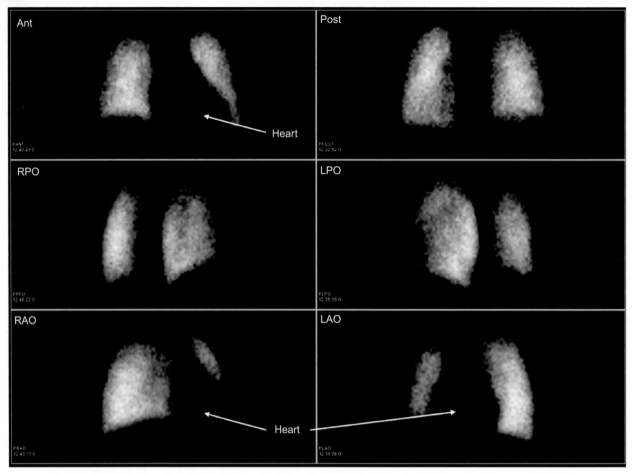

Fig. 8.1 A lung perfusion scan in a pregnant patient with a suspected PE. The images show a normal distribution of radionuclide, which effectively excludes a PE. *Ant*, Anterior; *LAO*, left anterior oblique; *LPO*, left posterior oblique; *Post*, posterior; *RAO*, right anterior oblique; *RPO*, right posterior oblique.

MYOCARDIAL PERFUSION SCAN

- Myocardial perfusion scans are specialised tests used to show the distribution of blood flow within the myocardium.
- ^{99m}TC sestamibi or $^{201}Thallium$ are the common radiopharmaceuticals. These are administered IV and taken up by myocytes proportionally to their perfusion. A gamma camera is used to detect the distribution of the radionuclide.
- Two studies are performed. A resting study shows the baseline perfusion. The stress study shows myocardial perfusion during exercise or after the administration of a pharmacological stressing agent such as adenosine.
- Infarcts appear as perfusion deficits on both the rest and stress studies whereas ischaemia will result in a defect in only the stress images.
- The site and size of infarcts and ischaemia can be identified.
- A separate nuclear medicine test can also be used to calculate the left ventricular ejection fraction. This is achieved by labelling the patient's red blood cells with a radionuclide and measuring the volume of red blood cells within the different chambers of the heart during different parts of the cardiac cycle. It is frequently used to monitor left ventricular function in patients receiving cardiotoxic chemotherapy.

GENITOURINARY SCANS

- Nuclear imaging can be used to measure renal function and assess the volume of the renal cortex.
- ^{99m}Tc DTPA (diethylenetriaminepentaacetic acid) and ^{99m}Tc MAG3 (methyl-acetyl-gly-gly-gly) can both be used to assess the split renal function (i.e. the proportion each kidney contributes to overall renal function). ^{99m}Tc MAG3 is better for patients with renal failure.
- ^{99m}Tc DTPA allows measurement of glomerular filtration rate.
- ^{99m}Tc MAG3 does not measure glomerular filtration, instead it measures the effective renal plasma flow.
- The radiopharmaceuticals are given IV and images are obtained for 30 minutes.

- ^{99m}Tc DMSA (dimercaptosuccinic acid) is used to assess the cortex. It is given IV and the patient imaged after 2 hours. The radionuclide binds to the cortex and will show areas of cortical loss/scarring as filling defects (photopenic). Such abnormalities are commonly found in pyelonephritis and its main use is for imaging children with suspected pyelonephritis.

BONE IMAGING

- The main type of bone imaging uses ^{99m}Tc phosphonates as the radionuclide (for example methylene diphosphonate (MDP)).
- Bone uptake depends mainly on osteoblastic activity but also on blood flow.

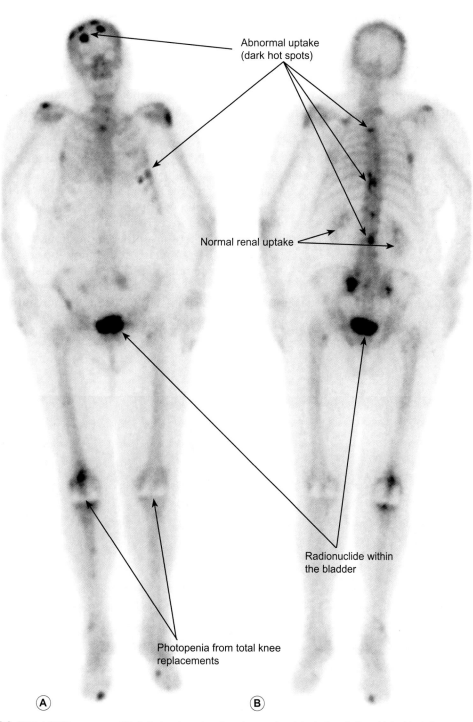

Abnormal uptake (dark hot spots)

Normal renal uptake

Radionuclide within the bladder

Photopenia from total knee replacements

(A)   (B)

Fig. 8.2 ^{99m}Tc MDP bone scan. **(A)** Anterior view showing abnormal uptake in the skull and left-sided ribs. **(B)** Posterior view showing abnormal uptake in the thoracolumbar spine. The patient was known to have breast cancer and these findings are in keeping with bone metastases. Bilateral total knee replacements appear as photopenic areas (with no uptake). *MDP*, Methylene diphosphonate.

- The radiopharmaceutical is given IV and the patient is imaged a few hours later (Fig. 8.2).
- It is useful for detecting bone metastases and is used in the staging of some tumours, such as prostate and breast cancer. It is also useful for identifying osteomyelitis and occult fractures.
- Degenerative changes (usually both sides of a joint, often symmetrical) and uptake within the soft tissues, particularly the kidneys, are common 'normal' findings.
- Asymmetric areas of markedly increased uptake are suspicious.
- Most bone metastases are osteoblastic in nature and appear as dark hot spots (due to high levels of uptake). Some tumours, such as renal cell carcinoma and thyroid cancer, result in osteolytic metastases and cause a resultant light cold spot (due to low levels of uptake) – these are easily overlooked.
- Marrow tumours, such as myeloma and lymphoma, are often not apparent on bone scans.
- Patients with diffuse osseous bone metastases (usually due to prostate cancer) can have a 'superscan' appearance. This is where there is diffuse increased uptake throughout the entire skeleton and results in a high ratio of bone to soft tissue tracer accumulation.

PET/CT

- The main indication for PET/CT is the staging of malignancies (Fig. 8.3).

- Tumours have increased glycolysis and upregulate glucose transporters. ^{18}FDG is a glucose analogue which competes with glucose for the glucose transporters. Once in the cells, it becomes partially metabolised and trapped inside the cell.
- ^{18}FDG depends not only on the glucose transporters but also peritumoral blood flow. Its uptake is not specific to malignant tumours and can occur in benign tumours and inflammatory cells. Conversely, not all malignant tumours will be 'PET positive', particularly those <1 cm in diameter.
- Patients are fasted before their scan (to reduce glucose levels and thus competition for the glucose transporters). The patients are then imaged 60 minutes after the IV injection of ^{18}FDG. A CT is usually performed to allow anatomical localisation of any abnormality and permit attenuation correction of the PET scan (the details of this are beyond the scope of this book).
- PET/CT is most commonly used in the assessment of patients with potentially curable lung tumours. Its role is to identify any other sites of disease which are not apparently on CT and that might preclude curative treatment.
- There are other indications for PET/CT, such as assessment and follow-up of lymphoma (lymphoma deposits often persist after treatment and PET/CT is used to see if they are still metabolically active) and detecting local recurrence of colorectal cancer.

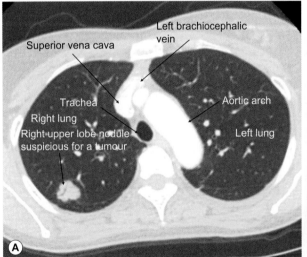
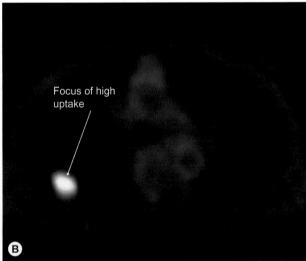

Fig. 8.3 Axial CT and PET images. **(A)** This contrast-enhanced CT shows a right upper lobe nodule which is suspicious for a malignancy. **(B)** PET performed in the same patient shows this nodule has increased uptake of FDG, indicating it is metabolically active. This is highly suggestive of malignancy. *CT*, Computed tomography; *FDG*, Fluorine-18 (^{18}F) combined with deoxyglucose; *PET*, positron emission tomography.

Fluoroscopy

Erin Visser and Bryan Dalton

9

Chapter Outline

WHAT IS FLUOROSCOPY?

Fluoroscopy (screening) uses X-rays and contrast material to produce images. The patient stands or lies on the screening table. The patient and X-ray camera are positioned and a series of low-dose X-rays are taken, often before, during and after the administration of contrast material.

Two types of images can be taken when screening (Fig. 9.1). Fluoroscopic imaging allows multiple images to be taken in quick succession. They are of lower quality than formal X-ray exposures as they use less radiation. The greyscale used is the opposite to standard X-rays, with high-attenuating material and structures, such as bone, appearing as dark areas, and low-attenuating substances, such as gas, appearing as light areas.

Formal X-ray exposures can also be acquired. These are like a normal X-ray in appearance (using the standard greyscale) and provide a more detailed image, but use a higher radiation dose and cannot be performed in quick succession. Usually a combination of these types of imaging are used during fluoroscopic studies.

The type of contrast used depends on the examination being performed. Most contrast material, such as barium, is **positive contrast** – it attenuates the X-rays significantly more than tissues and organs, and therefore appears dark on fluoroscopic imaging and bright on formal X-rays. Positive contrast materials can be water-soluble (e.g. gastrografin) or non-water soluble (e.g. barium). Barium produces the best images but is only safe for use inside the gastrointestinal tract. Water-soluble contrast, on the other hand, is safe for use almost everywhere in the body, including the

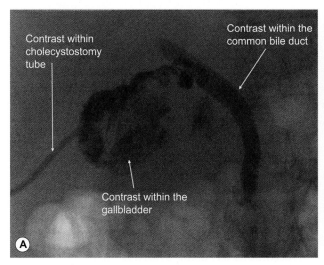

Contrast within cholecystostomy tube

Contrast within the common bile duct

Contrast within the gallblader

(A)

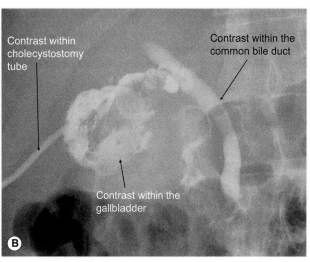

Contrast within cholecystostomy tube

Contrast within the common bile duct

Contrast within the gallblader

(B)

Fig. 9.1 Examples of a fluoroscopic and formal X-ray exposure from a cholecystostomy tubogram. **(A)** This image demonstrates that high-attenuation material, such as the contrast within the gallblader and common bile duct, are dark on fluoroscopic images and the edges of structures, such as the gallblader, are not particularly sharp. **(B)** This formal X-ray exposure performed in the same patient shows the usual greyscale we expect in X-rays, with high-contrast structures and material appearing white. Notice how the edges of the gallblader and common bile duct are better defined compared with the fluoroscopic image.

peritoneal cavity. Water-soluble contrast is therefore used for examinations where there may be leakage from the gastrointestinal tract (e.g. if the patient has a suspected viscus perforation) and for 'tubograms' (when contrast is injected into an iatrogenic tube, such as a surgical drain, urinary catheter or nasogastric tube).

Air or gas can be used as a **negative contrast** material (it attenuates the X-rays much less than tissues and organs). A double-contrast examination uses both a positive contrast material and air.

IONISING RADIATION

Fluoroscopy uses ionising radiation. The dose depends on the body part being examined, the length of the examination and whether fluoroscopic images or formal X-ray exposures are acquired. Several techniques can be used to reduce the dose, including restricting the field of view to the area of interest and reducing the frame rate. Even with these techniques, fluoroscopy can sometimes result in a significant radiation dose – a barium swallow gives approximately 2 mSv of radiation, which is similar to a CT of the head, and a barium enema uses 5 to 10 mSv of radiation, which is similar to a CT of the abdomen and pelvis.

Fluoroscopy can also result in a significant radiation exposure to the operators. The operators should use appropriate protective equipment, such as lead coats, leaded glasses and thyroid shields, dosimeter badges, and stand as far from the patient and X-ray machine as possible.

INDICATIONS

There are a variety of indications for fluoroscopy. Some previously common fluoroscopic tests, such as barium enemas and meals, have been superseded by other investigations such as endoscopy. The most frequently performed tests are barium swallows and tubograms. Some of the main indications are discussed later but further details can be found in the Royal College of Radiologist's guidelines (making the best use of clinical radiology services/iRefer).

CONTRAINDICATIONS

The patient should be sufficiently mobile to be transferred to and from the screening table. Additionally, they must be mobile and cooperative enough for the examination to be performed. For example, it is not appropriate to request a barium swallow on a patient who is drowsy as there is a significant risk of aspiration.

The other contraindications are related to the dose of ionising radiation and if there are better alternative

tests, such as CT colonography or colonoscopy rather than barium enema and endoscopy rather than barium meal.

SPECIFIC SCANS (INDICATIONS AND BASIC INTERPRETATION)

CONTRAST SWALLOW

- The term contrast swallow encompasses both barium and water-soluble contrast swallows.
- The main indications for contrast swallows are dysphagia, pain on swallowing, assessment of tracheo-oesophageal fistulae, detection of oesophageal perforation and postoperative assessment for anastomotic leaks (Figs 9.2–9.4).
- Endoscopy has largely replaced contrast swallows for the investigation of peptic ulcer disease and upper gastrointestinal haemorrhage. It is complementary to contrast swallows for the assessment of other oesophageal pathologies.
- A barium swallow produces the most comprehensive assessment of the oesophagus but is contraindicated if a viscus perforation or leak is suspected; in these cases, water-soluble contrast is used (gastrografin).
- The examination can be performed with the patient lying flat or standing (the choice is usually due to operator preference but may be influenced by patient mobility). The patient swallows a mouthful of contrast while fluoroscopy is performed. This is repeated with the patient in different positions to allow a complete assessment of the entire oesophagus.
- Contrast swallows can demonstrate various pathologies including pharyngeal pouches, strictures, extrinsic compression, achalasia (failure of the lower oesophageal sphincter to relax), hiatal hernias, reflux and perforations/leaks.

> **❶ KEY POINT**
>
> It is important to warn patients who undergo imaging with barium about its side effects. These include constipation (due to its high density) and white-coloured stools. Such side effects are temporary and are reduced by drinking plenty of fluids.

BARIUM FOLLOW-THROUGH

- Barium follow-through examinations are used to assess the small bowel.
- In the past, they were mainly used to assess inflammatory bowel disease, but this is now usually accomplished using MRI. The main indications are diarrhoea, malabsorption and partial obstruction. They are contraindicated in complete obstruction and suspected perforation (water-soluble contrast could be used in this scenario).

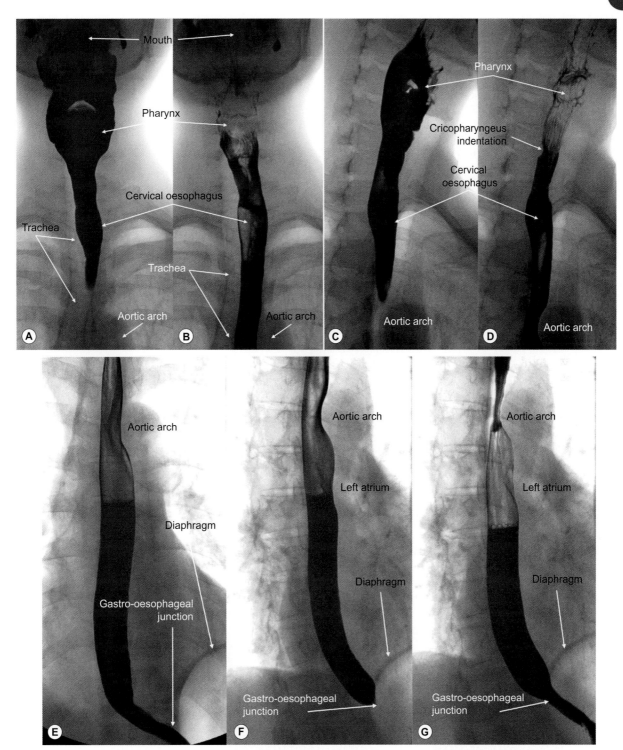

Fig. 9.2 Selected images from a normal barium swallow examination. **(A)** and **(B)** AP views of the pharynx and cervical oesophagus. **(C)** and **(D)** Lateral views of the pharynx and cervical oesophagus. The normal indentations from cricopharyngeus and the aortic arch are labelled. **(E)** Normal AP view of the mid and lower oesophagus showing the aortic arch indentation and the position of the gastroesophageal junction. **(F)** and **(G)** Oblique views of the mid and lower oesophagus with the normal indentations of the aortic arch and left atrium labelled.

- The patient is given barium to drink and images of the abdomen are obtained at different points as the barium transits through the small bowel. It is important for the barium to reach the caecum as the terminal ileum is a common site for pathology.

- Pathologies which can be demonstrated on barium follow-through include strictures, fistulae, extrinsic masses and mucosal abnormalities.

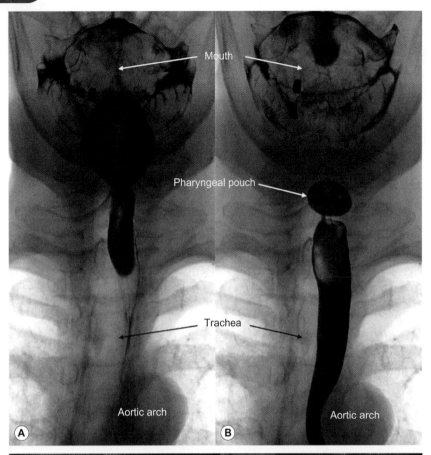

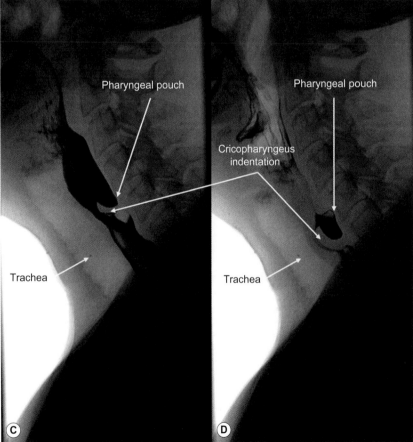

Fig. 9.3 Selected images from a barium swallow examination of the pharynx and cervical oesophagus. **(A)** and **(B)** The AP view shows an abnormal midline collection of barium in the pharynx. **(C)** and **(D)** The lateral view confirms a posterior pharyngeal pouch.

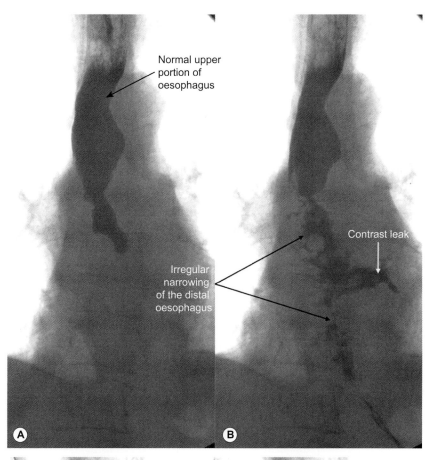

Normal upper portion of oesophagus

Contrast leak

Irregular narrowing of the distal oesophagus

A   B

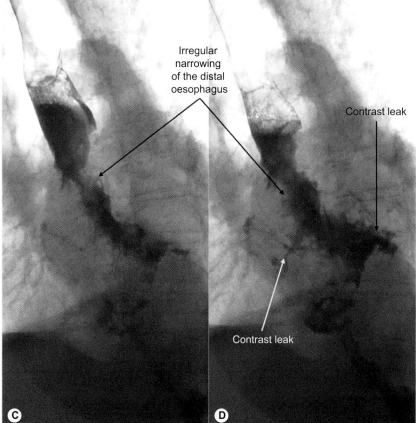

Irregular narrowing of the distal oesophagus

Contrast leak

Contrast leak

C   D

Fig. 9.4 Selected images from a water-soluble swallow examination of the lower oesophagus. (A and B) The AP and (C and D) oblique views show an irregular narrowing of the distal oesophagus. In addition, there is evidence of contrast leakage from the oesophagus into the surrounding tissues. These findings are highly suspicious of a perforated distal oesophageal tumour.

CONTRAST ENEMA

- The barium enema is a double-contrast examination (barium as the **positive contrast agent** and air as a **negative contrast agent**). It requires the patient to be relatively mobile as they have to manoeuvre to ensure the barium coats the entire colon. It uses high doses of radiation. Barium enema has almost been completely replaced by colonoscopy and CT colonoscopy and is rarely, if ever, performed.
- Water-soluble contrast enemas (Fig. 9.5) are used to assess some colonic strictures (e.g. prior to stenting of colon cancer) and to identify fistulae. They can be used to confirm a sigmoid volvulus or identify perforations/anastomotic leaks. A catheter is inserted into the rectum (the balloon may be inflated to keep it in place) and water-soluble contrast is run into the colon under gravity. The patient is manoeuvred to encourage the contrast to opacify the part of the bowel of concern and X-rays are taken with the patient in different positions to permit a thorough assessment.

TUBOGRAMS

- Tubograms refer to examinations where water-soluble contrast is injected into/through an iatrogenic tube or line, such as an NG tube, surgical drain or catheter (Fig. 9.6).
- There are various indications for tubograms:
  - To check to see if the line or tube is blocked (e.g. a central line which won't aspirate or flush).
  - To assess the position of the tip of a device (e.g. to ensure the tip of a PEG (percutaneous endoscopic gastrostomy) is within the stomach).
  - The size and shape of a collection in which a drain lies can be assessed.
  - Leaks, perforations and fistulae can be identified (e.g. a cystogram where contrast is instilled into the bladder via a catheter can identify leaks after prostate surgery or traumatic bladder injury and can outline colovesical fistulae).
- The technique varies slightly depending on the examination being performed but generally a control set of images are obtained before any contrast is administered, then a series of fluoroscopic images are taken during and after the administration of contrast. The patient may be manoeuvred to allow better assessment of any area of interest.

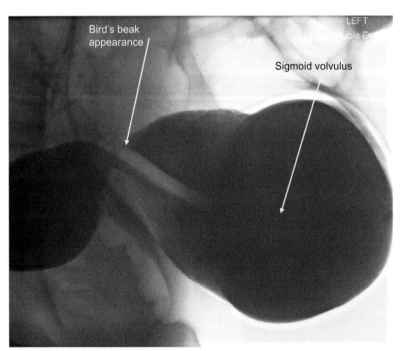

Fig. 9.5 Water-soluble enema showing the typical bird's beak appearance of a sigmoid volvulus.

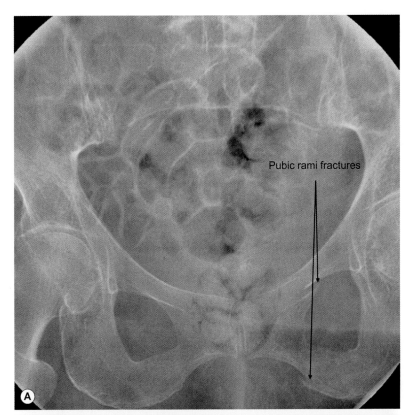

Pubic rami fractures

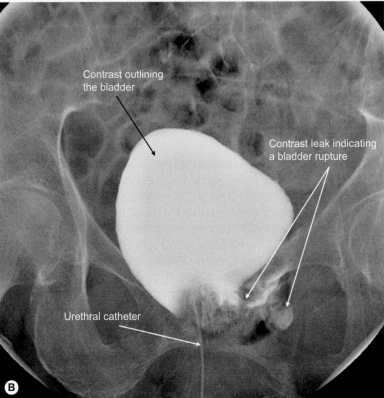

Contrast outlining the bladder

Contrast leak indicating a bladder rupture

Urethral catheter

Fig. 9.6 Water-soluble cystogram. **(A)** This pelvic X-ray exposure clearly shows left-sided superior and inferior pubic rami fractures. **(B)** Water-soluble contrast has been instilled into the bladder via a urethral catheter. This image demonstrates a leak of contrast from the left inferolateral aspect of the bladder, adjacent to the pubic rami fractures, indicating a traumatic bladder rupture.

Chapter Outline

INTRODUCTION

WHAT IS INTERVENTIONAL RADIOLOGY?

Interventional radiology (IR) involves the use of medical imaging to perform minimally invasive procedures safely and effectively. Many surgical techniques have now been replaced by the precise and noninvasive therapy achieved by these procedures. With significant advancements in technology and increased availability of high-quality imaging modalities, interventional radiologists (IRs) now play a vital role in the modern delivery of patient care. IRs can access locations throughout the body and hence can provide treatment for a multitude of conditions that affect different organ systems. In this chapter, the major procedures performed by IRs will be discussed in the context of the conditions being treated. The list of conditions and procedures discussed in this chapter are not exhaustive with respect to the role of IRs.

PRINCIPLES OF IR PROCEDURES

IRs perform minimally invasive procedures that are highly technical and require careful interpretation of different imaging modalities. Fluoroscopy, ultrasound and computed tomography are necessary for a wide range of IR procedures. IRs therefore require a solid foundation of diagnostic radiology knowledge in order to become competent in performing different procedures under accurate imaging guidance. IRs must be aware of the risks of routinely being exposed to ionising radiation and should actively take steps to minimise exposure during image-guided procedures.

Similar to surgery, forward planning is critical to ensure IR procedures are safely performed. Prior to all IR procedures, adequate patient preparation is necessary and informed consent must always be obtained. Screening blood tests, including a full blood count, renal function tests and coagulation profile, are usually performed to establish any factors that can increase the risk of complications during the procedure. Sedation can be used to relax patients and is an important consideration for extended procedures. Prophylactic analgesia should always be considered, especially for procedures that are predicted to be painful.

There is a wide variety of essential equipment that IRs must become familiar with in order to competently perform many procedures. Commonly used IR equipment includes guidewires, catheters, sheaths, angioplasty balloons and stents. Regardless of the procedure, the initial step in every IR procedure is gaining access. Once access is achieved, for most IR procedures, guidewires are inserted and directed towards the target location. Further equipment such as catheters can then be advanced over the guidewire to perform interventions inside the body.

THE SELDINGER TECHNIQUE

Establishing safe and effective vascular access is a fundamental aspect of achieving technical success with endovascular procedures. The choice of artery or vein for vascular access is crucial and is highly dependent on the type of procedure being performed. The Seldinger technique is the most commonly used method of gaining safe vascular access. Fig. 10.1 illustrates the key steps of the Seldinger technique.

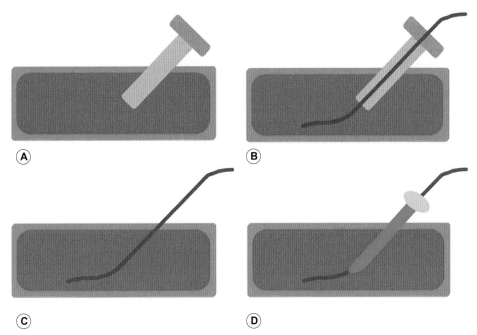

Fig. 10.1 The Seldinger technique. **(A)** A vascular access needle with a hollow core is advanced into the lumen of the vessel. **(B)** Once a bleed back is seen in the needle, a guidewire is introduced through the needle into the vessel. **(C)** The needle can then be removed, leaving the guidewire. **(D)** An introducer sheath is inserted over the guidewire to provide a stable conduit through which catheters, balloons or stents can be easily placed under imaging guidance.

IMAGE-GUIDED DRAINS

Image-guided drains are indicated for treatment of accessible fluid collections and are an alternative to surgical intervention in most cases. Ultrasound or CT imaging is generally used to safely guide drainage procedures. Ultrasound presents an advantage over CT because the position of the needle or catheter can be monitored in real time.

Samples of fluid collected can be sent for diagnostic tests to determine the contents of the fluid and the likely cause of the collection. Diagnostic studies can include microbiological, cytological, biochemical and histopathological analysis. The inserted drain should be monitored regularly to ensure that it does not become displaced or blocked. Drainage output should also be documented daily.

INTRATHORACIC COLLECTIONS

Thoracentesis (also known as a pleural tap) is needle aspiration of fluid from a pleural effusion.

- A thoracentesis can be performed to drain a volume of pleural fluid to relieve symptoms of a pleural effusion (Fig. 10.2). The pleural fluid obtained can also be investigated for diagnostic purposes.
- The intercostal neurovascular bundle is located along the lower edge of each rib. Therefore, the needle must be placed over the upper edge of the rib to avoid damage to the neurovascular bundle.

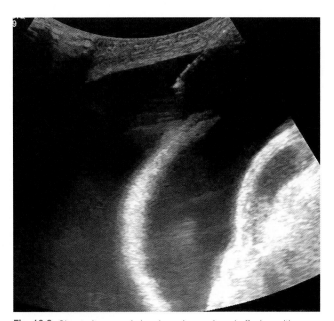

Fig. 10.2 Chest ultrasound showing a large pleural effusion with a collapsed lung. A thoracentesis needle is advanced into the pleural space. (Courtesy Dr Ram Kishore Reddy Gurajala.)

A chest drain (also known as an intercostal catheter) can be inserted into the pleural space to drain air, fluid, blood or pus from the chest.

- The chest drain is connected to an underwater seal suction apparatus below the patient. A chest X-ray is performed shortly after drain insertion to confirm correct tube placement.

- A chest drain can be used to resolve pneumothoraces that are recurrent, large, traumatic, bilateral or under tension.
- A chest drain can also be inserted to drain symptomatic or recurrent pleural effusion. Some clinicians advise against draining in excess of 1.5 L of pleural fluid in 24 hours due to the potential risk of reexpansion pulmonary oedema. However, there is currently a lack of evidence that the risk of reexpansion pulmonary oedema is proportional to the volume of fluid removed.

ABDOMINAL AND PELVIC COLLECTIONS

Image-guided percutaneous drainage of abdominal and pelvic collections is one of the most commonly performed interventional procedures.

- Common fluid collections include purulent fluid, blood, bile, urine, lymph and pancreatic secretions.
- Fluid can be drained to determine if it is infected or sterile. Abscesses are a common source of sepsis and can be amenable to percutaneous drainage. This is commonly performed in postoperative patients.
- Fluid from visceral organs such as the liver, spleen and pancreas can accumulate in various spaces and be treated with percutaneous drainage. The optimal drainage point can be marked by ultrasound.
- Ascites refers to fluid within the peritoneal cavity and it can be drained percutaneously by paracentesis for diagnostic and therapeutic purposes. A diagnostic paracentesis should be performed in all patients with new-onset ascites. Therapeutic paracentesis is a first-line therapy in patients with tense ascites and treatment-refractory ascites, especially when diuretics become ineffective, or their side effects prevent their continued use.

PERICARDIAL EFFUSION

- Pericardial fluid can be withdrawn for diagnostic purposes to investigate the cause of an effusion.
- Pericardiocentesis is also performed to urgently drain pericardial fluid to manage haemodynamically unstable patients with cardiac tamponade.

IMAGE-GUIDED BIOPSIES

Image-guided biopsies can be performed to allow histological analysis of various lesions located in various parts of the body. These procedures do carry small, common risks of bleeding and infection, in addition to specific risks associated with each type of biopsy. They have largely replaced exploratory laparotomy as a method of tissue diagnosis.

Ultrasound is typically used as it is relatively inexpensive and provides real-time localisation of structures especially if they are located superficially. Ultrasound can also be performed at the bedside, so is especially useful in the intensive care setting. However, ultrasound does not effectively visualise through air and bone due to poor sound transmission. CT can be used to give better visualisation of bone and air-filled structures such as the lungs and bowel loops. Other techniques such as MRI or PET-guided biopsy are occasionally performed; however, they are limited by availability and cost.

Most image-guided biopsies can be performed as an outpatient procedure with a short recovery period. When considering the ideal route of the biopsy, the shortest route from the skin to the lesion should be taken whilst avoiding vital structures.

LIVER

Liver biopsies are usually performed under ultrasound guidance. It may be targeted or nontargeted:

- Targeted liver biopsies are used to sample discrete focal lesions such as cancer.
- Non-targeted liver biopsies are useful to identify the cause and stage of liver disease.

A liver biopsy can be performed with the percutaneous approach or transjugular approach:

- The percutaneous approach is a reliable and accurate method of sampling liver tissue. It is important to avoid crossing the pleural space as this could increase the risk of pneumothorax. If ascites is present, they should drain prior to biopsy to reduce the distance to the liver. The liver is a highly vascular organ; hence, the risk of haemorrhage must also be considered.
- The transjugular approach is generally reserved for patients with uncorrectable coagulopathy, who have concomitant ascites or in those who need pressure assessments.
- Specific risks of liver biopsies include injury to bile ducts or gallbladder increasing the risk of biloma and biliary peritonitis.

RENAL

- Renal biopsies can be performed under ultrasound and CT guidance (Fig. 10.3).
- They are commonly performed to establish the cause of intrinsic renal disease if present or to diagnose the cause of a renal mass.
- Specific risks of renal biopsies include damage to the biliary system and renal collection system.

ADRENAL

- Adrenal biopsies are usually performed under CT guidance (Fig. 10.4).
- They can be performed to diagnose the nature of an adrenal mass that remains indeterminate after imaging.
- A specific risk of adrenal biopsy is damage to the adjacent kidney.

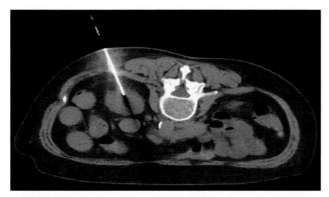

Fig. 10.3 Axial slice from a CT of the abdomen. A biopsy of the right kidney is being performed under CT guidance for assessment of intrinsic renal disease. (Courtesy Dr Ram Kishore Reddy Gurajala.)

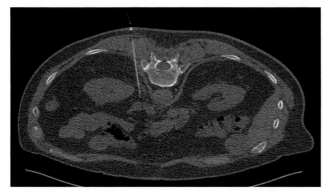

Fig. 10.4 Axial slice from a CT of the abdomen. A biopsy of the right adrenal gland is being performed under CT guidance for assessment of an adrenal lesion. (Courtesy Dr Ram Kishore Reddy Gurajala.)

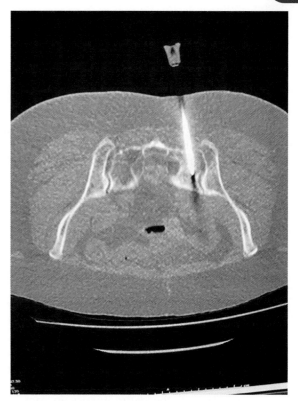

Fig. 10.5 Axial slice from a CT of the pelvis. A biopsy of the sacral bone is being performed under CT guidance for assessment of a bone lesion. (Courtesy Dr Aamer Iqbal)

THORACIC

- Thoracic biopsies are usually performed under CT guidance.
- They are performed to diagnose the cause of suspicious lesions in the lung, pleura and mediastinum.
- Specific risks of thoracic biopsies include pneumothorax, pulmonary haemorrhage and air embolism.

BONE

- Bone biopsies are typically performed under CT or fluoroscopic guidance (Fig. 10.5).
- They are commonly used in bone infections and malignancy.
- A specific risk of bone biopsy is damage to the adjacent neurovascular structures. For vertebral biopsies, the risk of damage to the spinal cord must also be considered.

ARTERIAL INTERVENTIONS

PERIPHERAL ARTERIAL DISEASE

Revascularisation therapy is indicated:
- In peripheral arterial disease (PAD) where patients continue to experience functional impairment

from intermittent claudication symptoms despite employment of conservative measures.
- In patients with features of critical limb ischaemia such as rest pain, ulceration and gangrene.

There are various modalities available for revascularisation therapy. The choice of modality depends on several factors such as the location and morphology of disease, patient preferences and comorbidities. Percutaneous transluminal angioplasty (PTA) is the primary endovascular strategy for dilating vascular occlusions. Various types of angioplasty balloons can be inserted into different vessels depending on the dimension of the balloons. Stents can be inserted with angioplasty to increase arterial patency and reduce the risk of reocclusion. PTA is used when the occlusion affects a single arterial segment. It is generally the first-line option in patients with aortoiliac disease.

ACUTE LIMB ISCHAEMIA

- Acute limb ischaemia is a serious limb-threatening condition that is managed initially with intravenous heparin. Urgent revascularisation is needed to restore perfusion.
- Intraarterial catheter-directed thrombolysis is an endovascular procedure that can be performed acutely. It involves inserting a catheter directly into

a thrombus so that thrombolytic agents can be delivered and the thrombus removed.

- Other minimally invasive procedures such as mechanical thrombectomy have also been used to treat acute limb ischaemia.

ACUTE MESENTERIC ISCHAEMIA

- Endovascular strategies can be employed in certain patients with acute mesenteric ischaemia. It is considered in patients who are hemodynamically stable and do not have features of advanced intestinal ischemia.
- Endovascular strategies for acute mesenteric ischaemia include catheter-directed thrombolysis, mechanical thrombectomy and angioplasty with or without stenting.

AORTIC ANEURYSMS

- EVAR of AAA can be performed as an elective procedure or as an emergency procedure if there is a known or suspected rupture.
- Thoracic aortic endovascular aneurysmal repair (TEVAR) is used to treat thoracic aortic aneurysms.
- Endovascular repair procedures involve placing a stent-graft through the entire aneurysm sac. This acts as a channel for blood to flow through the aneurysm and reduces the pressure on the aneurysm sac.
- Endovascular repair is less invasive compared to open surgical repair; however, there is a higher rate of re-intervention.
- For EVAR, significant oversizing of the graft can cause branch vessels to be inadvertently occluded. Undersizing the graft can lead to inadequate AAA repair and the requirement for further interventions. The graft should ideally extend from below the renal arteries to the iliac bifurcation.
- A common complication of endovascular repair is an endoleak where blood persistently leaks back into the aneurysm sack following the procedure. This can expand the aneurysm sac and potentially lead to rupture.
- Patients who have had an EVAR require lifelong imaging surveillance to assess the AAA diameter, graft morphology and to actively monitor for complications such as endoleak.

AORTIC DISSECTION

- TEVAR can be used to treat patients with an aortic dissection that does not involve the ascending aorta. This type of aortic dissection is classified as a Stanford B aortic dissection.
- A stent-graft is placed to cover the intimal tear in the aorta. This will enhance blood flow into the true aortic lumen and promote thrombosis of the false lumen.
- TEVAR can only be performed in patients who have suitable anatomy to allow adequate thoracic aortic access.

HEPATIC INTERVENTIONS

PORTAL HYPERTENSION

- In patients who have treatment-refractory variceal haemorrhage due to portal hypertension, a transjugular intrahepatic portosystemic shunt (TIPSS) can be placed (Fig. 10.6).
- The TIPSS procedure involves creating an artificial shunt between the portal and systemic venous circulation to reduce portal pressure. It can be a definitive treatment for portal hypertension in appropriately selected individuals.
- After the TIPSS procedure, pressure measurements and venography are performed to assess if the required portosystemic pressure gradient has been achieved and if further shunt dilation is necessary.
- Relative and absolute contraindications of TIPSS include hepatic encephalopathy, advanced liver failure and heart failure.
- Other indications for TIPSS include treatment-refractory ascites, hepatic hydrothorax and Budd–Chiari syndrome.

LIVER TRANSPLANT

- Patients who have had a liver transplant are at risk of complications which can be managed by endovascular procedures.

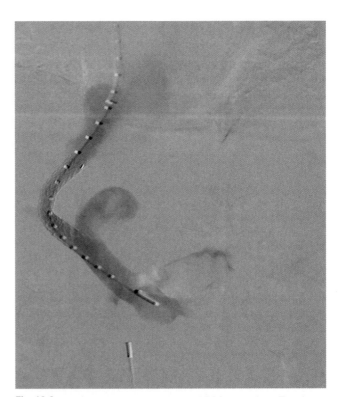

Fig. 10.6 Right hepatic venography of a TIPSS procedure. The shunt is placed from the main hepatic vein to the main portal vein. *TIPSS,* Transjugular intrahepatic portosystemic shunt. (Courtesy Dr Ram Kishore Reddy Gurajala.)

- Hepatic artery stenosis is a relatively common complication following liver transplantation. Reduced perfusion through the hepatic artery is concerning in liver transplantation and can lead to hepatocellular necrosis, biliary injury and graft failure. An angioplasty with or without a stent can be inserted to open the hepatic artery.
- Other procedures can be employed depending on the presentation including biliary interventions, drainages and hepatic interventions.

BILIARY INTERVENTIONS

BILIARY OBSTRUCTION/LEAK

- Patients with an infected, obstructed biliary obstruction or biliary leak require urgent drainage.
- Percutaneous biliary procedures have become less frequent as endoscopic techniques have matured. ERCP is the preferred method to drain the biliary system. However, ERCP may not be feasible due to a patient's anatomy. For example, if there is malignant obstruction of the biliary ducts or if they have had gastric bypass surgery.
- Percutaneous transhepatic cholangiography (PTC) and percutaneous transhepatic biliary drainage (PTBD) can be considered when ERCP is not feasible (Fig. 10.7).
- PTC is a minimally invasive technique to image the biliary system. The PTC technique facilitates the passage of a catheter to drain the biliary system and is referred to as PTBD.
- The major complications of PTC and PTBD include haemobilia, infection and damage to surrounding structures.

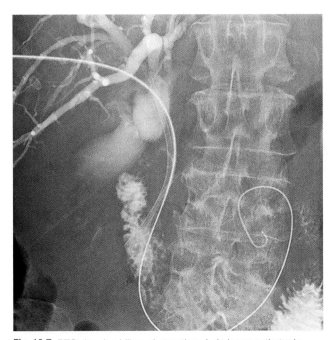

Fig. 10.7 PTC showing biliary obstruction. A drainage catheter is inserted to drain the biliary obstruction (PTBD). *PTBD*, Percutaneous transhepatic biliary drainage; *PTC*, percutaneous transhepatic cholangiography. (Courtesy Dr Praveen Eadala.)

ACUTE CHOLECYSTITIS

- In patients with acute cholecystitis, treatment typically involves conservative management and early laparoscopic cholecystectomy. For patients who are not suitable for acute surgery or have developed complications such as gallbladder empyema, a percutaneous cholecystostomy should be considered.
- A percutaneous cholecystostomy involves placing a catheter directly into the gallbladder to drain bile (Fig. 10.8). The drain is left in place until a tract has formed around it or a cholecystectomy can be safely performed at a later date.

GASTROINTESTINAL INTERVENTIONS

NUTRITIONAL SUPPORT

- For patients who have impaired oral intake and have an increased risk of aspiration, enteral feeding can be provided. Enteral feeding refers to feeding via the gastrointestinal tract.
- A gastrostomy tube can be inserted to provide long-term enteral nutrition. It can also be used for gastric decompression.
- Gastrostomy tubes can be inserted surgically, endoscopically or radiologically.
- Radiologically inserted gastrostomy (RIG) tubes require the stomach to be insufflated with air using a nasogastric tube. The stomach is punctured between the lesser and greater curvature of the stomach to reduce damage to vasculature. The stomach is fastened to the anterior abdominal wall. Serial dilators can then be used to dilate the puncture hole and allow a gastrostomy tube to be inserted and secured to the skin with sutures.

GASTROINTESTINAL STENTING

- Gastrointestinal stents can be placed endoscopically or under fluoroscopic guidance.
- For patients who have dysphagia from an unresectable or inoperable oesophageal carcinoma, symptomatic relief can be provided by inserting an oesophageal stent. A common complication of oesophageal stents is stent migration.

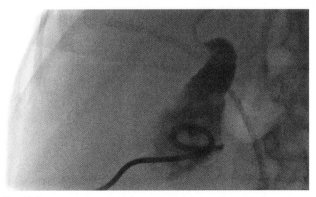

Fig. 10.8 Fluoroscopic image showing a percutaneous cholecystostomy inserted into the gallbladder. (Courtesy Dr Ram Kishore Reddy Gurajala.)

- For patients who have emergency bowel obstruction due to colorectal cancer, symptomatic relief can be provided by inserting a colorectal stent. Colorectal stents are typically used in the palliative setting. They do not significantly affect the activities of daily living compared to if stomas are inserted.

GENITOURINARY INTERVENTIONS

OBSTRUCTIVE UROPATHY

- Obstructive uropathy refers to any obstruction of the urinary tract.
- External urinary drainage can be performed by percutaneous nephrostomy (PCN) to treat obstructive uropathy. This can treat any hydronephrosis and reduce the risk of subsequent septicaemia and loss of renal function.
- PCN can allow urinary diversion to allow healing of a urinary fistula or leak. It can also be performed to allow access for certain procedures such as extracorporeal shock wave lithotripsy and antegrade ureteral stenting.
- The safest place to access the kidney for PCN is in the avascular plane of Brodel, just posterior to the lateral border of the kidney. This area has a relative paucity of vessels. Urinary drainage should be carefully monitored to evaluate if decompression has been achieved.
- Antegrade ureteral stenting can be inserted when long-term ureteric drainage is required and can be used to replace a nephrostomy tube that has already been inserted. They drain from the renal pelvis to the native bladder.

SUPRAPUBIC CATHETER

- Patients with acute urinary retention should ideally receive urethral catheterisation.
- A suprapubic catheter can be inserted to treat urinary retention for patients where urethral catheterisation is not feasible. For example, if a patient has urethral trauma.
- It can be performed under ultrasound guidance if needed.

RENAL ARTERY STENOSIS

- Renal artery stenosis (RAS) is a cause of renovascular hypertension and renal failure.
- The reasons for RAS are various and commonly include atherosclerotic disease and vasculitis. RAS can also occur as a complication of renal transplantation.
- Angioplasty with or without stenting can be performed to treat RAS.

NEUROLOGICAL INTERVENTIONS

ACUTE ISCHAEMIC STROKE

- The mainstay of management of acute ischaemic stroke is urgent revascularisation to reperfuse salvageable brain tissue and minimise the extent of infarction.

- Revascularisation can be achieved by thrombolysis or by mechanical thrombectomy. The benefit of both therapies is highly time-dependent.
- Thrombolysis is performed with a synthetic tissue plasminogen activator.
- Thrombolysis is currently licensed in patients who present within four and a half hours of symptom onset. Thrombolysis has limited benefit in patients who present beyond this timeframe.
- There are a number of contraindications to thrombolysis such as evidence of intracranial haemorrhage.
- Mechanical thrombectomy is an endovascular procedure to retrieve a thrombus from a vessel under guidance of angiography. A range of devices are available to retrieve the clot.
- Mechanical thrombectomy is used in carefully selected patients. Its use depends on the location of the stroke and the potential for the procedure to salvage brain tissue.
- Mechanical thrombectomy can be combined with thrombolysis if there are no contraindications and if within the licensed timeframe.
- Mechanical thrombectomy can have better outcomes than thrombolysis in patients with large-vessel occlusions, especially in the anterior circulation.

ANEURYSMAL SUBARACHNOID HAEMORRHAGE

- Subarachnoid haemorrhage (SAH) caused by rupture of a cerebral aneurysm is an emergency that requires urgent treatment. Aneurysms can be secured by an endovascular procedure known as coiling. An alternative approach is microsurgical clipping which is performed by neurosurgeons.
- Endovascular coiling is generally preferred to microsurgical clipping for aneurysmal SAH to minimise the risk of rebleeding. Platinum microcoils are inserted into the aneurysm lumen using a catheter. The coils interrupt blood flow and induce clot formation to close off the aneurysmal sac.

CAROTID ARTERY STENOSIS

- Significant carotid artery stenosis can increase the risk of a transient ischaemic attack and ischaemic stroke.
- Carotid artery stenting (CAS) can be performed in patients who are not suitable for carotid endarterectomy or are at increased risk of perioperative complications. It has the potential to offer similar benefits to carotid endarterectomy with lower procedural risk and at a lower cost.

MUSCULOSKELETAL INTERVENTIONS

JOINT INJECTIONS

- Joint injections can be performed for interventional purposes such as injecting intraarticular steroids for severe joint pain.

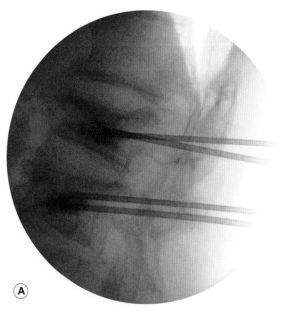
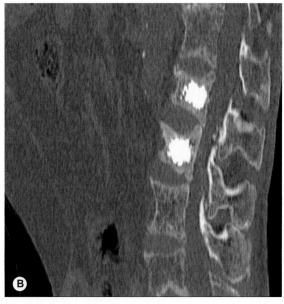

Fig. 10.9 Vertebroplasty. **(A)** Fluoroscopic image showing vertebroplasty needles advanced into the L1 and L2 vertebral bodies. **(B)** Sagittal slice from a CT of the lumbar vertebrae. Vertebroplasty has been performed and bone cement has been injected into the L1 and L2 vertebral bodies. (Courtesy of Dr Radhesh Lalam.)

- Joint aspirations can also be performed for diagnostic purposes to determine the cause of a joint effusion.

VERTEBRAL FRACTURES

- Vertebral compression fractures commonly occur in patients with decreased bone density due to osteoporosis or malignancy.
- Vertebroplasty and kyphoplasty procedures may be performed in patients who have progressive pain despite conservative treatment with analgesia and bracing.
- Vertebroplasty is performed to stabilise the vertebral column and involves the injection of bone cement into fractured vertebra (Fig. 10.9).
- Kyphoplasty involves inserting a balloon into the vertebral body. Bone cement is injected to restore the lost height from the vertebral compression fracture.
- Kyphoplasty reduces kyphotic deformation and is especially useful in patients suffering from severe vertebral collapse.

BLEEDING INTERVENTIONS

- Embolisation refers to a minimally invasive technique to occlude bleeding blood vessels. Various embolisation materials are available depending on the clinical situation.

TRAUMA

- Embolisation is an important aspect of managing many traumatic injuries.
- In abdominal trauma, arteries supplying the spleen, liver and kidneys can all be accessed sub-selectively and embolisation can be performed to manage any haemorrhage.
- Splenic injuries were previously managed by a splenectomy. Splenic artery embolisation allows spleen function to be maintained. Preserving the spleen is useful to reduce the risk of encapsulated bacterial infections.
- Hepatic injuries can result in significant haemorrhage as the liver has a dual blood supply. Embolisation management has an advantage over surgical management as surgery has a risk of causing further haemorrhage when the liver is being mobilised.
- In pelvic trauma, embolisation is the treatment of choice for hemodynamically significant haemorrhage. It is often preferred to surgical management as multiple, small arterial branches are usually involved in pelvic trauma which can be difficult to recognise intraoperatively.

POSTPARTUM HAEMORRHAGE

- Uterine artery embolisation can be a lifesaving procedure for women with postpartum haemorrhage. It is especially considered when uterotonic medications have failed or there is uncontrolled bleeding.
- Uterine artery embolisation has the advantage of preserving the patient's fertility as there is collateral blood supply to the uterus by ovarian arteries.

GASTROINTESTINAL BLEEDING

- Angiography and embolisation are important aspects of managing bleeding from arteries supplying the gastrointestinal tract (Fig. 10.10).

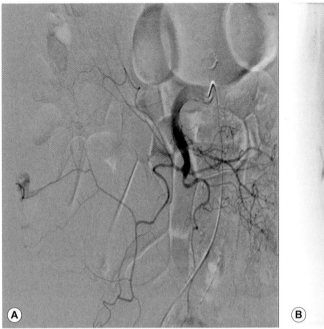
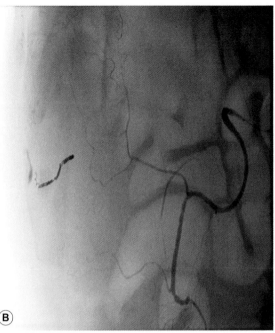

Fig. 10.10 GI bleeding. **(A)** Arteriogram showing extravasation of contrast. **(B)** Arteriogram done after embolisation with microcoils and no further bleeding. (Courtesy Dr Ram Kishore Reddy Gurajala.)

- For upper GI bleeding, treatment is usually performed by endoscopy. Embolisation can be performed if endoscopic measures fail.
- For lower GI bleeding, embolisation is an important aspect of managing active bleeding as access is usually difficult with endoscopy.

GASTRIC VARICES

- Gastric varices can occur as a complication of portal hypertension.
- A balloon-occluded retrograde transvenous obliteration procedure (BRTO) can be performed to treat treatment-refractory gastric variceal haemorrhage. It is especially considered in patients who have uncontrollable encephalopathy, isolated gastric varices and in those who have contraindications to TIPSS.

HAEMOPTYSIS

- Massive haemoptysis often occurs due to abnormalities in the bronchial circulation.
- Bronchial artery embolisation (BAE) can be performed to treat massive haemoptysis.
- The spinal arteries are located close to the bronchial arteries. It is therefore important to monitor for neurological symptoms after BAE as the spinal arteries can be inadvertently blocked.

EPISTAXIS

- Severe epistaxis may occur in patients with hypertension or bleeding disorders, or following severe traumatic injury.

- Embolisation of the internal maxillary artery can be performed as an alternative to surgical ligation for severe epistaxis.

VENOUS INTERVENTIONS

DEEP VEIN THROMBOSIS

- DVT can lead to fatal complications such as pulmonary embolism and post-thrombotic syndrome (PTS).
- Long-term anticoagulation forms the mainstay of management of DVTs; however, in many cases, its use is not sufficient to prevent complications.
- Catheter-directed thrombolysis (CDT) can be performed to prevent complications of an acute DVT. Venous access is ideally performed under ultrasound guidance to reduce the risk of puncturing an artery. The presence of thrombolytic agents in the artery can significantly increase the risk of bleeding.
- Recombinant tissue plasminogen activator (rt-PA) is the thrombolytic agent of choice. It has a short half-life and is mostly eliminated by the liver.
- CDT is performed for patients with symptomatic proximal DVT who exhibit anatomic and/or clinical progression during anticoagulation therapy.
- CDT can be performed as an adjunct to anticoagulant therapy to enable quicker symptom relief and prevent PTS in patients with symptomatic proximal DVT. Patients with iliofemoral DVT are especially considered for CDT as it can be highly effective.
- Mechanical thrombectomy can also be performed and combined with CDT to remove the DVT.

OTHER INTERVENTIONS

UTERINE FIBROIDS

- The majority of uterine fibroids are identified incidentally, and treatment is often not necessary.
- Uterine artery embolisation can be performed to reduce the size of uterine fibroids and relieve symptoms.

PELVIC VENOUS CONGESTION

- Pelvic venous congestion syndrome refers to chronic pelvic pain caused by retrograde flow through incompetent valves in ovarian veins. These veins have a similar pathology to varicose veins.
- Ovarian vein embolisation is an effective treatment for pelvic venous congestion.

VASCULAR MALFORMATIONS

- Vascular malformations can be embolised to reduce the size of the malformation and the risk of bleeding.
- It is typically performed in high-flow lesions where there is an abnormal connection between the arterial and venous systems.

VARICOCELE

- A varicocele refers to an enlargement and tortuosity of the pampiniform plexus in the scrotum.
- Gonadal vein embolisation can be performed for symptomatic varicoceles.

INFERTILITY

- Fallopian tube disease is a common cause of female infertility.
- In appropriate conditions, Fallopian tube recanalisation can be performed to reopen a proximal fallopian tube occlusion.

PULMONARY EMBOLISM

- CDT has also become a novel therapy for the management of a massive PE.
- To prevent a PE, an IVC filter can be inserted to trap venous emboli. The IVC filter is released into the vena cava and is typically deployed inferior to the lowest renal veins. Most IVC filters have hooks so that they can be held in the vena cava and prevent migration.
- IVCs act to filter the blood but do not prevent the formation of a new thrombus. They are commonly used in patients with a contraindication to anticoagulation.

VARICOSE VEINS

- Endovenous thermal ablation can be performed in patients who have symptomatic varicose veins that do not respond to conservative measures.
- Endovenous thermal ablation involves using laser or high-frequency radio waves over an affected vein to seal it off and prevent further blood flow. Blood will then be diverted to other veins with proper valve functioning.
- Sclerotherapy can also be used for varicose veins and involves injecting a chemical irritant to ablate the varicose veins.

DIALYSIS FISTULAE AND GRAFTS

- Long-term haemodialysis can be facilitated by surgically creating an anastomosis between an artery and a vein to create safe, large-bore vascular access for haemodialysis.
- The use of native vessels to create an anastomosis is called an arteriovenous fistula (AVF). Alternatively, prosthetic materials can be used to create an AV graft (AVG).
- Endovascular procedures can be performed to maintain the function of haemodialysis access. Stenosis is a common complication in both AVFs and AVGs and can be managed by angioplasty.

MAY–THURNER SYNDROME

- May–Thurner syndrome occurs when the left common iliac vein is compressed against the lumbar vertebrae by the overlying right common iliac artery.
- These patients are at risk of developing an iliofemoral DVT.
- Venous percutaneous transluminal angioplasty (PTA) and stenting can be performed to recanalise an occluded vein.
- Venous PTA is also indicated in other causes of venous stenosis such as in superior vena cava obstruction or Budd–Chiari syndrome.

CENTRAL VENOUS ACCESS

- Central venous catheters (CVCs) can be inserted under image guidance with greater reliability and cost-effectiveness to surgical placement.
- The tip of the CVC is ideally placed at or below where the superior vena cava meets the right atrium (cavoatrial junction).
- CVCs allow intravenous access to be maintained long term. This allows intravenous medications to be delivered for an extended period, frequent blood transfusions and sampling to be performed. Central venous access also allows rapid fluid resuscitation.
- Medications that are harmful to peripheral veins can be safely administered with CVCs. This includes chemotherapy and total parenteral nutrition.
- There are four main types of CVC: PICC lines, non-tunnelled central catheters, tunnelled central catheters and implantable ports.

PERIPHERALLY INSERTED CENTRAL CATHETER

- PICC lines are percutaneously inserted into the basilic, brachial or cephalic veins and then advanced into the central veins.
- They are frequently used for patients requiring central venous access for short durations; however, insertion requires an accessible peripheral vein.
- PICC lines have advantages over traditional CVCs such as being more cost-effective and being more safely inserted as there are no vital organs in the arms.

TUNNELLED CENTRAL CATHETER

- Tunnelled central catheters provide a more long-term method of central venous access compared to nontunnelled central catheters.
- Tunnelled central catheters enter the skin at one location and enter the central vein at a different location (Fig. 10.11). A tunnel is created subcutaneously between these two points and provides separation between the external portion of the catheter and where the catheter enters the central vein (venotomy site). A catheter is pulled through the created tunnel towards the venotomy site. Blunt dissection is used to ensure there is no skin or fibrous tissue between the catheter and venotomy site.

- The tunnel improves the stability of the device and can therefore be used long term. It also reduces the risk of infection.

NONTUNNELLED CENTRAL CATHETER

- Nontunnelled central catheters are percutaneously inserted directly into a central vein such as the internal jugular vein. The external portion of the catheter directly overlies the venous access site (Fig. 10.11).
- Nontunnelled central catheters are only used for short-term central venous access such as in the intensive care setting where emergency access may be needed.

IMPLANTABLE PORTS

- Implantable ports consist of a catheter attached to a mechanical reservoir (Fig. 10.11).
- Implantable ports are inserted using a similar method to the tunnelled central venous catheter. The reservoir is buried entirely under the skin inside a subcutaneous pocket. It is connected to a tunnelled catheter that is inserted into a central vein.
- The reservoir has a self-healing silicone surface that can be repeatedly accessed. A Huber needle can be used to puncture through the skin to access the port.

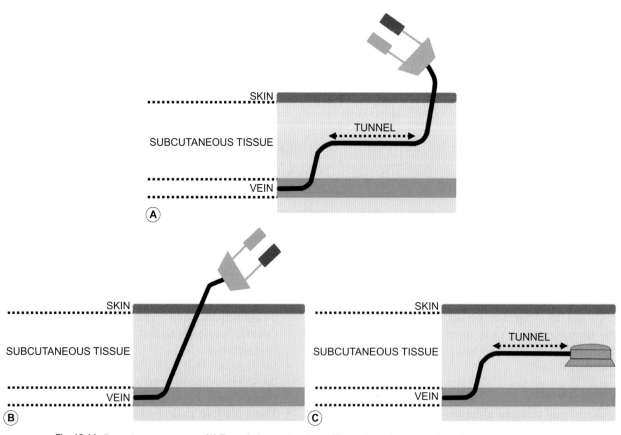

Fig. 10.11 Central venous access. **(A)** Tunnelled central catheter. The catheter is passed through a subcutaneous tunnel before it enters the central vein. **(B)** Nontunnelled central catheter. The catheter is inserted directly into the vein. **(C)** Implantable port. The port is embedded in the subcutaneous tissue and is then advanced into the central vein.

- Implantable ports have the advantage of being completely internalised; hence, the infection risk is lower. Unlike other CVCs where the external portion needs to be kept dry, they also allow patients to undertake daily activities more easily, such as showering.

VENOUS SAMPLING

- Venous sampling is a diagnostic procedure that is performed, for example to localise abnormal hormone secretion in different endocrine disorders.
- Adrenal vein sampling is an investigation for suspected primary hyperaldosteronism (Fig. 10.12). It helps differentiate unilateral disease and bilateral disease. It is an invasive procedure with minimal risk of bleeding. It should only be performed for patients in whom surgery is desired and feasible.
- Inferior petrosal vein sampling is performed in suspected Cushing's syndrome to evaluate for an adrenocorticotropic hormone (ACTH)-secreting pituitary adenoma. The ACTH levels in the inferior petrosal veins are compared to levels from a peripheral vein.
- Parathyroid vein sampling can be performed to identify a functional parathyroid adenoma. It is typically done when a parathyroid adenoma cannot be localised accurately on imaging.

- Ovarian vein sampling can be performed in patients with excessive androgens, where imaging is unable to locate the source.

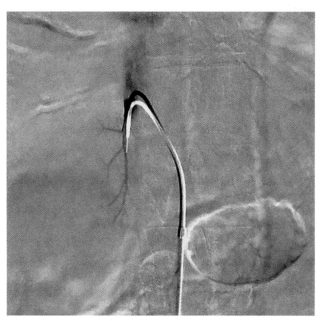

Fig. 10.12 Catheter in the right adrenal vein which drains directly into the IVC. (Courtesy Dr Ram Kishore Reddy Gurajala.)

Chapter Outline

Cases 11.1–11.58 cover bonus X-rays. Cases 11.1–11.17 are chest X-rays (Cases 11.1–11.12 standard and Cases 11.13–11.17 advanced), Cases 11.18–11.29 are abdominal X-rays (Cases 11.18–11.23 standard and Cases 11.14–11.29 advanced) and Cases 11.30–11.58 are orthopaedic X-rays (Cases 11.30–11.46 standard and Cases 11.47–11.58 advanced).

BONUS CHEST X-RAYS

CASE 11.1

An 18-year-old male presents to the A&E department with shortness of breath, following an episode of sudden onset left-sided pleuritic chest pain. There is no history of trauma.

He is a slim, tall, healthy young man. His clinical examination is unremarkable, but he is still mildly dyspnoeic. You request a chest X-ray for further assessment.

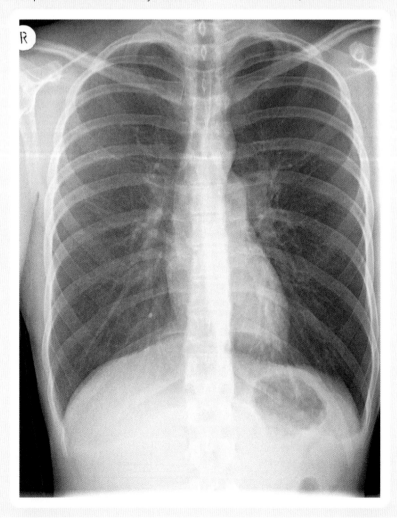

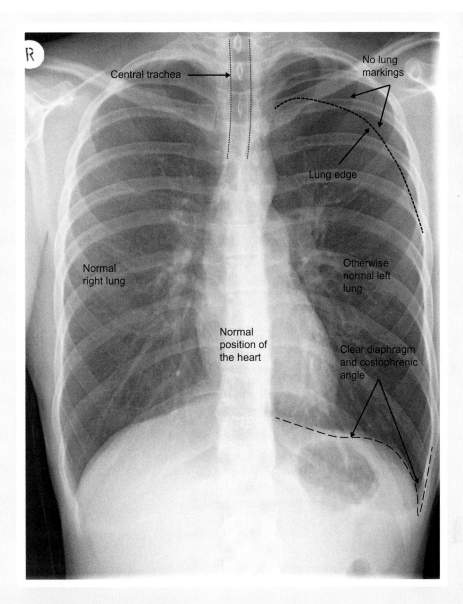

Central trachea →

No lung markings

Lung edge

Normal right lung

Otherwise normal left lung

Normal position of the heart

Clear diaphragm and costophrenic angle

🔍 PRESENT YOUR FINDINGS

- This is a PA chest X-ray of an adult.
- There are no patient identifiable data on the X-ray. I would like to confirm the patient's name, date of birth and the date and time the X-ray was performed.
- The patient is well centred, there is satisfactory inspiratory achievement and the X-ray is adequately penetrated.
- The most striking abnormality is the asymmetry of the apices, with a lung edge visible at the left apex. There are no lung markings visible peripheral to this. The findings are consistent with a left apical pneumothorax.
- There is no evidence of a mediastinal shift.
- The lungs are clear, with no masses, nodules, consolidation or collapse visible.

- The heart is not enlarged and the cardiac and mediastinal contours are normal.
- Both hemidiaphragms and the costophrenic angles are clearly demarcated.
- No free subdiaphragmatic gas is seen.
- There is no abnormality of the imaged soft tissues or skeleton; in particular, there are no rib fractures.

IN SUMMARY – This chest X-ray shows a small left apical pneumothorax. As the patient is mildly symptomatic, he should be admitted for observation and supplementary oxygen if required. The pneumothorax is probably too small to attempt aspiration or drainage, and it should resolve with conservative measures.

CASE **11.2**

A 40-year-old woman has presented to A&E with increased breathlessness and left-sided pleuritic chest pain. She had no significant past medical history but takes the oral contraceptive pill. She returned from a holiday in Australia 3 days ago. Clinical examination reveals a raised respiratory rate. A chest X-ray was requested to look for any lung pathology.

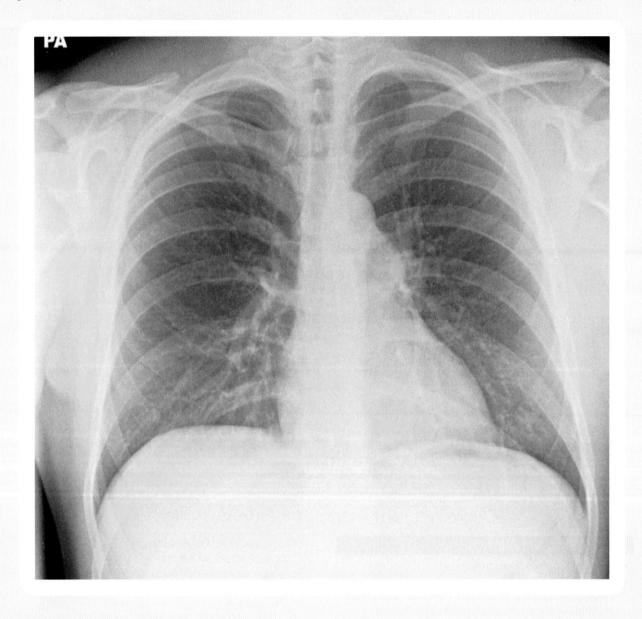

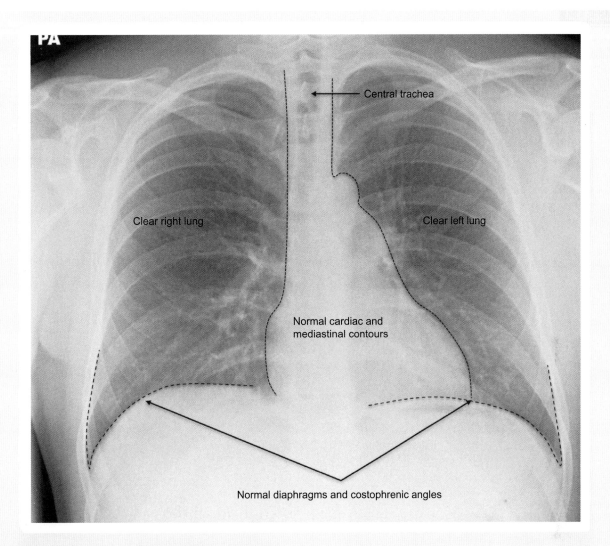

PA

Central trachea

Clear right lung

Clear left lung

Normal cardiac and
mediastinal contours

Normal diaphragms and costophrenic angles

PRESENT YOUR FINDINGS

- This is a PA chest X-ray in an adult.
- There are no patient identifiable data on the X-ray.
  I would like to confirm the patient's name and date of
  birth and the date and time the X-ray was performed.
- The patient is well centred. There is adequate inspiratory effort and satisfactory penetration.
- The trachea is central.
- The lungs are clear, with no masses, nodules, consolidation or collapse visible.
- The heart is not enlarged and the cardiac and mediastinal contours are normal.

- Both hemidiaphragms and the costophrenic angles are clearly demarcated.
- No free subdiaphragmatic gas is seen.
- There is no abnormality of the imaged soft tissues or skeleton.

IN SUMMARY – This is a normal chest X-ray showing no obvious abnormality. If there is clinical suspicion of pulmonary embolus, a CTPA should be considered.

CASE **11.3**

A 60-year-old woman presents to A&E with severe abdominal pain. She recently injured her back and has been using a lot of analgesia. On examination, she is unwell with a peritonitic abdomen. PR examination is unremarkable. You request an erect chest X-ray to look for evidence of a perforation.

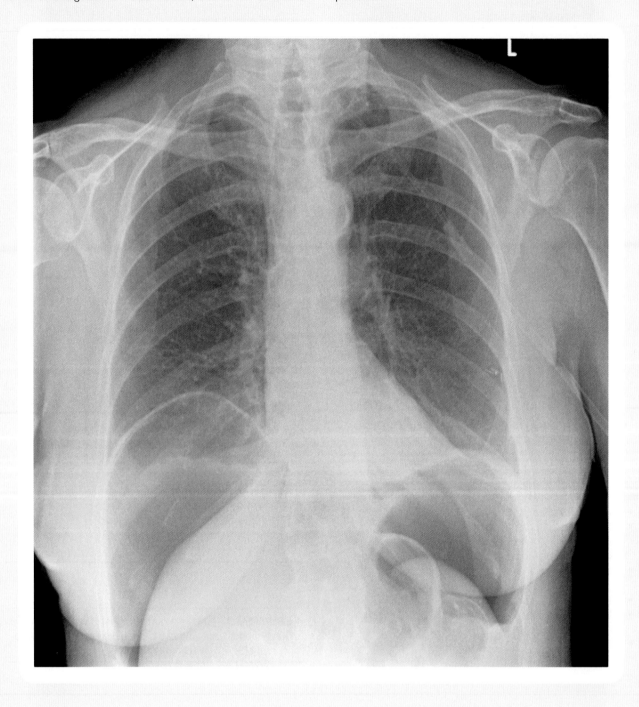

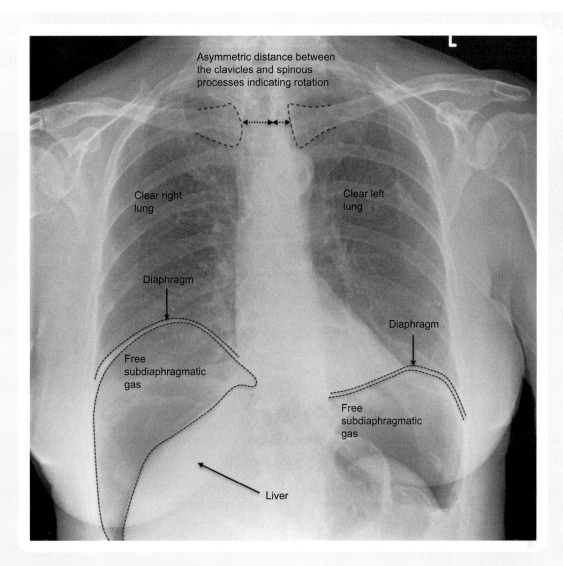

Asymmetric distance between the clavicles and spinous processes indicating rotation

L

Clear right lung

Clear left lung

Diaphragm

Diaphragm

Free subdiaphragmatic gas

Free subdiaphragmatic gas

Liver

🔍 PRESENT YOUR FINDINGS

- This is an AP erect chest X-ray of an adult.
- There are no patient identifiable data on the X-ray. I would like to confirm the patient's name and date of birth and the date and time the X-ray was performed.
- The patient is slightly rotated to the right. There is adequate inspiratory achievement and penetration.
- The most striking abnormality is the large pneumoperitoneum.
- The trachea is central.
- The lungs are clear, with no masses, nodules, consolidation or collapse visible.
- The heart is not enlarged and the cardiac and mediastinal contours are normal.

- Both hemidiaphragms and the costophrenic angles are clearly demarcated.
- There is no abnormality of the imaged soft tissues or skeleton.

IN SUMMARY – This chest X-ray shows a large volume of free subdiaphragmatic gas. Given the history and examination, it is most likely secondary to perforation, possibly of a peptic ulcer from use of non steroidal anti inflammatory drugs. The patient should be made nil by mouth, given adequate analgesia and fluid resuscitated as necessary. An urgent referral to the general surgeons is required. A contrast-enhanced CT of the abdomen and pelvis could be considered to identify the site of the perforation.

CASE **11.4**

A 74-year-old man presents with gradually increasing breathlessness. He is a lifelong smoker. Apart from a 'smoker's cough', which he has had for several months, he is otherwise well. On examination, he has oxygen saturations of 86% on room air, an increased respiratory rate and reduced air entry on the left with a dull percussion note. You request a chest X-ray for further assessment.

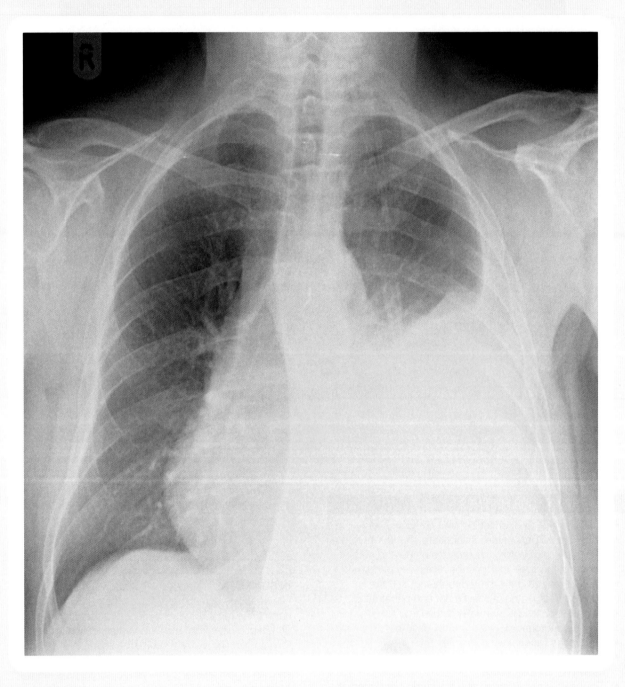

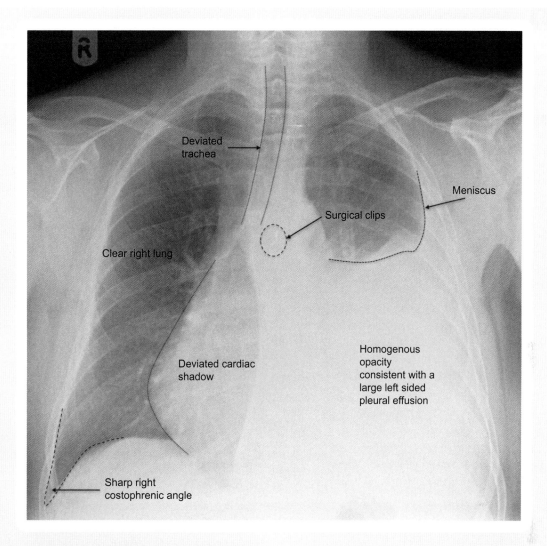

Deviated trachea

Meniscus

Surgical clips

Clear right lung

Deviated cardiac shadow

Homogenous opacity consistent with a large left sided pleural effusion

Sharp right costophrenic angle

PRESENT YOUR FINDINGS

- This is a PA chest X-ray of an adult.
- There are no patient identifiable data on the X-ray. I would like to confirm the patient's name and date of birth and the date and time the X-ray was performed.
- The patient is not rotated, there is satisfactory inspiratory achievement and the X-ray is adequately penetrated.
- The most striking abnormality is the large homogeneous opacity projected over the lower two-thirds of the left lung. A meniscus is visible superolaterally. These findings are consistent with a large pleural effusion.
- There is associated mediastinal shift to the right.
- The right lung shows no area of consolidation and no lobar collapse or pulmonary masses/nodules. The visible left lung is also clear.
- There are two surgical clips projected over the origin of the left main bronchus.

- There is no free subdiaphragmatic gas.
- No skeletal or soft tissue abnormalities are identified.

IN SUMMARY – This chest X-ray shows a large left-sided pleural effusion, which has caused a right-sided mediastinal shift. The differential diagnosis for this is initially wide; however, given the clinical findings, I am concerned there is an underlying malignancy. I would ask the patient about the nature of the previous thoracic surgery. Routine bloods are required to assess for evidence of infection. I would start the patient on supplementary oxygen. A chest drain should be inserted to help relieve the symptoms and a sample of the pleural fluid should be sent for analysis (cytology, biochemistry, microbiology). A post procedural chest X-ray will be required. Depending on the results of the above, further imaging in the form of a CT may be helpful.

CASE 11.5

A 57-year-old patient who has a previous diagnosis of laryngeal cancer is admitted with increasing dysphagia. As part of his initial management, you try to pass an NG tube, but you are unable to aspirate anything back. You therefore request a chest X-ray to assess its position.

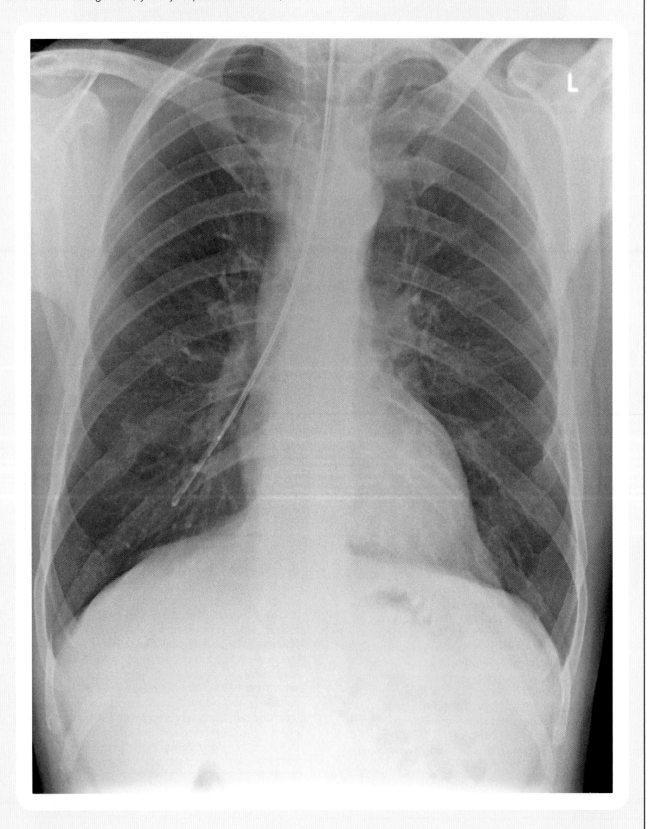

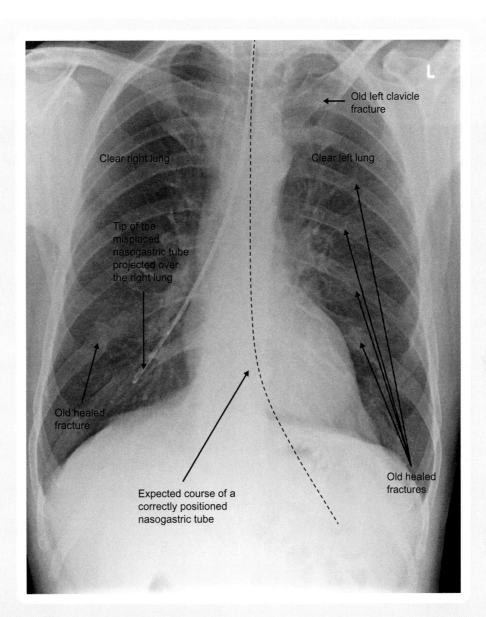

Old left clavicle
fracture

Clear right lung

Clear left lung

Tip of the
misplaced
nasogastric tube
projected over
the right lung

Old healed
fracture

Old healed
fractures

Expected course of a
correctly positioned
nasogastric tube

L

🔍 PRESENT YOUR FINDINGS

- This is a PA chest X-ray of an adult.
- There are no patient identifiable data on the X-ray. I would like to confirm the patient's name and date of birth, and the date and time the X-ray was performed.
- The patient is well centred. There is adequate inspiratory achievement and penetration.
- The most striking abnormality is the inappropriate placement of the NG tube. The NG tube is projected over the right main bronchus, with its tip in the right lung. The NG tube must be resited before use.
- The trachea is central and the cardiac and mediastinal contours are unremarkable.

- The lungs are clear, showing no area of consolidation, lobar collapse or pulmonary masses/nodules.
- The costophrenic angles are sharp, with no evidence of pleural effusion.
- No free subdiaphragmatic gas is evident.
- There are old healed fractures of the medial end of left clavicle, the 4th, 5th, 6th and 7th ribs on the left, and the 7th rib on the right. No other skeletal or soft tissue abnormalities are identified.

IN SUMMARY – This chest X-ray shows a misplaced NG tube, which needs to be resited before use, and multiple healed fractures.

CASE **11.6**

A 65-year-old female is in the high-dependency unit. She suffered a subarachnoid haemorrhage 2 days ago. She has since had the culprit aneurysm coiled. You are reviewing her as she has become dyspnoeic and hypoxic. She has an increased respiratory rate. Chest examination is largely unremarkable. You request a portable chest X-ray for further assessment.

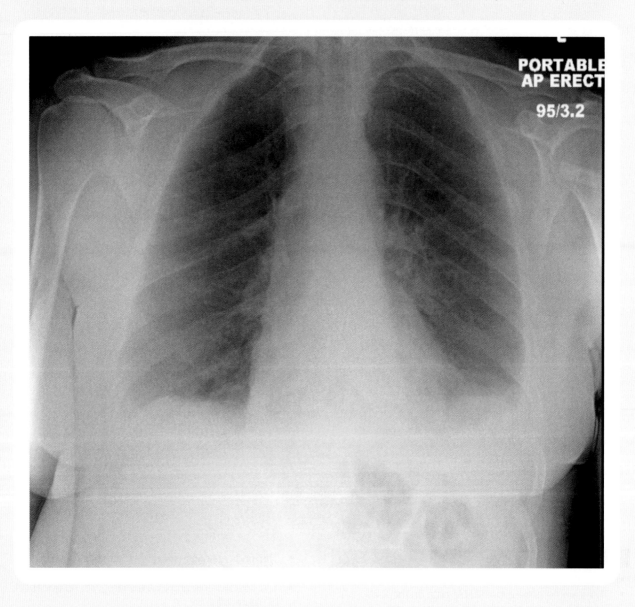

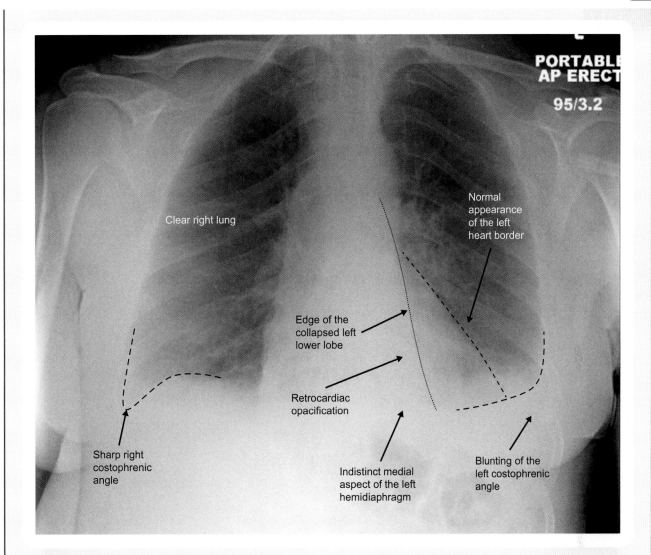

Clear right lung

Normal appearance of the left heart border

Edge of the collapsed left lower lobe

Retrocardiac opacification

Sharp right costophrenic angle

Indistinct medial aspect of the left hemidiaphragm

Blunting of the left costophrenic angle

PORTABLE AP ERECT

95/3.2

PRESENT YOUR FINDINGS

- This is a portable AP erect chest X-ray in an adult.
- There are no patient identifiable data on the X-ray. I would like to confirm the patient's name and date of birth and the date and time the X-ray was performed.
- The patient is slightly rotated. There is adequate inspiratory achievement. It is slightly underpenetrated but otherwise technically adequate.
- There is a dense left-sided retrocardiac opacity with a linear edge. This results in the appearance of a double left heart border. The medial aspect of the left hemidiaphragm is not visible, indicating the pathology is within the left lower lobe. These findings are in keeping with a left lower lobe collapse.
- The lungs are otherwise clear, with no consolidation or masses/nodules.
- There is blunting of the left costophrenic angle, suggestive of a small pleural effusion.

- The right costophrenic angle and hemidiaphragm are sharply defined.
- Allowing for patient rotation, the cardiac and mediastinal contours are unremarkable.
- There is no evidence of free subdiaphragmatic air. No skeletal or soft tissue abnormalities are identified.

IN SUMMARY – This chest X-ray shows a left lower lobe collapse. There is also a small left-sided pleural effusion. The cause of the lobar collapse is most likely due to mucous plugging. Review of previous chest X-rays would be useful to ensure this is a new finding. The patient should be treated with chest physiotherapy and supplementary oxygen. Follow-up chest X-ray to ensure the changes are resolving is also required.

CASE 11.7

A 50-year-old female presents to hospital with increasing breathlessness on exertion and chest pain. Examination reveals slightly muffled heart sounds, a raised jugular venous pulse and a clear chest. You request a chest X-ray.

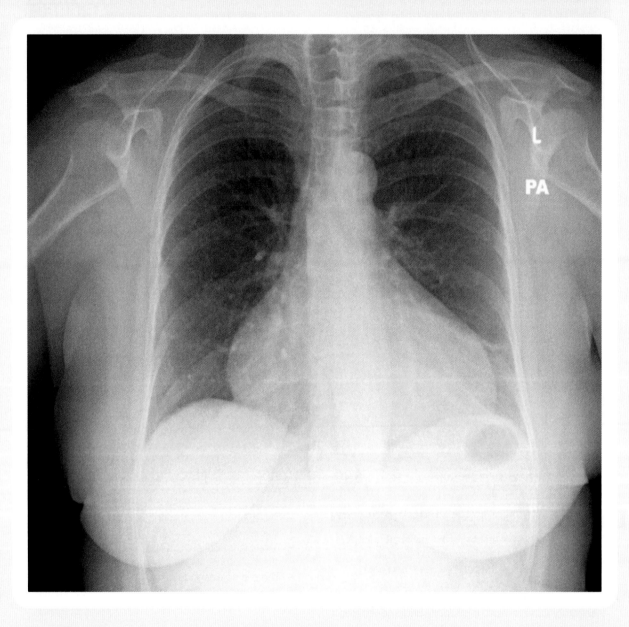

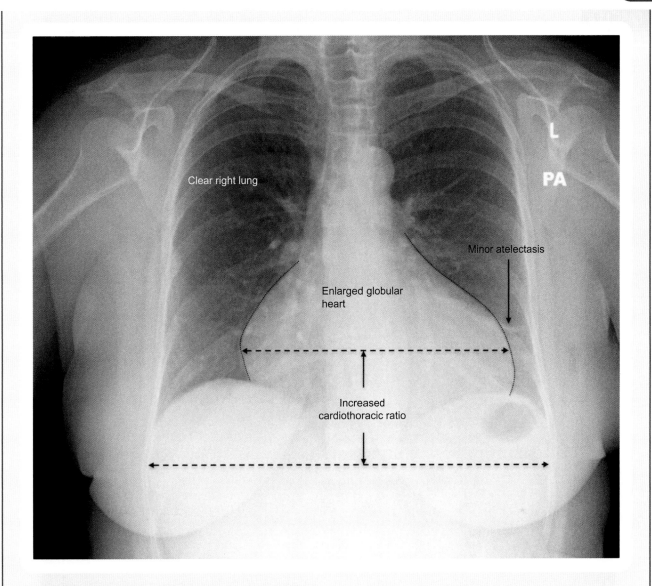

Clear right lung

Minor atelectasis

Enlarged globular
heart

Increased
cardiothoracic ratio

L

PA

PRESENT YOUR FINDINGS

- This is a PA chest X-ray of an adult.
- There are no patient identifiable data on the X-ray. I would like to confirm the patient's name and date of birth and the date and time the X-ray was performed.
- The patient is slightly rotated to the right. There is satisfactory inspiratory achievement and adequate penetration.
- The most striking abnormality is an enlarged heart, with a cardiothoracic ratio of >50%. It also has a globular appearance, in keeping with a pericardial effusion.
- Apart from minor left basal atelectasis, the lungs are clear, with no consolidation, lobar collapse or pulmonary masses/nodules.
- The costophrenic angles are sharp, with no evidence of pleural effusion.

- Allowing for the patient's rotation, the trachea appears central.
- There is no free subdiaphragmatic gas.
- No skeletal or soft tissue abnormalities are identified.

IN SUMMARY – This chest X-ray shows a large globular-shaped heart, in keeping with a pericardial effusion. The differential diagnosis of a pericardial effusion is large. Blood tests, including full blood count (to look for infection), U&Es (to look for renal failure) and thyroid function tests (to look for hypothyroidism), should be performed. An ECG will be required to assess for evidence of ischaemia and pericarditis. I would discuss further investigations and management with cardiology, including an echocardiogram. Since she is symptomatic, she may require a therapeutic pericardiocentesis.

CASE 11.8

A 76-year-old female in a nursing home was admitted with small bowel obstruction. The nurses on the ward have inserted an NG tube to decompress the small bowel. It was easy to pass the NG tube, but it was not possible to aspirate anything from it. The nurses have informed you and you request a chest X-ray to check its position.

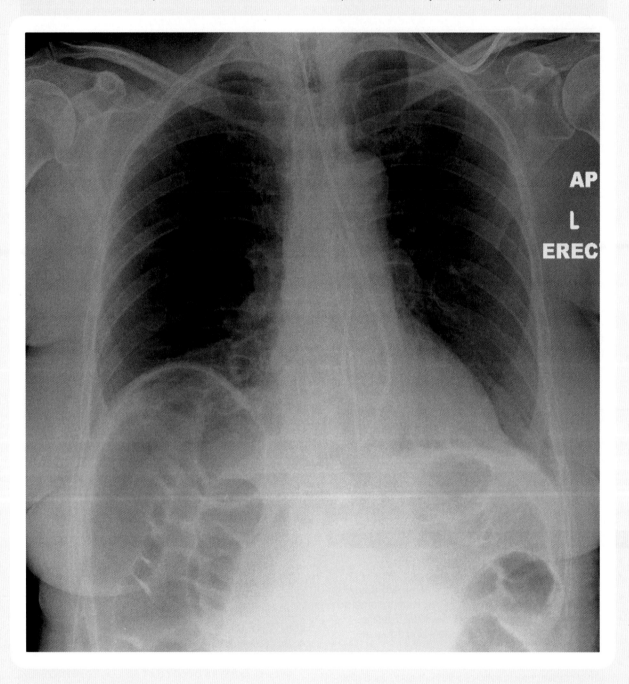

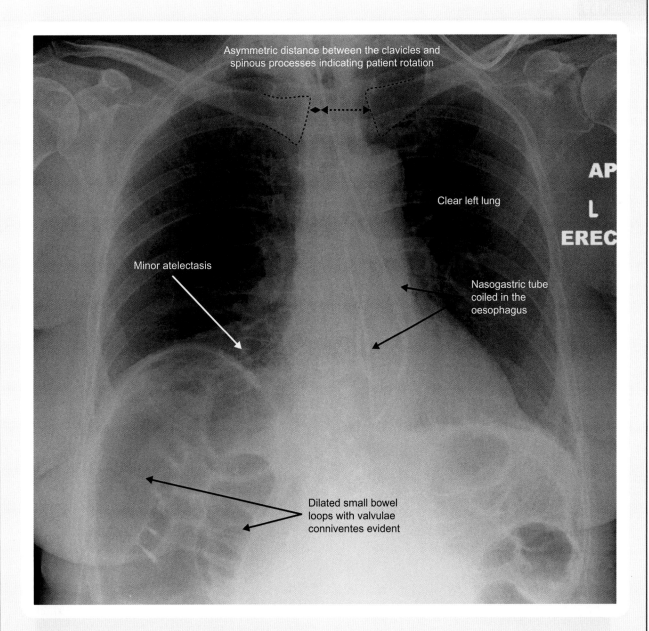

Asymmetric distance between the clavicles and spinous processes indicating patient rotation

AP
L
EREC

Clear left lung

Minor atelectasis

Nasogastric tube coiled in the oesophagus

Dilated small bowel loops with valvulae conniventes evident

🔍 PRESENT YOUR FINDINGS

- This is an AP erect chest X-ray of an adult.
- There are no patient identifiable data on the X-ray. I would like to check the patient's name and date of birth and the date and time the X-ray was performed.
- The patient is slightly rotated to the left. There is adequate inspiratory achievement and penetration.
- The NG tube is coiled in the oesophagus. It should be withdrawn completely and reinserted.
- Apart from some minor atelectasis in the right lower zone, the lungs are clear.
- The costophrenic angles are sharp, with no evidence of pleural effusion.
- Allowing for patient rotation, the trachea is central and the cardiac and mediastinal contours are unremarkable.

- Multiple distended gas-filled loops of bowel noted below the hemidiaphragm. Valvuae conniventes are evident, suggesting small bowel obstruction.
- There is no evidence of free subdiaphragmatic air.
- No skeletal or soft tissue abnormalities are identified.

IN SUMMARY – This chest X-ray shows the NG tube is coiled in the oesophagus and needs resiting. A follow-up chest X-ray following re-insertion may be required if there is no aspirate from the tube. The patient also has dilated small bowel loops, which are seen under the right hemidiaphragm - a formal abdominal X-ray would be helpful.

CASE **11.9**

A 35-year-old homeless man presents with breathlessness and a productive cough. On examination, he has a raised temperature and increased inspiratory rate. There are crackles at the left base. You request a chest X-ray for further assessment.

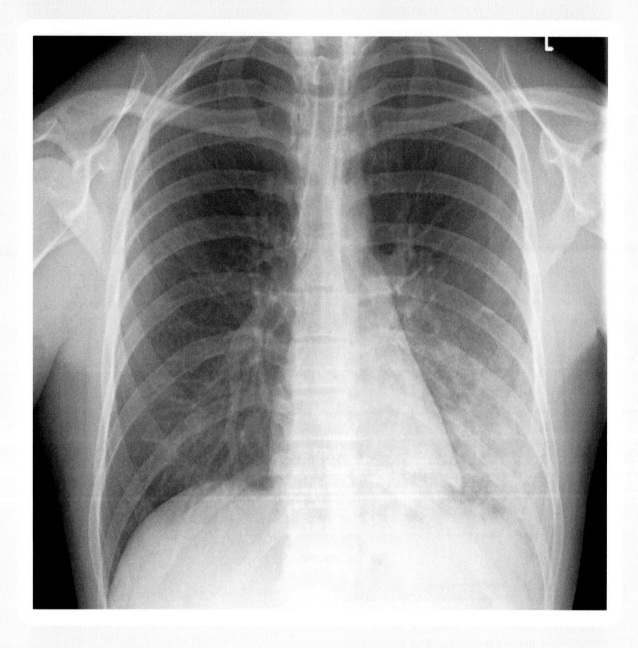

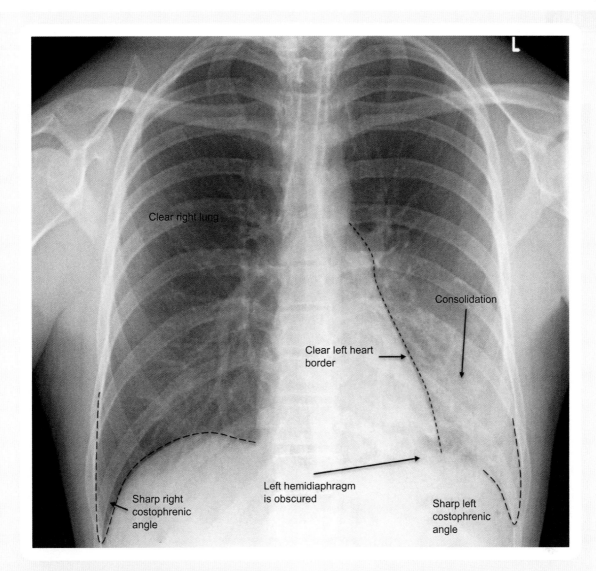

Clear right lung

Consolidation

Clear left heart border

Left hemidiaphragm is obscured

Sharp right costophrenic angle

Sharp left costophrenic angle

🔍 PRESENT YOUR FINDINGS

- This is a PA chest X-ray of an adult.
- There are no patient identifiable data on the X-ray. I would like to confirm the patient's name and date of birth and the date and time the X-ray was performed.
- The patient is well centred. There is satisfactory inspiratory achievement and adequate penetration, but the top of the lung apices are cut off.
- The most striking abnormality is the patchy airspace opacification in the left lower zone. This obscures the left hemidiaphragm; however, the left heart border remains clear. The findings are consistent with left lower lobe consolidation.
- The remaining lungs are clear.

- The cardiac and mediastinal contours are normal.
- The costophrenic angles are sharp, with no evidence of pleural effusion.
- There is no free subdiaphragmatic gas.
- No skeletal or soft tissue abnormalities are identified.

IN SUMMARY – This chest X-ray shows left lower lobe consolidation. Given the clinical findings, the most likely cause for this is community-acquired pneumonia. The patient should be assessed using the CURB-65 clinical scoring system and treated with appropriate antibiotics. A follow-up chest X-ray should be performed in 4-6 weeks following the commencement of treatment to ensure resolution of the pneumonia.

CASE **11.10**

A 7-year-old girl is brought into A&E by her father. She has developed a cough and fever. On examination, she has some crackles in the right mid and lower zones. You request a chest X-ray for further assessment.

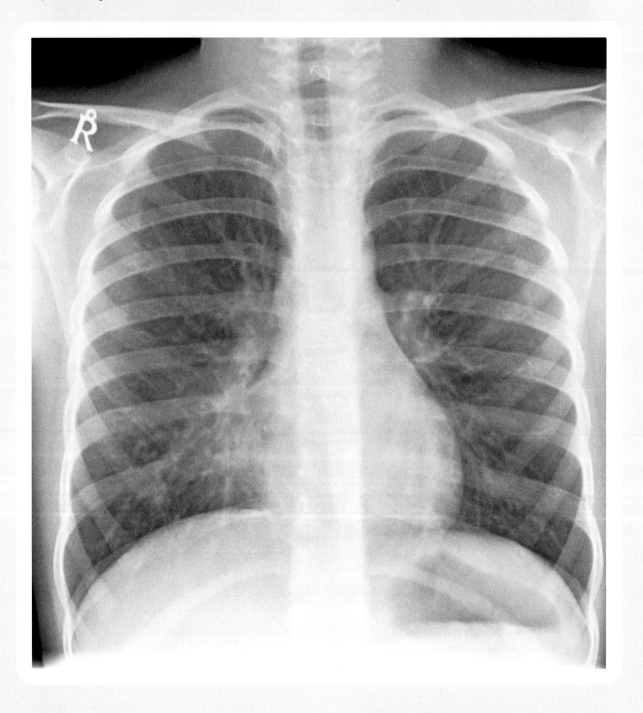

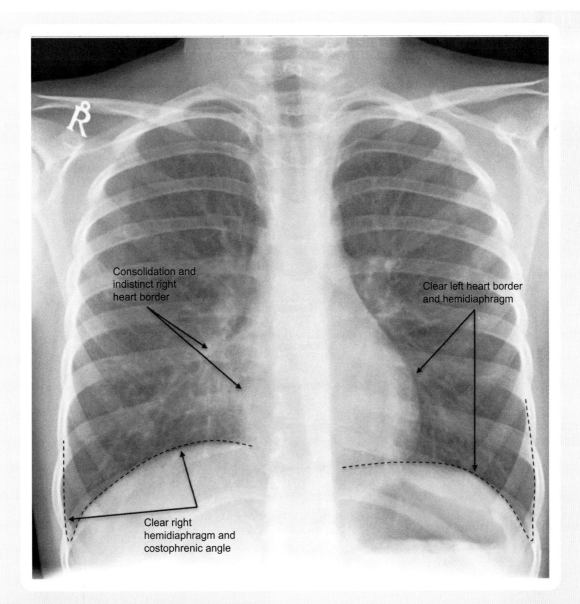

Consolidation and
indistinct right
heart border

Clear left heart border
and hemidiaphragm

Clear right
hemidiaphragm and
costophrenic angle

PRESENT YOUR FINDINGS

- This is a PA chest X-ray of a child.
- There are no patient identifiable data on the X-ray. I would like to confirm the patient's name and date of birth and the date and time the X-ray was performed.
- The patient is not rotated. There is satisfactory inspiratory achievement and adequate penetration.
- The most striking abnormality is the patchy airspace opacification identified in the right mid zone of the lung. The right heart border is indistinct but the right hemidiaphragm remains clear, implying right middle lobe consolidation.
- The cardiomediastinal contours are otherwise normal.

- The left lung is clear, with no consolidation, lobar collapse or pulmonary masses/nodules.
- The costophrenic angles are sharp, with no evidence of pleural effusion.
- There is no free subdiaphragmatic gas.
- No skeletal or soft tissue abnormalities are identified.

IN SUMMARY – This chest X-ray shows right middle lobe consolidation, which is most likely due to pneumonia given the clinical history. The patient should be treated with appropriate antibiotics. A follow-up chest X-ray should be requested 4-6 weeks following the commencement of treatment to ensure resolution of the pneumonia.

CASE **11.11**

A 39-year-old man with known asthma presents to the A&E department for the third time this month with worsening shortness of breath. The patient is hypoxic and tachycardic, with reduced air entry on the right. You request a portable chest X-ray in the resuscitation room.

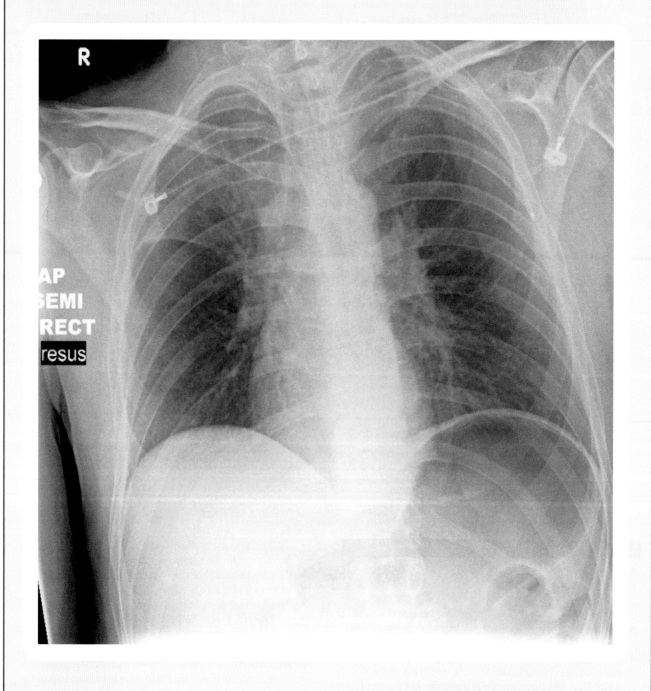

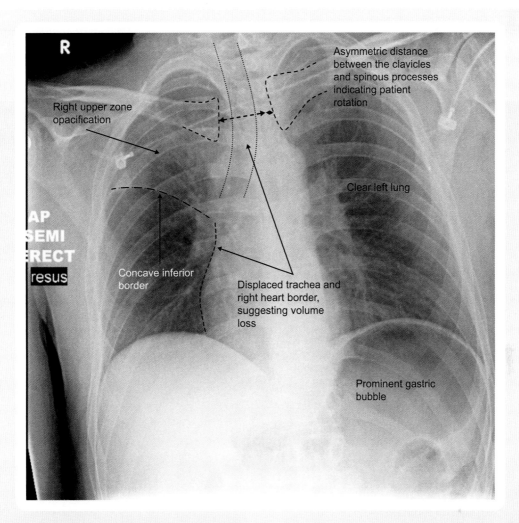

R

Right upper zone opacification

Asymmetric distance between the clavicles and spinous processes indicating patient rotation

Clear left lung

AP
SEMI
ERECT
resus

Concave inferior border

Displaced trachea and right heart border, suggesting volume loss

Prominent gastric bubble

🔍 PRESENT YOUR FINDINGS

- This is a portable AP chest X-ray in an adult.
- There are no patient identifiable data on the X-ray. I would like to check the patient's name and date of birth and the date and time the X-ray was performed.
- The patient is leaning towards the right. He is also rotated to the right. There is inadequate inspiratory achievement, but satisfactory penetration.
- The most striking abnormality is the increased opacification in the right upper zone. This has a concave inferior border. There is volume loss in the right upper zone, as shown by the deviation of the trachea and mediastinum (more than would be expected for the patient's rotation). These findings are in keeping with a right upper lobe collapse.
- The cause for the collapse is not clearly identified. In particular, there is no obvious mass.

- The left lung is clear, with no consolidation, lobar collapse or pulmonary masses/nodules.
- The costophrenic angles are sharp, with no evidence of pleural effusion.
- There is no evidence of free subdiaphragmatic air. However, there is a prominent gastric bubble.
- No skeletal or soft tissue abnormalities are identified.

IN SUMMARY – This chest X-ray shows right upper lobe collapse. The cause is not clearly shown, but given the patient is young and asthmatic, I think it is most likely due to mucous plugging. The patient should be treated for an acute exacerbation of asthma, as well as having chest physiotherapy. A follow-up X-ray following appropriate treatment should be requested to ensure resolution of the lobar collapse. If the collapse persists, then we should consider a CT of the chest to assess for an alternative cause of the lobar collapse, such as a malignancy.

CASE 11.12

An 80-year-old male patient is admitted with confusion and a fever. Examination is difficult but you think there are some right-sided crackles. A chest X-ray is requested for further assessment of these findings.

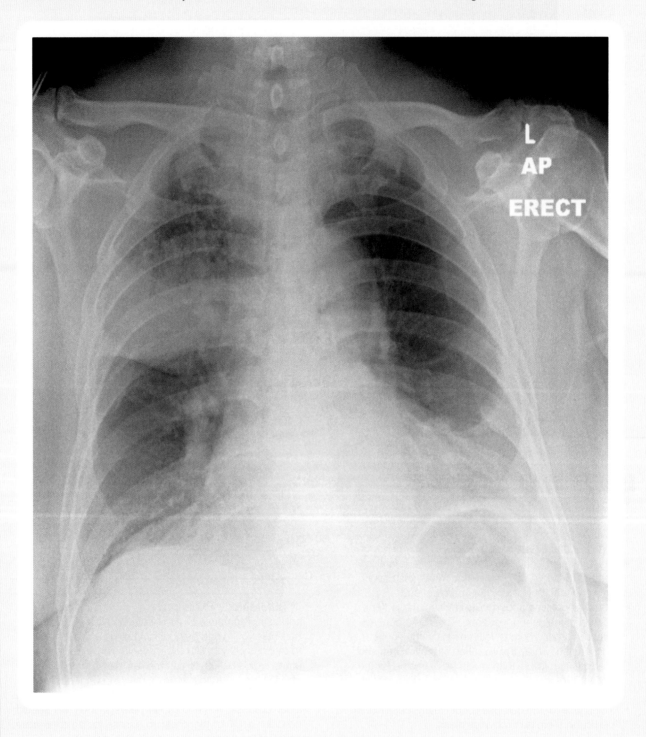

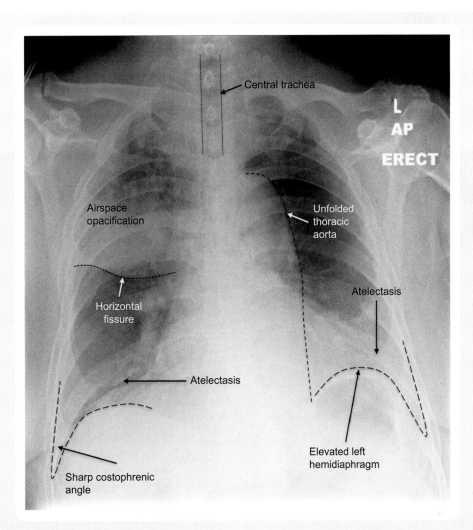

Central trachea

L
AP
ERECT

Airspace
opacification

Unfolded
thoracic
aorta

Horizontal
fissure

Atelectasis

Atelectasis

Elevated left
hemidiaphragm

Sharp costophrenic
angle

PRESENT YOUR FINDINGS

- This is an AP erect chest X-ray of an adult.
- There are no patient identifiable data on the X-ray. I would like to check the patient's name and date of birth and the date and time the X-ray was performed.
- The patient is not rotated. There is satisfactory inspiratory achievement and penetration.
- The most striking abnormality is the patchy airspace opacification identified in the right upper lobe of the lung. The inferior margin of this consolidation is outlined by the horizontal fissure. It is important to note that the right heart border is clear, implying that the right middle lobe is not affected and there is no evidence of associated volume loss, mitigating against lobar collapse.
- There is bibasal atelectasis, but the lungs are otherwise clear.
- The costophrenic angles are sharp, with no evidence of pleural effusion.

- The left hemidiaphragm is elevated.
- There is mild unfolding of the thoracic aorta, but the cardiac and mediastinal contours are otherwise unremarkable.
- There is no free subdiaphragmatic gas.
- No skeletal or soft tissue abnormalities are identified.

IN SUMMARY – This chest X-ray shows right upper lobe consolidation, in keeping with community-acquired pneumonia. The severity of the pneumonia should be assessed with the CURB-65 scoring system and appropriate antibiotics commenced. The patient may also need supplementary oxygen and fluids. A follow-up chest X-ray should be requested in 4-6 weeks following the commencement of treatment to ensure resolution of the pneumonia. The left hemidiaphragm is elevated. This may be related to the left basal atelectasis; however, I would like to review previous X-rays to see if this is a new or longstanding finding.

ADVANCED CHEST X-RAYS

CASE 11.13

A 73-year-old woman with background COPD presents to A&E with a productive cough, increasing shortness of breath and a fever. Clinical examination reveals reduced air entry and some crackles in the right lung. A chest X-ray is performed.

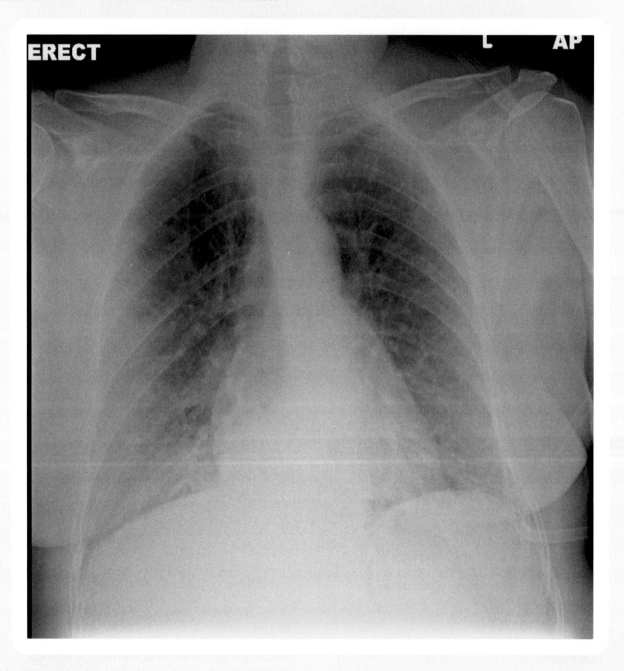

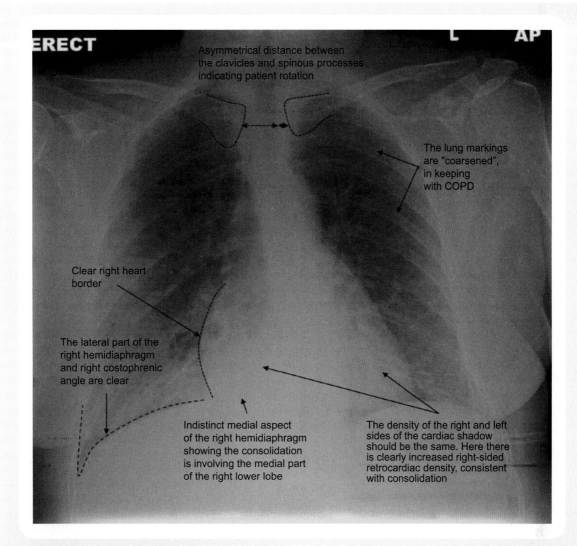

Asymmetrical distance between the clavicles and spinous processes indicating patient rotation

The lung markings are "coarsened", in keeping with COPD

Clear right heart border

The lateral part of the right hemidiaphragm and right costophrenic angle are clear

Indistinct medial aspect of the right hemidiaphragm showing the consolidation is involving the medial part of the right lower lobe

The density of the right and left sides of the cardiac shadow should be the same. Here there is clearly increased right-sided retrocardiac density, consistent with consolidation

PRESENT YOUR FINDINGS

- This is an AP erect chest X-ray of an adult.
- There are no patient identifiable data on the X-ray. I would like to confirm the patient's name and date of birth and date and time the X-ray was performed before making any further assessment.
- The patient is slightly rotated to the right, and the X-ray is underpenetrated. It is otherwise a technically adequate examination with a satisfactory inspiratory achievement and no areas cut off.
- The most striking abnormality is increased density in the right lower zone. This is most notable behind the right side of the cardiac shadow. The medial aspect of the right hemidiaphragm is obscured but the right heart border is clear, indicating there is right lower lobe consolidation.
- Elsewhere in the lungs, there are coarsened lung markings in keeping with COPD but no other areas

of consolidation and no lobar collapse or pulmonary masses/nodules.
- Allowing for the rotation, the trachea, mediastinal and cardiac contours, and hila are unremarkable.
- The costophrenic angles are sharp, with no evidence of pleural effusion.
- There is no free subdiaphragmatic gas.
- No skeletal or soft tissue abnormalities are noted.

IN SUMMARY – This chest X-ray shows right lower lobe consolidation with background changes of COPD. Given the clinical findings, these changes are consistent with right lower lobe pneumonia. A follow-up chest X-ray in 4-6 weeks after appropriate antibiotic treatment should be considered to ensure resolution of the pneumonic changes.

CASE 11.14

A 73-year-old man has presented to A&E with severe abdominal pain. He has a past history of hypertension, diabetes and osteoarthritis. He is taking a variety of medications, including metformin, lisinopril and ibuprofen. On examination, he is tachycardic, with peritonism in his upper abdomen. You request a chest X-ray as part of your assessment.

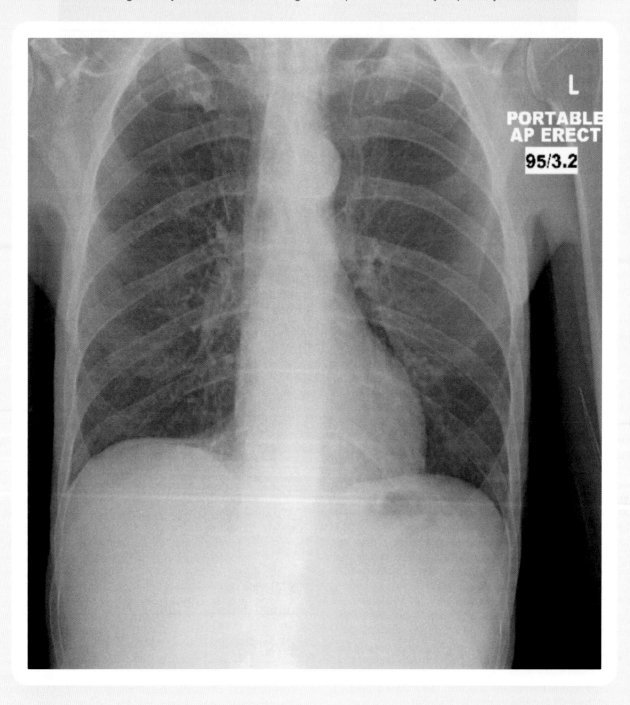

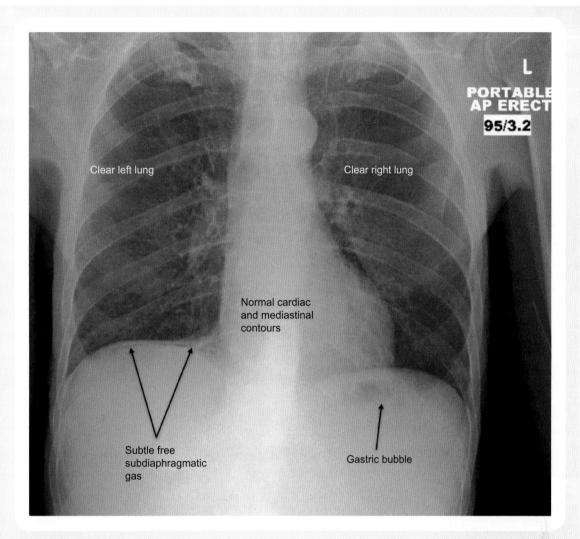

Labels on image:
- Clear left lung
- Clear right lung
- L
- PORTABLE AP ERECT
- 95/3.2
- Normal cardiac and mediastinal contours
- Subtle free subdiaphragmatic gas
- Gastric bubble

🔍 PRESENT YOUR FINDINGS

- This is a portable AP erect chest X-ray of an adult.
- There are no patient identifiable data on the X-ray. I would like to confirm the patient's name and date of birth and the date and time the X-ray was performed.
- The lung apices and clavicles have not been included in the X-ray. The patient appears well centred and there is adequate inspiratory achievement and penetration.
- The trachea is central.
- The lungs are clear, with no masses, nodules, consolidation or collapse visible.
- The heart is not enlarged and the cardiac and mediastinal contours are normal.
- Both hemidiaphragms and the costophrenic angles are clearly demarcated.

- There is a very subtle slither of free air underneath the right hemidiaphragm. The air under the left hemidiaphragm represents the gastric bubble.
- There is no abnormality of the imaged soft tissues or skeleton.

IN SUMMARY – This chest X-ray shows free subdiaphragmatic gas, most likely related to a perforation. The patient should be made nil by mouth, have routine bloods performed, given appropriate analgesia and fluid resuscitation and referred urgently to the general surgeons. The site of perforation may be a peptic ulcer, given that the patient is on long-term ibuprofen; however, a CT of the abdomen and pelvis with IV contrast may be required for further assessment, in which case his metformin should be withheld.

CASE **11.15**

A 4-year-old boy is brought in by his mother with a cough and fever. On examination, he is pyrexial, with an increased respiratory rate. Chest examination is difficult but you think there may be left-sided crackles. You request a chest X-ray for further assessment.

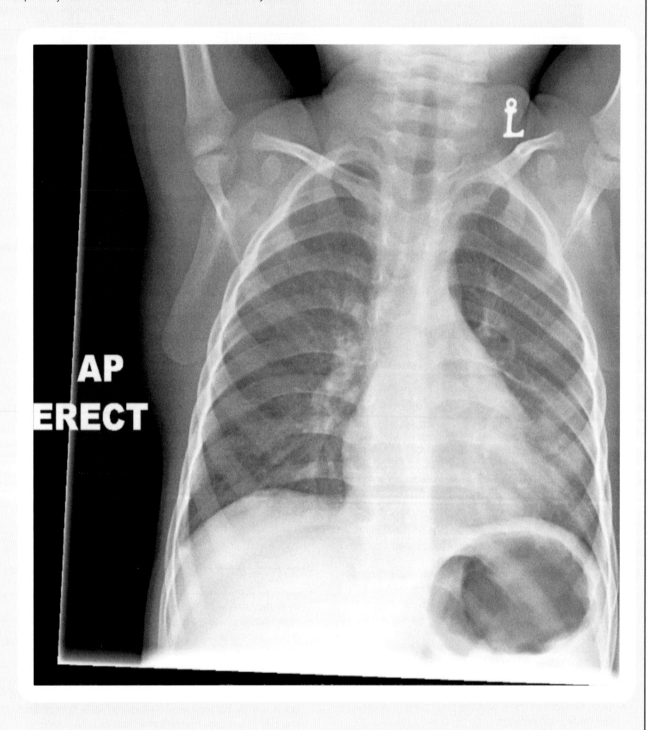

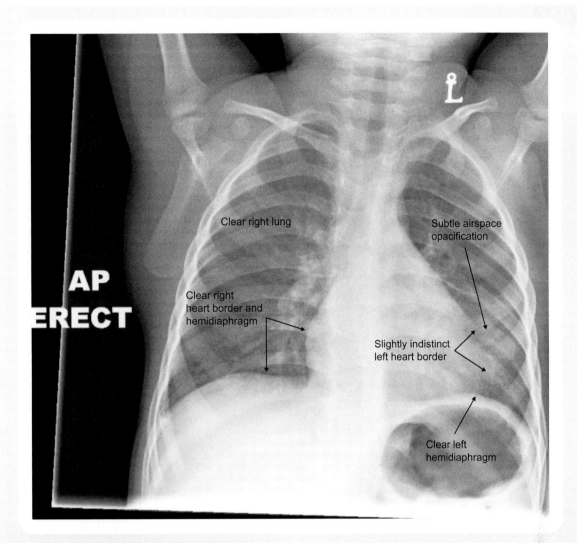

Clear right lung

Subtle airspace opacification

Clear right heart border and hemidiaphragm

Slightly indistinct left heart border

AP ERECT

Clear left hemidiaphragm

PRESENT YOUR FINDINGS

- This is an AP erect chest X-ray of a child.
- There are no patient identifiable data on the X-ray. I would like to confirm the patient's name and date of birth and the date and time the X-ray was performed.
- The patient is slightly rotated (as demonstrated by the asymmetrical appearance of the clavicles). There is satisfactory inspiratory achievement and penetration.
- There is subtle airspace opacification obscuring the left heart border. The left hemidiaphragm remains clear. These findings are in keeping with lingula consolidation.
- The cardiomediastinal contours are otherwise normal.

- The right lung is clear, with no area of consolidation, lobar collapse or pulmonary masses/nodules.
- The costophrenic angles are sharp, with no evidence of pleural effusion.
- There is no free subdiaphragmatic gas.
- No skeletal or soft tissue abnormalities are identified.

IN SUMMARY – This chest X-ray shows consolidation within the lingula. Given the clinical findings, the most likely cause is pneumonia. He should be treated with appropriate antibiotics and paracetamol (to lower his temperature).

CASE **11.16**

A 60-year-old male smoker patient presents to his GP with a 3-month history of a worsening cough and unintentional weight loss. There was no history of haemoptysis. Physical examination was unremarkable; in particular, there was no finger clubbing or chest signs. The GP requests a chest X-ray for further assessment.

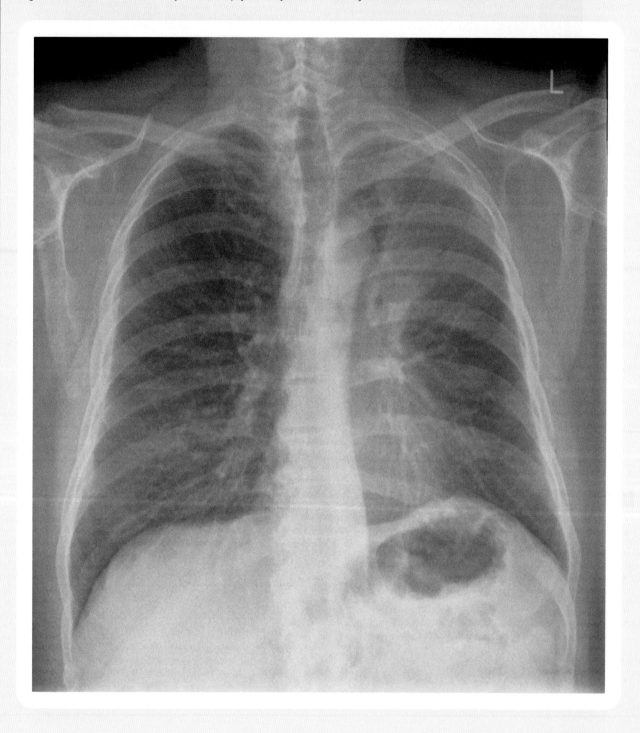

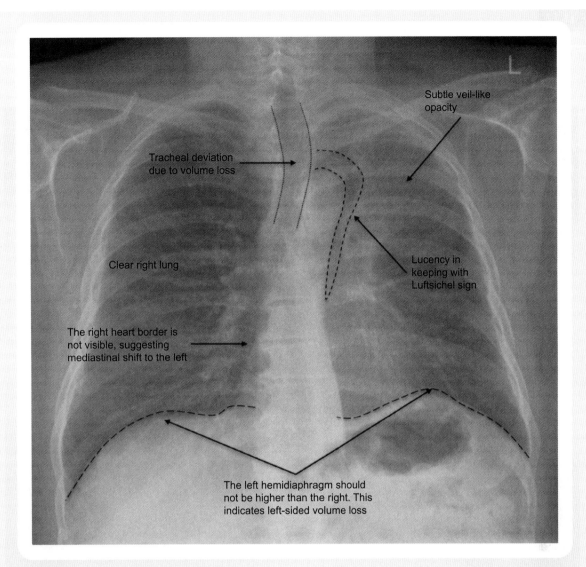

Tracheal deviation due to volume loss

Subtle veil-like opacity

Clear right lung

Lucency in keeping with Luftsichel sign

The right heart border is not visible, suggesting mediastinal shift to the left

The left hemidiaphragm should not be higher than the right. This indicates left-sided volume loss

🔍 PRESENT YOUR FINDINGS

- This is a PA chest X-ray of an adult.
- There are no patient identifiable data on the X-ray. I would like to check the patient's name and date of birth and the date and time the X-ray was performed.
- The patient is not rotated. There is satisfactory inspiratory achievement and adequate penetration.
- Compared to the right upper zone, there is a subtle increased opacification over the left upper zone. It is difficult to define its inferior extent and it could be described as having a veil-like appearance. There is evidence of volume loss, with deviation of the trachea and mediastinum to the left and slight elevation of the left hemidiaphragm. These findings are in keeping with left upper lobe collapse.
- The cause of the left upper lobe collapse is not visible.

- There is a curved lucent area in the left upper zone, adjacent to the lateral aspect of the aortic shadow. This is in keeping with compensatory hyperexpansion of the left lower lobe and known as the 'Luftsichel' sign.
- The right lung shows no other areas of consolidation, lung collapse or pulmonary masses/nodules.
- The costophrenic angles are sharp, with no evidence of pleural effusion.
- There is no free subdiaphragmatic gas.
- No skeletal or soft tissue abnormalities are identified.

IN SUMMARY – This chest X-ray shows a left upper lobe collapse. The cause of this is not apparent, but given the smoking history and weight loss, I am concerned there is an underlying bronchogenic malignancy. CT of the chest and abdomen with IV contrast is appropriate for further assessment.

CASE **11.17**

A 12-year-old boy with asthma presents with a 1-day history of pleuritic chest pain. He requires oxygen at paediatric A&E and it is thought that he has a pneumothorax. A chest X-ray is performed.

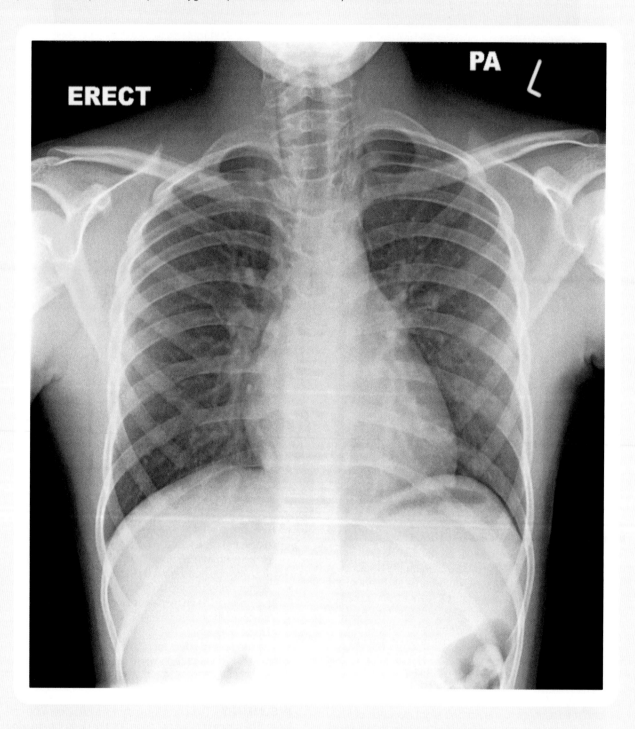

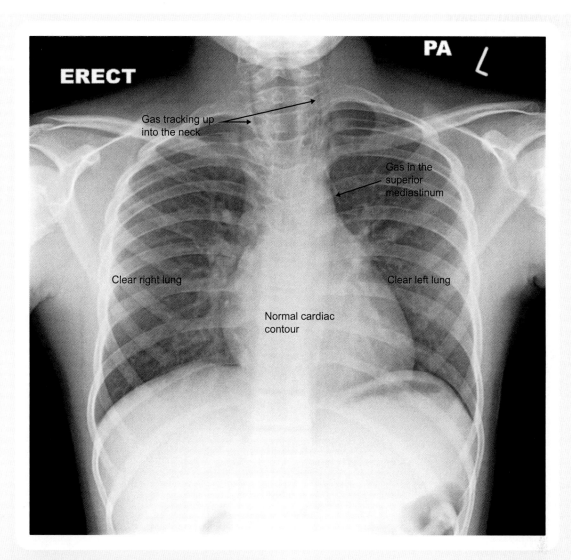

ERECT

PA

Gas tracking up
into the neck

Gas in the
superior
mediastinum

Clear right lung

Clear left lung

Normal cardiac
contour

🔍 PRESENT YOUR FINDINGS

- This is a PA chest X-ray of a child.
- There are no patient identifiable data on the X-ray. I would like to check the patient's name and date of birth and the date and time the X-ray was performed.
- The patient is slightly rotated to the left. There is satisfactory inspiratory achievement and adequate penetration.
- The most striking abnormalities are the lucent lines projected over the superior mediastinum and neck. These are in keeping with gas within the mediastinum.
- There is no evidence of pneumothorax or pneumopericardium.
- The lungs are clear.

- The costophrenic angles are sharp, with no evidence of pleural effusion.
- The cardiomediastinal contours are within normal limits.
- There is no free subdiaphragmatic gas.
- No skeletal or soft tissue abnormalities are identified; in particular, there is no surgical emphysema or rib fractures.

IN SUMMARY – This chest X-ray shows a pneumomediastinum, which is relatively common in asthmatics. There are no other significant findings on the chest X-ray. The patient needs to be urgently reviewed. The pneumomediastinum may not need specific management, though it can be a sign of sinister pathology (e.g. oesophageal perforation).

BONUS ABDOMINAL X-RAYS

A 70-year-old woman, who has a past history of ischaemic heart disease, hypertension and obesity, presents with ongoing intermittent episodes of upper abdominal pain, nausea and constipation. Her abdominal X-ray is shown here.

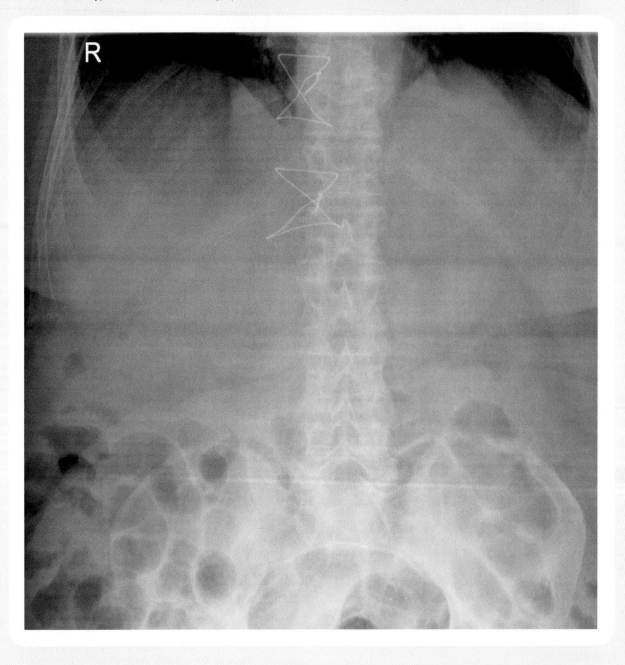

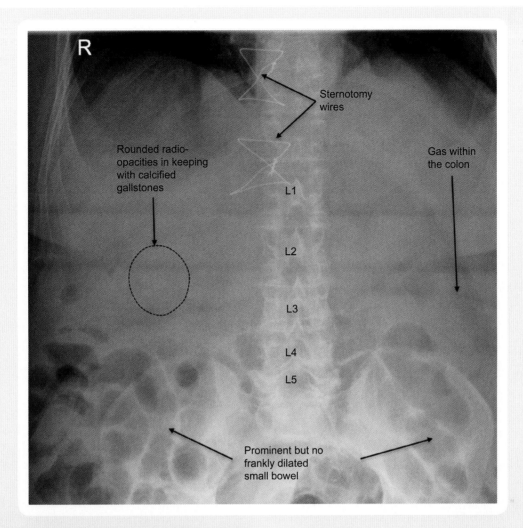

R

Sternotomy
wires

Rounded radio-
opacities in keeping
with calcified
gallstones

Gas within
the colon

L1

L2

L3

L4

L5

Prominent but no
frankly dilated
small bowel

🔍 PRESENT YOUR FINDINGS

- This is a supine AP abdominal X-ray of an adult.
- There are no patient identifiable data on the X-ray. I would like to confirm the patient's name, date of birth and the date and time that the X-ray was performed before making any further assessment.
- The lower pelvis, hernial orifices and flanks are not completely imaged. The X-ray is therefore technically inadequate.
- There are some prominent gas-filled loops of small bowel in the lower half of the imaged abdomen. These are not frankly dilated.
- Some gas is visible in the large bowel but the lower pelvis is not fully included, therefore I am unable to ascertain whether there is gas in the rectum.
- There is no evidence of definite obstruction and no features of perforation or mucosal oedema.
- There are at least four small round radio-opacities projected over the right upper quadrant at the level

of L2/3. Given their position, they are in keeping with gallbladder calculi.
- No abnormality of the other visible abdominal organs is evident.
- Midline sternotomy sutures are in situ.
- No major skeletal or soft tissue abnormality is visible.

IN SUMMARY – This abdominal X-ray shows prominent small bowel loops (meaning the diameter is the 'upper limit of normal') but no perforation, mucosal oedema or definite obstruction. There are calcified gallstones present, which may partly account for the patient's symptoms. The lower half of the abdomen has not been imaged. The differential diagnosis for this lady remains wide. I would like to assess the patient to determine whether her presentation may be related to gallstone pathology. Routine blood tests and a chest X-ray should be performed. Depending on the above, an ultrasound to assess the gallbladder and biliary tree may be appropriate.

CASE **11.19**

A 34-year-old woman presents to A&E with lower abdominal pain and nausea. She has recently had an IUCD inserted by her GP. On examination with a speculum, the strings of the IUCD were not visible, and an ultrasound scan could not identify the IUCD within the uterine cavity. An abdominal X-ray has subsequently been performed.

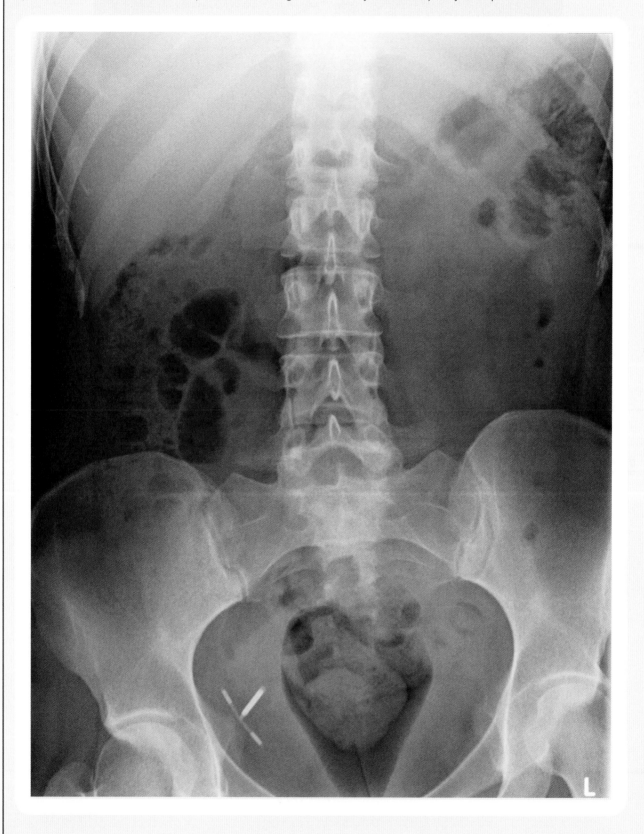

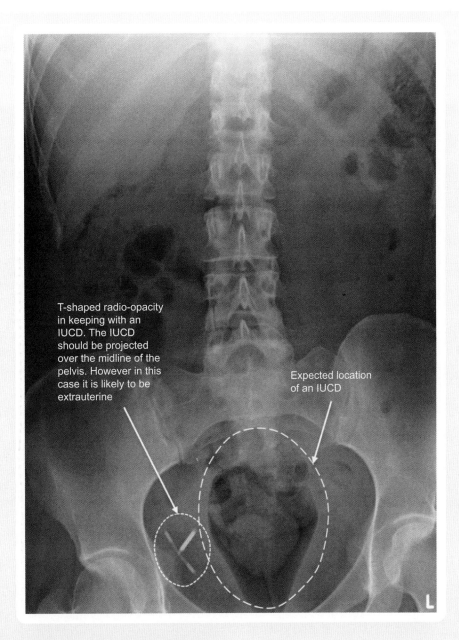

T-shaped radio-opacity in keeping with an IUCD. The IUCD should be projected over the midline of the pelvis. However in this case it is likely to be extrauterine

Expected location of an IUCD

L

🔍 PRESENT YOUR FINDINGS

- This is a supine AP abdominal X-ray of an adult.
- There are no patient identifiable data on the X-ray. I would like to confirm the patient's name, date of birth and time that the X-ray was performed before making any further assessment.
- The hemidiaphragms and hernial orifices are not completely imaged. The X-ray is therefore technically inadequate; however, the salient abnormality is displayed.
- Within the pelvis, a T-shaped radiopaque object is projected to the right of the midline and is in keeping with an IUCD. Its position, coupled with the clinical and ultrasound examinations, suggests it is outside the uterus.

- The bowel gas pattern is normal, with no plain X-ray evidence of obstruction, perforation or mucosal oedema.
- There is no obvious abnormality of the visible solid abdominal organs.
- No major skeletal or soft tissue abnormality is evident.

IN SUMMARY – This abdominal X-ray shows an IUCD projected over the right side of the pelvis. Its position, coupled with the clinical and ultrasound examinations, suggests it has migrated outside the uterus. There is a risk of infection and damage to adjacent organs, such as the bowel or bladder. An urgent gynaecology review is required.

CASE 11.20

A 55-year-old man who has diabetes and hypertension presents with severe central abdominal pain with associated vomiting. He has not passed a bowel movement or flatus for the past 24 to 48 hours. His abdominal X-ray is shown here.

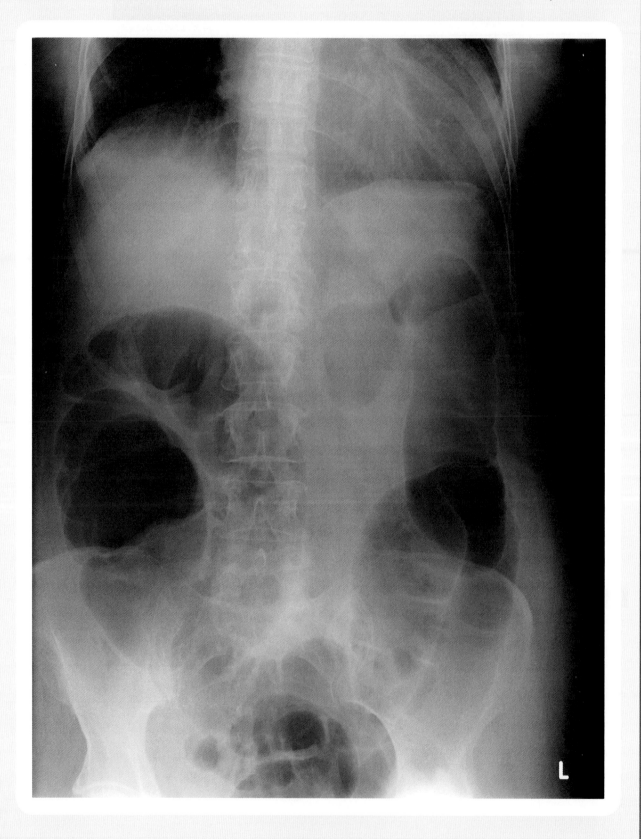

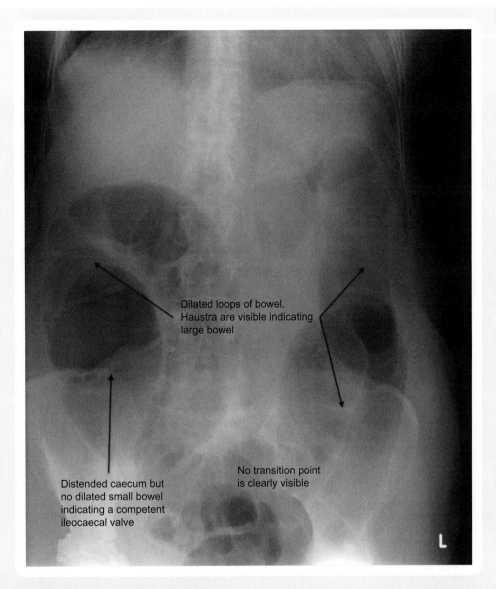

Dilated loops of bowel.
Haustra are visible indicating
large bowel

Distended caecum but
no dilated small bowel
indicating a competent
ileocaecal valve

No transition point
is clearly visible

L

PRESENT YOUR FINDINGS

- This is a supine abdominal X-ray of an adult.
- There are no patient identifiable data on the X-ray. I would like to confirm the patient's name, date of birth, date and time that the X-ray was performed before making any further assessment.
- The hernial orifices are not completely imaged. The X-ray is therefore technically inadequate.
- The most striking abnormality is markedly dilated loops of large bowel within the whole abdomen. The site of obstruction is difficult to identify on this X-ray and the rectum is not clearly seen.
- There is no dilatation of the small bowel, suggesting the ileocaecal valve is competent.
- There is no X-ray evidence of perforation or mucosal oedema.
- There is no obvious abnormality of the solid abdominal organs.
- No major skeletal or soft tissues abnormality can be identified.

IN SUMMARY – This abdominal X-ray shows large bowel dilatation with no evidence of perforation. This site of obstruction is not clearly identifiable and the ileo caecal valve appears competent. My differential diagnosis includes mechanical bowel obstruction (malignancy, inflammatory or ischaemic strictures) and functional obstruction. I would ensure routine blood tests and an erect chest X-ray have been performed, make the patient nil by mouth and consider commencing IV fluids. An urgent surgical review is required, with a view to requesting a CT abdomen and pelvis with contrast to investigate for a potential cause of obstruction.

CASE 11.21

A 50-year-old man with no significant past medical history presents to A&E with generalised abdominal pain and nausea. He has not opened his bowels for 4 days. His abdominal X-ray is shown here.

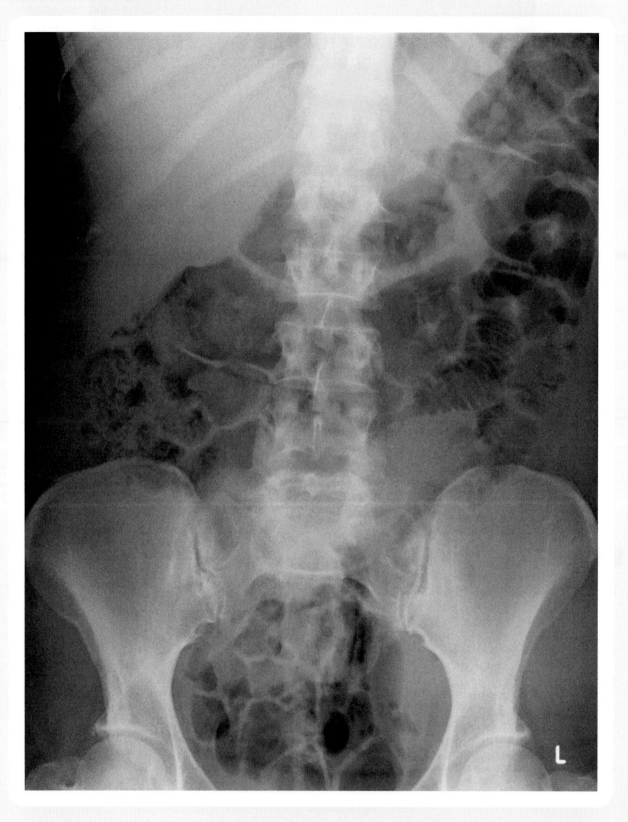

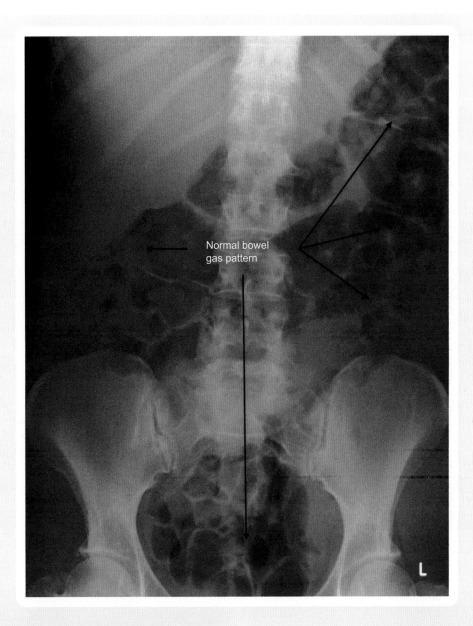

Normal bowel
gas pattern

L

PRESENT YOUR FINDINGS

- This is a supine AP abdominal X-ray of an adult.
- There are no patient identifiable data on the X-ray. I would like to confirm the patient's name, date of birth and the date and time that the X-ray was performed before making any further assessment.
- The hemidiaphragms, hernial orifices and flanks are not completely imaged. The X-ray is therefore technically inadequate.
- The bowel gas pattern is normal, with no X-ray evidence of obstruction, perforation or mucosal oedema.

- There is no obvious abnormality of the visible solid abdominal organs.
- No major skeletal or soft tissues abnormality is visible.

IN SUMMARY – This is a normal abdominal X-ray with no features to explain the presenting symptoms. The differential diagnosis for this patient's presentation remains wide. Clinical assessment (history and examination) along with routine blood tests and an erect chest X-ray should help to guide further management.

CASE 11.22

A 32-year-old man, who has had previous abdominal sur-gery, presents with central abdominal pain and bilious vomiting. His abdomen is diffusely tender and peritonitic. His abdominal X-ray is shown here.

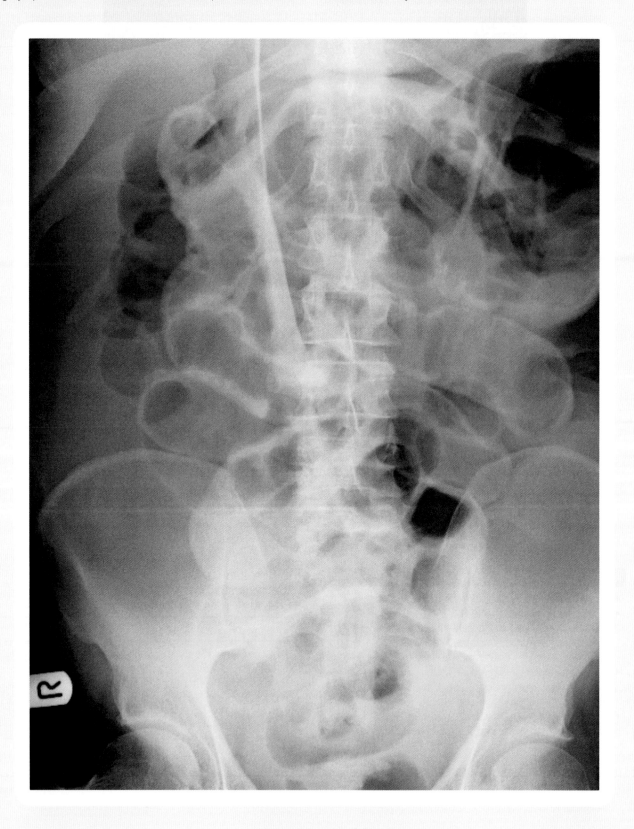

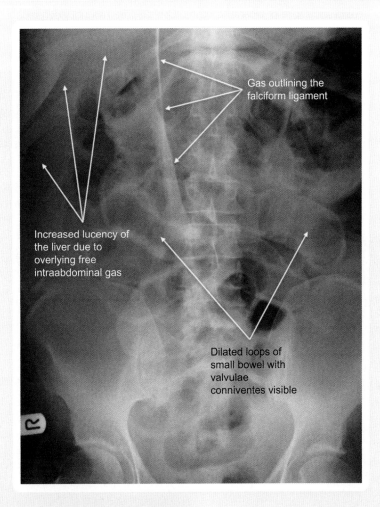

Gas outlining the
falciform ligament

Increased lucency of
the liver due to
overlying free
intraabdominal gas

Dilated loops of
small bowel with
valvulae
conniventes visible

PRESENT YOUR FINDINGS

- This is a supine abdominal X-ray of an adult.
- There are no patient identifiable data on the X-ray. I would like to confirm the patient's name, date of birth and the date and time that the X-ray was performed before making any further assessment.
- The hemidiaphragms, hernial orifices and flanks are not completely imaged. The X-ray is therefore technically inadequate.
- The most striking abnormality is that there are several loops of gas-filled dilated small bowel in the centre of the X-ray.
- The large bowel is not obviously seen, which supports the suspicion of complete small bowel obstruction with collapsed distal large bowel.
- The falciform ligament is clearly visible and the liver appears hyperlucent. These findings are consistent with free intraabdominal gas.

- There is no evidence of mucosal oedema.
- No major skeletal or soft tissues abnormality is identified.

IN SUMMARY – This abdominal X-ray shows small bowel obstruction with evidence of pneumoperitoneum. There is a wide differential diagnosis for small bowel obstruction, but given the previous surgery one must consider adhesions. The pneumoperitoneum may be secondary to the small bowel obstruction, or conversely, the small bowel dilatation may represent a functional obstruction secondary to peritioneal contamination following a perforation. The patient should be nil by mouth, have an NG inserted to decompress the small bowel, commenced on IV fluid and given appropriate analgesia. I would arrange for an urgent surgical review. A CT of the abdomen and pelvis will probably be required for further assessment.

CASE **11.23**

A 35-year-old man is being treated for a flare of ulcerative colitis. Clinically, he has not been responding well and a repeat abdominal X-ray has been performed.

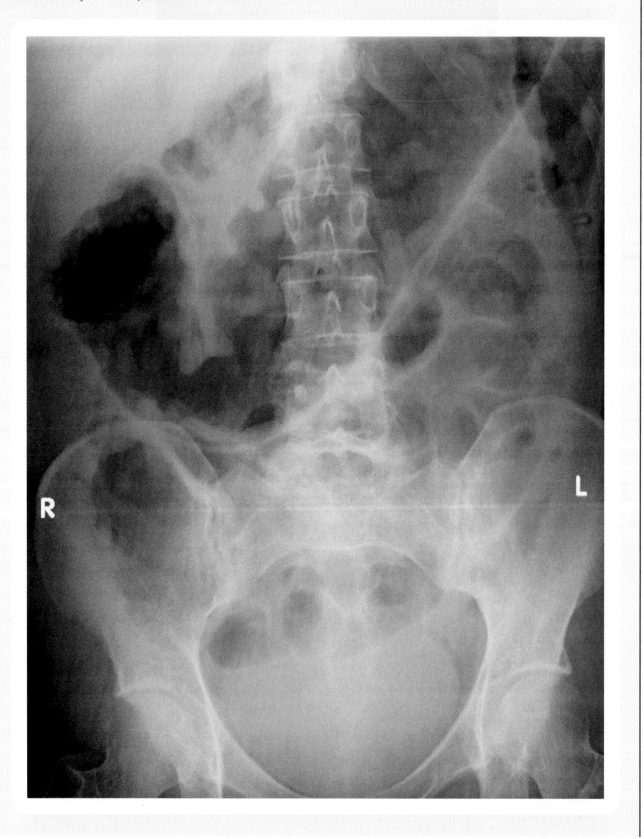

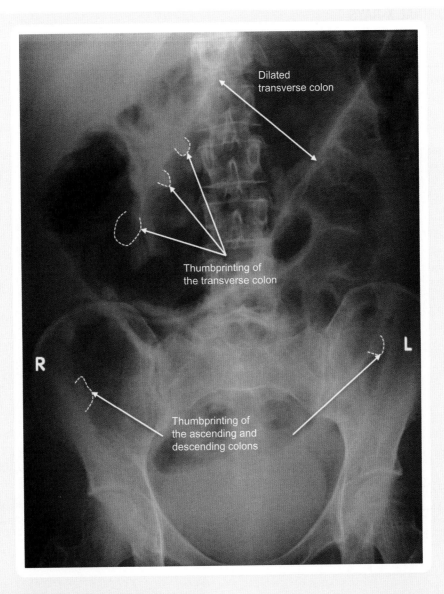

Image labels:
- Dilated transverse colon
- Thumbprinting of the transverse colon
- Thumbprinting of the ascending and descending colons
- R
- L

PRESENT YOUR FINDINGS

- This is a supine AP abdominal X-ray of an adult.
- There are no patient identifiable data on the X-ray. I would like to confirm the patient's name, date of birth and the date and time that the X-ray was performed before making any further assessment.
- The hemidiaphragms, hernial orifices and flanks are not completely imaged. The X-ray is therefore technically inadequate; however, the salient abnormality is displayed.
- The most striking abnormality is a markedly dilated, abnormal transverse colon with loss of the normal haustral markings.
- There is thumbprinting within the transverse colon, as well as the ascending and descending colon. No gas is visible in the rectum.
- There is no X-ray evidence of perforation.
- There is no obvious abnormality of the visible abdominal organs.
- No major skeletal or soft tissues abnormalities are identified. In particular, the sacroiliac joints appear normal.

IN SUMMARY – This abdominal X-ray is grossly abnormal. The findings are consistent with marked mucosal oedema and toxic dilatation of the transverse colon, in keeping with the history of inflammatory bowel disease. This patient requires urgent medical and surgical review. He should be made nil by mouth with IV fluid resuscitation and electrolyte replacement. A decision regarding continued medical management versus surgical treatment (colectomy) should be made by senior doctors.

ADVANCED ABDOMINAL X-RAYS

CASE 11.24

A 65-year-old man, who has recently been diagnosed with advanced bladder cancer, was admitted to hospital 6 days ago with urinary obstruction. He has not opened his bowels for the last 5 days and has developed abdominal pain. An abdominal X-ray has been performed.

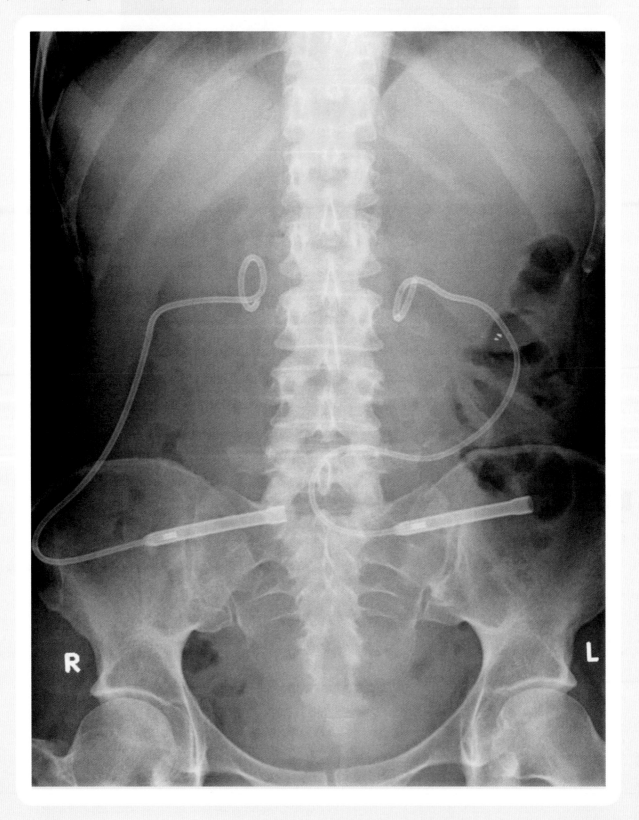

Continue

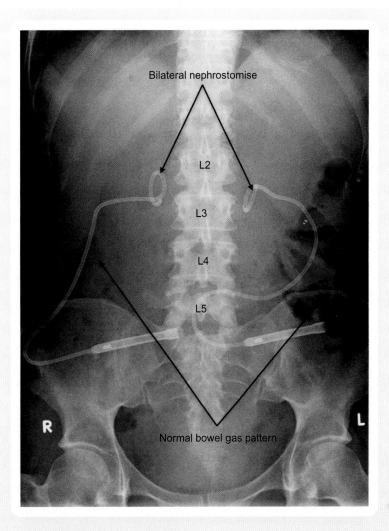

Bilateral nephrostomise

L2

L3

L4

L5

R

L

Normal bowel gas pattern

PRESENT YOUR FINDINGS

- This is a supine AP abdominal X-ray of an adult.
- There are no patient identifiable data on the X-ray. I would like to confirm the patient's name, date of birth and date and time that the X-ray was performed before making any further assessment.
- The hernial orifices are not completely imaged; therefore the film is technically inadequate.
- There are bilateral radio-opaque tubes in situ, each of which has a coiled end projected over the transverse processes of L2/3. These are consistent with bilateral nephrostomy catheters and were presumably recently inserted to relieve the urinary obstruction.
- The bowel gas pattern is normal, with no plain X-ray evidence of obstruction, perforation or mucosal oedema.
- There is no obvious abnormality of the visible solid abdominal organs.
- No skeletal or soft tissues abnormalities are identified.

IN SUMMARY – This abdominal X-ray shows bilateral renal nephrostomies in situ but no evidence of bowel obstruction, perforation or mucosal oedema. The cause of the patient's symptoms is not demonstrated; however, my differential diagnosis includes potential nephrostomy complications such as catheter obstruction, displacement or urinary leakage, and other causes of an acute abdomen. I would like to examine the patient, in particular looking for evidence of peritonism and displacement/obstruction of the nephrostomies. An erect chest X-ray and routine bloods, including renal function and inflammatory markers, should be performed. I would discuss the patient with my seniors, as further imaging such as a CT or fluoroscopic nephrostograms may be required.

CASE 11.25

A 74-year-old woman, who has a past history of ischaemic heart disease, atrial fibrillation and COPD, presents with a 10-hour history of severe central abdominal pain. She has had a few episodes of diarrhoea but no vomiting. Her abdominal X-ray is shown here.

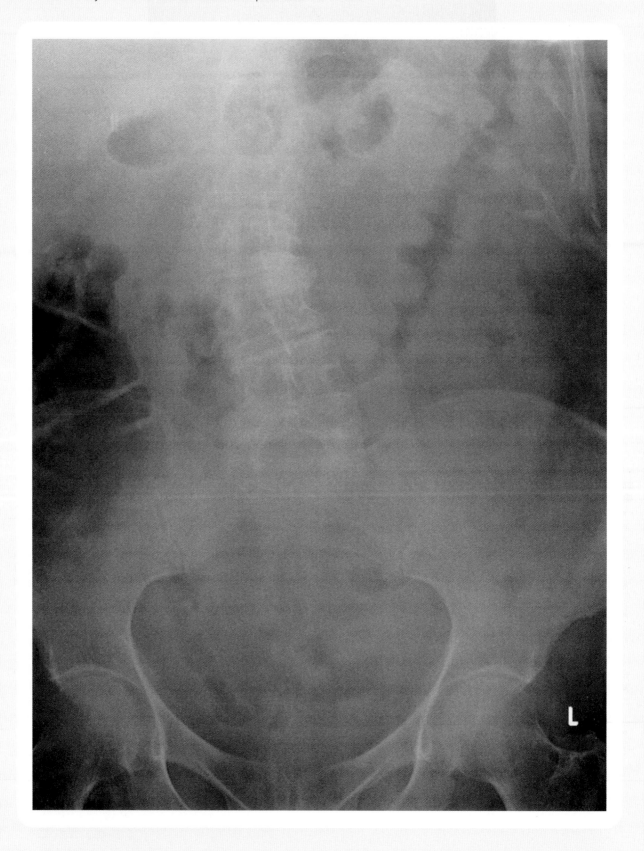

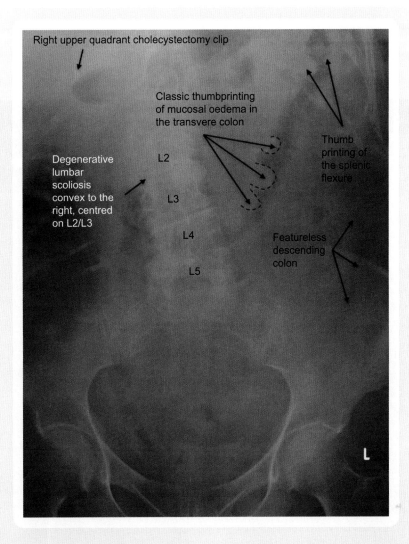

Right upper quadrant cholecystectomy clip

Classic thumbprinting of mucosal oedema in the transvere colon

Thumb printing of the splenic flexure

Degenerative lumbar scoliosis convex to the right, centred on L2/L3

L2

L3

L4

L5

Featureless descending colon

L

🔍 PRESENT YOUR FINDINGS

- This is a supine abdominal X-ray of an adult.
- There are no patient identifiable data on the X-ray. I would like to confirm the patient's name, date of birth and date and time that the X-ray was performed before making any further assessment.
- The hemidiaphragms, hernial orifices and flanks are not completely imaged. The X-ray is therefore technically inadequate.
- The most striking abnormality is marked mucosal oedema and thumbprinting affecting the transverse colon and extending to the splenic flexure.
- There is no toxic dilatation.
- The descending colon is empty and featureless. Elsewhere, the bowel gas pattern is unremarkable, with no plain X-ray evidence of obstruction or perforation.
- There is a surgical clip projected over the right upper quadrant, in keeping with a previous cholecystectomy. No obvious abnormality of the solid abdominal organs is evident.

- There is no obvious abnormality of the visible solid abdominal organs.
- A degenerative lumbar scoliosis convex to the right centred on L2/3 is present. No other skeletal or soft tissues abnormality is visible.

IN SUMMARY – This abdominal X-ray shows marked mucosal oedema of the transverse colon. There is no evidence of toxic dilatation currently. My differential diagnosis for mucosal oedema includes ischaemic, infective (such as Clostridium diffi cile) and infl ammatory causes. Other possibilities include malignancy and haemorrhage; however, given the clinical details and the watershed distribution of the colitis, ischaemia would be highest on my differential. Routine bloods, a serum lactate and stool samples should be acquired. Urgent discussion with the general surgeons is needed, and a CT of the abdomen and pelvis with contrast (arterial and portal venous phases) should be considered.

CASE 11.26

A 2-day-old premature neonate develops abdominal distension and bloody stools. On examination, the abdomen feels tense and there are decreased bowel sounds. His abdominal X-ray is shown here.

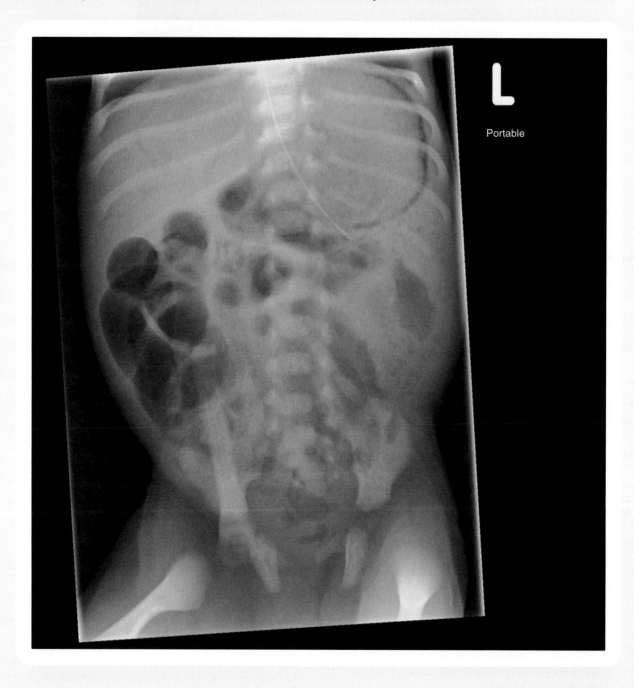

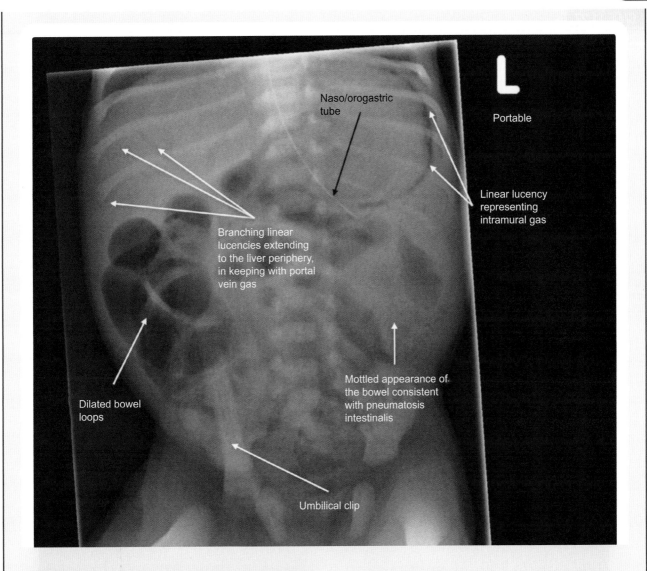

Naso/orogastric tube

Portable

Linear lucency representing intramural gas

Branching linear lucencies extending to the liver periphery, in keeping with portal vein gas

Dilated bowel loops

Mottled appearance of the bowel consistent with pneumatosis intestinalis

Umbilical clip

PRESENT YOUR FINDINGS

- This is a portable supine AP abdominal X-ray of a neonate.
- There are no patient identifiable data on the X-ray. I would like to confirm the patient's name, date of birth and the date and time that the X-ray was performed before making any further assessment.
- The X-ray is technically adequate.
- There are multiple abnormalities demonstrated. There are dilated loops of bowel within the right side of the abdomen. At this age, differentiation between the small and large bowel is difficult on X-rays.
- The bowel in the left flank has a mottled appearance and a linear lucency is evident in the left upper quadrant. These findings are consistent with pneumatosis intestinalis with intramural gas in the stomach.
- Linear gas patterns projected over the liver are present. The linear gas patterns most likely represent gas within the portal venous system as they

extend out towards the liver periphery/edge (as opposed to pneumobilia in which the gas is central within the liver).
- There is no evidence of pneumoperitoneum.
- A naso/orogastric tube is in situ, with its tip in the stomach, and an umbilical clip is present projected over the right lower quadrant.

IN SUMMARY – This abdominal X-ray shows dilated bowel loops, pneumatosis intestinalis and portal venous gas. These findings, in combination with the clinical presentation, are in keeping with necrotising enterocolitis. There is no evidence of pneumoperitoneum. The patient should be made nil by mouth and IV fluid commenced. Routine bloods including inflammatory markers, as well as blood cultures, should be taken. IV antibiotics in accordance with local guidelines should be started and an urgent surgical review arranged.

CASE 11.27

A 70-year-old man has an abdominal X-ray for vague abdominal pain and symptoms of altered bowel habit. His X-ray is shown here.

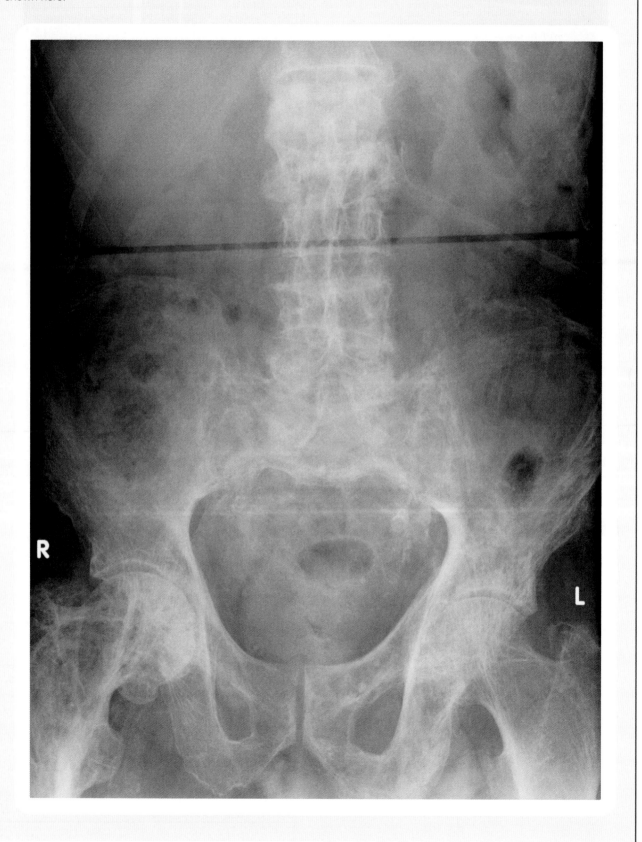

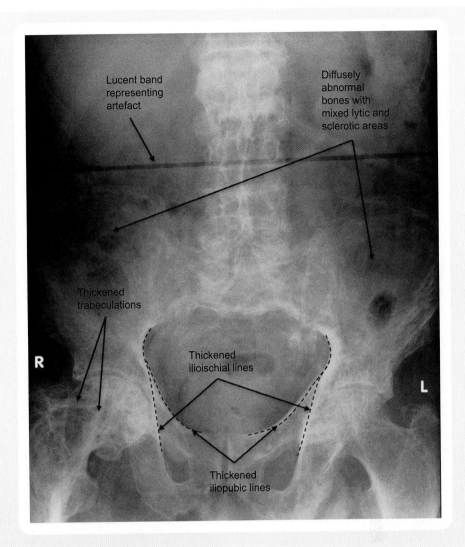

Lucent band representing artefact

Diffusely abnormal bones with mixed lytic and sclerotic areas

Thickened trabeculations

Thickened ilioischial lines

R

L

Thickened iliopubic lines

🔍 PRESENT YOUR FINDINGS

- This is a supine AP abdominal X-ray of an adult.
- There are no patient identifiable data on the X-ray. I would like to confirm the patient's name, date of birth and the date and time that the X-ray was performed before making any further assessment.
- The hemidiaphragms and flanks are not completely imaged. The X-ray is therefore technically inadequate.
- The most striking abnormality is the diffusely abnormal bones. The pelvis and imaged femori are expanded with a mixed lytic and sclerotic pattern. There is thickening of the iliopubic and ilioischial lines and of the trabeculations. The spine appears to be involved as well but is difficult to assess on this projection.

- The bowel gas pattern is normal and there is no X-ray evidence of obstruction, perforation or mucosal oedema.
- No obvious abnormality of the solid abdominal organs is visible.
- There is a thin horizontal lucent line running transversely across the image which is du e to artefact.

IN SUMMARY – The bones are diffusely abnormal, particularly the pelvis and femori. The appearances are classical for Paget disease which is a chronic bone disorder characterised by excessive and disorganised bone remodelling. I would review the patient's routine blood tests and expect to see elevated levels of alkaline phosphatase (ALP) to be in keeping with Paget disease. No cause for the patient's abdominal symptoms is demonstrated and further investigations should be guided by the history and examination.

CASE 11.28

A 35-year-old man, who has no significant past medical history, presents with abdominal pain and vomiting. His bowels have not opened for 3 days. He has been feeling generally unwell for a few weeks. Clinically, there is a mass within his abdomen. An abdominal X-ray is performed as obstruction is felt likely.

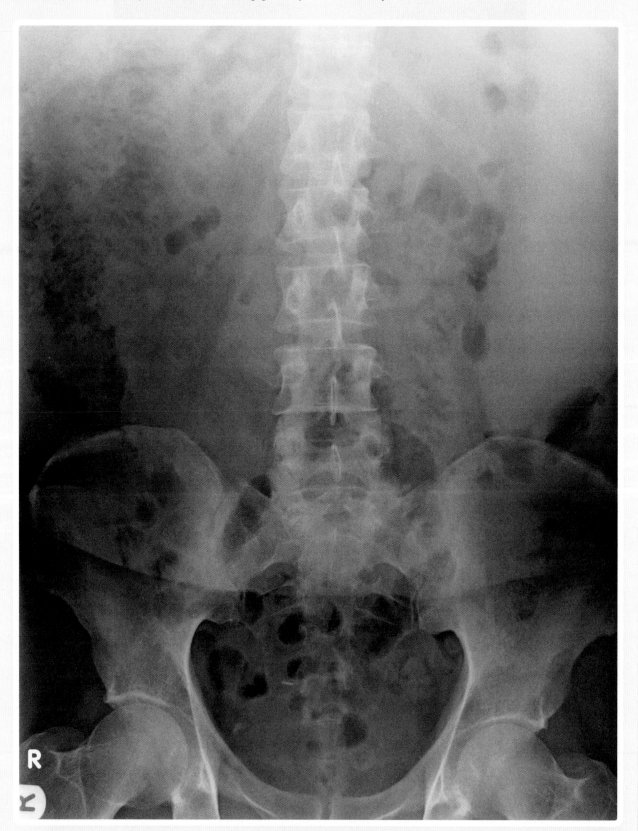

Continue

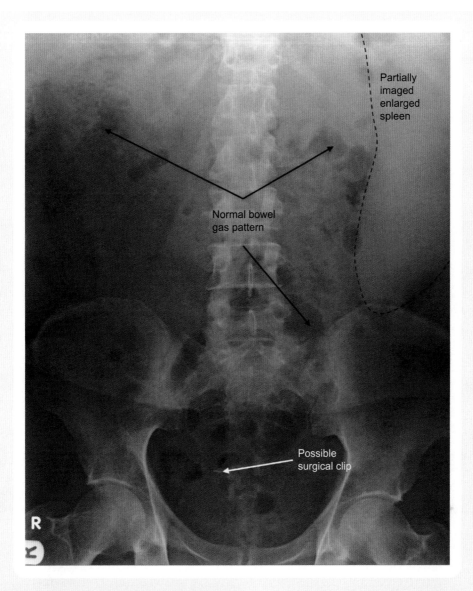

Partially imaged enlarged spleen

Normal bowel gas pattern

Possible surgical clip

R

PRESENT YOUR FINDINGS

- This is a supine AP abdominal X-ray of an adult.
- There are no patient identifiable data on the X-ray. I would like to confirm the patient's name, date of birth and the date and time that the X-ray was performed before making any further assessment.
- The hemidiaphragms and hernial orifices are not completely imaged. The X-ray is therefore technically inadequate; however, the salient abnormality is displayed.
- The most striking abnormality is a large homogeneous region of increased radiodensity in the left upper quadrant. This extends inferiorly to the level of the iliac crest. It is in keeping with a partially imaged enlarged spleen.
- The bowel gas pattern appears normal, with no X-ray evidence of obstruction, perforation or mucosal oedema.

- A small linear radio-opacity is projected over the pelvis. This may represent a surgical clip or may be on the patient's skin or clothing.
- No skeletal abnormality is visible.

IN SUMMARY – This abdominal X-ray shows a markedly enlarged spleen extending from the left upper quadrant down to the level of the pelvis. There are no other signifi cant findings. My differential diagnosis for massive splenomegaly includes lymphoma and malaria. Myelofi brosis and chronic myeloid leukaemia are other possibilities but they are uncommon in a patient of this age. Other causes for splenomegaly to consider are portal hypertension, haemoglobinopathies and infective causes such as infectious mononucleosis and TB. A full history including medication, family history and travel history are all important for helping to narrow the differential. Routine as well as specialised blood tests will also be integral to obtaining the diagnosis. Further imaging will be determined by the likely underlying diagnosis.

CASE 11.29

A 40-year-old man is recovering from colorectal surgery 5 days ago. He has ongoing central abdominal pain, vomiting and no bowel movement since his operation. His abdominal X-ray is shown here.

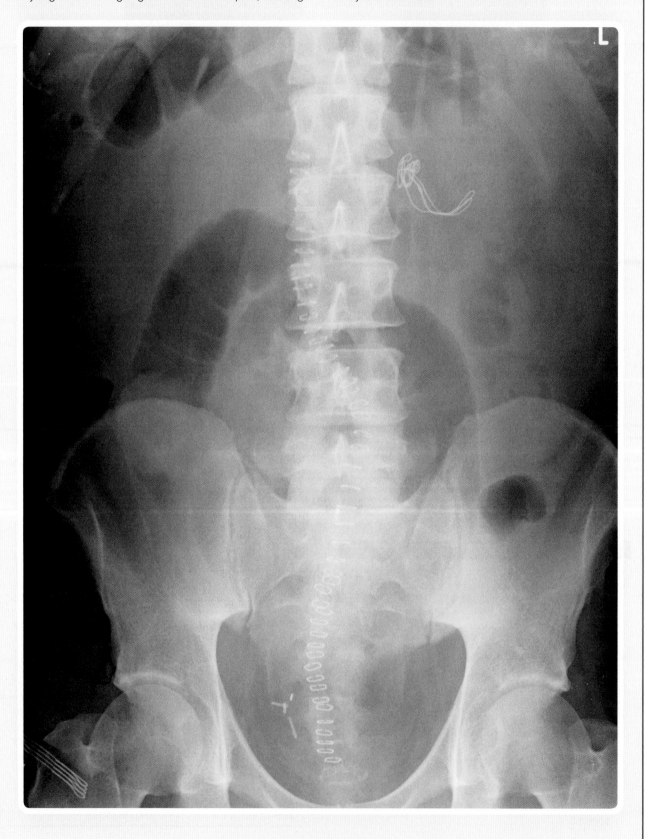

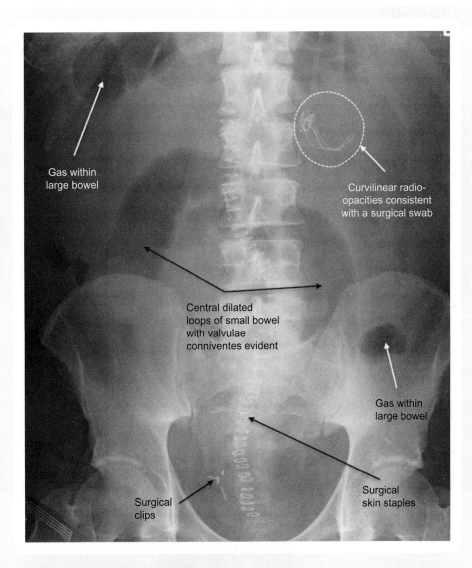

Gas within
large bowel

Curvilinear radio-
opacities consistent
with a surgical swab

Central dilated
loops of small bowel
with valvulae
conniventes evident

Gas within
large bowel

Surgical
clips

Surgical
skin staples

PRESENT YOUR FINDINGS

- This is a supine AP abdominal X-ray of an adult.
- There are no patient identifiable data on the X-ray. I would like to confirm the patient's name, date of birth and date and time that the X-ray was performed before making any further assessment.
- The hemidiaphragms and hernial orifices are not completely imaged. The X-ray is therefore technically inadequate.
- The most striking abnormality is the central dilated loops of small bowel. No distinct cut-off point is visible. Some gas is seen within the nondilated colon, suggesting the small bowel obstruction is either an early obstruction or incomplete.
- There are characteristic curvilinear radio-opacities projected over the left upper quadrant which are highly suspicious of a surgical swab. This may be on the patient's skin; however, I am concerned it represents an intraabdominal swab mistakenly left in situ.
- Abdominal surgical staples project along the midline of the abdomen and radiopaque surgical clips project

over the right pelvis. These features are in keeping with the history of recent surgery.
- No plain X-ray evidence of pneumoperitoneum or mucosal oedema is visible.
- No obvious abnormality of the solid abdominal organs is evident.
- No skeletal or soft tissues abnormalities are apparent.

IN SUMMARY – This abdominal X-ray shows dilated small bowel loops with features of a possible intra abdominal surgical swab. I would like to examine the patient to determine whether the swab is on the patient's skin. The differential diagnosis for this post operative small bowel obstruction is between a mechanical obstruction, possibly related to the surgical swab and any associated inflammatory reaction, and a functional obstruction (ileus). I would obtain routine bloods, commence IV fluids and insert an NG tube to help decompress the GI tract. The patient should be nil by mouth, and I would contact the patient's surgical team for urgent assessment and possible intervention.

BONUS ORTHOPAEDIC X-RAYS

CASE 11.30

A 22-year-old man punched another person whilst intoxicated. He has presented to A&E with pain in his right little finger.

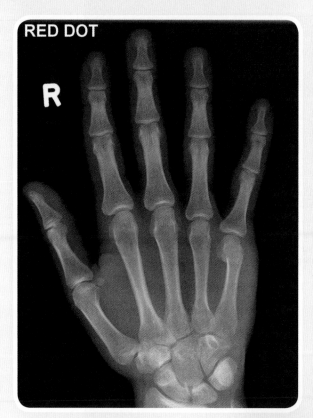

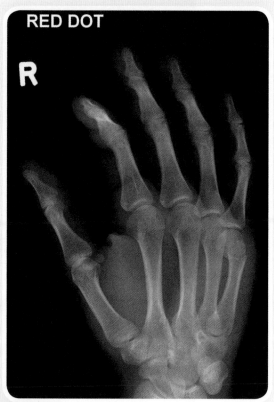

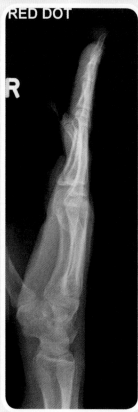

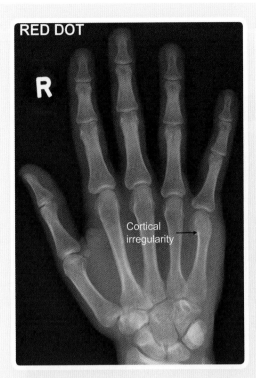

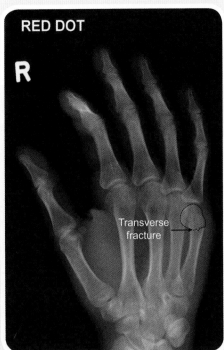

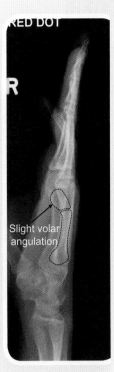

RED DOT

R

Cortical irregularity

RED DOT

R

Transverse fracture

RED DOT

R

Slight volar angulation

🔍 PRESENT YOUR FINDINGS

- These are AP, oblique and lateral X-rays of the right hand of a skeletally mature patient.
- There are no patient identifiable data on the X-rays. I would like to confirm the patient's name, date of birth and date and time that the X-rays were performed before making any further assessment.
- The X-rays are technically adequate, with no important areas cut off.
- There is a simple, transverse fracture through the neck of the 5th metacarpal. Volar angulation of the distal fracture fragment is present. No shortening.

- Overlying soft tissue swelling is evident.
- The rest of the bones are normal, with no other fracture visible and no areas of bone destruction, lucency or abnormal bone texture.

IN SUMMARY – These X-rays show a minimally angulated fracture through the neck of the 5th metacarpal. The fracture is consistent with a punch injury. Treatment options are determined by the degree of functional impairment and include conservative management with buddy strapping of the 5th digit or operative reduction and fixation.

CASE **11.31**

A 14-year-old boy presents to A&E with pain over the lateral aspect of his foot following an inversion injury. He is tender over the base of the 5th metatarsal but able to weight bear. X-rays have been performed for further assessment.

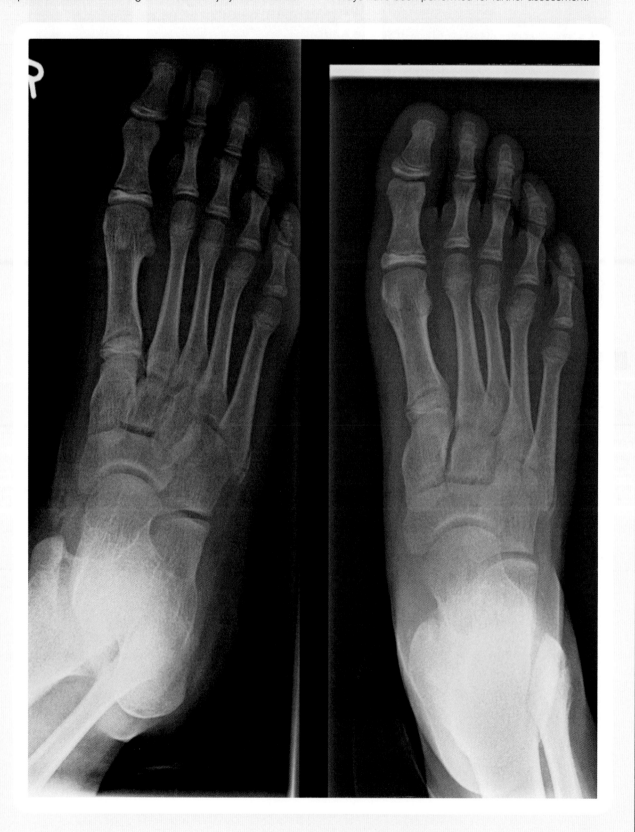

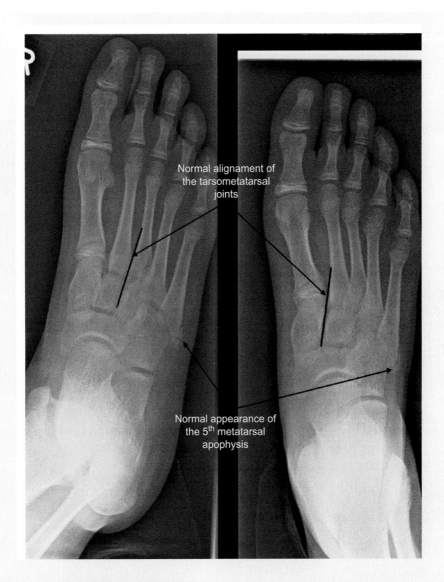

Normal alignament of
the tarsometatarsal
joints

Normal appearance of
the 5th metatarsal
apophysis

PRESENT YOUR FINDINGS

- These are frontal and oblique X-rays of the right foot of a skeletally immature patient.
- There are no patient identifiable data on the X-rays. Confirmation of the patient's name and date of birth, and the date and time when the X-rays were performed is required before making any further assessment.
- The X-rays are technically adequate, with no important areas cut off.

- Normal appearance of the bones with no fracture visible.
- The alignment of the right midfoot is normal.
- No areas of bone destruction, lucency or abnormal bone texture are visible.
- The soft tissues are unremarkable.

IN SUMMARY – These X-rays show a normal right foot with no acute bony injury visible.

CASE **11.32**

A 57-year-old man was knocked off his bicycle by a car. He developed pain around his left shoulder and rib cage and felt winded. He was brought to A&E by ambulance. He is tender around the left shoulder girdle but able to move his arm. An X-ray of his shoulder has been performed.

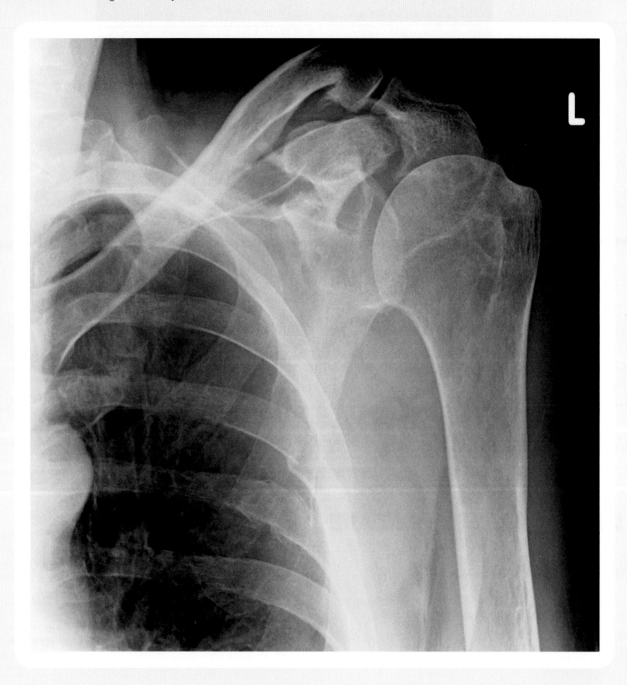

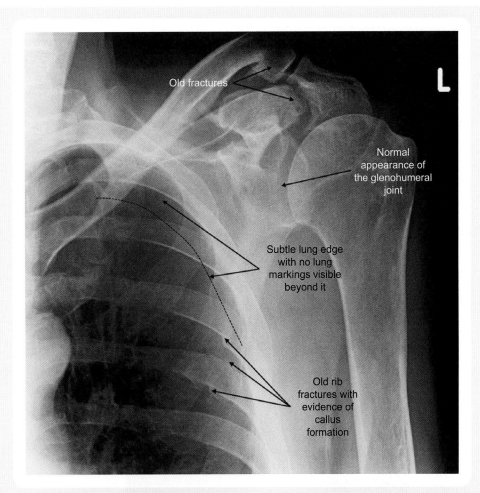

Old fractures

L

Normal
appearance of
the glenohumeral
joint

Subtle lung edge
with no lung
markings visible
beyond it

Old rib
fractures with
evidence of
callus
formation

PRESENT YOUR FINDINGS

- This is an AP X-ray of the left clavicle and shoulder in a skeletally mature patient.
- There are no patient identifiable data on the X-ray. I would like to confirm the patient's name, date of birth and the date and time the X-ray was performed before making any further assessment.
- The X-ray is adequately exposed but I would also like to see a 'second' view of the left shoulder.
- There are old fractures of the lateral aspect of the clavicle and the coracoid.
- In addition, old healed fractures of the left 5th and 6th ribs are evident.
- I cannot see any acute fracture. The left glenohumeral joint appears to be intact although I would like to review a 'second' view of the shoulder to confirm this.

- No areas of bone destruction, lucency or abnormal bone texture.
- There is a small left apical pneumothorax visible in the imaged lung, no other lung abnormality.
- The soft tissues are unremarkable.

IN SUMMARY – This X-ray shows a small apical left-sided pneumothorax and old fractures of the left clavicle, coracoid and 5th and 6th ribs. The cause of the pneumothorax is not visible. I would like to request a PA chest X-ray for further assessment of the pneumothorax and to look for any acute rib fractures. Additionally, I would like to review a second view of the left shoulder to ensure there is no dislocation.

CASE 11.33

A 42-year-old woman fell off her bike, landing on her right elbow. It is tender on palpation, with a reduced range of movement. X-rays of the elbow have been performed.

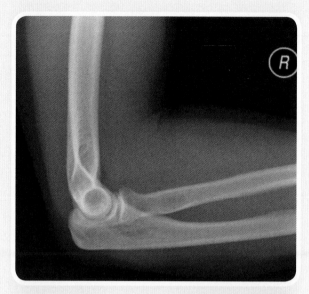

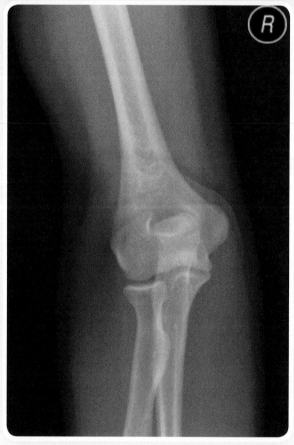

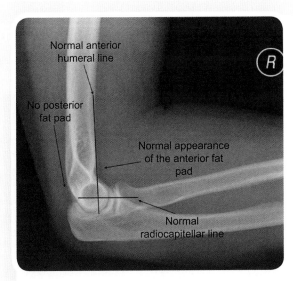

Normal anterior humeral line

No posterior fat pad

Normal appearance of the anterior fat pad

Normal radiocapitellar line

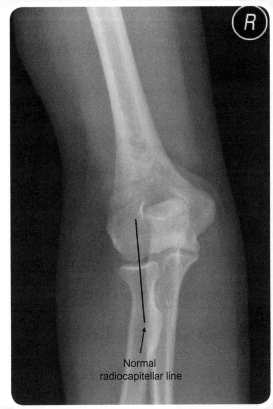

Normal radiocapitellar line

PRESENT YOUR FINDINGS

- These are lateral and frontal X-rays of the right elbow of a skeletally mature patient.
- There are no patient identifiable data on the X-rays. Confirmation of the patient's name and date of birth, and the date and time when the X-rays were performed is required before making any further assessment.
- The X-rays are technically adequate with no important areas cut off.

- There is normal alignment of the elbow joint.
- No fracture or joint effusion is visible.
- No areas of bone destruction, lucency or abnormal bone texture.
- The soft tissues are unremarkable.

IN SUMMARY – These X-rays show a normal right elbow with no evidence of a fracture, effusion or dislocation.

CASE 11.34

An 11-year-old girl presents with progressive left hip pain and a limp which has worsened over the last few days. She is systemically well, with no fever, but is finding it painful to bear weight. A pelvic X-ray is performed.

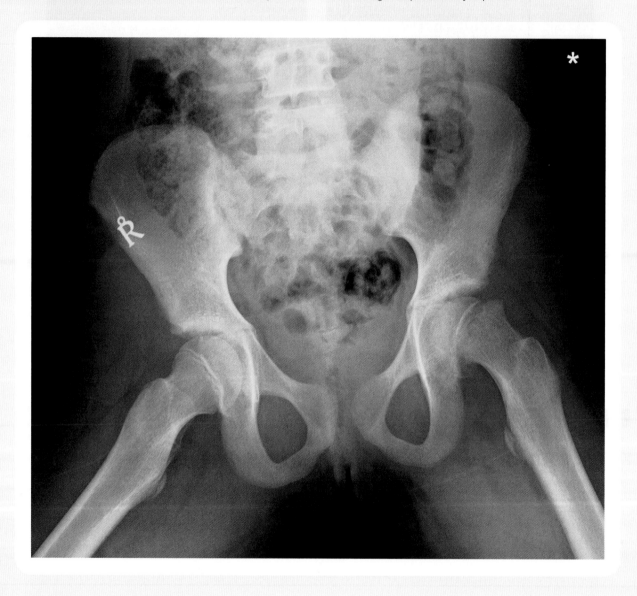

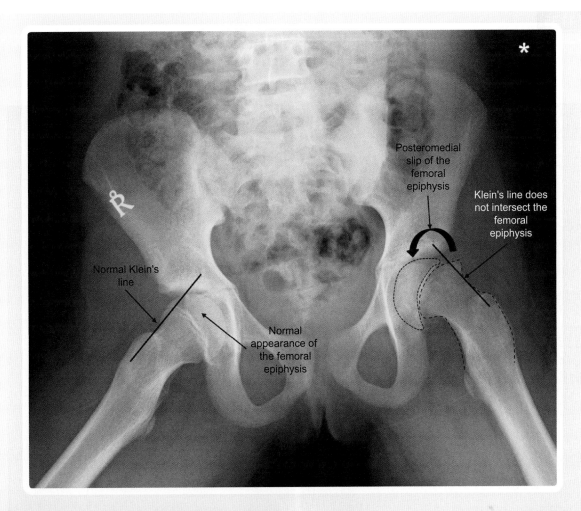

Posteromedial
slip of the
femoral
epiphysis

Klein's line does
not intersect the
femoral
epiphysis

Normal Klein's
line

Normal
appearance
of the femoral
epiphysis

PRESENT YOUR FINDINGS

- This is a 'frog leg' lateral X-ray of the hips in a skeletally immature patient.
- There are no patient identifiable data on the X-ray. I would like to confirm the patient's name, date of birth and the date and time the X-ray was performed before making any further assessment.
- The X-ray is adequately exposed, with no important areas cut off.
- There is abnormal alignment of the left epiphysis with respect to the femoral metaphysis. The epiphysis has slipped medially, with irregularity of the physis. These

findings are in keeping with a slipped upper femoral epiphysis.
- No other fracture or bony abnormality is visible. In particular, the right upper femoral epiphysis appears normal.
- No significant abnormality of the soft tissues is evident.

IN SUMMARY – This X-ray demonstrates a left slipped upper femoral epiphysis. The right upper femoral epiphysis appears normal. The patient should be referred to orthopaedics as it will require operative fixation. The right hip may be prophylactically fixed at the same time.

CASE **11.35**

A 45-year-old has fallen over whilst running for a bus. She is unsure how she landed on her foot but is unable to weight bear. She is tender over the mid and forefoot. X-rays have been performed.

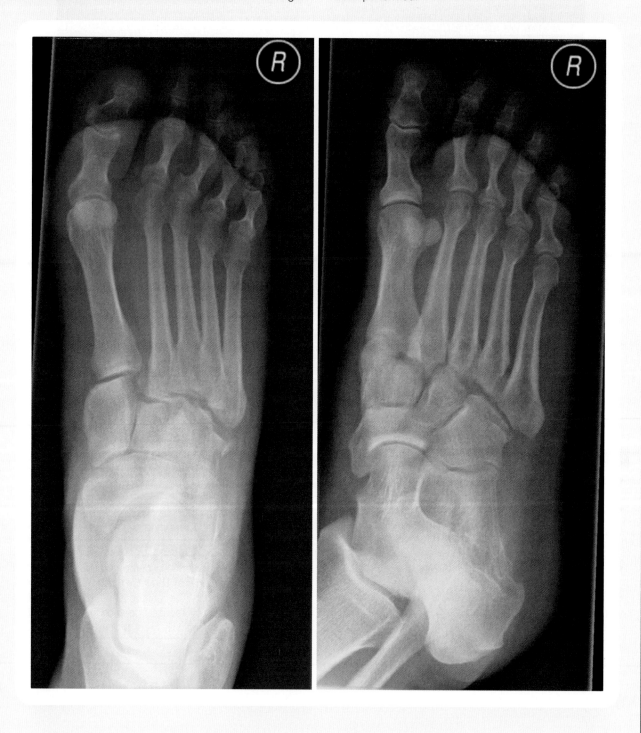

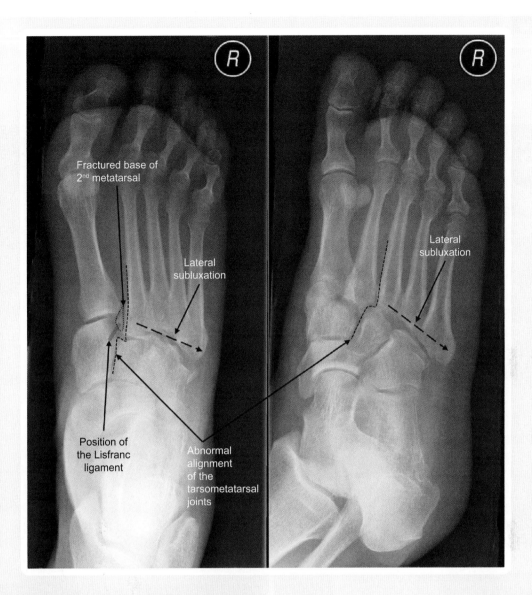

Fractured base of 2nd metatarsal

Lateral subluxation

Lateral subluxation

Position of the Lisfranc ligament

Abnormal alignment of the tarsometatarsal joints

PRESENT YOUR FINDINGS

- These are frontal and oblique X-rays of the right foot.
- There are no patient identifiable data on the X-rays. Confirmation of the patient's name and date of birth, and the date and time when the X-rays were performed is required before making any further assessment.
- The X-rays are technically adequate, with no important areas cut off.
- There is loss of the normal alignment of the 2nd metatarsal with the middle cuneiform and the 3rd metatarsal with the lateral cuneiform – the 2nd to 5th metatarsals have subluxed laterally.
- There is a small vertical fracture at the base of the 2nd metatarsal visible on the AP view. There is minor medial displacement of the small fracture fragment but no significant angulation or shortening. This is

consistent with an avulsion fracture at the insertion of the Lisfranc ligament on the base of the 2nd metatarsal.
- No other dislocation or fracture is evident.
- No areas of bone destruction, lucency or abnormal bone texture are visible.
- The soft tissues are unremarkable.

IN SUMMARY – These X-rays show a fracture at the base of the 2nd metatarsal, and dislocation of the 2nd-5th tarso-metatarsal joints (Lisfranc injury). Such injuries are unstable and urgent orthopaedic referral is required. The patient may require a CT of the foot for further assessment of the fracture/fractures prior to operative fixation.

CASE **11.36**

A 60-year-old woman has tripped on the pavement. She landed on her outstretched right hand. Her right wrist is swollen, tender on palpation and she has a reduced range of movement. She works as a secretary and is right-hand dominant. You request X-rays for further assessment.

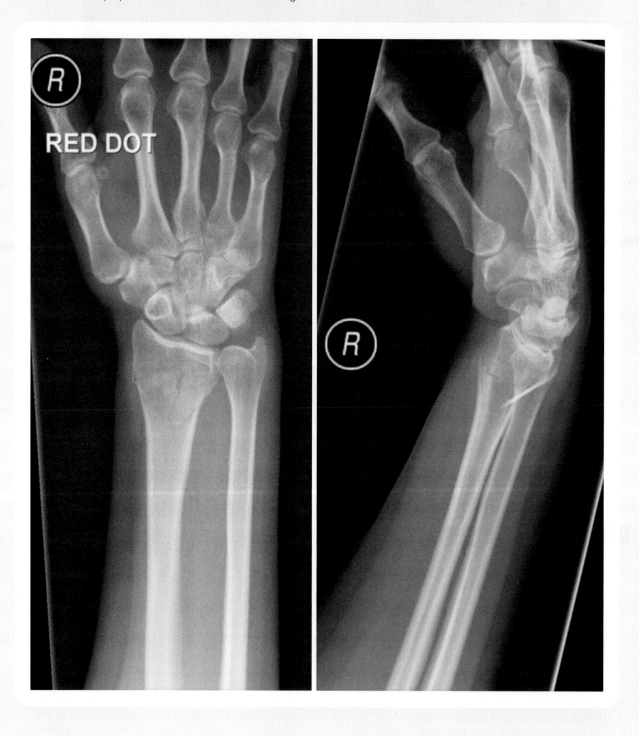

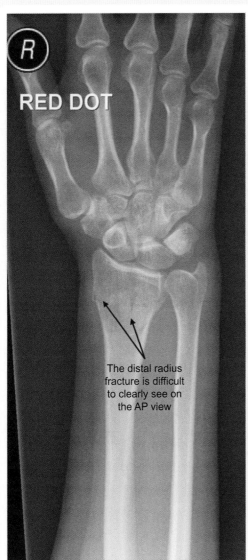

RED DOT

The distal radius fracture is difficult to clearly see on the AP view

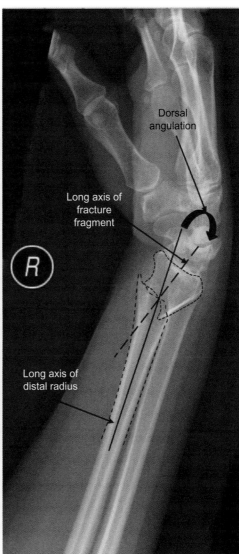

Dorsal angulation

Long axis of fracture fragment

Long axis of distal radius

PRESENT YOUR FINDINGS

- These are AP and lateral X-rays of the right wrist in a skeletally mature patient.
- There are no patient identifiers on the X-rays. I would like to confirm the patient's name and date of birth, and the date and time the X-rays were performed before making any assessment.
- The X-rays are adequately exposed with no important areas cut off.
- There is a simple transverse fracture through the distal radius. A small amount of dorsal angulation is visible on the lateral view. There is no significant displacement, rotation or shortening.
- No other fracture is visible.

- Alignment of the carpal bones is normal.
- No areas of bone destruction, lucency or abnormal bone texture are visible.
- There is some soft tissue swelling on the dorsal aspect of the right wrist, but no significant soft tissue abnormality.

IN SUMMARY – These X-rays show a distal radial fracture with mild dorsal angulation. Given the patient's job, it would be appropriate to reduce this fracture into a better position. Repeat X-rays following manipulation and casting are required, and the patient should be referred to the fracture clinic.

CASE 11.37

A 40-year-old man was playing football when he was tackled and fell over his right ankle. He felt immediate pain around the lateral aspect of his ankle and was unable to weight bear. He has come to A&E department for assessment.

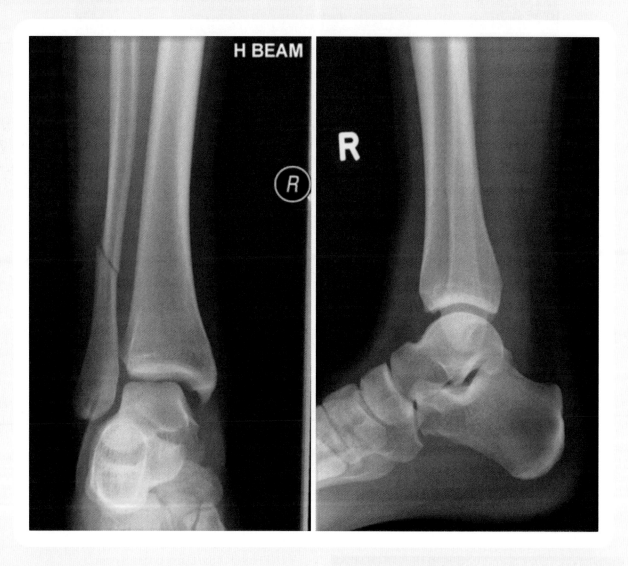

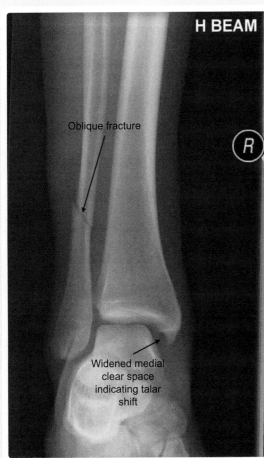

H BEAM

Oblique fracture

Widened medial
clear space
indicating talar
shift

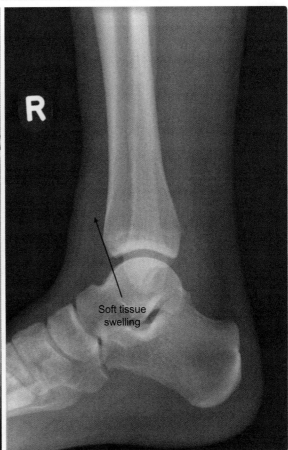

R

Soft tissue
swelling

PRESENT YOUR FINDINGS

- These are AP and lateral X-rays of the right ankle in a skeletally mature patient.
- There are no patient identifiable data on the X-rays. I would like to confirm the patient's name and date of birth, and the date and time the X-rays were performed before making any further assessment.
- The X-rays are adequately exposed with no important areas cut off.
- There is an oblique fracture through the distal third of the fibula. The fracture is minimally displaced and proximal to the syndesmosis. There is no shortening.

- There is widening of the medial joint space indicating talar shift (implying rupture of the deltoid ligaments).
- No other fractures are visible.
- No areas of bone destruction, lucency or abnormal bone texture are evident.
- There is some subtle soft tissue swelling over the fracture but no other significant abnormality of the soft tissues.

IN SUMMARY – These X-rays show a right Weber C ankle fracture with talar shift. This is an unstable injury which will require surgical fixation. The ankle should be put into a cast and the patient referred to orthopaedics.

CASE 11.38

A 54-year-old woman fell, 'going over' her left ankle. Her ankle and lateral aspect of the foot are painful on weight bearing and palpable. There is some soft tissue swelling over the lateral aspect of the foot.

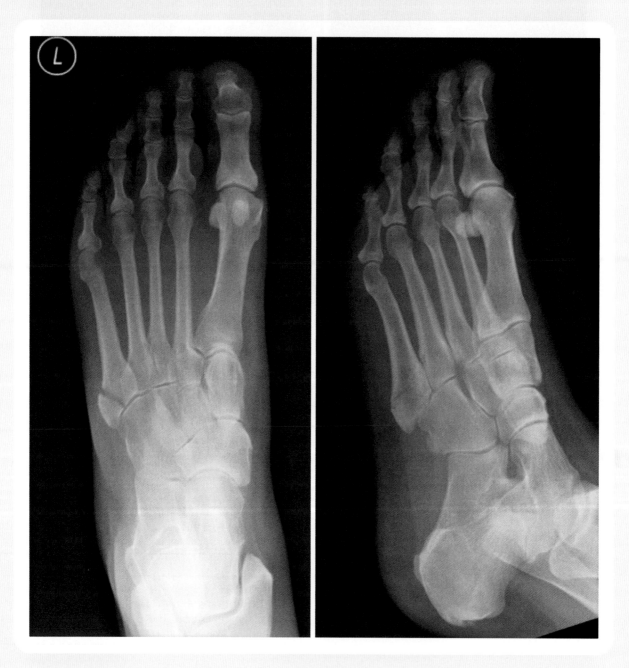

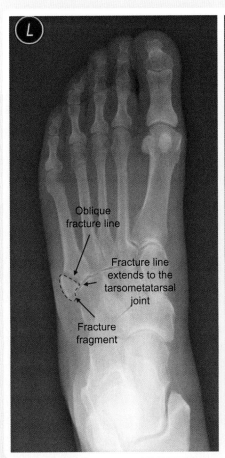

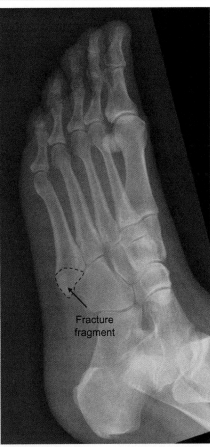

Oblique fracture line

Fracture line extends to the tarsometatarsal joint

Fracture fragment

Fracture fragment

PRESENT YOUR FINDINGS

- These are AP and oblique X-rays of the left foot in a skeletally mature patient.
- There are no patient identifiable data on the X-rays. I would like to confirm the patient's name and date of birth, and the date and time the X-rays were performed before making any further assessment.
- The X-rays are adequately exposed, with no important areas cut off.
- There is a minimally displaced oblique fracture through the base of the 5th metatarsal. This extends to the tarsometatarsal joint surface. There is no shortening.

- No other fracture is visible.
- Alignment of the midfoot is normal.
- No areas of bone destruction, lucency or abnormal bone texture are evident.
- There is no significant abnormality of the soft tissues.

IN SUMMARY – These X-rays show a fracture through the base of the 5th metatarsal. Given its appearance, it is consistent with an avulsion fracture (at the site of the insertion point of peroneus brevis). The patient should be fitted with a walking boot and referred to the fracture clinic.

CASE **11.39**

A 24-year-old man attends A&E after falling off his motorbike. He complains of a painful right knee and is unable to weight bear. X-rays of the knee have been performed.

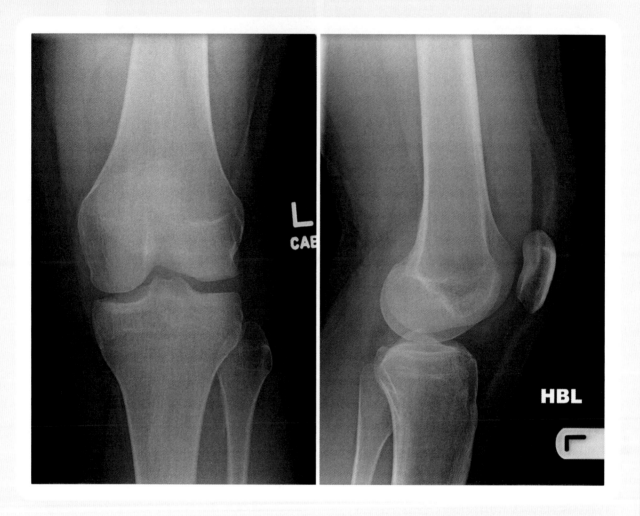

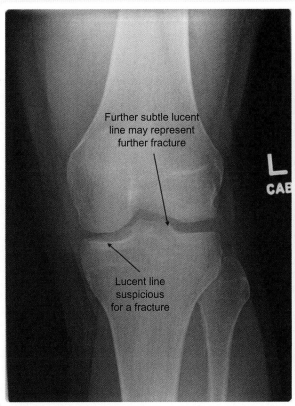

Further subtle lucent line may represent further fracture

L
CAE

Lucent line suspicious for a fracture

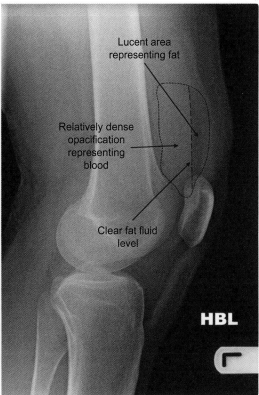

Lucent area representing fat

Relatively dense opacification representing blood

Clear fat fluid level

HBL

🔍 PRESENT YOUR FINDINGS

- These are horizontal beam lateral and frontal X-rays of the right knee of a skeletally mature patient.
- There are no patient identifiable data on the X-rays. Confirmation of the patient's name and date of birth, and the date and time when the X-rays were performed is required before making any further assessment.
- The X-rays are technically adequate, with no important areas cut off.
- The most obvious abnormality is the large knee effusion visible on the lateral view. This has a fluid-fluid level and is consistent with a lipohaemarthrosis.
- The underlying fracture is difficult to see but there is a lucent line in the medial tibial plateau visible on the frontal view which is suspicious for a fracture. Additionally there may be a fracture of the tibial spine.
- No other fractures are visible.
- Alignment of the knee is normal.
- No areas of bone destruction, lucency or abnormal bone texture are evident.

IN SUMMARY – These X-rays show a lipohaemarthosis with likely fractures of the medial tibial plateau and possible tibial spine. Referral to orthopaedics is required with a view to requesting a CT for further assessment of the fracture fragments prior to possible fracture fixation.

CASE **11.40**

A 34-year-old man fell and landed on his left shoulder. He is in a great deal of pain and unable to move his shoulder.

There is an obvious deformity of the left shoulder on clinical assessment. You request an X-ray for further assessment.

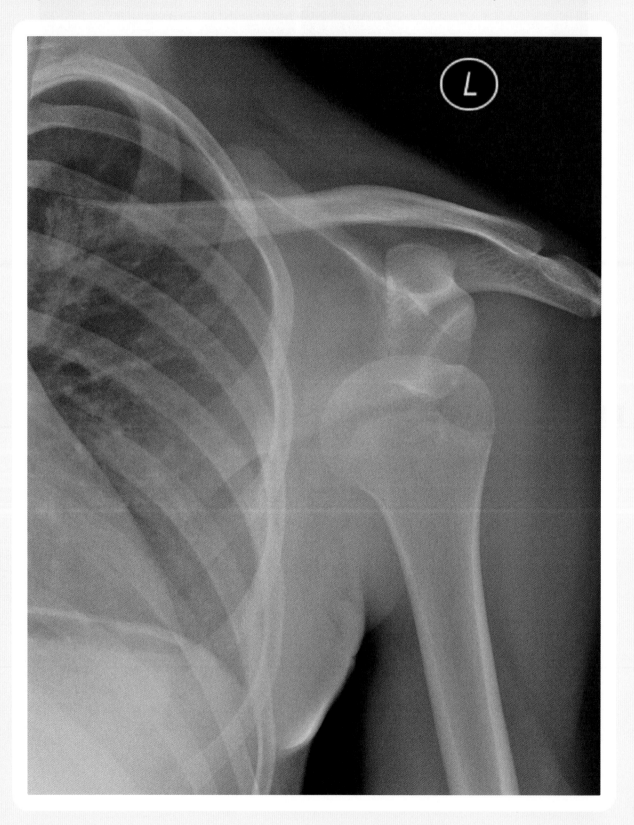

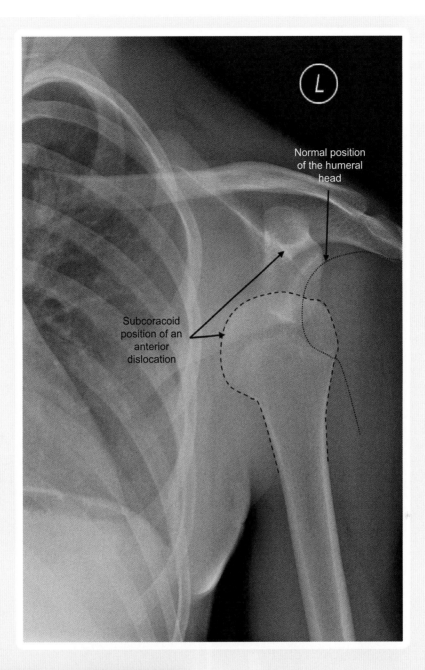

Normal position of the humeral head

Subcoracoid position of an anterior dislocation

🔍 **PRESENT YOUR FINDINGS**

- This is an AP X-ray of the left shoulder.
- There are no patient identifiable data on the X-ray. I would like to confirm the patient's name and date of birth, and the date and time when the X-ray was performed before making any further assessment.
- The X-ray is technically adequate, with no important area cut off.
- The left humeral head has an abnormal subcoracoid position, consistent with an anterior dislocation.
- No fracture is visible.

- No areas of bone destruction, lucency or abnormal bone texture are evident.
- The acromioclavicular joint appears normal on this nondedicated, single view.
- The visible left lung appears normal.
- No significant abnormality of the soft tissues is visible.

IN SUMMARY – This X-ray shows an anterior shoulder dislocation. No associated fracture is visible. The patient should have the shoulder relocated under sedation. A postreduction X-ray is required to confirm relocation of the glenohumeral joint and assess for any fractures.

CASE **11.41**

A 22-year-old man was a passenger in a road traffic accident. He had to be extracted from the car by the fire service and complained of severe pain in his left thigh. His leg was splinted by the ambulance crew. X-rays of the left femur were performed in A&E.

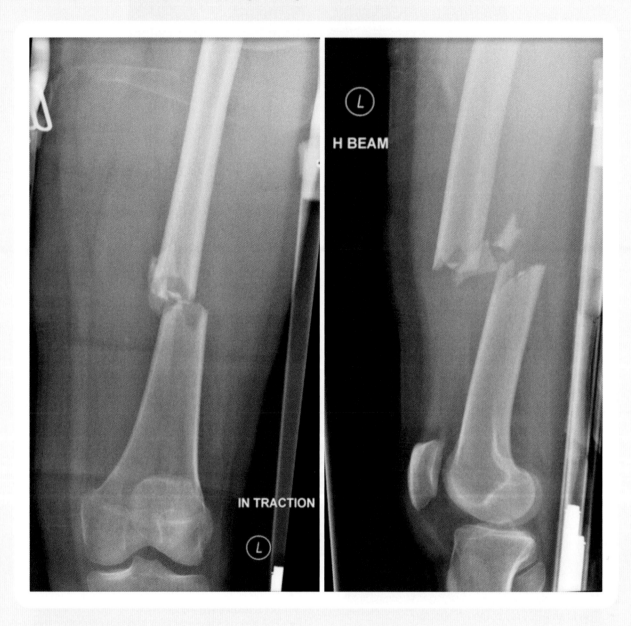

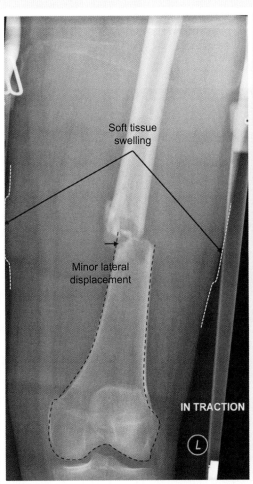

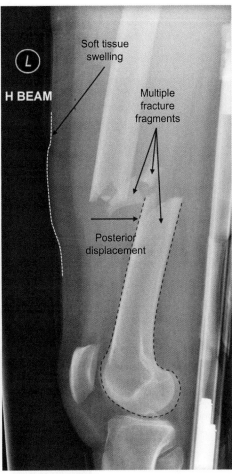

PRESENT YOUR FINDINGS

- These are AP and lateral X-rays of the left femur in a skeletally mature patient.
- There are no patient identifiable data on the radiograph. I would like to confirm the patient's name and date of birth, and the date and time the X-rays were performed before making any further assessment.
- The X-rays are adequately penetrated with no important areas cut off.
- The patient has been imaged with the left femur in traction.
- There is a comminuted transverse fracture involving the middle third of the femur.

- There is marked posterior displacement of the largest fracture fragment with minor lateral displacement. No significant angulation, rotation or shortening is present.
- Normal appearance of the partially imaged knee joint.
- No areas of bone destruction, lucency or abnormal bone texture are evident.
- There is some soft tissue swelling overlying the fracture but no X-ray evidence of this being an open fracture.

IN SUMMARY – These X-rays show a displaced, comminuted left mid shaft femoral fracture. The patient should have been assessed along the ATLS guidelines (ABCDE). I would check the distal neurovascular status of the limb. An attempt to reduce the fracture under sedation in A&E should be considered; however, this patient will require operative fixation.

CASE **11.42**

A 72-year-old woman slipped on ice injuring her right shoulder. It is swollen and tender on palpation, with a reduced range of movement. X-rays of the right shoulder have been performed.

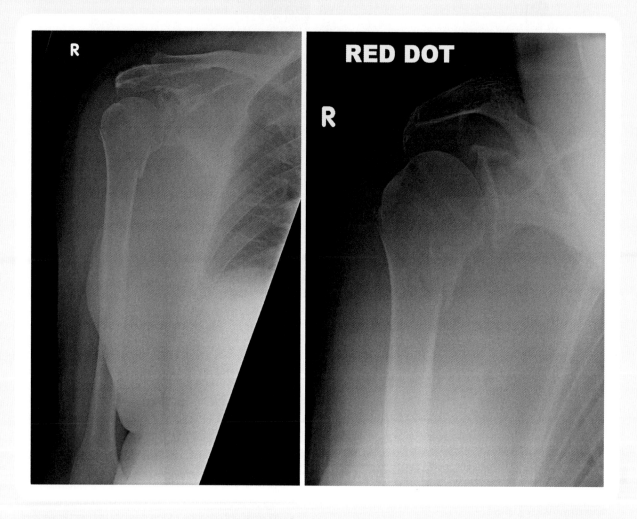

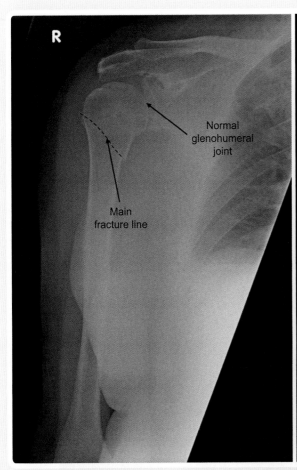

R

Normal
glenohumeral
joint

Main
fracture line

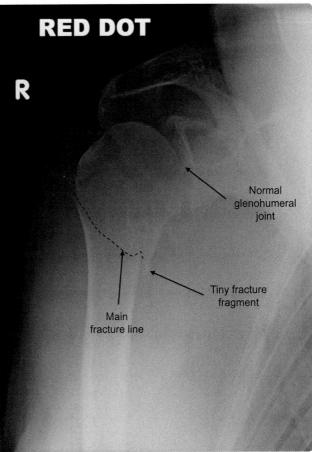

RED DOT

R

Normal
glenohumeral
joint

Tiny fracture
fragment

Main
fracture line

🔍 PRESENT YOUR FINDINGS

- These are AP and apical oblique X-rays of the right shoulder in a skeletally mature patient.
- There are no patient identifiable data on the X-rays. I would like to confirm the patient's name and date of birth, and the date and time the X-rays were performed before making any further assessment.
- The X-rays are adequately penetrated, with no important areas cut off.
- There is a minimally displaced oblique fracture through the right surgical neck of the humerus. There is no shortening. It appears to be a comminuted fracture.

- No other fracture is visible.
- The glenohumeral joint is intact and the acromioclavicular joint appears normally aligned.
- No areas of bone destruction, lucency or abnormal bone texture are evident.
- The imaged right lung is clear.
- The soft tissues are unremarkable.

IN SUMMARY – These X-rays show a minimally displaced, comminuted fracture through the right humeral surgical neck. The patient should be treated with a sling and referred to the fracture clinic.

CASE **11.43**

A 12-year-old girl fell off a trampoline, injuring her left forearm. Assessment in A&E reveals tenderness and swelling over the mid forearm. She is having difficulty moving the arm. You request X-rays of the forearm for further assessment.

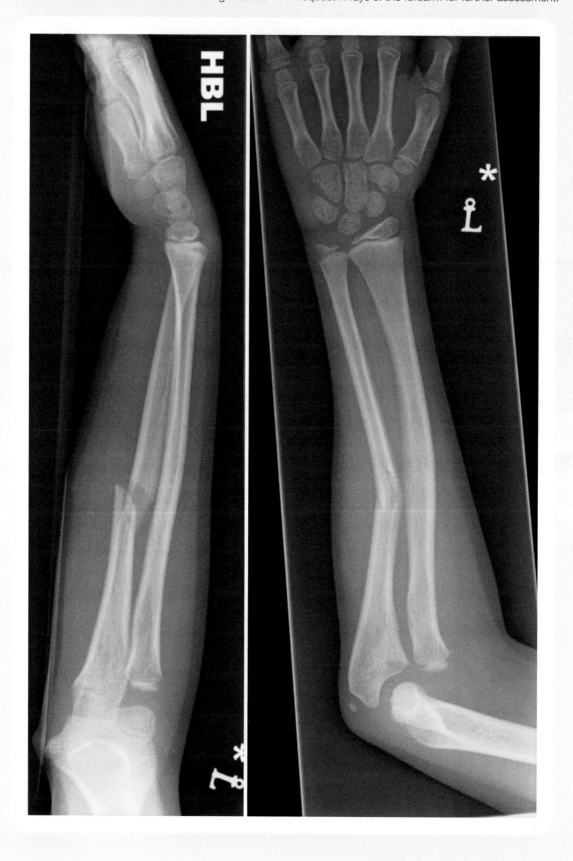

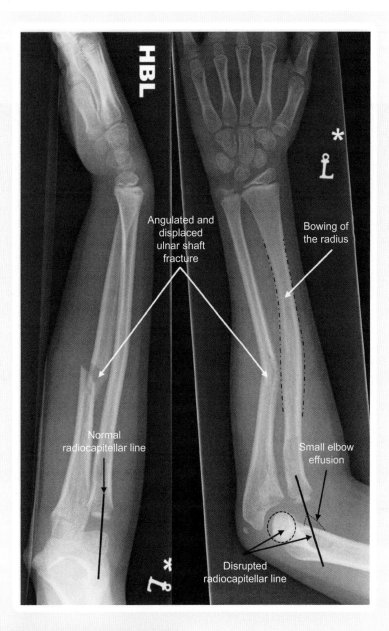

Angulated and displaced ulnar shaft fracture

Bowing of the radius

Normal radiocapitellar line

Small elbow effusion

Disrupted radiocapitellar line

🔍 PRESENT YOUR FINDINGS

- These are AP and lateral X-rays of the left forearm in a skeletally immature patient.
- There are no patient identifiers on the X-rays. I would like to confirm the patient's name and date of birth, and the date and time the X-rays were performed before making any further assessment.
- The X-rays are adequately exposed, with no important areas cut off.
- There is a fracture through the mid shaft (diaphysis) of the ulna. There is ulnar and dorsal angulation and dorsal displacement of the distal fragment. No shortening is apparent.
- In addition, there is disruption of the radiocapitellar line on the AP view, indicating anterior dislocation of the radial head.

- There is a possible small elbow joint effusion.
- There is bowing of the mid radius, in keeping with a plastic deformity (children's bones are flexible and may bend/bow rather than break following trauma). No other fracture is visible.
- No areas of bone destruction, lucency or abnormal bone texture are visible.
- Apart from small elbow effusion associated with the fracture, the soft tissues are unremarkable.

IN SUMMARY – These X-rays show a displaced ulnar shaft fracture with associated anterior dislocation of the radial head. These findings are consistent with a Monteggia fracture. The patient should be referred to orthopaedics for consideration of operative fixation.

CASE 11.44

A 37-year-old woman with epilepsy has been brought into A&E following a seizure. She is complaining of pain in her right shoulder. She is unable to move the shoulder. You request X-rays for further assessment.

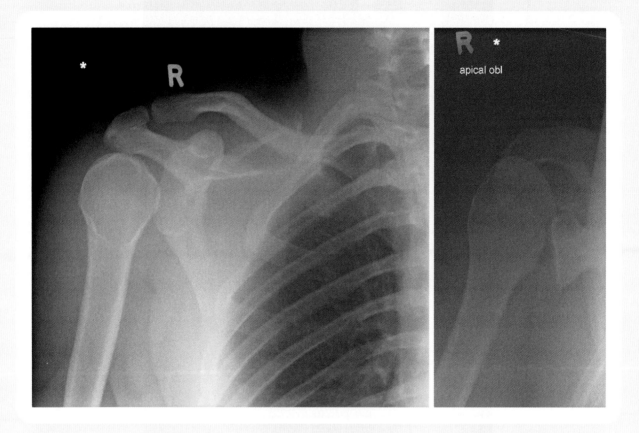

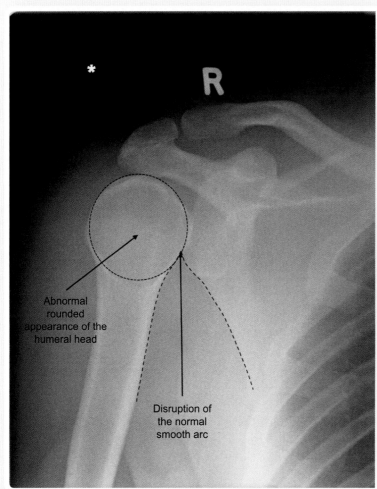

Abnormal rounded appearance of the humeral head

Disruption of the normal smooth arc

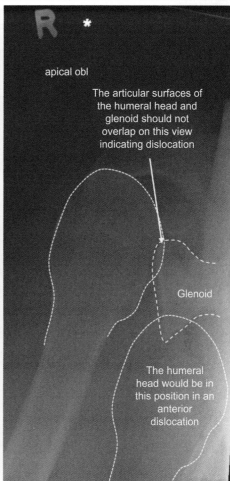

apical obl

The articular surfaces of the humeral head and glenoid should not overlap on this view indicating dislocation

Glenoid

The humeral head would be in this position in an anterior dislocation

🔍 PRESENT YOUR FINDINGS

- These are frontal and apical oblique X-rays of the right shoulder of a skeletally mature patient.
- There are no patient identifiable data on the X-rays. I would like to check the patient's name and date of birth, and the date and time when the X-rays were performed before making any further assessment.
- The X-rays are technically adequate, with no important areas cut off.
- The left humeral head has an abnormal rounded appearance on the frontal X-ray. In addition, the normal smooth arc connecting the medial aspect of the proximal humerus and the lateral part of the scapula is disrupted. These findings are in keeping with a posterior shoulder dislocation, which is confirmed on the apical oblique view.
- There is no fracture.
- No areas of bone destruction, lucency or abnormal bone texture are evident.
- The soft tissues and imaged lung are unremarkable.

IN SUMMARY – These X-rays show a posterior shoulder dislocation. An attempt should be made to relocate the shoulder under sedation. A postreduction X-ray is needed to assess the relocation and identify any fractures.

CASE 11.46

During your final examination you are asked to assess a 60-year-old lady's hands. She has had painful and sore hands for several years and is struggling to perform activities of daily living. After your clinical assessment, you tell the examiner you would request an X-ray for further assessment.

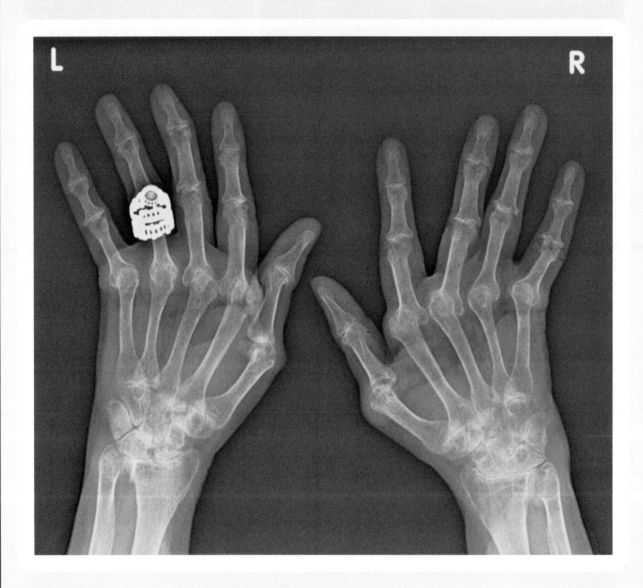

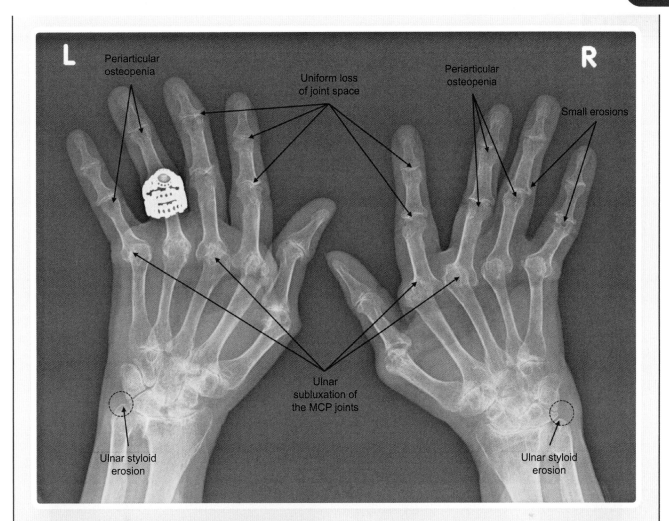

L

Periarticular
osteopenia

Uniform loss
of joint space

Periarticular
osteopenia

Small erosions

R

Ulnar
subluxation of
the MCP joints

Ulnar styloid
erosion

Ulnar styloid
erosion

🔍 PRESENT YOUR FINDINGS

- This is a PA X-ray of both hands in a skeletally mature patient.
- There are no patient identifiable data on the X-ray. I would like to confirm the patient's name and date of birth, and the date and time the X-ray was performed before making any further assessment.
- The X-ray is adequately exposed, with no important areas cut off. There is a metallic artefact from a ring projected over the proximal interphalangeal joint of the left fourth finger.
- There are bilateral, symmetrical abnormalities.
- The metacarpophalangeal joints are predominantly affected, with marked ulnar subluxation evident.
- There is uniform loss of joint space.

- There is periatricular osteopenia, most notably around the interphalangeal joints.
- There are erosions of the ulnar styloids bilaterally as well as some of the interphalangeal joints.
- The soft tissues appear unremarkable. In particular, there is no significant soft tissue swelling, which goes against acute inflammation/synovitis.

IN SUMMARY – The X-ray shows a bilateral, symmetrical erosive arthropathy predominantly involving the metacarpophalangeal joints. The differential diagnoses for an erosive arthropathy include psoriatic arthritis, Reiter syndrome and gout; however, the radiographic appearances are typical of rheumatoid arthritis.

CASE 11.46

A 46-year-old woman tripped whilst walking her dog, injuring her right wrist. She presents to A&E complaining of pain around the wrist. On examination, there is some mild swelling over the dorsum of the wrist and associated tenderness. X-rays of the right wrist have been performed.

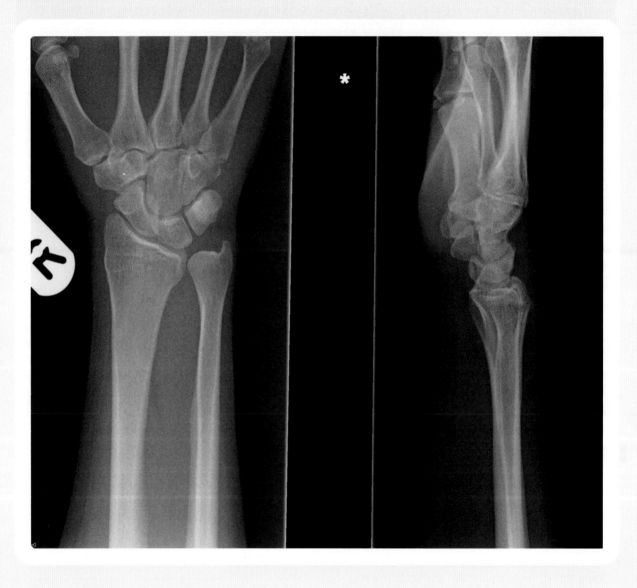

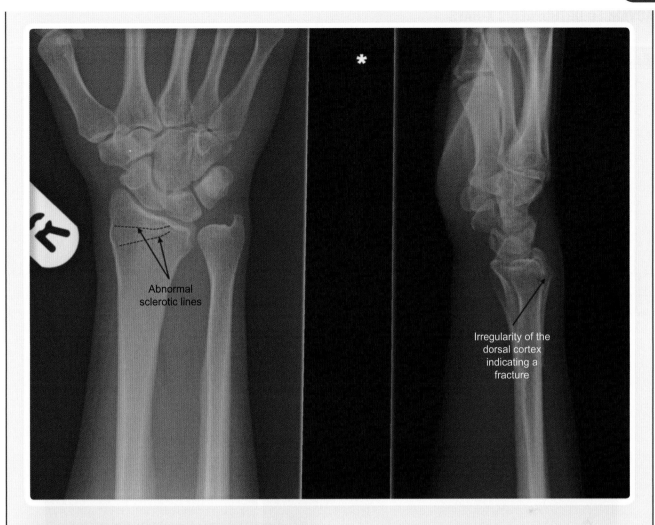

Abnormal
sclerotic lines

*

Irregularity of the
dorsal cortex
indicating a
fracture

🔍 PRESENT YOUR FINDINGS

- These are AP and lateral X-rays of the right wrist in a skeletally mature patient.
- There are no patient identifiers on the X-rays. I would like to confirm the patient's name and date of birth, and the date and time the X-rays were performed before making any further assessment.
- The X-rays are adequately exposed, with no important areas cut off.
- There is a subtle sclerotic line in the distal radius visible on the AP view. The dorsal cortex of the distal radius is irregular on the lateral X-ray.

- No other fracture is visible.
- There is a normal alignment of the carpal bones.
- No areas of bone destruction, lucency or abnormal bone texture are evident.
- There is mild soft tissue swelling dorsally around the fracture.

IN SUMMARY – These X-rays show a minimally displaced distal radius fracture. Given its good position, it is not necessary to attempt manipulation/reduction. Therefore the patient should be treated with a cast or splinting and referred to the fracture clinic.

ADVANCED ORTHOPAEDIC X-RAYS

CASE 11.47

A 62-year-old woman fell whilst shopping, injuring her right leg. She is very sore in the mid shaft of her right leg and unable to weight bear. She has been brought into A&E by ambulance. She is very tender on palpation of the right thigh and unable to move the leg. She is distally neurovascularly intact. X-rays of the right femur have been performed.

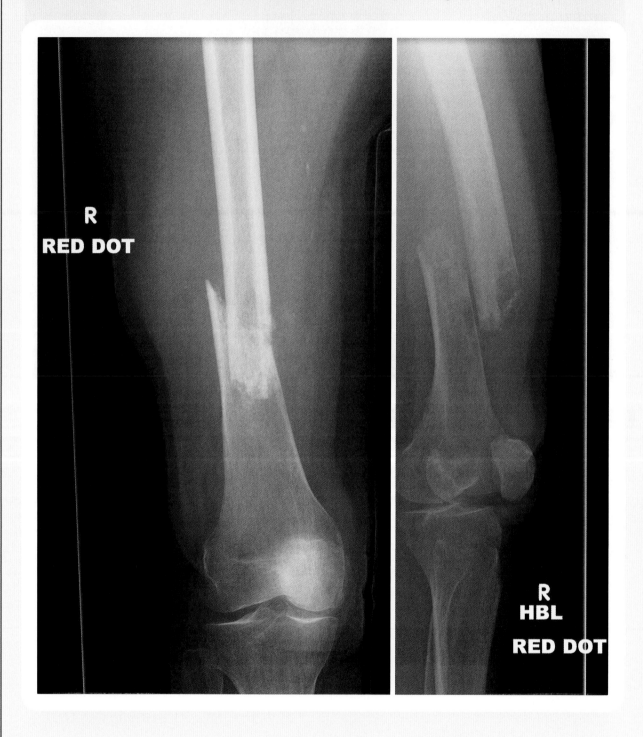

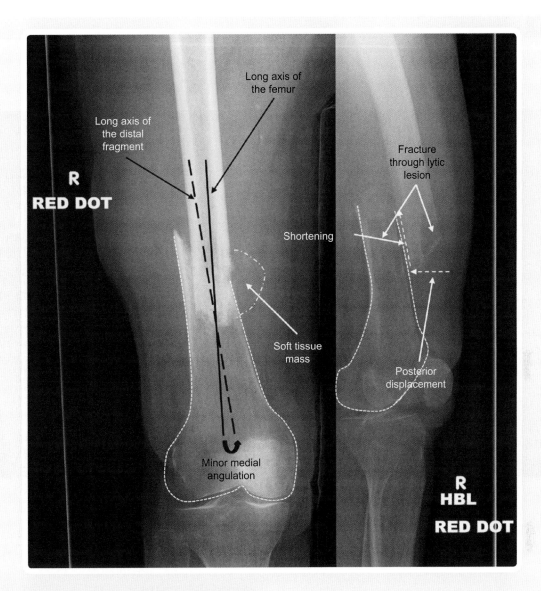

Long axis of
the femur

Long axis of
the distal
fragment

R
RED DOT

Shortening

Soft tissue
mass

Minor medial
angulation

Fracture
through lytic
lesion

Posterior
displacement

R
HBL
RED DOT

PRESENT YOUR FINDINGS

- These are AP and lateral X-rays of the right femur in a skeletally mature patient.
- There are no patient identifiable data on the X-rays. I would like to confirm the patient's name and date of birth, and the date and time the X-rays were performed before making any further assessment.
- The X-rays are adequately penetrated, although the proximal femur has not been included.
- There is a transverse fracture through the distal third of the right femoral shaft.
- There is significant posterior displacement and shortening with minor medial angulation. Normal alignment of the right knee joint is evident.
- At the site of the fracture, there is a heterogenous but predominantly lytic bone lesion. There is evidence of cortical destruction and a possible soft tissue mass. These findings are suggestive of an aggressive bone lesion.

- No other fracture or dislocation is visible.
- There is soft tissue swelling over the shaft of the right femur.

IN SUMMARY – These X-rays show a displaced pathological fracture of the right shaft of the femur. An attempt at reducing and splinting the fracture should be made under sedation. Adequate analgesia should be prescribed. Further X-rays of the entire femur will be required to look for further bone lesions prior to surgical fixation. Given the age of the patient, the underlying bone lesion is most likely a metastasis, with the two most likely primaries in a female being breast and lung cancer. The patient will require a full history and examination, including a breast exam, routine bloods and a chest X-ray. Further imaging will be guided by the above but will likely involve a CT for staging.

CASE 11.48

A 47-year-old woman slipped on her way to work and landed on her left clavicle and shoulder. She is tender on palpation of the left clavicle, with a normal range of movement in the shoulder. An X-ray is performed.

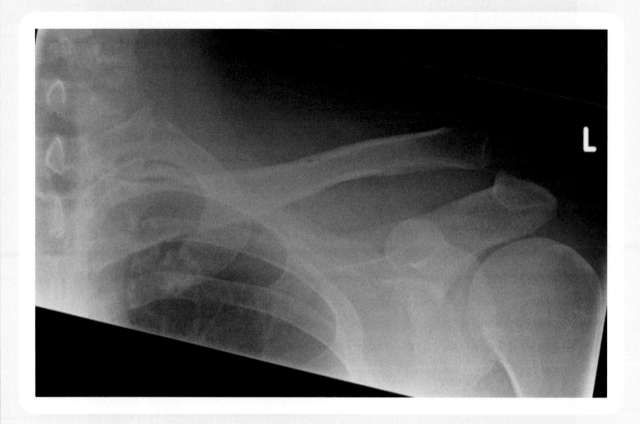

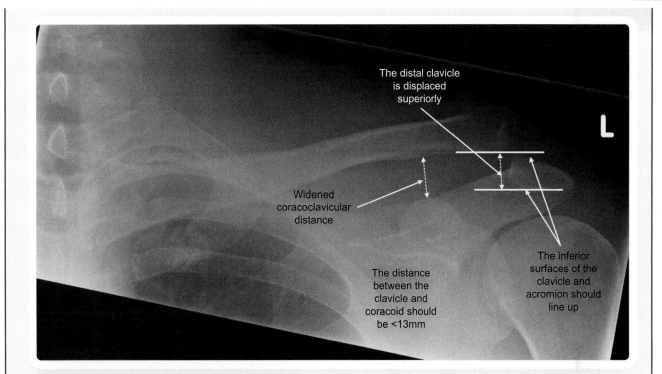

The distal clavicle
is displaced
superiorly

L

Widened
coracoclavicular
distance

The distance
between the
clavicle and
coracoid should
be <13mm

The inferior
surfaces of the
clavicle and
acromion should
line up

🔍 PRESENT YOUR FINDINGS

- This is a single frontal view of the left clavicle in a skeletally mature patient.
- There are no patient identifiable data on the X-ray. I would like to confirm the patient's name and date of birth, and the date and time when the X-ray was performed before making any further assessment.
- The X-ray is technically adequate, with no important area cut off.
- The alignment of the left acromioclavicular joint is abnormal and the clavicular-coracoid distance is increased.
- There is no fracture or glenohumeral joint dislocation visible on this single view.

- There is a normal alignment of the shoulder joint.
- These are no areas of bone destruction, lucency or abnormal bone texture.
- The visualised left lung apex is clear.
- There is some soft tissue swelling superiorly to the left ACJ. The soft tissues are otherwise unremarkable.

IN SUMMARY – This X-ray shows a disruption of the left acromio clavicular joint. Management includes placing the left arm in a collar and cuff and referring the patient to the fracture clinic.

CASE **11.49**

A 29-year-old man was playing tennis when he sustained an inversion injury and presented to A&E with a painful right ankle and foot. The lateral view of his ankle X-ray is shown below.

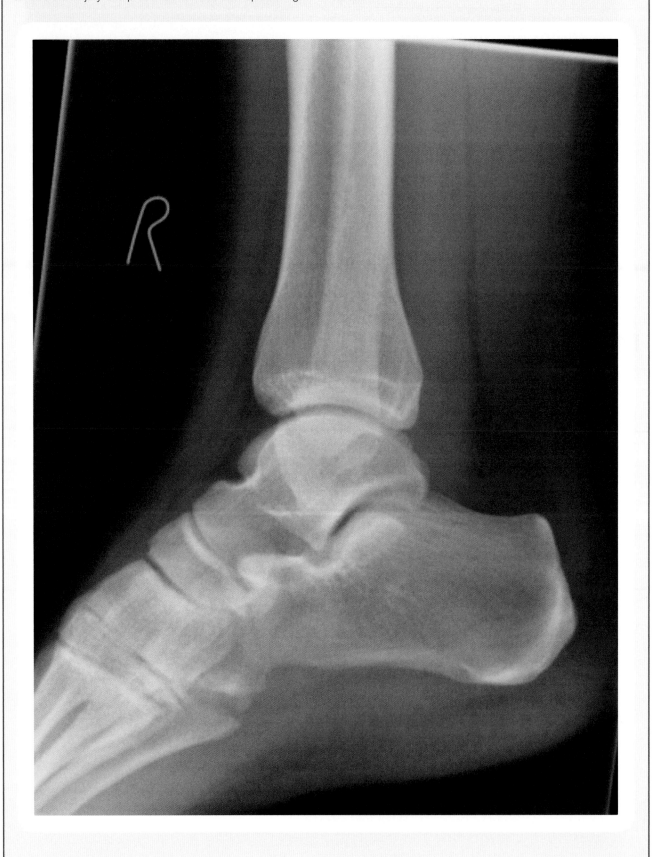

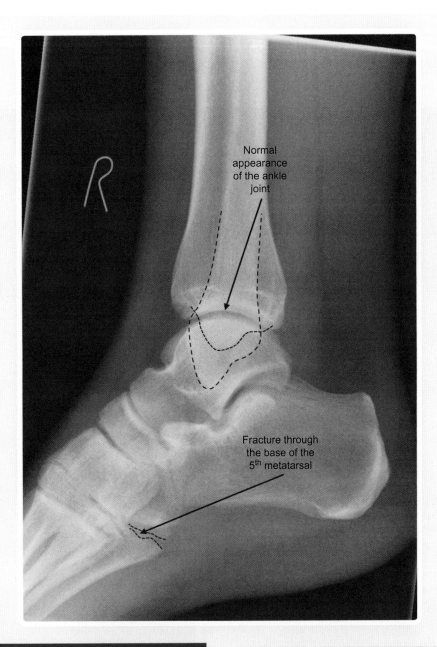

Normal
appearance
of the ankle
joint

Fracture through
the base of the
5th metatarsal

🔍 PRESENT YOUR FINDINGS

- This is a lateral X-ray of the right ankle in a skeletally mature patient.
- No patient identifiable data are present on this X-ray. I would like to confirm the patient's name, date of birth and date and time the X-ray was performed before making any further assessment.
- The X-ray is technically adequate, with no important areas cut off.
- There is a minimally displaced transverse fracture at the base of the 5th metatarsal. It is not possible to fully assess the fracture on this single ankle X-ray – AP and oblique X-rays of the foot are required.
- No other fractures are visible.

- The ankle joint appears normal on this single view.
- There are no areas of bony destruction/lucency or abnormal texture.
- No significant abnormality of the soft tissues is evident.

IN SUMMARY – This lateral X-ray shows a minimally displaced fracture at the base of the 5th metatarsal. This is in keeping with an avulsion fracture (at the peroneus brevis tendon insertion site). It requires further assessment on formal foot X-rays. I would also like to assess the AP ankle X-ray to complete my assessment of the ankle. Treatment of this type of fracture usually involves fitting a walking boot and referring the patient to the fracture clinic.

CASE **11.50**

A 48-year-old woman trapped the tip of her right index finger in a door. It is tender but there is no significant soft tissue swelling. You request X-rays to exclude an underlying fracture.

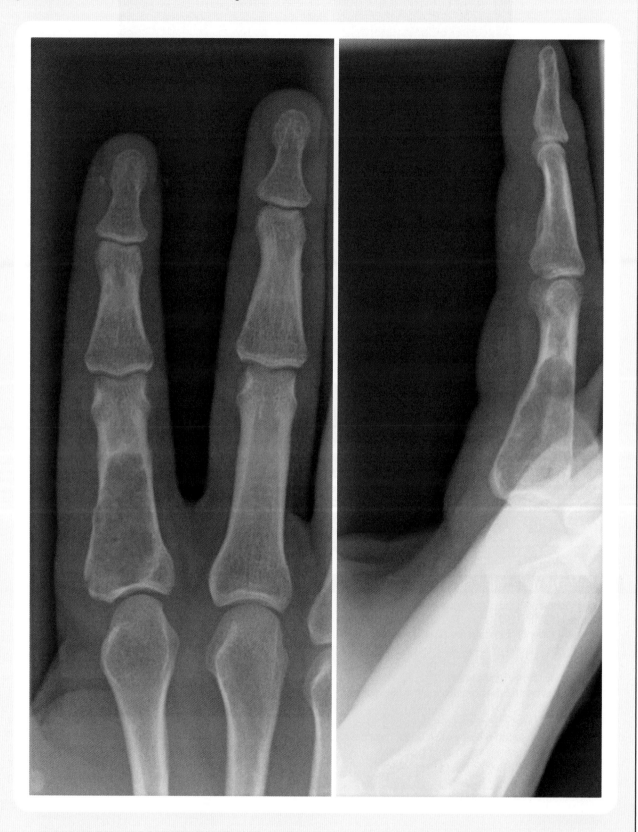

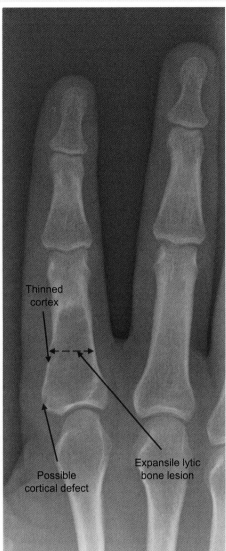
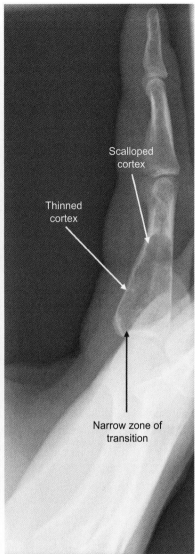

Scalloped
cortex

Thinned
cortex

Thinned
cortex

Possible
cortical defect

Expansile lytic
bone lesion

Narrow zone of
transition

PRESENT YOUR FINDINGS

- These are AP and lateral X-rays of the right index finger in a skeletally mature patient.
- There are no patient identifiable data on the X-rays. I would confirm the patient's name and date of birth, and the date and time the X-ray was performed before making any further assessment.
- The X-rays are adequately exposed, with no important areas cut off.
- The distal phalanx has a normal appearance, with no fracture visible.
- There is a well-defined lytic lesion within the proximal phalanx. It is slightly expansile (the bone is widened at the site), has a narrow zone of transition (the transition zone from normal to abnormal bone) and is causing thinning of the cortex, with a scalloped (series of curved projections) internal cortical surface (endosteal

scalloping). The adjacent cortex is largely intact and there is no soft tissue mass. There is no periosteal reaction. The findings are in keeping with a benign, slow growing bone lesion.
- There is a possible defect in the cortex at the base (radial aspect), which may represent a pathological fracture.
- The alignment of the finger joint is normal.
- No other bone lesions are visible.
- The soft tissues are unremarkable.

IN SUMMARY – These X-rays show a benign bone lesion within the proximal phalanx of the right index finger. The location, combined with the appearances, is in keeping with an enchondroma. There is a possible pathological fracture at the base. I would discuss this patient with orthopaedics.

CASE 11.51

A 6-year-old boy fell over whilst playing. He is complaining of a sore wrist. It is slightly swollen, tender on palpation, with a reduced range of movement. X-rays of the forearm/wrist have been performed.

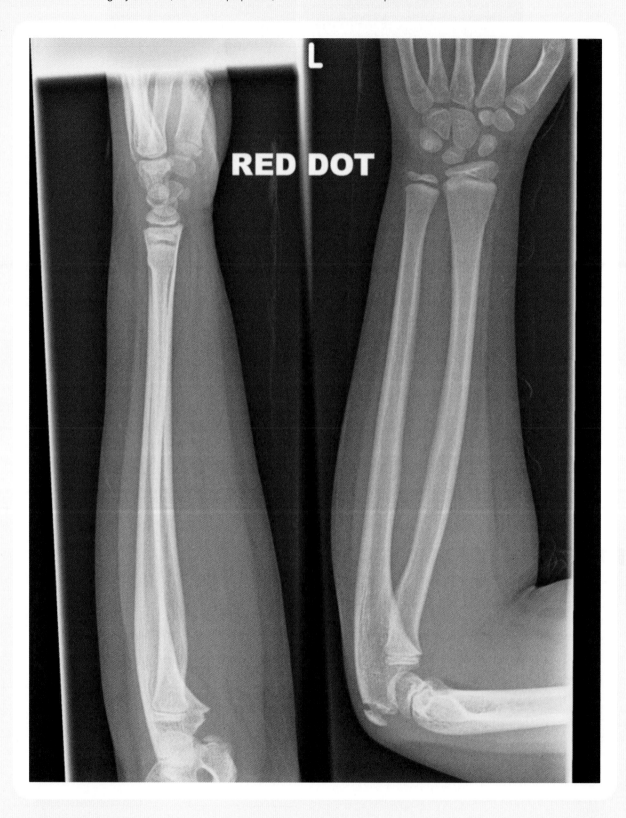

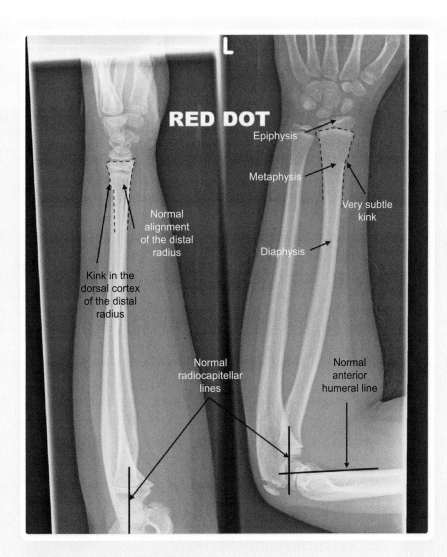

RED DOT

Epiphysis

Metaphysis

Very subtle kink

Diaphysis

Normal alignment of the distal radius

Kink in the dorsal cortex of the distal radius

Normal radiocapitellar lines

Normal anterior humeral line

🔍 PRESENT YOUR FINDINGS

- These are lateral and AP X-rays of the left forearm in a skeletally immature patient.
- There are no patient identifiable data on the X-rays. I would like to confirm the patient's name and date of birth, and the date and time the X-rays were performed before making any further assessment.
- The X-rays are adequately exposed, with no important areas cut off.
- There is a buckling of the dorsal cortex of the distal radial metaphysis. This is most clearly seen on the lateral view of the wrist. There is no cortical break visible. Alignment of the distal radius is normal. No shortening is evident.

- No other fractures are visible, in particular the distal ulnar appears normal and there is no evidence of a Salter–Harris fracture.
- No areas of bone destruction, lucency or abnormal bone texture are evident.
- Articulation of the partially imaged elbow is normal. There is no elbow joint effusion.
- There is minor soft tissue swelling related to the fracture but no other significant soft tissue abnormality.

IN SUMMARY – These X-rays show a distal radial metaphyseal buckle fracture. The patient should be treated with a splint or a cast and referred to the fracture clinic.

CASE **11.52**

An 84-year-old man is found on the floor next to his bed by the care home staff. He is unable to weight bear and brought to hospital. His left lower limb is shortened. An X-ray of the hips has been performed.

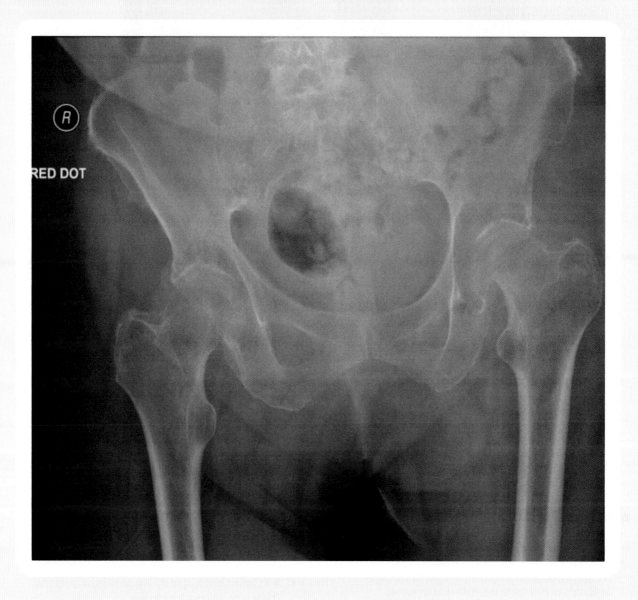

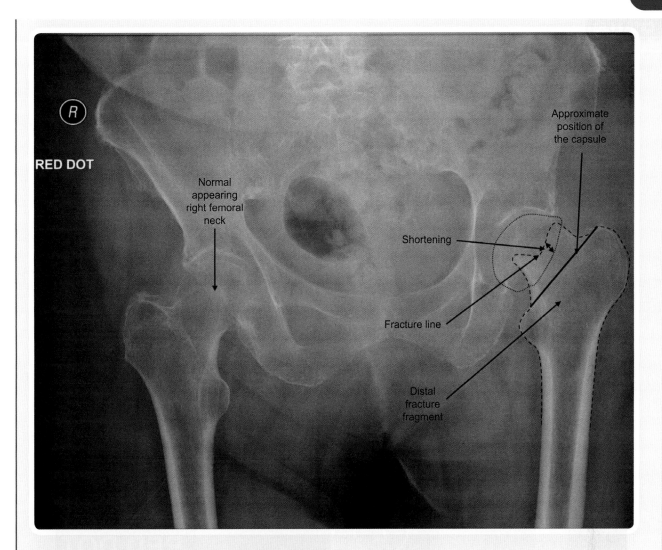

Normal
appearing
right femoral
neck

Approximate
position of
the capsule

Shortening

Fracture line

Distal
fracture
fragment

RED DOT

R

🔍 PRESENT YOUR FINDINGS

- This is an AP X-ray of the pelvis in a skeletally mature patient.
- There are no patient identifiable data on the X-ray. I would like to confirm the patient's name and date of birth, and the date and time the X-ray was performed before making any further assessment.
- The X-ray is adequately exposed, with no important areas cut off.
- There is a simple transverse transcervical fracture through the left femoral neck. There is medial displacement but no significant angulation visible on this single AP view. Additionally, there is shortening and overlap at the fracture site.

- No other fracture is visible with normal alignment of the right hip.
- No areas of bone destruction, lucency or abnormal bone texture are evident.
- There are minor degenerative changes at both hip joints.
- The soft tissues are unremarkable.

IN SUMMARY – This X-ray shows a displaced intracapsular fracture of the left femoral neck. I would like to request a lateral X-ray to complete the radiological assessment of the fracture. The patient should be referred to orthopaedics as he will require surgical fixation in the form of a hip prosthesis.

CASE 11.53

A 52-year-old woman slipped on some ice and injured her left wrist. It is slightly swollen and tender on palpation, with a reduced range of movement. She is very tender on the dorsum of her left wrist and X-rays have been performed.

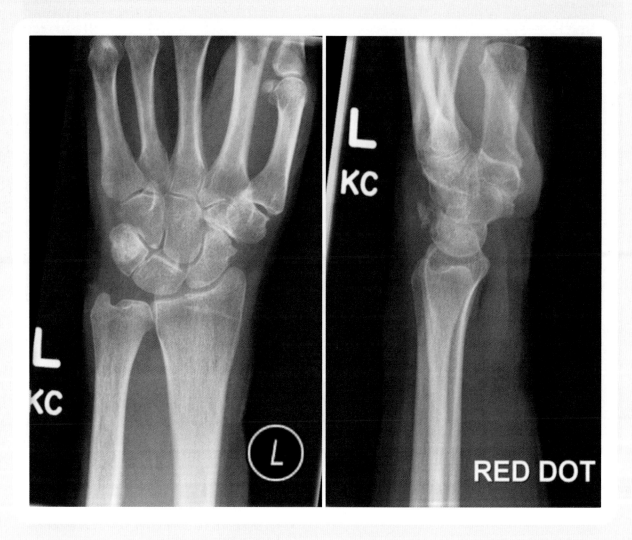

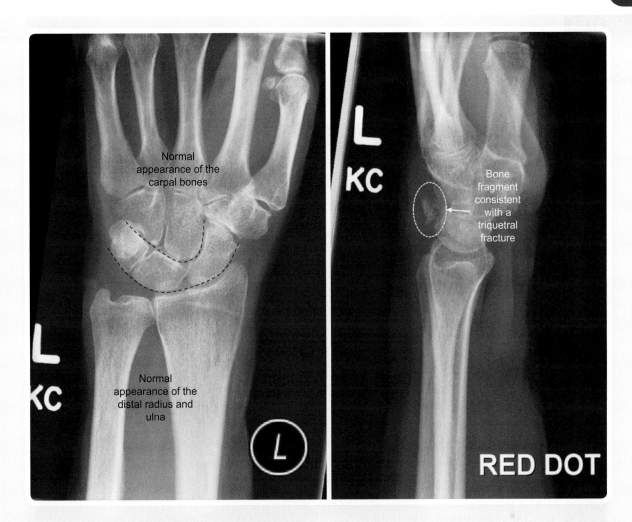

Normal
appearance of the
carpal bones

Bone
fragment
consistent
with a
triquetral
fracture

Normal
appearance of the
distal radius and
ulna

RED DOT

🔍 PRESENT YOUR FINDINGS

- These are lateral and AP X-rays of the left wrist of a skeletally mature patient.
- There are no patient identifiable data on the X-rays. Confirmation of the patient's name and date of birth, and the date and time when the X-rays were performed is required before making any further assessment.
- The X-rays are technically adequate, with no important areas cut off.
- There is a small bone fragment overlying the dorsal aspect of the proximal row of carpal bones visible on the lateral view. Given its location, this is in keeping with a triquetral fracture. There is no associated soft tissue swelling.
- No other fracture is apparent.
- Alignment of the wrist joint and carpal bones is normal.
- No areas of bone destruction, lucency or abnormal bone texture are evident.

IN SUMMARY – These X-rays show a triquetral fracture. Management will involve immobilisation with a cast and referral to the fracture clinic.

CASE **11.54**

A 54-year-old woman slipped walking along the super-market aisle, injuring her left ankle. She attends A&E and explains that she inverted her ankle and has been struggling to weight bear since. She is tender over the lateral malleolus and there is obvious swelling. X-rays of the left ankle had been requested.

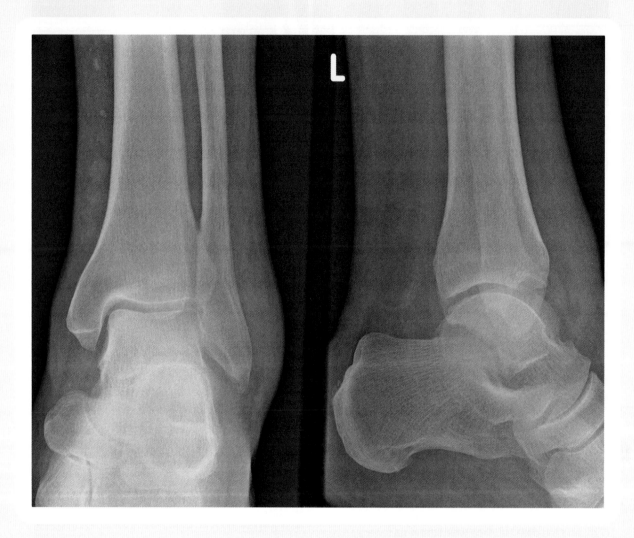

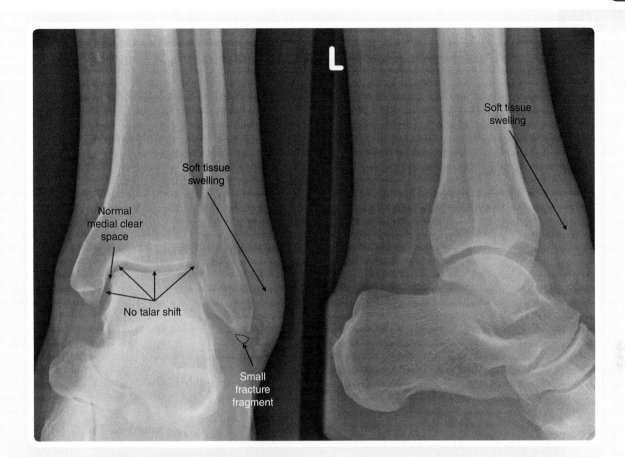

Soft tissue
swelling

Soft tissue
swelling

Normal
medial clear
space

No talar shift

Small
fracture
fragment

L

PRESENT YOUR FINDINGS

- These are AP and lateral X-rays of the left ankle in a skeletally mature patient.
- There are no patient identifiers on the X-rays. I would like to confirm the patient's name and date of birth, and the date and time the X-rays were performed before making any further assessment.
- The X-rays are adequately exposed with no important areas cut off.
- There is soft tissue swelling anterolaterally around the ankle joint.
- A small fracture can be seen at the tip of the lateral malleolus.

- There is a normal alignment of the ankle mortise.
- No other fracture is visible.
- No areas of bone destruction, lucency or abnormal bone texture are evident.

IN SUMMARY – These X-rays show a small fracture at the distal tip of the left lateral malleoli (Weber A) with associated soft tissue swelling. The rest of the ankle joint appears normal. The patient should be treated with a cast and referred to the fracture clinic.

A 34-year-old woman slipped on some ice and injured her right elbow. It is slightly swollen, tender on palpation, with a reduced range of movement. X-rays of the elbow have been performed.

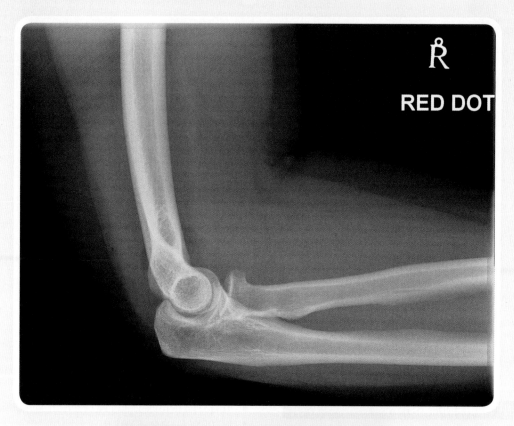

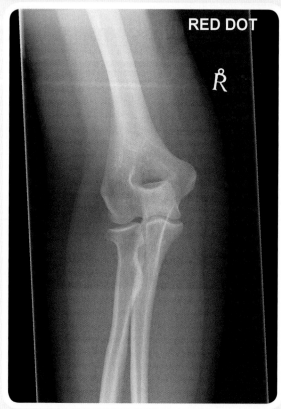

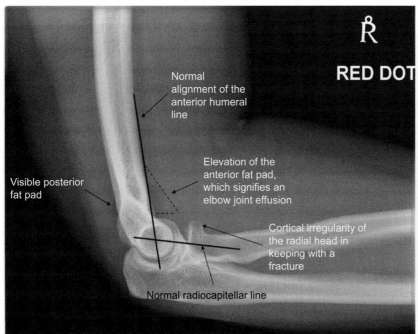

Normal
alignment of the
anterior humeral
line

Elevation of the
anterior fat pad,
which signifies an
elbow joint effusion

Visible posterior
fat pad

Cortical irregularity of
the radial head in
keeping with a
fracture

Normal radiocapitellar line

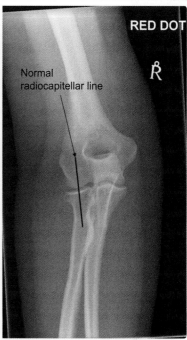

RED DOT

Ř

Normal
radiocapitellar line

PRESENT YOUR FINDINGS

- These are lateral and AP X-rays of the right elbow in a skeletally mature patient.
- There are no patient identifiable data on the X-rays. I would like to confirm the patient's name, date of birth and date and time the X-rays were performed before making any further assessment.
- The X-rays are adequately exposed, with no important areas cut off.
- The anterior fat pad is elevated, in keeping with an elbow effusion. A posterior fat pad is also visible.
- There is subtle cortical irregularity around the radial head consistent with an undisplaced radial head fracture.

- Alignment of the elbow joint (radiocapitellar and anterior humeral lines).
- No other fracture is visible.
- No areas of bone destruction, lucency or abnormal bone texture are evident.
- The soft tissues are unremarkable.

IN SUMMARY – These X-rays show an undisplaced radial head fracture with an associated elbow effusion. The patient should be treated with a sling and referred to the fracture clinic.

CASE 11.56

A 28-year-old man fell off his motorbike, injuring his right ankle. He sustained no other significant injuries. His right ankle, however, is extremely painful. X-rays of the ankle have been performed.

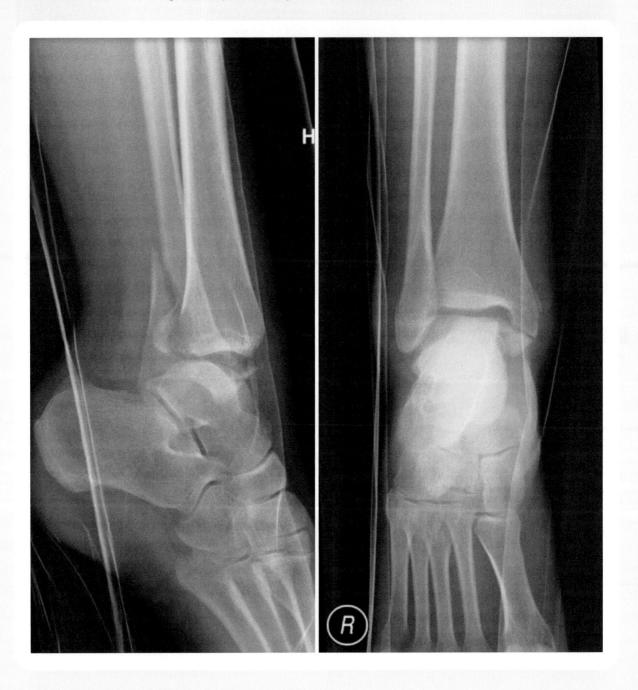

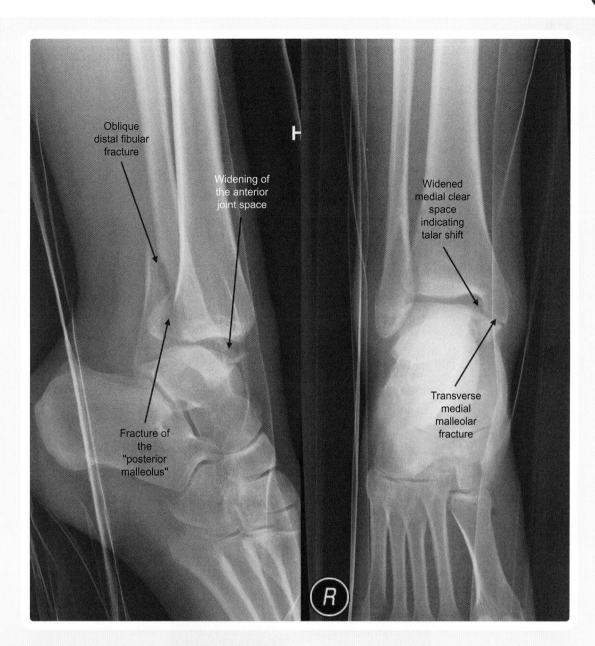

Oblique distal fibular fracture

Widening of the anterior joint space

Widened medial clear space indicating talar shift

Fracture of the "posterior malleolus"

Transverse medial malleolar fracture

H

R

PRESENT YOUR FINDINGS

- These are AP and lateral X-rays of the right ankle in a skeletally mature patient.
- There are no patient identifiable data on the X-rays. I would like to confirm the patient's name and date of birth, and the date and time the X-rays were performed before making any further assessment.
- The X-rays are adequately exposed, with no important areas cut off.
- There is a minimally displaced oblique fracture through the distal fibula, a minimally displaced transverse fracture through the medial malleolus and a fracture involving the 'posterior malleolus'.

- There is talar shift, and widening of the anterior ankle joint space visible on the lateral X-ray. There is no shortening or rotation.
- No areas of bone destruction, lucency or abnormal bone texture are visible.
- There is soft tissue swelling overlying the medial and lateral malleoli.

IN SUMMARY – These X-rays show a 'trimalleolar' fracture of the right ankle with associated talar shift and subluxation of the ankle joint. This is an unstable injury to the ankle which will require open reduction and internal fixation. Referral to orthopaedics is therefore required, following manipulation in the A&E department.

CASE 11.57

A 76-year-old woman fell in the bathroom and was found on the floor the next day by her son. He called an ambulance and she was taken to A&E. She is complaining of pain in the left hip. You request X-rays of the left hip.

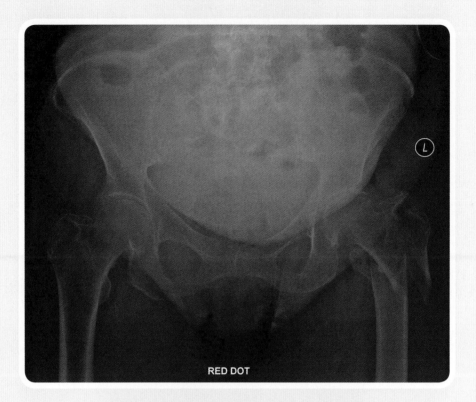

RED DOT

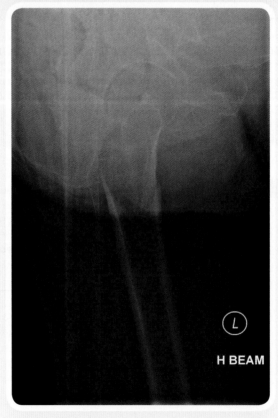

H BEAM

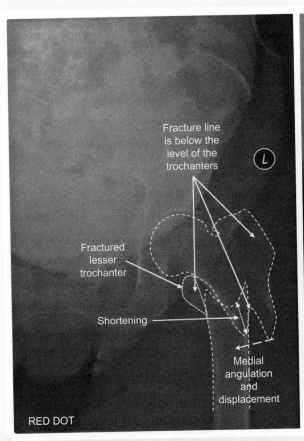

Fracture line
is below the
level of the
trochanters

Ⓛ

Fractured
lesser
trochanter

Shortening

Medial
angulation
and
displacement

RED DOT

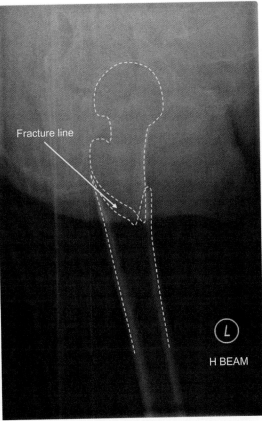

Fracture line

Ⓛ

H BEAM

PRESENT YOUR FINDINGS

- These are AP and lateral X-rays of the left hip in a skeletally mature patient.
- There are no patient identifiers on the X-rays. I would like to confirm the patient's name and date of birth, and the date and time the X-rays were performed before making any further assessment.
- The X-rays are adequately exposed, with no important areas cut off.
- There is a displaced fracture through the proximal left femur. The fracture is in a subtrochanteric position. There is shortening at the fracture site, with medial angulation and displacement of the main distal fragment.
- Additionally, there is a minimally displaced vertical fracture involving the left lesser trochanter. There

is a small amount of angulation of this fracture fragment.
- Normal alignment of the left hip joint can be seen.
- No other fracture is visible.
- No areas of bone destruction, lucency or abnormal bone texture are evident.
- The soft tissues are unremarkable.

IN SUMMARY – These X-rays show a displaced left sub-trochanteric femoral fracture (extracapsular), with an additional fracture involving the lesser trochanter. The patient should be referred to orthopaedics for operative management of the fracture. She will also need a full history and examination to identify any other injuries, as well as routine blood tests, including creatinine kinase and renal function, as she has been lying on the floor over night.

CASE 11.58

A 6-year-old girl slipped in the playground and injured her right elbow. It is slightly swollen, tender on palpation, with a reduced range of movement. X-rays of the elbow have been performed.

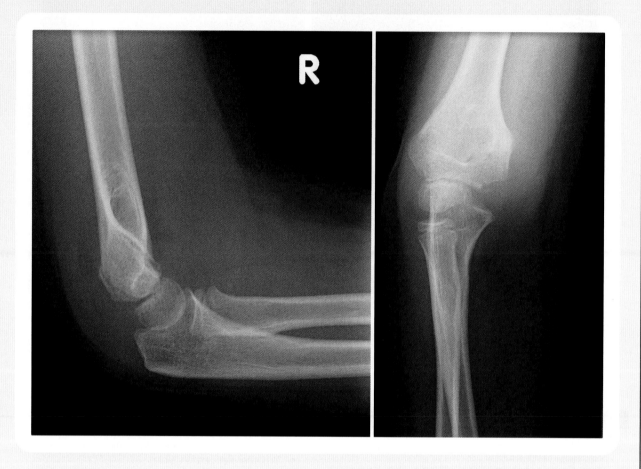

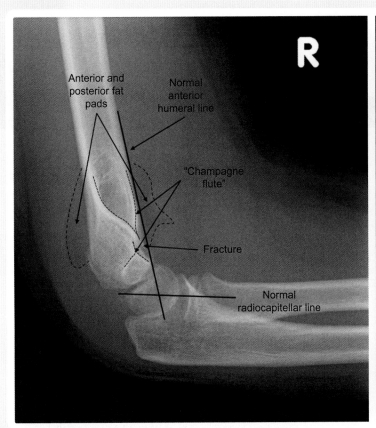

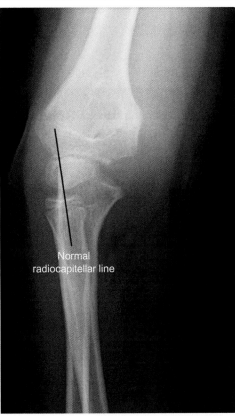

PRESENT YOUR FINDINGS

- These are AP and lateral X-rays of the right elbow of a skeletally immature patient.
- There are no patient identifiers on the X-rays. I would like to confirm the patient's name and date of birth, and the date and time the X-rays were performed before making any further assessment.
- The X-rays are adequately penetrated, with no important areas cut off.
- There is elevation of the anterior fat pad and the presence of a posterior fat pad, indicating an elbow effusion.
- Whilst the anterior humeral line is normal, there is a subtle supracondylar fracture with no significant posterior angulation or shortening. This is evident when

assessing the 'stem of the champagne flute' in the distal humerus.
- No other fracture is visible.
- No areas of bone destruction, lucency or abnormal bone texture are evident.
- Articulation of the elbow joint is normal.
- No significant abnormality of the soft tissues is evident.

IN SUMMARY – These X-rays show a minimally displaced supracondylar fracture with an associated elbow effusion. The patient should be treated with a collar and cuff and referred to the fracture clinic.

CASE INDEX

BONUS ORTHOPAEDIC X-RAYS

INDEX

Note: Page numbers followed by *f* indicate figures, *t* indicate tables and *b* indicate boxes.

A

AAA. *See* Abdominal aortic aneurysm
ABCDD mnemonic, chest X-ray assessment
  airway, 8
  breathing, 8–9
  cardiac and mediastinum, 9–10, 10*f*
  delicates, 10
  diaphragm, 10, 11*f*
ABCDE assessment, pelvic fracture, 347
ABCDEF mnemonic, pulmonary oedema chest X-ray assessment, 13–14
Abdominal aorta, abdominal X-ray assessment, 141*f*
Abdominal aortic aneurysm (AAA)
  abdominal X-ray, 222*b*–226*b*
  causes, 225
  clinical findings, 225
  computed tomography angiography, 427*f*
  diameter, 225
  management, 225–226
  rupture imaging, 226
Abdominal collections, 462
Abdominal computed tomography
  colonoscopy, 424*f*
  haematuria, 426*f*
  haemorrhage, 422*f*
  indications, 420
  renal tract calculi, 425*f*
  sepsis, 421*f*
  trauma, 421*f*
  tumour staging, 423*f*
Abdominal ultrasound, 445*f*
Abdominal X-ray
  adequacy, 137
  case examples
    abdominal aortic aneurysm, 222*b*–226*b*, 224–226
    ankylosing spondylitis, 232*b*–236*b*, 234–236
    bone metastasis, 227*b*–231*b*, 229–231
    bowel ischaemia, 177*b*–182*b*, 179–182, 520*f*, 521*f*

Abdominal X-ray (*Continued*)
    colitis, 171*b*–176*b*, 173–176
    constipation, 183*b*–187*b*, 185–187
    duodenal atresia, 242*b*–246*b*, 244–246
    foreign body ingestion, 237*b*–241*b*, 239–241
    gallstones, 193*b*–198*b*, 195–198, 506*f*, 507*f*
    inflammatory bowel disease, 516*f*, 517*f*
    intrauterine contraceptive device migration, 508*f*, 509*f*
    large bowel obstruction, 154*b*–159*b*, 156–159, 510*f*, 511*f*
    necrotising enterocolitis, 247*b*–252*b*, 248–252, 522*f*, 523*f*
    nephrostomy complications, 518*f*, 519*f*
    Paget's disease, 524*f*, 525*f*
    pancreatitis, 205*b*–210*b*, 206–210
    pneumoperitoneum, 165*b*–170*b*, 166–170, 514*f*, 515*f*
    renal calculi, 199*b*–204*b*, 200–204
    sigmoid colon volvulus, 160*b*–164*b*, 161–164
    small bowel obstruction, 148*b*–153*b*, 149–153, 528*f*, 529*f*
    splenic artery aneurysm, 216*b*–221*b*, 217–221
    splenomegaly, 188*b*–192*b*, 189–192, 526*f*, 527*f*
    uterine fibroid, 211*b*–215*b*, 212–215
  checklist, 142*t*
  dose, 146, 408
  indications, 146
  normal findings, 143*b*–147*b*, 145–147, 512*f*, 513*f*
  projection, 137
  small/large bowel differences, 145
  systematic review, 137–138
Abscess. *See* Lung abscess; Pancreatic abscess
Achilles tendon, rupture, 404*b*
Acute cholecystitis, 465, 465*f*
Acute ischaemic stroke, 466
Acute limb ischaemia, 463–464
Acute mesenteric ischaemia, 464
Acute pancreatitis
  causes, 208
  complications, 209–210
  management, 209
  pleural effusion induction, 43

Acute pancreatitis (*Continued*)
  ultrasound for gallstones, 209
Adhesions, small bowel obstruction, 152
Adrenal biopsy, 462–463, 463*f*
Advance Trauma Life Support (ATLS), 347, 373
AIN. *See* Anterior interosseous nerve
Alcoholism
  acute pancreatitis, 208
  chronic pancreatitis, 208
  lung abscess risk factor, 101–102
Allergy, contrast agents, 408
AMPLE assessment, 348
Anal fissure, constipation, 186
Anaphylaxis, breathlessness, 21
Anatomical snuff box, pain and scaphoid fracture, 323
Aneurysmal subarachnoid haemorrhage, 466
Ankle
  medial clear space, 405
  orthopaedic X-ray
    assessment, 279*f*
    fracture with talar shift, 544*f*, 545*f*
    malleolar fracture case examples, 401*f*, 402*f*, 403–406, 578*f*, 579*f*, 582*f*, 583*f*
    Ottawa Ankle Rules, 404
    Weber classification of lateral malleolus fractures, 404–405
  talar shift, 405
  triplane fracture, 318–319
Ankle jerk, spinal injury assessment, 294
Ankylosing spondylitis
  abdominal X-ray, 232–235
  clinical presentation, 235
  extra-spinal joint involvement, 236
  hepatic fibrosis, 236
  treatment, 236
Anterior interosseous nerve (AIN)
  fracture, 312
  testing, 329
Aortic aneurysms, 464
Aortic dissection, 464
Aortic dissection, chest computed tomography, 419*f*
Appendicitis, foreign body ingestion, 374
Arterial interventions
  acute limb ischaemia, 463–464
  acute mesenteric ischaemia, 464